Feline
Behavioral Health
and Welfare

Feline Behavioral Health and Welfare

Edited by

Ilona Rodan, DVM, DABVP (Feline Practice)
Founder, Cat Care Clinic
Feline-Friendly Consultations
Cat Behavior Consultations
Madison, Wisconsin

Sarah Heath, BVSc, DipECAWBM(BM), CCAB, MRCVS
European Veterinary Specialist in Behavioural Medicine
  (Companion Animals)
Behavioural Referrals Veterinary Practice
Upton, Chester, United Kingdom

ELSEVIER

ELSEVIER

3251 Riverport Lane
St Louis, MO 63043

FELINE BEHAVIORAL HEALTH AND WELFARE   978-1-4557-7401-2

Notice

Knowledge and best practice in this field are constantly changing. As new research and experience broaden our understanding, changes in research methods, professional practices, or medical treatment may become necessary.

Practitioners and researchers must always rely on their own experience and knowledge in evaluating and using any information, methods, compounds, or experiments described herein. In using such information or methods they should be mindful of their own safety and the safety of others, including parties for whom they have a professional responsibility.

With respect to any drug or pharmaceutical products identified, readers are advised to check the most current information provided (i) on procedures featured or (ii) by the manufacturer of each product to be administered, to verify the recommended dose or formula, the method and duration of administration, and contraindications. It is the responsibility of practitioners, relying on their own experience and knowledge of their patients, to make diagnoses, to determine dosages and the best treatment for each individual patient, and to take all appropriate safety precautions.

To the fullest extent of the law, neither the Publisher nor the authors, contributors, or editors, assume any liability for any injury and/or damage to persons or property as a matter of products liability, negligence or otherwise, or from any use or operation of any methods, products, instructions, or ideas contained in the material herein.

Library of Congress Cataloging-in-Publication Data

Feline behavioral health and welfare / edited by Ilona Rodan, Sarah E. Heath.
       p. cm.
    Includes bibliographical references and index.
    ISBN 978-1-4557-7401-2 (pbk. : alk. paper) 1. Cats–Behavior. 2. Cats–Behavior therapy. I. Rodan, Ilona, editor. II. Heath, Sarah, 1964-, editor.
    [DNLM: 1. Behavior, Animal–physiology. 2. Cats. 3. Animal Welfare. 4. Behavior Control–methods. 5. Behavioral Symptoms–therapy. SF 446.5]
    SF446.5.F447 2015
    636.8'083–dc23
                                                                2015021780

Vice President and Publisher: Loren Wilson
Content Strategy Director: Penny Rudolph
Content Development Manager: Jolynn Gower
Content Development Specialist: Brandi Graham
Publishing Services Manager: Jeffrey Patterson
Project Manager: Tracey Schriefer
Designer: Margaret Reid

Printed in the United States of America
Last digit is the print number: 9   8   7   6   5   4   3

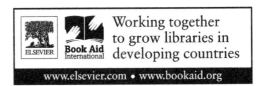

I dedicate this book to my late parents, Susan and Kenneth Rodan, who taught me to love all animals and to care for those in need while allowing them to maintain species-specific behaviors; to my husband, Barry Ganetzky, for his incredible support and patience during the past 2 years; and to my daughter Rebecca, son-in-law David, and granddaughter Leora, for being the wonderful family that they are.

Ilona Rodan

I dedicate this book to my family and friends and also to all my pets and patients past and present who have taught me so much about the art of veterinary medicine.

Sarah Heath

Cats are not small dogs.
Barbara Stein

Cats are not small people. We need to allow cats to be cats!
Ilona Rodan

The veterinary disciplines of feline internal medicine and behavioral medicine are inextricably linked, and in this first edition of *Feline Behavioral Health and Welfare,* authors from both of these fields have come together with colleagues from other specialties, such as pain management and neurology, to address the importance of feline behavior in veterinary practice and the interplay between behavior and disease.

ORGANIZATION

The aim of this book is to improve the quality of care that feline patients receive during their visit to the veterinary practice and maximize the benefits of the relationship between cats and their owners.

In Part 1, the book starts by looking at the importance of behavior in a veterinary practice setting and considers the implications for feline welfare, for example in terms of lack of adequate veterinary care; lack of understanding of feline physical, social, and emotional needs; and risk of relinquishment and euthanasia.

The section that follows explores the issue of normal feline behavior and encourages better understanding of social interactions and communication styles. Information about feline learning processes also provides important background knowledge that lays the foundation for a better understanding of feline patients.

Parts 3 and 4 focus on the need to prevent behavior problems, both in the home setting and in the veterinary practice. Practical advice for clients regarding pet selection is combined with information about the provision of adequate healthcare for cats in both a physical and an emotional sense. Prevention of behavior-related problems in the veterinary practice is addressed over three chapters covering the overall veterinary experience and the specific contexts of the consulting room and the hospitalization area.

In the following section, the interplay between behavior and disease is explored. Changes in behavior are often the key to owners recognizing illness, pain, or stress and can also be important tools in the diagnostic process. Stress as a risk factor for disease has now been well recognized in feline patients, and the first chapter in this section looks at this issue. Obesity is a medical problem of great concern to feline practitioners and owners and this book explores the link between obesity and behavior in terms of both etiology and potential management. Pain is commonly found to be involved in cases that present as behavioral concerns, and experts from the field of veterinary pain management have provided in-depth consideration of the issues associated with the recognition and management of acute and chronic pain in feline patients. The specific condition of feline orofacial pain syndrome is also discussed.

When dealing with behavior cases, it is important to have a good understanding of the emotional motivations that are involved, and in Part 6 of the book, the first chapter is dedicated to this important topic. An overview of some of the tools that can be used when managing and treating behavior cases is given in the chapters on pheromones, drugs, and nutraceuticals.

In the last two sections of the book, the focus is on dealing with behavior that is considered to be problematic first within the veterinary context and secondly within the home. The veterinary section concentrates on providing a cat-friendly approach to the consultation and gives practical advice on handling fearful, painful, and behaviorally challenging feline patients.

The final section begins with a review of those normal feline behaviors that can be undesirable within the home and offers practical advice for owners on how to deal with these. The remaining chapters concentrate on the two most commonly presented feline behavior problems of house soiling and aggression and the distressing issue of behavioral change in the senior cat.

To accompany the book, client handouts are provided to support the veterinary profession in educating cat owners.

Key Information

- The relevance of behavior to feline health and welfare
- Normal feline behavior and how it affects provision of resources within a domestic environment
- Important client concerns and barriers to feline veterinary visits
- Feline emotions and how to recognize and manage negative emotional states within the veterinary practice
- The interplay between behavior and disease
- The tools that are available to assist in the management and treatment of behavioral cases
- Commonly encountered behavioral challenges, including house soiling and aggression

INTENDED AUDIENCE

This book is principally written for primary veterinary practitioners who work with cats regardless of the type of practice, and other members of the veterinary team including veterinary technicians/nurses. It is also an important resource for veterinary students, behavior residents, and veterinary technician students and those preparing for the behavior specialty. It is hoped that behavior and other veterinary specialists will also find the focus on feline behavior and welfare interesting and enlightening.

This book would not have been possible without our outstanding authors. Recruitment of international authors was important to provide a global perspective on feline behavioral health and welfare. Additionally, authors specializing in behavior, feline medicine, pain management, and other fields were chosen to ensure the emotional, social, and physical aspects of feline welfare were all included. Tremendous thanks goes to all of them. We would like to specifically acknowledge the contribution from our colleague, Sophia Yin, who tragically died while the book was in production. Her contribution to animal welfare was significant and she will be sadly missed. While it is customary to edit a multiple-author book into a common style, you will note that one of Sophia's chapters (Chapter 5) has been left in her original writing style as a mark of respect.

We are also grateful to several colleagues for their help in editing certain chapters, and they include Irene Rochlitz, Margie Scherk, Andrew Sparkes, and Clare Wilson. Thanks also goes to Gaille Perry for pictures she provided.

We would also like to thank Penny Rudolph, Brandi Graham, and Tracey Schriefer from Elsevier for all their support and commitment throughout the writing and editing stages.

We hope that this book will make a positive contribution to the understanding of our feline patients and will help to improve the welfare of cats within the veterinary practice and at home.

Ilona Rodan
Sarah Heath

In addition to thanking my family to whom I dedicate this book, I also wish to thank the veterinary team at the Cat Care Clinic, our clients, and especially all the cats who have helped teach me about feline behavior and welfare over the past three decades. Thanks also to the American Association of Feline Practitioners for helping me become the best feline practitioner possible and a leader in veterinary medicine. Enormous thanks also goes to my best friend, Eliza Sundahl, who emotionally supported me throughout the long process of writing and editing. I am also forever grateful to veterinary behaviorists, especially Sarah Heath, as well as Karen Overall, Gary Landsberg, and Debbie Horwitz, who taught and mentored me during the past 18 + years, accepting me as a nonbehaviorist with a passion to help veterinarians understand cats and to prevent behavior problems. Last, but certainly not least, my gratitude goes to coeditor Sarah Heath for her incredible knowledge of feline behavior, her patience and ability to write, her perseverance and dedication despite her health problems and treatments, and for her friendship.

Ilona Rodan

The writing and editing for this book has been a struggle as it has coincided with a period of ill health. My treatment for breast cancer has been a hard journey and this book has been a companion along the way. That companionship has not always been easy but I am glad we have made it to the end of the publication process. I would like to thank Ilona for her patience when I have been unable to contribute and when health and hospital visits have prevented me from responding as promptly as she would have liked. Ilona has been a true friend and I thank her for her personal support as well. I would like to acknowledge all of those who have been beside me on my cancer journey and have shown me so much love and support. There are too many to mention all by name but in particular I would like to thank my sons Matthew and David, my daughter-in-law Emma, grandchildren Ethan and Beth, and all my wonderful friends including Rachel Dean, Christine Neilson, Ann Parry, Tiny DeKeuster, John Robinson, Dorothy Cummins, Allison German, Jill McPherson, Laura Borromeo, Clare Hemmings, Karin Fairhurst, and Jane Trundle. Thanks also to all the staff at my practice for their help in supporting me over this difficult time and to Chris Fozzard, who will always be someone special to me. Above all I would like to thank the wonderful staff of the NHS (Clatterbridge Cancer Centre and the Countess of Chester Hospital) and Macmillan Cancer Support who have quite literally saved my life.

Sarah Heath

Martha Cannon, BA, VetMB, DSAM(Fel)
Oxford Cat Clinic
Oxford, Oxfordshire, UK
The Cat in the Veterinary Practice
The Cat in the Consulting Room
Housing Cats in the Veterinary Practice

Rachel Casey, BVMS, PhD, DipECAWBM, CCAB, MRCVS
Senior Lecturer in Companion Animal Behaviour and Welfare
School of Clinical Veterinary Science
University of Bristol
Bristol, UK
Human-Directed Aggression in Cats

Sagi Denenberg, DVM, MACVSc(Behaviour)
Behaviour Consultant
North Toronto Veterinary Behaviour Specialty Clinic
Thornhill, Ontario, Canada
Behavior Problems of the Senior Cat

Theresa L. DePorter, DVM, MRCVS, DipECAWBM
Oakland Veterinary Referral Services
Bloomfield Hills, Michigan
Use of Pheromones in Feline Practice
Tools of the Trade: Psychopharmacology and Nutrition

Alexander German, BVSc(Hons), PhD
Reader in Small Animal Medicine
Department of Obesity and Endocrinology
School of Veterinary Science
University of Liverpool
Neston, Merseyside, UK
Feline Obesity

Richard Gowan, BVSC(Hons), MACVSc(Feline Medicine)
The Cat Clinic
Melbourne, Victoria, Australia
Chronic Pain and Behavior

Sarah Heath, BVSc, DipECAWBM(BM), CCAB, MRCVS
European Veterinary Specialist in Behavioural Medicine (Companion Animals)
Behavioural Referrals Veterinary Practice
Upton, Chester, UK
Feline Behavior and Welfare
Feline Obesity
Feline Orofacial Pain Syndrome

Understanding Emotions
Providing Feline-Friendly Consultations
Handling the Cat that is in Pain
Intercat Conflict

Debra F. Horwitz, DVM, Diplomate ACVB
Veterinary Behaviorist
Veterinary Behavior Consultations
St. Louis, Missouri
Pet Selection
Tools of the Trade: Psychopharmacology and Nutrition

Isabelle Iff, Dr.med.vet., DipECVAA, CertVetAc (IVAS), LicAc(BAWMA), MRCVS
Anaesthetist and Instructor
Veterinary Anaesthesia School For Technicians (VASTA)
Veterinary Anaesthesia Services
Zurcherstrasse, Winterthur, Switzerland
Chronic Pain and Behavior

Christos Karagiannis, DVM, MSc, MRCVS
Resident ECAWBM
Animal Behaviour, Cognition and Welfare Group
School of Life Sciences
University of Lincoln
Lincoln, Lincolnshire, UK
Stress as a Risk Factor for Disease
Understanding Emotions

Gary M. Landsberg, BSc, DVM, DACVB, DECVBM-CA
Veterinary Behaviourist
North Toronto Animal Clinic;
Director of Veterinary Affairs
CanCog Technologies
Toronto, Ontario, Canada
Tools of the Trade: Psychopharmacology and Nutrition
Behavior Problems of the Senior Cat

Jacqueline M. Ley, BVSc(Hons), PhD (Psychology), FANCVS(Veterinary Behaviour), DECAWBM
Registered Specialist in Veterinary Behaviour
Animal Behaviour Consultations
Narre Warren, Victoria, Australia
Feline Communication
Normal Social Behavior
Normal but Unwanted Behavior in Cats

Susan Little, DVM, DABVP(Feline)
President
American Association of Feline Practitioners
Hillsborough, New Jersey;
Owner, Bytown Cat Hospital,
Ottawa, Ontario, Canada
Providing Appropriate Healthcare

Amy L. Pike, BS(Zoology), DVM
Resident
Veterinary Behavior Consultations
St. Louis, Missouri
Pet Selection

Sheilah A. Robertson, BVMS(Hons), PhD
Assistant Director
Animal Welfare Division
American Veterinary Medical Association
Schaumburg, Illinois
Acute Pain and Behavior

Ilona Rodan, DVM, DABVP(Feline Practice)
Founder, Cat Care Clinic
Feline-Friendly Consultations
Cat Behavior Consultations
Madison, Wisconsin
Importance of Feline Behavior in Veterinary Practice
Feline Behavior and Welfare
The Cat in the Veterinary Practice
The Cat in the Consulting Room
Housing Cats in the Veterinary Practice
Providing Feline-Friendly Consultations
Handling the Cat that is in Pain

Clare Rusbridge, BVMS, PhD, DECVN, MRCVS
Chief of Neurology
Fitzpatrick Referrals
Eashing, Surrey, UK;
Reader In Veterinary Neurology
School of Veterinary Medicine
University of Surrey
Guildford, Surrey, UK
Feline Orofacial Pain Syndrome

Kersti Seksel, BVSc(Hons), MRCVS. MA(Hons),
 FACVSc, DACVBM, DECAWBM
Adjunct Senior Lecturer
School of Animal and Veterinary Sciences
Charles Sturt University
Wagga Wagga, NSW, Australia
Providing Appropriate Behavioral Care
House Soiling Problems

Eliza Sundahl, DVM, DABVP(Feline)
KC Cat Clinic
Kansas City, Missouri
Overland Park, Kansas
Providing Feline-Friendly Consultations

Sophia Yin[†], DVM, MS, DACVB
Department of Animal Science
University of California
Davis, California;
Premier Pet Behavior Consultant;
Behavior Consultant
San Francisco Veterinary Specialists
San Francisco, California;
President
CattleDog Publishing
Davis, California
Feline Learning
Handling the Challenging Cat

[†]Deceased.

CONTENTS

Introduction

Importance of Feline Behavior in Veterinary Practice

Ilona Rodan

INTRODUCTION

The growing popularity of the cat as a pet has led to many benefits, including increased feline safety and length of life. Cats are beloved companions, with the majority of cat owners considering them to be family members.[1,2] Many cat owners adopt a cat that needs a home and provide them with love, food, and comfort. The majority of today's cats live longer lives due to safer environments and advances in feline medical care.[3] This all sounds great, but do most cats truly have a great life? Are cat owners and veterinary professionals really doing the best for the cat?

The sad reality is that millions of pet cats receive little or no veterinary care and suffer significant levels of unrecognized pain and illness.[4,5] Other cats endure boredom and stress due to inadequate feline environments and stressful social situations.[6,7] Feline stressors negatively impact physical health, resulting in a range of recurrent physical conditions.[8,9] Add to that the relinquishment and euthanasia each and every year of millions of cats that were once beloved companions because of undesirable or abnormal behaviors[10,11] and it would appear that the cat is not getting the best possible care despite its popularity.

The good news is that most of the problematic issues facing the domestic cat can be prevented or addressed if we understand cats as pets as well as patients. The vast majority of problems that owners and veterinarians encounter with cats do not occur out of feline malice, but rather due to a lack of understanding of the cat, its normal behaviors, and its needs. The cat is a paradox—although fairly adaptable and social animals, cats have retained many of the behaviors of their wild ancestors.[12,13]

Veterinarians have a unique opportunity to vastly improve the cat's physical and emotional health and to enhance the relationship between them and their people. In turn this will improve feline welfare and benefit the veterinary profession as they gain more satisfaction from their feline work. Behavior and physical health are closely intertwined, making the need to address behavior essential in all aspects of feline healthcare. Incorporating behavior into each and every appointment is the key to optimizing feline veterinary care and to keeping cats healthy, content, and remaining in their homes.

CHALLENGES IN FELINE PRACTICE

There are four major challenges for the veterinary profession in the context of striving to provide an optimal level of feline healthcare. The first challenge is the lack of regular veterinary care and the resulting late presentation of cats with physical disease or behavioral health issues. A large number of cats do not receive routine preventative healthcare and never see a veterinarian unless they are sick. As a result of the cat's ability to mask signs of illness and pain, these animals are often presented with advanced disease that is often unable to be treated. Some cats do come to the practice for preventive treatment through vaccination, worming, and flea treatment as kittens, but their owners never bring them back for booster vaccinations or repeated preventive treatments. For many, this lack of ongoing veterinary care is a result of poor client education and awareness, but for others there may be specific reasons for client reluctance to return, such as the stress of bringing a cat to the veterinary practice. Infrequent feline visits can be frustrating for veterinary personnel, who are seeking to provide a high standard of care, and can lead to decreasing levels of job satisfaction. In addition, there are financial implications for the veterinary practice as a result of poor levels of feline attendance. This can indirectly affect the quality of feline care that can be provided due to lack of ability to invest in practice development and staff selection.

The second challenge in feline practice is the prevalence of stress-associated illness. In many cases the physical signs are identified and treated without any understanding of the influence of stress and behavioral factors on the condition. As a result, resolution is temporary and recurrence is a familiar outcome. True resolution is not possible without addressing the environmental and social needs of the cat in a consistent and predictable fashion, and therefore, behavioral knowledge is essential for the feline practitioner.

The third challenge is the incidence of behavioral issues in the feline population and the risk of cats being relinquished or euthanized because of behavior problems, normal but undesirable feline behaviors, or incompatibility with other cats in the household. It is also important to remember those cats that remain in the same household but suffer from unrecognized stress, pain, and even illness and fail to receive appropriate veterinary intervention.

The fourth challenge is that, although veterinary professionals strive to provide the best healthcare for their feline patients, many are poorly equipped to deal with the behavioral factors that are such an important component of the preceding three challenges. Behavioral medicine is a relatively young veterinary discipline and many veterinary schools still fail to provide specific education in this field. The fact that there are considerable differences between feline and human social behavior and communication makes intuitive interaction more of a challenge. As a result, there can be significant problems in terms of appropriate handling in the veterinary context. Failing to see things from a feline perspective can result in restraint methods that induce fear and lead to escalating levels of feline aggression which is not only detrimental to the cat but also to practice personnel. Improving veterinary education in the field of behavioral medicine is perhaps one of the major challenges facing the profession.

The aim of this book is to address the behavioral issues that are so fundamentally important in relation to feline veterinary practice and explain how a better understanding of feline behavior can help to improve the physical and emotional health of feline patients (Box 1-1) as well as increase owner and veterinary team satisfaction when living and working with cats.

LACK OF VETERINARY CARE

Although the majority of owners consider their cats to be family members, many fail to understand the importance of regular veterinary care. A lack of understanding of normal feline behavior leads to many

---

BOX 1-1 Problems Associated with Poor Understanding of Feline Behavior

Medical Problems
- Lack of preventive care due to:
  - Poor recognition of value
  - Stress surrounding the veterinary experience
- Increase in preventable diseases, such as:
  - Diabetes mellitus
  - Intestinal parasites
  - External parasites
  - Dental disease
- Lack of recognition and prevention of painful conditions, such as:
  - Appendicular degenerative joint disease
  - Axial degenerative joint disease
  - Oral disease—resorptive lesions, periodontal disease
- Stress-associated sickness behavior—feline idiopathic cystitis
- Obesity epidemic
- Lack of recognition of behavioral signs of pain and illness, such as:
  - Subtle changes in behavior
  - Loss of normal behaviors
  - Abnormal behaviors
- Stress surrounding the veterinary visit
- Difficulty differentiating illness or pain from fear on exam findings
  - Tachycardia
  - Increased respiratory rate
- Increased temperature
- Tension or aggression making it difficult to perform a comprehensive examination
- Pupillary dilation
- Difficulty differentiating illness or pain from fear on laboratory findings
  - White coat hypertension
  - Stress hyperglycemia +/− glucosuria
  - Mature neutrophilia and lymphopenia
  - Lymphocytosis
  - Alkaline urine +/− struvite crystals
- Advanced disease or pain due to the client's inability to recognize the subtle signs of illness and pain
- Decreased feline welfare associated with sickness
- Early death

Behavioral Problems
- Lack of understanding of normal feline behavior
- Lack of understanding of feline social and emotional needs
- Lack of appropriate resources for cats
- Inadequate distribution of resources in relation to number of cats within home
- Inadequate prevention of behavior problems
- Decreased feline welfare
- Behavior problems
- Surrender and relinquishment to shelters
- Early death

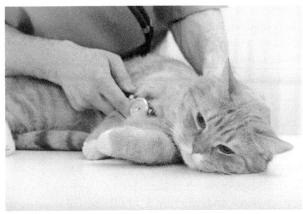

FIGURE 1-1 Since cats show only subtle signs of illness and pain, many cat owners assume they are healthy and bring them to the veterinarian only when disease is advanced or when behavior problems occur. (Copyright © iStock.com)

misconceptions. The fact that cats are often acquired at little or no cost can lead to a perception that they are low cost, low maintenance pets.[5] When cats are apparently healthy and are kept in an indoor environment that is considered to be free of disease risk, owners do not see any reason to visit the veterinary practice. The fact that many owners consider veterinary visits stressful for both the cat and themselves compounds this.[4,5,14]

A further complication in the battle to convince owners to provide their cats with regular veterinary attention is the fact that feline signs of pain and illness are often very subtle and many owners simply do not recognize that the pet is in need of assistance (Figure 1-1). When cats display undesirable behaviors, owners will often attribute this behavior to being "old" or spiteful rather than considering the possibility of pain or illness as an underlying cause.

As a result of all of these factors, the veterinary profession faces a huge challenge in trying to ensure that cats are given the veterinary care that they deserve.

Between 2001 and 2011, there has been an almost 15% decline in the number of feline veterinary visits in the United States despite the growing number of pet cats and cats considered to be family members.[1,5] In 2011, only 55.1% of cat owners took their cat to the veterinarian at least once, as compared with 81.3% of dogs.[1] If both dogs and cats live in the same home, the dogs go to the veterinarian almost twice as often as the cats.[4] Of the cats receiving veterinary care on an annual or more frequent basis, only 48% received wellness or preventive care.[5] The decline in feline healthcare negatively impacts pet cats, cat owners, and the veterinary care that practices provide.

Major efforts have been taken since 2006 by most American veterinary organizations that work with cats (American Association of Feline Practitioners [AAFP], American Animal Hospital Association [AAHA], and the American Veterinary Medical Association [AVMA]) to increase awareness of the need for regular feline healthcare. Tremendous support has been provided by industry to complete surveys and to increase veterinary awareness and cat owner education. Despite all of this, there continues to be a decline in feline veterinary visits. Comparing 2011 with 2006, the number of cat-owning households in the United States that did not take their cat to the veterinarian increased by a staggering 24%.[1] Despite similar awareness campaigns driven by International Cat Care in the UK and Europe, there is no reason to believe that cats receive better healthcare in other countries.

In order to address this problem, the veterinary profession needs to be aware of the issues that are contributing to this decline in feline healthcare and become educated in the role of behavior-related misunderstandings. This will enable them to educate not only clients, but also veterinary practice staff in ways that will decrease feline stress and increase client compliance with the goal of regular veterinary visits.

Owners Think Cats are Self-Sufficient and Convenient to Own

In a study of almost 2000 cat owners, 81% believe that cats are self-sufficient and healthy and therefore require little care.[5] Another report indicated that 57% of cat owners said that cats were convenient and easy to maintain, whereas dog, fish, and bird owners indicated that these pets needed more care to maintain.[15] Unfortunately, some of the popularity of the cat has occurred because cats are considered "low maintenance" pets. With changing human lifestyles, such as both adult family members working, and more apartment and condominium dwellers, the "low maintenance" or "independent" cat is considered easier to care for than the dog.[4]

Cats are Often Acquired Through Impulse Adoptions or as "Free Cats"

The majority of cats enter people's homes as impulse acquisitions and with no education about their needs (Figure 1-2). Of those who acquired new cats, 59% of people did not expect to get a cat, and 69% adopted a cat at no cost. This differs dramatically from dogs who were adopted after thoughtful consideration and at a cost.[5] There are two significant problems here—the misconception of cats adopted at little or no cost being "low cost" pets and the lack of education about the necessary level of veterinary and home care. When a cat shows up on someone's doorstep, or is given to someone as a present or through rehoming, cat owners receive little to no education about the associated care and expenses of owning a cat.

Many people have unrealistic expectations when they acquire a cat, resulting in 54% of newly adopted cats

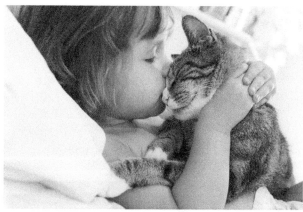

FIGURE 1-2 Many adoptions are unplanned, with a cat showing up on a doorstep or when free kittens are available for adoption. Often these cats are adopted without advice about home and veterinary care, which may result in their surrender. (Copyright © iStock.com)

being returned within the first 2 weeks post-adoption.[16] Initially excited to bring home a new pet, owners felt they had no option but to return the pet. They also felt a sadness and a sense of failure, with 41.4% indicating that they would not adopt another pet in the near future.[16] Most realized that they needed to devote more time, thought, and planning to both the consideration and the process of adoption. Others indicated that they needed to learn more about cat behavior.[16]

Owners Underestimate the Need for Regular Veterinary Care

In some countries, such as the United States and Australia, there has been a push to keep cats indoors with the goals of increased safety for the cat and prevention of destruction of wildlife. The problem with this is two-fold—first, clients do not think indoor cats need healthcare, and second, unless the home environment meets the needs of the cat, stress can lead to behavior problems and recurrent health problems which may lead owners to relinquish or euthanize a once beloved cat. Interestingly, veterinary visits in the United States started to decline after 2001 which was the same year that the American Veterinary Medical Association (AVMA) developed a position statement to keep cats indoors.[17] The goals of that position statement were to increase life expectancy and reduce injury, disease, and zoonoses,[17] but other factors such as behavioral needs and quality of life also need to be considered. Cat owners often assume that due to the indoor lifestyle of their cat, it will be protected from disease, injury, and parasites, and therefore there will be no need for veterinary care. This misunderstanding leaves indoor cats vulnerable, and since the majority of pet cats have non-infectious health conditions that impair their quality of life,[18] the decline in veterinary visits has been associated with a significant increase in cats with preventable diseases. U.S. studies have identified a 10% increase in dental disease, 13% increase in internal parasites, 16% increase in flea and tick infestation, and a 16% increase in diabetes mellitus.[19] With almost 60% of cats in the United States being overweight or obese, the increase in diabetes mellitus comes as no surprise.[20]

Cat owners are often very devoted to their pets and often expect that they will be able to tell if their cats are sick because of the bond they share with them. However, cats are particularly skilled at masking the signs of illness, and many health conditions go unrecognized until they are advanced and difficult to treat or manage. Painful and common conditions, such as dental disease and degenerative joint disease, are often not recognized by owners; without regular veterinary visits there is no opportunity for the veterinary profession to detect them in the early stages. Even when disease has been identified, many owners find the administration of medication is a real challenge and they may opt to euthanize cats with advanced disease, or keep cats at home without analgesia or other treatments, unable to accept the welfare effects of their decision.

Owners and Cats Experience Stress in Association With the Veterinary Visit

The stress of the veterinary experience is a major factor in the lack of preventive healthcare for cats and in the delays for many sick cats in gaining access to veterinary care. In one survey 58% of owners said their cat *hates* going to the veterinarian, and 37.6% said that just thinking about taking their cat to the veterinarian is stressful.[14] It is not only the fear-related behavior of the cat within the practice setting which is disturbing for owners, but also the related behavioral challenges at home before and after the consultation, such as chasing the cat to get it into the carrier, listening to the howling in the car, cleaning up the urine and feces in the carrier on arrival at the veterinary practice, and then dealing with the hostility from other household cats when the cat returns from the visit. A consultation that lasts for five to thirty minutes in the veterinary practice can result in stress for the owner over a matter of days to weeks. Clients need specific advice from the veterinary practice as to how to minimize this stress (see Chapters 9 and 20).

STRESS-RELATED DISEASES

The negative impact of chronic stress on the physical health of humans is well recognized. More recently, awareness of feline stressors leading to physical health problems in cats has been well documented.[8,9,21] Although cats do not always express overt signs of stress, it is important for owners and veterinary practices to be aware of how feline stress can be associated with suboptimal environmental and social conditions.

There is a strong link between feline stress and the chronic pain syndrome, feline idiopathic cystitis

(FIC).[8,9,22] Also called feline interstitial cystitis, it is the most common cause of feline lower urinary tract disease, with 54%-64% of cats presenting with lower urinary tract signs having idiopathic disease.[23] FIC was initially considered a disease of the bladder alone, but it is now recognized that the response is activated in the brain by the hypothalamic stress response system.[9]

Co-morbid disorders commonly occur in combination with FIC and affect organs such as the skin, gastrointestinal tract, or immune system.[24] The combination of multiple affected body systems, signs that wax and wane in severity, and that the cats show a favorable response to environmental enrichment has led to the identification of these cases as "Pandora Syndrome."[24]

In addition to the well-documented contribution of stress to cases of feline lower urinary tract disease, stress has also been shown to have other negative health effects. For instance, stress decreases food intake and increases incidence of upper respiratory infections in cats in humane shelters.[21]

Stress-related diseases can occur in the home, the veterinary practice, and the humane society. Stressors include unfamiliar environments and individuals, and a lack of predictability and sense of control. For example, a hospitalized cat may have a perception of poor predictability and a lack of sense of control if there are inconsistencies in caretakers, feeding and cleaning routines, or periods of light and dark.[9]

Studies indicate a significant decrease in the frequency of signs of stress-related diseases with environmental enrichment, familiarity, and a sense of control (Figure 1-3).[8,22] Interestingly, there was also a decrease in fear and upper respiratory infections.[8] Based on this information, it is necessary for veterinarians to address environmental stressors and consider how to improve the environment and offer predictability for the cat.

For more information about what causes stress in cats in the home environment, see Chapter 2. For more detailed information about stress as a risk factor for physical disease, see Chapter 12.

RELINQUISHMENT AND EUTHANASIA OF PET CATS

A significant proportion of adopted cats do not remain in their original home for life. Many apparently healthy cats are rehomed, released to enter the stray cat population, surrendered to shelters, and/or euthanized (Figures 1-4 and 1-5). While many of the reasons that owners give for these decisions relate to the behavior or characteristics of the cat, changes in the owners' circumstances, for example a housing or relationship change, are also offered as reasons why a cat needs to leave its present home. Euthanasia due to behavior problems is the number one cause of death of adult cats

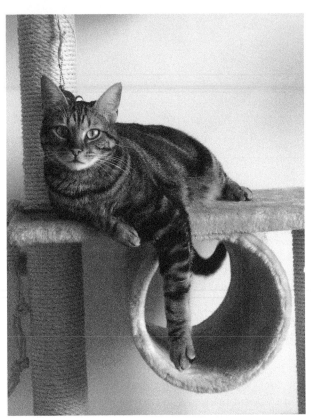

FIGURE 1-3 Vertical space enriches the environment by providing a safe perch from which the cat can monitor the environment. (Copyright © iStock.com)

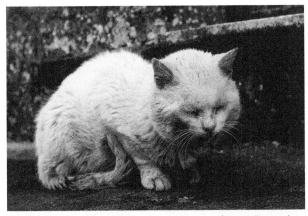

FIGURE 1-4 Once beloved cats are often released to enter the stray cat population because people worry that they will be euthanized if surrendered to a shelter. However, these cats may not be able to properly fend for themselves among feral cats, and their welfare is often poor. (Copyright © iStock.com)

in the United States,[25] with millions of cats being euthanized each year because of behavior problems. House soiling is the most commonly reported behavior problem to result in surrender,[10,11] and the second is a newly adopted cat not getting along with existing cats in the household.[11,26,27] The third most common cause is

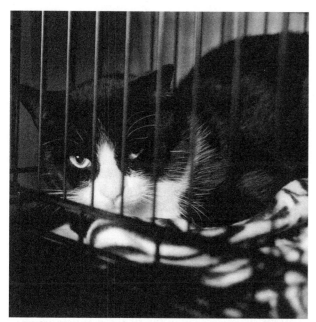

FIGURE 1-5 Cats are often surrendered to shelters because of either undesirable behaviors or attributes, behavior problems, or changes in owner circumstances. (Copyright © iStock.com)

aggression towards people.[11] Cat to human aggression is a common public health issue. One study indicated that 15% of cats were relinquished to shelters because of aggression towards people.

There is an association between owners' misconception that their cat misbehaves to spite them and relinquishment.[10] In one study, 65.8% of the cat owners relinquishing a cat thought that their cat eliminated outside the litter box or destroyed furniture to spite them.[10] Client education is needed to explain that spite is not a feline motivation for these behaviors. Cats are also surrendered as a result of normal but undesirable feline behaviors, such as scratching, and because of unrealistic owner expectations which lead to the perception that their cat is "needing too much attention", "unfriendly", "disobedient", "too active", or having other undesirable traits.[11]

Many cat owners cannot face the decision processes necessary to organize the rehoming or euthanasia of their pet and instead they prefer to release their cat to the outdoors. This addition to the stray cat population is reported in many countries but may be even more of a problem in those countries where it is illegal to euthanize a pet that is not physically ill.[28] Releasing pet cats into the stray population has a number of implications both in terms of the welfare of the cat, which is not adapted to a stray lifestyle and may be prone to injury and infectious disease, and the welfare of the wildlife population which may be exposed to increased threat from an increasing stray cat population. [26]

FELINE BEHAVIORAL ISSUES COMMONLY ASSOCIATED WITH RELINQUISHMENT OR EUTHANASIA

House Soiling (see Chapter 24)

In a study of 1286 feline relinquishments to 12 different shelters, house soiling was the cause of relinquishment in approximately 40% of the cats.[11] These included cats surrendered for reasons which were classified as either behavioral or mixed, with behavior being a possible component in the mixed category.[11]

Many of the cats surrendered or euthanized for house soiling are older or physically ill.[10] Owners who erroneously thought the cat house soiled in order to spite them were more likely to surrender or euthanize their cat.[10] Many cats with inappropriate elimination may have an underlying medical problem that is undiagnosed or a litter box aversion, either of which can be effectively treated by veterinarians, thus reducing the euthanasia of cats. Referral to a behaviorist for more challenging problems will further reduce these numbers.

Intercat Conflict (see Chapter 26)

In the same study, relinquishment was found to be associated with the number of pets in the household, as well as the introduction of new cats to the home environment. Often the new cat had been adopted to be a friend for the already existing cat(s). In order to reduce the levels of relinquishment for these reasons, owners need to develop an understanding of feline social behavior and environmental needs for each cat. This will assist them in making appropriate adoption decisions and, if they decide to go ahead with adoption, will assist them in carrying out appropriate introductions of new cats.

Aggression Towards Humans (see Chapter 27)

Aggression directed towards humans is less frequently reported in cats than in dogs, but it is still a serious and common behavior problem as well as a public health concern.[29] The incidence varies from 12% to 47% of all behavior problems reported by cat owners.[30] In a U.S. study of 12 shelters and more than 1000 cats, 15% of cats surrendered for behavior problems were due to aggression towards people.[11]

Aggression that occurs in association with being handled or played with is the most frequently reported, and a survey in the United States indicated that redirected aggression is also common, most often occurring when an outdoor cat is seen through a window by an indoor cat, or a cat is startled by noise.[31,32] Self-protection or defensive aggression in a fearful cat is another reported form of cat aggression towards family members.[29,31] Most cat aggression towards humans in the home occurs towards family members,[29,31] and one study indicated that it occurs more frequently towards women and children.[31]

Client education about how to handle and play with cats is essential to prevent these problems. Dissuading clients from approaching an aroused cat is also important to prevent unexpected and serious bite or scratch injuries.

Normal but Undesirable Behaviors (see Chapter 23)

Many causes of surrender are not related to a behavior problem at all, but rather normal cat behavior that owners find undesirable.[10,26,27] For example, scratching is normal behavior, but cats are commonly surrendered for furniture destruction and marking behaviors, which are also normal but often unacceptable in an indoor context. Once again, client education is essential so that owners can learn how to redirect undesirable behaviors to appropriate areas or alter the cat's home environment to ensure that behaviors are no longer displayed in that context.

Old Age (see Chapter 25)

One U.S. study identified two categories of cats surrendered to shelters, with older or sick cats being surrendered for euthanasia, and younger cats being surrendered for adoption.[10] Of those being surrendered for euthanasia 59% were seniors, at least 8 years of age or older, and over 20% were 16 years of age or older (Figure 1-6).[10] Many of these cats had been in their owner's possession for a considerable period of time and been regarded as beloved pets and family members and yet at end of their lives, a decision was made to surrender them to a shelter, with all of the unfamiliar stimuli that it presents for the cat, rather than take them to a veterinary practice to seek a diagnosis and potential treatment or request a veterinarian to come to the cat's home to offer euthanasia in a comfortable home environment.

Owner's Personal Issues

Another significant reason for surrender is change in the owner's personal circumstances which results in the cat being considered an "inconvenience"; these include a change in housing, arrival of a new baby or housemate, divorce, or the desire to travel.[33] It may be hard for veterinary professionals, who have devoted their lives to helping animals, to comprehend that the cat becomes a disposable "thing" when it is no longer convenient. Preadoption counseling, understanding the responsibilities of living with a cat, and helping potential owners anticipate how they will handle future situations helps prevent some of these situations (see Chapter 6).

INCORPORATING BEHAVIOR INTO FELINE PRACTICE

Veterinarians have a great opportunity to improve the uptake of veterinary care for pet cats and reduce levels of relinquishment and euthanasia by providing a holistic approach that encompasses not only the physical health of patients, but also their psychological and emotional health (Figure 1-7). It is important to recognize that behavioral issues are of major concern for clients,[1] and education of potential adopters and current cat owners about the nature of the cat and its needs will not only increase owner appreciation of their pet, but also of the veterinary profession and the importance of providing regular healthcare.

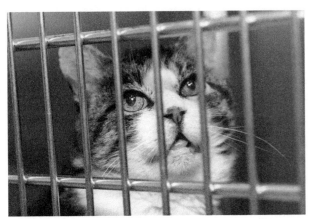

FIGURE 1-6   Many of the cats surrendered to shelters are senior cats that have been with the owners for many years before surrender. (Copyright © iStock.com)

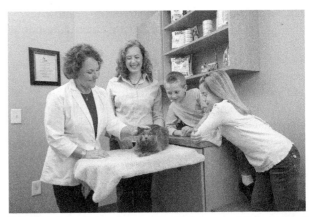

FIGURE 1-7   Educating both adults and children about their cat's veterinary and home care can prevent both medical and behavioral problems.

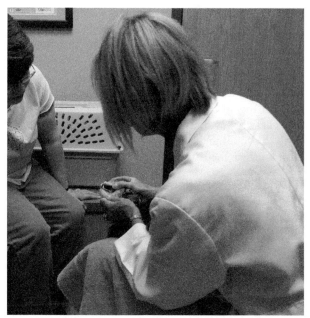

FIGURE 1-8 Each veterinary consultation provides an opportunity to teach clients about their cat's needs and how to maintain or improve their physical and emotional health, both during veterinary visits and in the home environment. (Courtesy D. Echelberry & M. Miller)

Client education can occur in a variety of ways within the veterinary practice. Information can be imparted during consultations (Figure 1-8), but it is also possible to educate via websites and social media, in presentations to cat owners, and through working with shelters.

In order to offer the best possible level of client education, it is important for members of staff to learn about normal feline behavior and understand the importance of meeting basic feline needs through providing appropriate environments both at home and in the practice.

Preadoption Counseling

Adding preadoption counseling as a service in the veterinary practice can help to provide people with realistic expectations of living with a cat and help them set up the environment for successful adoption. In other situations, it can persuade clients that it is not the best time for them to adopt a cat. People with cats already in the household should be educated about the possibility of a new cat not being accepted by the other cat(s) and helped to decide if they will be able to accept such a situation. See Chapter 6 for more information.

If preadoption counseling has not occurred, all the information should be covered during the first visits. Unfortunately, this can be a more difficult approach as the client has already set up the home as they feel appropriate, and being told that they need to make changes may be difficult for them to accept, especially when no problems have been noted. The client may already have issues, such as furniture scratching or

children getting scratched or bitten, and more detailed advice will then be necessary to ensure that these issues are addressed as soon as possible. Staff will need more training to offer appropriate advice and more time will need to be allocated for these appointments to effectively care for the cat's needs and to help the client understand why the cat is behaving in this manner.

Incorporation of Behavior into Every Veterinary Visit

Behavioral knowledge has a role to play in all feline consultations, not only in terms of ensuring that cats are handled in the most effective and welfare friendly manner, but also in terms of gathering an accurate history which will assist in the pursuit of a definitive diagnosis. A change in behavior occurs when cats are ill, in pain, or stressed. Subtle changes such as a change in appetite, a decline in grooming, or an inability to get to the litter box will often be the instigator for a visit to the veterinary practice.

Since the signs of feline illness are often subtle, it can be beneficial to ask open-ended questions[34] during all feline consultations with a view to gathering important information about the cat's behavior.

There is a strong correlation between the behavior and physical health of the cat and combining behavioral and medical questioning will help veterinarians to reach a more accurate diagnosis in many feline cases.

Addressing Behavior Problems in Primary Practice

Many feline behavior problems have underlying medical causes or occur in combination with other health issues.[9] The accurate diagnosis of those medical issues is therefore the first step for any case of a cat presenting with behavior problem(s) and thorough history-taking, clinical examination, and diagnostic workup will be needed for every case. In some cases the presenting behavior problem may resolve as a result of the treatment for the medical problem, but in many cases the behavioral issues also need to be addressed. A good example is the cat that usually eliminates in litter box (es) even though it finds them undesirable—either too small, dirty, or an offensive type of litter—but starts to select a more comfortable or desirable toileting location when it is suffering from a urinary tract disease. Despite successful treatment of the medical problem, the cat may continue to eliminate in the more desirable area and client education about normal feline toileting behavior and advice about how to provide suitable toileting facilities will also be needed to resolve the problem completely (see Chapter 24). The behavioral advice can be incorporated into the treatment plan for the cat at their initial appointment, during a follow-up behavior consultation appointment, or follow-up appointments to reassess the medical problem.

SUMMARY

As cats increase in popularity, there is a growing challenge to the veterinary profession to provide adequate and appropriate healthcare for the feline population. Many cats fail to receive regular healthcare, and increasing awareness of feline behavior is vital if veterinary practices are to offer an environment which reduces feline stress and encourages clients to bring their pets to the veterinary practice more regularly.

Behavior and physical health are closely intertwined, making the need to address behavior within feline practice essential. Incorporating behavior into primary practice increases client awareness of the cat's physical, social, and environmental needs, setting up the client(s) and cat(s) for success. It also increases client awareness to contact the veterinary practice with any concerns about their cat's behavior as early as possible. This will not only help to avoid the development of behavior problems but also increase the early detection of disease.

REFERENCES

1. American Veterinary Medical Association. *U.S. pet ownership & demographics sourcebook.* 2012; https://www.avma.org/KB/Resources/Statistics/Pages/Market-research-statistics-US-Pet-Ownership-Demographics-Sourcebook.aspx. Accessed December 12, 2014.
2. Taylor P, Funk C, Craighill P. *Gauging family intimacy: dogs edge cats (dads trail both).* Pew Research Center; 2006.
3. Gunn-Moore D. Considering older cats. *J Sm Anim Pract Age.* 2006;47:430–431.
4. Lue TW, Pantenburg DP, Crawford PM. Impact of the owner-pet and client-veterinarian bond on the care that pets receive. *JAVMA.* 2008;232:531–540.
5. Bayer HealthCare. *Veterinary care usage study III: Feline findings;* 2012. http://www.bayerdvm.com/show.aspx/news-release-bvcus-iii-feline-findings. Accessed January 7, 2015.
6. Heath SE. Behaviour problems and welfare. In: Rochlitz I, ed. *The welfare of cats.* Dordrecht: Springer; 2005:91–118.
7. Ellis SH, Rodan I, et al. AAFP and ISFM Feline Environmental Needs Guidelines. *J Feline Med Surg.* 2013; 15:219–230.
8. Buffington CA, Westropp JL, Chew DJ, Bolus RR. Clinical evaluation of multimodal environmental modification (MEMO) in the management of cats with idiopathic cystitis. *J Feline Med Surg.* 2006;8:261–268.
9. Stella JL, Lord LK, Buffington CAT. Sickness behaviors in response to unusual external events in healthy cats and cats with feline interstitial cystitis. *J Am Vet Med Assoc.* 2011;238:67–73.
10. Kass PH, New Jr JC, Scarlett JM, Salman MD. Understanding animal companion surplus in the United States: relinquishment of nonadoptables to animal shelters for euthanasia. *J Applied Anim Welfare Sci.* 2001;4:237–248.
11. Salman MD, Hutchison J, Ruch-Gallie R. Behavioral reasons for relinquishment of dogs and cats to 12 shelters. *J Applied Anim Welfare Sci.* 2000;3:93–106.
12. Driscoll CA, Menotti-Raymond M, Roca AL, et al. The Near Eastern origin of cat domestication. *Science.* 2007;317:519.
13. Bradshaw JWS, Casey RA, Brown SL. *The behaviour of the domestic cat.* ed 2. CABI Publ; 2012.
14. Bayer HealthCare LLC. *Brakke Consulting, and the National Commission of Veterinary Economics Issues;* 2011.
15. American Pet Products Association's 2009–2010 National Pet Owners Survey. http://www.americanpetproducts.org/. 2010.
16. Shore ER. Returning a recently adopted companion animal: adopters' reasons for and reactions to the failed adoption experience. *J Applied Anim Welfare Sci.* 2005;8:187–198.
17. AVMA animal welfare position statement, free-roaming, owned cats. https://www.avmª.org/News/JAVMANews/Pages/s071501e.aspx.
18. Sturgess K: Disease and welfare. In: Rochlitz I, editor: *The welfare of cats.* Dordrecht: Springer; 2007:205–225.
19. *Banfield Pet Hospital: State of pet health 2011 report, vol 1.* Portland, Ore: Banfield Pet Hospital; 2011. http://www.banfield.com/Banfield/files/bd/bd826667-067d-41e4-994d-5ea0bd7db86d.pdf.
20. Association for Pet Obesity Prevention: http://www.petobesityprevention.com/.
21. Tanaka A, Wagner DC, Kass PH, Hurley KF. Associations among weight loss, stress, and upper respiratory tract infection in shelter cats. *J Am Vet Med Assoc.* 2012; 240:570–576.
22. Stella J, Croney C, Buffington CAT. Effects of stressors on the behavior and physiology of domestic cats. *Appl Anim Behav Sci.* 2013;143:157–163.
23. Defauw PAM, et al. Risk factors and clinical presentation of cats with feline idiopathic cystitis. *J Feline Med Surg.* 2011;13:967–975.
24. Buffington CAT. Idiopathic cystitis in domestic cats—beyond the lower urinary tract. *J Vet Intern Med.* 2011; 25:784–796.
25. Patronek GJ, Dodman NH. Attitudes, procedures, and delivery of behavior services by veterinarians in small animal practice. *J Am Vet Med Assoc.* 1999;215:1606–1611.
26. Fournier AK, Geller ES. Behavior analysis of companion-animal overpopulation: a conceptualization of the problem and suggestions for intervention. *Behav Social Issues.* 2004;13:51–68.
27. New JC, Salman MD, King M, Scarlett JM, Kass PH, Hutchison JM. Characteristics of shelter-relinquished animals and their owners compared with animals and their owners in U.S. pet-owning households. *J Applied Anim Welfare Sci.* 2000;3:179–201.
28. Slater ML, Di Nardo A, Pediconi O, et al. Free-roaming dogs and cats in central Italy: Public perceptions of the problem. *Pre Vet Med.* 2008;84:27–47.
29. Palacio J, León-Artozqui M, Pastor-Villalba E, Carrera-Martín F, García-Belenguer S. Incidence of and risk factors for cat bites: a first step in prevention and treatment of feline aggression. *J Feline Med Surg.* 2007; 9:188–195.
30. Ramos D, Mills DS. Human directed aggression in Brazilian domestic cats: owner reported prevalence, contexts and risk factors. *J Feline Med Surg.* 2009;11:835–841.
31. Amat M, Manteca X, Le Brech S, Ruiz de la Torre JL, Mariotti VM, Fatjó J. Evaluation of inciting causes,

alternative targets, and risk factors associated with redirected aggression in cats. *J Am Vet Med Assoc.* 2008; 233:586–589.

32. Curtis TM. The more common causes for human-directed aggression in cats include play, fear, petting intolerance, and redirected aggression. *Vet Clin North Am Small Anim Pract.* 2008;38:1131–1143.

33. Scarlett JM, Salman MD, New JG, Kass PH. Reasons for relinquishment of companion animals in U.S. animal shelters: selected health and personal issues. *J Appl Anim Welf Sci.* 1999;2:41–57.

34. Dysart LMA, Coe JB, Adams CL. Analysis of solicitation of client concerns in companion animal practice. *J Am Vet Med Assoc.* 2011;238:1609–1615.

Feline Behavior and Welfare

Ilona Rodan and Sarah Heath

INTRODUCTION

Veterinarians and other veterinary professionals have a duty to protect animal welfare and to make it a major focus in their daily work. The goals are to provide the best healthcare for their patients and to enhance the quality and length of the relationship between people and their pets. However, until recently, veterinary training has tended to focus on welfare only from the perspective of physical health. Because cats are sentient beings,[1,2] which are conscious, have feelings, and are therefore able to suffer, a comprehensive approach to the welfare of feline patients needs to be adopted by all veterinary professionals. A lack of understanding of cats, their normal behaviors, and their needs negatively impacts their welfare. Many behavior problems are related to poor welfare situations that go unrecognized until unwanted behaviors occur.

Adequate healthcare in terms of physical health is not a guarantee of good welfare, and, although cat owners may think that they provide the best possible life for their cats and even talk about their cats as being spoiled or pampered, some well-loved cats have poor welfare. When people have minimal knowledge of another species, it is common to think about what is best for that species from the human point of view (anthropomorphism), which can often result in compromised welfare despite good intentions.

Addressing welfare sounds easier than it actually is. It is important to recognize that feline needs differ significantly from those of dogs and humans and to acknowledge that even a domestic cat that lives exclusively indoors is more similar to its African Wildcat ancestor than to other pets or humans. When considering the welfare implications of any interactions with cats, it is important to consider the situation from a feline perspective. One might consider the example of a hungry and cold street cat that is taken into a loving home, and provided with nutritious meals and a warm bed. On the one hand, the cat was starving and cold outdoors, but it had its own familiar territory and was able to express a range of normal feline behaviors. Moving the cat into a home, and treating it as a member of the family, may seem like a wonderful and caring act. However, the cat may be fearful of people and of the unfamiliar indoor environment. This fear may take weeks or months to subside and it is possible that the cat will never learn to cope in its new surroundings. In order to determine the welfare outcome of a decision, it is important to consider the individual cat and to determine if its needs are being met. As this example illustrates, the cat could experience poor welfare in both situations and it might be better to find a compromise that allows the cat to continue to live independently but offers some form of outdoor shelter and the provision of food. In this way its physical and mental health and welfare can be optimized.

Primary veterinarians who see feline patients—regardless of practice type—have the opportunity and the responsibility to educate clients about all aspects of feline welfare. Negative welfare issues occur frequently and can be prevented or addressed by incorporating client education about feline behavior into veterinary appointments.

There is a common saying that cats are not small dogs. Today, a lot of people consider their cats to be their "children" or lifelong companions, but cats are not small people either. Addressing cats' emotional, social, and physical needs, and allowing them to perform their normal behaviors in an enriched environment ensures good feline welfare.

THE CONNECTION BETWEEN BEHAVIOR AND WELFARE

Animal welfare is defined as how an animal copes with the conditions in which it lives.[3-5] Good welfare is concerned with allowing animals to engage in their normal behaviors and addressing their species-specific needs. When a cat's needs are not met, it affects both their physical and psychological health. When cats cannot engage in their normal behaviors, unwanted behaviors often occur. In fact, behavior changes and problems are important indicators of feline welfare[6] and vital indicators of the need for veterinary care. Behavior problems are a common cause of breakdown of the bond between owner and pet and subsequent surrender to a shelter or request for euthanasia.[7] It is essential, therefore, to meet cats' needs and allow them to express their natural behaviors to prevent stress and undesirable behavior and to improve feline health and welfare.

THE HUMAN–CAT RELATIONSHIP AND ITS IMPACT ON FELINE WELFARE

Ensuring animal welfare is a human responsibility[2,8] and veterinarians have an obligation to teach cat owners about the welfare needs of their feline companions. Changes in feline welfare are related to changes in the relationship between people and cats over time. While many of those changes, especially during the last century, have benefited cats, there are some individuals for whom cats' closer interaction with humans has not been entirely positive. Understanding past and current human–cat relationships can make it easier to recognize the issues involved.

History of the Human–Cat Relationship

The history of *Felis catus* and its welfare are directly related to human history. Cats and people have lived together for approximately 10,000 years, when *Felis catus* evolved from *Felis sylvestris lybica* (Figures 2-1 and 2-2).[9,10] The human–cat relationship has changed greatly over the centuries, with cats first deified by the Egyptians, then demonized during the Middle Ages, and now owned as a very popular pet. The increasing popularity of the cat has both positive and negative impacts on welfare. Understanding normal feline behaviors in the context of the original mutualistic relationship and how it evolved helps to identify the strengths of the initial relationship and some of the weaknesses seen today.

The history of people and cats through the centuries is fascinating. As people adapted from being

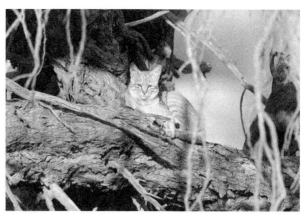

FIGURE 2-2 The African wildcat, *Felis sylvestris lybica*, the ancestor to *Felis catus*, uses high perches to monitor its environment and to protect itself. Note that the African wildcat is often colored so as to be well camouflaged in its environment. (Copyright © iStock.com)

hunter-gatherers to cultivators approximately 10,000 years ago, their crops attracted rodents, which in turn attracted cats. The proximity of cats to human settlements was mutually beneficial by protecting the food supply of both species. In contrast to the human–dog relationship—a much older relationship with genetic selection to address human needs (e.g., hunting and herding dogs)—farmers found the innate behaviors of cats highly desirable, and the human–cat relationship did not require genetic modification.[11] As a result, the behavior of the domestic cat today is not significantly different from that of its wild ancestors.[11]

Until approximately 50 to 60 years ago, the cat's primary function remained the control of rodent populations. Most cats were free to make the most of their access to a warm and comfortable indoor environment while continuing to hunt for their food and have the opportunity to perform other natural behaviors in an outdoor context.

From Utilitarian Relationships to Cats as Family Members

Over the last century, changing human lifestyles have led to changes in the relationship between people and cats. As urbanization has increased, the popularity of the cat has also increased.[12] The cat is now the most popular pet in many countries (Box 2-1). With urbanization and the dispersion of human family units, pets have often replaced extended families and provided a continuing outlet for the human need to nurture.[13] As people began to work longer hours, spend less time at home, and live in more compact dwellings, the cat appeared to be a good fit as a pet that is apparently convenient and easy to care for.

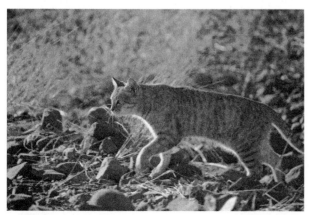

FIGURE 2-1 The pet cat, *Felis catus*, evolved from the African wildcat, *Felis sylvestris lybica*. (Copyright © iStock.com)

BOX 2-1	Countries Where Cats Were the Most Popular Pet in 2008

United States
Russia
United Kingdom
Canada
France
Ukraine
Germany
Italy
Netherlands
Turkey
Austria
Switzerland
Sweden
New Zealand

From Batson A: World Society for the Protection of Companion Animals (WSPCA) Global Companion Animal Ownership and Trade: Project Summary, June 2008. http://www.worldanimalprotection.org/

The development of cat litter in 1947 made indoor cat living more acceptable,[14] and by 1970, some veterinary organizations in the United States were recommending that cats be kept indoors to protect them from outdoor dangers and to protect from damage to wildlife. Cats went from being primarily appreciated for their hunting skills to being valued as well-loved pets. There was no longer any requirement to hunt to survive, but the instinct remained, and the very behavior that led to the relationship between humans and cats was now a potential source of tension.

As the relationship between humans and pets changed, the term *human–animal bond* was established, reflecting the importance of the relationship between owners and their pets. The vast majority of cat owners undoubtedly want to do the best for their beloved pets, but unfortunately, there is often a discrepancy between what people think is good for cats and what actually is. For example, people often acquire additional cats in the belief that they are providing a friend for their existing cat and, through a lack of understanding of normal feline social behavior, fail to understand the potential distress that the introduction of an unfamiliar cat into the household may cause (Figure 2-3, *A–G*). The potential impact of human lifestyles on the emotional state of domestic cats is often underestimated. Cats are territorial creatures, and familiarity and consistency associated with their environment is important for their security. Change is a common feature of human households, with people redecorating, renovating, and refurnishing on a regular basis, as well as changing both the human and animal composition of their households or physically changing territory by moving to a new home. These unintentional threats to territorial security, combined with the decreasing available territory in urban areas due to the diminishing size of housing plots and the increasing density of feline populations, have led to increasing pressure on the domestic cat, and many normal feline behaviors, such as hunting and marking, are actively discouraged in a domestic context.

The Relationship of Veterinary Professionals to Cats

Many veterinary professionals who work with cats recognize the uniqueness of the feline patient and find the nature and behaviors of cats fascinating. However, for others, working with feline patients is extremely challenging, and there are some members of the profession who admit to finding feline work unrewarding and even unpleasant.[15] In general, those who understand the cat and its fears, as well as how to address them in the veterinary environment, gain more pleasure from working with cats than those who do not.

One of the biggest challenges of veterinary practice is successful handling of the feline patient and unfortunately, many of the feline restraint methods that are still taught are fundamentally at odds with the natural behavior of the cat. As a result, they lead to an increase in feline fear and associated defensive behaviors, which in turn increase the potential for human injury and consequently the levels of anxiety in veterinary personnel when working with feline patients. The result of inadequate and sometimes inaccurate handling training is that some veterinary professionals understand very little about why the cat reacts as it does at the veterinary practice and therefore inaccurately label cats as aggressive or even malevolent. It is not unusual to hear veterinarians and technicians describe individual cats as "crabby," "evil," and "bad." Chapters 20, 21, and 22 describe respectful handling techniques to aid in handling cats in a way that reduces their fear and aggression.

There can be no doubt that cats have benefitted from increasing veterinary knowledge in terms of their medical care, and feline longevity has significantly increased as a result of improved therapies for both infectious and noninfectious diseases. Prevention of pain and advancement of pain management for acute and chronic conditions has also greatly improved the quality of life of feline patients (see Chapters 14 and 15). Veterinarians routinely collaborate with clients to support their goals for their beloved cats in terms of disease control and prevention, but it is also important to consider whether the goals of cat owners and veterinarians address the welfare needs of the cat.

In this chapter, we address the welfare issues associated with behavioral and physical health that primary veterinarians encounter on a daily basis but that are often unrecognized and consequently overlooked. Clinical scenarios commonly involve compromise of feline freedoms, such as freedom from pain and disease,

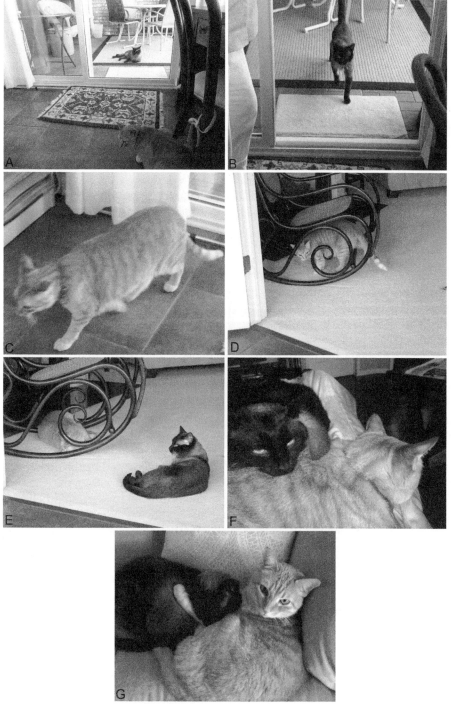

FIGURE 2-3   A–E, Most cats do not readily accept a new cat being added to a household. This adult Siamese was adopted after the death of the orange tabby's previous companion, which was also Siamese. Note the reaction of the fearful orange tabby to the new cat. **F, G,** Separating the cats, providing multiple resources in different locations, and synthetic feline pheromone analog diffusers helped to increase the orange tabby's sense of security. Gradual introductions increase familiarity over time. It took 4 months for these cats to sleep together (F) and 8 months for the orange tabby to be completely relaxed around the Siamese, likely due to the immediate initial introduction.

freedom to express most normal behaviors, and free-dom from fear and distress. Awareness of these issues is essential to understanding the solutions to these challenges.

ISSUES THAT CONTRIBUTE TO NEGATIVE FELINE WELFARE

Many cats live in stressful social situations and/or inadequate physical environments. When this happens, it can limit the cat's ability to perform normal feline behaviors and may lead to an inability to cope with the living situation, resulting in the potential for issues of fear and distress.

In some circumstances, failure to recognize the compromised welfare state of cats can be associated with the serious human mental health issue of hoarding. In hoarding situations, dozens to hundreds of cats may live surrounded by feces and urine—and even dead cats—and the hoarders may truly believe that they are doing the best for their cats. Detailed discussion of this condition is outside the scope of this book, but it is the duty of the veterinary professional to report these situations to appropriate authorities so that the animals and humans involved can receive appropriate care.

In other circumstances, the pressures on the cat are not obvious to the caring cat providers and veterinary professionals at an early stage. When left unresolved, the outcome is often behavior problems, the breakdown of the relationship between cats and owners, and even surrender to a shelter or euthanasia.

The Five Freedoms, initially written to address the welfare of livestock, have been recognized as essential to the welfare of pets as well, regardless of whether they are in the home environment, the veterinary practice, or a shelter.[16]

1. Freedom from Hunger and Thirst: by ready access to fresh water and a diet to maintain full health and vigor.
2. Freedom from Discomfort: by providing an appropriate environment, including shelter and a comfortable resting area.
3. Freedom from Pain, Injury, or Disease: by prevention or rapid diagnosis and treatment.
4. Freedom to Express Normal Behavior: by providing sufficient space, proper facilities, and company of the animal's own kind.
5. Freedom from Fear and Distress: by ensuring conditions and treatment that avoid mental suffering.

Issues related to all of these freedoms are covered in various chapters in this book. The focus of this chapter is the final three freedoms, which have a significant impact on the behavioral aspects of feline veterinary practice and need to be considered to prevent suffering and promote positive feline welfare.[3-5]

CONCERN FOR FELINE FREEDOMS

Freedom from Pain and Disease

Freedom from pain and disease through prevention, rapid diagnosis, and treatment is the welfare issue that most veterinarians recognize and strive to address. Unfortunately, millions of pet cats receive little or no veterinary care and suffer significant levels of unrecognized pain and illness.[15,17] It is not unusual for feline patients to go for periods of two years or more without any veterinary attention. When clients do not come to the practice and do not respond to routine reminders, it may be assumed that they have either moved away from the area or gone to another veterinary practice. When the client does eventually come to the practice, a recent decline in the cat's health is often reported, with the cat being well until then, thereby justifying to the client the choice not to come in earlier. These clients may apologize and will often explain that they are reluctant to visit the practice because it is a very stressful experience for both themselves and their pet. If their cat is elderly, they think that the health changes, especially aspects such as alterations in appetite and mobility, are inevitable changes associated with the aging process. They may believe that nothing can be done or that the difficulty of administering any necessary medication makes a visit to the veterinary practice unjustified. Eventually, the client feels compelled to bring the cat to the practice, and by the time this happens, obtaining an accurate history from the client can be a challenge. It can be difficult to ascertain whether the cat's deteriorating health has happened gradually over the previous months or more dramatically over recent days or weeks. When it is reported to the clients that the cat is now in an advanced state of disease, it is not uncommon for clients to have feelings of guilt related to their decision not to bring their cat in sooner.

The outcome may be positive for the cat and client if the condition can be treated and the cat's comfort and welfare restored. Many chronic conditions, such as degenerative joint disease, hyperthyroidism, and chronic kidney disease, can be controlled or stabilized. The client's respect and awareness of veterinary care then increases, and the client is more likely to return for appropriate follow-up care for the cat. If there is more than one cat in the household, the client is more likely to accept education about prevention and early detection of pain and illness for the other cats in the household.

Unfortunately, many outcomes are not positive. If a decision is made that the cat's condition is now too advanced to justify treatment, the client's guilt is further compounded by the decision to euthanize. It can be extremely difficult for a client to face the prospect of losing a much-loved pet, and a decision to pursue treatment, however difficult that may be for both the cat and the client, is often made. When clients need more time to come to terms with the seriousness of their pet's condition and to say their goodbyes, high-quality palliative or hospice care may be appropriate to safeguard feline welfare in the short term. However, discussion about the welfare of the pet, follow-up communications, and provision of a feline quality of life scale (see Box 7-4, Quality of Life Scale, in Chapter 7) can help to ensure the cat's welfare during this interim period and help the client to recognize when euthanasia is in the best interest of the patient to prevent its suffering and pain.

Client education about analgesia and nutritional and supportive care is also indicated, along with instructions on how to administer medications. If recommendations are not made or are unclear, poor welfare situations may result. One example is the difficulty in recognizing the subtle signs of pain and the client's concomitant decision to withhold analgesia. Another is inappetence as a factor in a disease state; many owners are reluctant to opt for medications or the placement of a feeding tube. Instead, they may opt to attempt to force-feed the cat with a syringe or force food into the cat's mouth, both of which can be painful for the cat and lead to the sensation of nausea. Offering multiple types of food or following the cat around with food can also lead it to experience nausea, food aversion, stress, and even avoidance of its owners. These well-meant attempts to offer nutrition can detrimentally affect the welfare of the cat, and avoiding these problems will prevent feline suffering. The decision to euthanize may be painful and emotionally challenging for the clients, but it may be the right decision and be in the interests of the welfare of their pet.

Advanced disease states on presentation and the associated dilemma of the end-of-life decision are potential threats to feline welfare, and chronic unrecognized disease is another. Clients' misconceptions that their pet will show obvious signs such as inappetence or lameness if they are experiencing dental or orthopedic conditions lead to unrecognized and therefore untreated pain from periodontal disease, oral resorptive lesions, and feline degenerative joint disease (DJD). The prevalence of DJD in cats has only recently been recognized within the veterinary profession. It is now acknowledged that, because the signs of the condition are very subtle on clinical examination, diagnosis is often delayed. Welfare considerations of chronic pain states cannot be ignored. The subject of chronic pain is dealt with in much more detail in Chapter 15. Information about the handling of painful patients is discussed in Chapter 21.

In contrast, clients often assume that cats with physical disabilities have poor welfare, but there are plenty of examples of cats that are born with leg deformities or are blind and live their lives with excellent welfare because

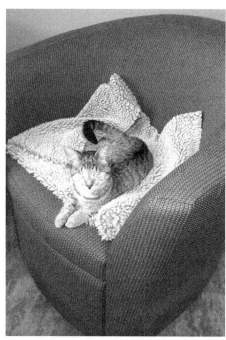

FIGURE 2-4 This blind cat (both eyes removed because of severe buphthalmos and corneal perforations secondary to congenital feline herpesvirus 1) is very content and able to climb everywhere. This photo was taken in a veterinary practice, where the cat did not know the environment.

they have strategies available to them that enable them to cope with their disabilities (Figure 2-4).

Freedom to Express Most Normal Behaviors

To enjoy good welfare, the cat should be able to engage in a range of its natural behaviors in a suitable environment with sufficient space, proper resources, and appropriate interactions with other animals.[3] Many innate feline behaviors, such as hunting, marking, scratching, climbing, and jumping, are undesirable to owners. Cats are often relinquished or euthanized for performing these instinctive behaviors, but some owners take the alternative approach of using techniques to prevent their pet from engaging in these behaviors. Keeping cats indoors to prevent hunting, performing onychectomy to prevent furniture destruction, and using a squirt gun to keep cats off counters are some of the recommendations that have been made by veterinary professionals to assist clients in their goal of keeping their pet. From a feline welfare perspective, however, these interventions limit the cat's ability to express innate behaviors and are therefore detrimental to its welfare.

A good example of the potential discrepancy between human and feline goals is onychectomy, or declawing. Although this procedure is illegal in a number of countries and controversial in others, many veterinary practices in the United States still perform declawing as a routine procedure. Outstanding surgical skills and excellent perioperative and postoperative analgesia may make the procedure acceptable to many from a purely clinical perspective, but the fact that it is designed to eliminate scratching from the behavioral repertoire of the cat raises some serious concerns from a welfare viewpoint. There are excellent alternatives to declawing, including client education about claw care and providing desirable scratching posts in appropriate places to prevent furniture scratching (Figure 2-5). More information on this topic is available in Chapter 8.

Another area in which the expression of normal feline behavior is often severely compromised is feeding. As solitary hunters, cats naturally eat multiple small meals every day, with each of these resulting from a short period of intense energy-consuming activity during which the cat chases, pounces, and catches its prey (Figure 2-6, A and B). In contrast, the domestic cat is usually provided with food once or twice daily, with the food presented in a bowl. If the cat lives in a multicat household, the owners will often feed the cats together and expect them to eat from the same bowl or in bowls positioned next to each other (Figure 2-7). Whereas communal eating is a sign of social cohesion in humans, the feeding process has no social significance for cats. The stress of eating in the company of other cats can lead to a range of behavioral consequences, including inappetence due to fear of close proximity to an unfamiliar or incompatible cat, and gorging and regurgitating due to the rapid consumption of food in an attempt to limit the time spent in close proximity to the other

cat. Both of these scenarios are indicative of poor welfare.

Innate feline toileting behavior is also frequently compromised in the domestic setting through the provision of inappropriate litter box facilities that are often poorly

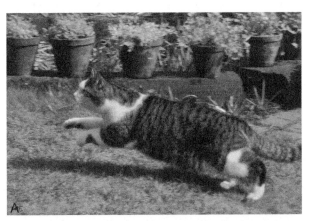

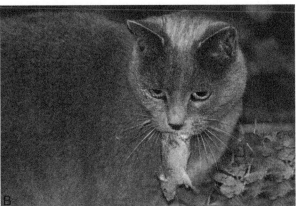

FIGURE 2-6   Cats are solitary hunters that eat many small meals each day to survive. They exert a lot of energy to chase, pounce on, and catch their prey. (Courtesy A. Dossche)

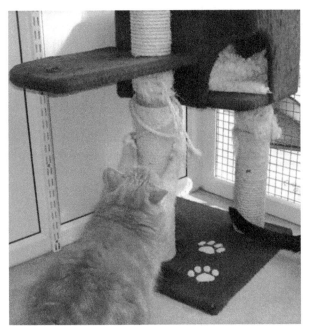

FIGURE 2-5   Scratching posts should be placed in areas where cats prefer to scratch, such as near a primary piece of furniture or where the scent profile changes (e.g., near a door or window). Providing a post that allows a cat to stretch fully is ideal. (Courtesy S. Ellis)

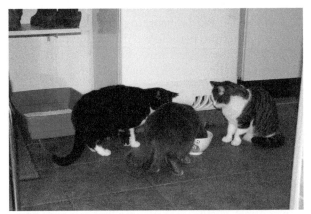

FIGURE 2-7   Feeding cats in close proximity to each other causes stress and competition for resources. Note that only one of the cats is eating while the others wait. The food dish is also close to the litter box, which is not compatible with normal feline behavior. (Courtesy A. Dossche)

maintained, inadequately cleaned, and positioned in inappropriate locations (Figures 2-8 and 2-9). This not only has a negative effect on the cat's welfare but also results in the onset of house soiling problems, which are one of the most common reasons that cats are surrendered or euthanized.

The way a cat is housed, whether for the short term (e.g., hospitalization or boarding) or the long term (at home), will have a significant impact on its welfare.[18,19] Cats cope with their environment by using a range of behaviors, including hiding and elevation (Figures 2-10 and 2-11). In the wild, they maintain their territory and reduce potential fights by dispersing or avoiding cats that are unfamiliar or threatening.[18] Often these coping strategies are not available to the cat in a domestic setting, and this is particularly true when the cat finds itself in unfamiliar situations or places (e.g., encountering someone unfamiliar in the home or being taken to the veterinary practice) or living in

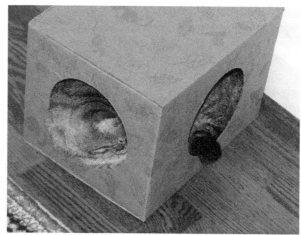

FIGURE 2-10   Instead of forcing interactions with the cat, providing hiding places big enough for only one cat to enter can help to increase their sense of security, especially in a new environment.

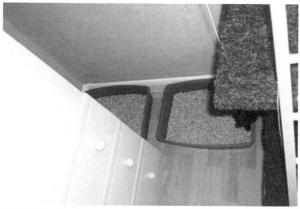

FIGURE 2-8   Cats prefer privacy when they toilet. It is not sufficient to provide one litter box per cat if the boxes are in close proximity, as in this case. These litter boxes are close together, so a cat may be blocked in the inner tray or prevented from getting to the box.

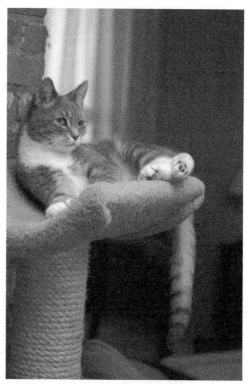

FIGURE 2-11   The vertical dimension is essential in the home environment. This cat monitors the environment from its safe perch, from which it can see who is approaching. It enables the cat to get away from dogs, a younger cat, small children, or anyone it prefers to avoid. (Courtesy D. Givin)

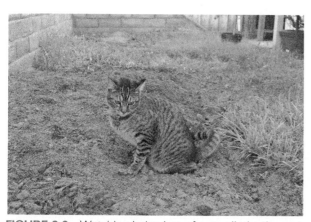

FIGURE 2-9   Watching behaviors of cats eliminating outdoors helps identify suitable indoor litter boxes. Cats need a suitable substrate and also a large enough space to turn around, scratch, and eliminate. (Copyright © iStock.com)

multicat households. Well-intentioned efforts by owners to introduce their cat to their friends and family can result in their cat being deprived of the opportunity to elevate and hide when faced with a stranger. Likewise, in multicat households, owners often encourage proximity between their cats through communal feeding or restriction of feline resting and hiding places, and the chronic stress that results can lead to a range of feline behavior problems. An understanding of natural feline behavior and communication will help owners to avoid these situations and provide feline-friendly homes that enable their cats to cope more effectively with life in a domestic context.

Freedom from Fear and Distress

Fear is a normal emotional response to potential threats, and perceptions of threats can be increased in unfamiliar situations or environments.[20] A perceived threat can be anything unfamiliar to the cat, such as a trip to the veterinary practice, a change in the home, or the presence of unfamiliar people or other pets. Fear can be induced by interactions that the cat finds oppressive, such as interactions with people who force the cat to be held, placed on a lap, or followed, instead of waiting until the cat is ready to interact (Figure 2-12). When fear is related to a perception rather than a reality of threat, it ceases to be adaptive and it is the veterinarian's responsibility to prevent mental suffering by offering appropriate advice to owners of these patients. Stress can be a normal result of fear, and both short term and long term stress can lead to poor feline welfare.[3,21] Overt aggression is a last resort as a feline defense strategy because it runs the risk of debilitating injury to both

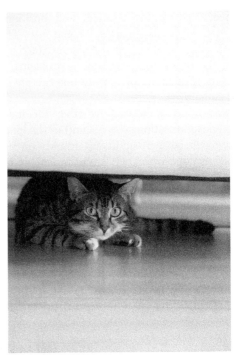

FIGURE 2-13 Feline signs of fear can be passive and subtle. Many cats prefer to avoid or hide rather than run away or fight. (Copyright © iStock.com)

parties. As a result, passive defense options of avoidance and inhibition are more likely to occur[22] and many fearful cats are inactive and quieter as a result of their negative emotional state (Figure 2-13).[23] This passive feline expression of fear and distress can delay detection and result in compromised welfare.

When fear and distress result in chronic stress, cats may cease to demonstrate normal behavior, such as by becoming inappetent or unkempt, but they may also demonstrate normal stress-related behaviors that are unacceptable to the humans with whom they live. For example, cats will often urine mark or urinate outside the litter box when stressed, leading to punishment by the owner or relinquishment, which increases the cat's stress further. Regardless of whether it is rehomed, sent to a shelter, or put outside permanently to enter the stray cat population, the cat's loss of the familiarity and security of its environment causes it fear and distress. As a social species, there is also the loss of the relationship with a person or persons, and possibly with other pets.

EXAMPLES OF IMPAIRMENT OF MULTIPLE FREEDOMS CONCURRENTLY

Clinical scenarios commonly involve compromise of more than one of the five freedoms. For example, a cat with unrecognized degenerative joint disease that is introduced to a new family dog may experience compromise of its freedom from pain and illness, but it may also compromise its freedom to express most normal

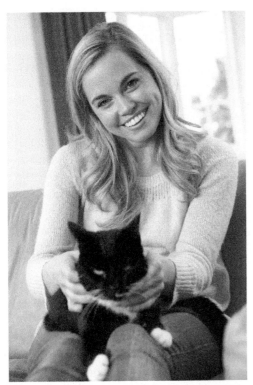

FIGURE 2-12 Forcing a cat to sit on a lap when it does not want to is stressful for the cat, and the contrast between the relaxed body language of the person and the tense body posturing of the cat illustrates the level of miscommunication between the species. (Copyright © iStock.com)

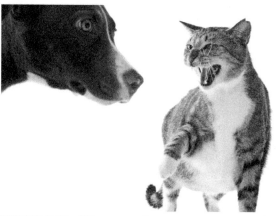

FIGURE 2-14 When a curious puppy comes to investigate, the fearful cat may first hiss and swat at the puppy. However, with time, the cat prefers to hide and get away from the dog. (Copyright © iStock.com)

behavior through not being able to jump up to elevated resting and hiding places, as well as its freedom from fear and distress through having to endure interaction with a puppy that it is scared of. If the cat tries to protect itself by hissing at the curious puppy (Figure 2-14), the owners may punish the cat, further adding to its fear and detracting from its welfare. To safeguard such a cat's welfare, the veterinarian needs not only to treat the painful joint disease but also to educate the client about feline environmental needs and social behavior.

VETERINARY PROFESSIONAL DUTY

The veterinary profession has only recently started to focus on the social and emotional needs of patients, with most veterinary education continuing to address primarily physical needs. Although concern for animal welfare is not new to the veterinary profession, most concerns have been focused on food, research, and zoo or other captive animals. Some countries have only recently revised their veterinary oaths to emphasize the welfare of all nonhuman animals. In 2014, the World Small Animal Veterinary Association (WSAVA) revised its oath to include welfare. Most veterinary organizations, including the major feline organizations, now have welfare statements to help veterinary professionals understand and meet the needs of a species so different from our own. Additionally, new organizations have been established specifically to promote the welfare of both pets and nonpets, the latter of which include the large feral cat population.

Welfare principles of different veterinary organizations include statements about treating animals with respect and dignity through use of species-appropriate handling techniques, providing an environment appropriate to the care of that species, and taking due consideration for species-typical behavior.[24] Animals should be cared for in ways that minimize their fear, pain, stress, and suffering. This is important, both in veterinary practices and at home.[24]

CONCLUSION

Poor feline welfare is frequently caused by a lack of understanding of the feline species, which stems from a fundamental difference between the social behaviors and communication systems of cats and people. This misunderstanding leads to unintentional restrictions of normal feline behavior that compromise feline welfare. The result is often the onset of behavior that is considered problematic or abnormal.[25] This book is designed to assist veterinarians and other veterinary professionals in recognizing what cats need in order to prevent or improve negative welfare situations while enhancing the human–animal bond.

ADDITIONAL RESOURCES

Ellis SL, Rodan I, Carney HC, et al: AAFP and ISFM feline environmental needs guidelines. *J Feline Med Surg* 15:219–230, 2013.

http://indoorpet.osu.edu/assets/documents/Herron10_EE_for_Indoor_Cats.pdf. Accessed January 7, 2015.

REFERENCES

1. American Animal Hospital Association position statement on animal sentience. https://www.aaha.org/professional/resources/sentient_beings.aspx#gsc.tab=0. Accessed January 27, 2015.
2. Sparkes AH, Bessant C, Cope K, et al. ISFM Guidelines on population management and welfare of unowned domestic cats (*Felis catus*). *J Feline Med Surg*. 2013;15:811–817.
3. Casey RA, Bradshaw JWS. The assessment of welfare. In: Rochlitz I, ed. *The welfare of cats*. Dordrecht, The Netherlands: Springer; 2005:23–46.
4. Bradshaw JWS, Casey RA, Brown SL. Cat welfare. In: *The behaviour of the domestic cat*. ed 2. 2012. Wallingford, UK: CABI; 2012:175–189.
5. American Veterinary Medical Association. Animal Welfare: What is It? https://www.avma.org/KB/Resources/Reference/AnimalWelfare/Pages/what-is-animal-welfare.aspx. Accessed January 27, 2015.
6. Health S. Behaviour problems and welfare. In: Rochlitz I, ed. *The welfare of cats*. Dordrecht, The Netherlands: Springer; 2007:91–118.

7. New JC, Salman MD, King M, et al. Characteristics of shelter relinquished animals and their owners compared with animals and their owners in U.S. pet-owning households. *J Appl Anim Welf Sci*. 2000;3:179–201.

8. American Veterinary Medical Association. Animal welfare is a human responsibility. https://www.avma.org/public/AnimalWelfare/Pages/default.aspx. Accessed July 14, 2013.

9. Driscoll CA, Macdonald DW, O'Brien SJ. From wild animals to domestic pets, an evolutionary view of domestication. *Proc Natl Acad Sci USA*. 2009;106(Suppl 1):9971–9978.

10. Driscoll CA, Clutton-Brock J, Kitchener AC, O'Brien SJ. The taming of the cat: genetic and archaeological findings hint that wildcats became housecats earlier—and in a different place—than previously thought. *Sci Am*. 2009;300 (6):68–75.

11. Bradshaw JWS, Casey RA, Brown SL. The cat: domestication and biology. In: *The behaviour of the domestic cat*. Wallingford, UK: CABI; 2012:1–15.

12. Heilig GK. *World Urbanization Prospects: The 2011 Revision. Presentation at the Center for Strategic and International Studies (CSIS)*; June 7, 2012. Washington, DC. http://esa.un.org/wpp/ppt/CSIS/WUP_2011_CSIS_4.pdf. Accessed January 7, 2015.

13. Neville PF. An ethical viewpoint: the role of veterinarians and behaviourists in ensuring good husbandry for cats. *J Feline Med Surg*. 2004;6:43–48.

14. Ed Lowe (businessman). Invention of kitty litter. http://en.wikipedia.org/wiki/Ed_Lowe_%28businessman%29#Invention_of_Kitty_Litter.

15. Bayer HealthCare. *Veterinary care usage study III: Feline findings*; 2012. http://www.bayerdvm.com/show.aspx/news-release-bvcus-iii-feline-findings. Accessed January 7, 2015.

16. Brambell FWR. *Report of the technical committee to enquire into the welfare of animals kept under intensive livestock husbandry systems*. London: Her Majesty's Stationery Office; 1965.

17. Lue TW, Pantenburg DP, Crawford PM. Impact of the owner-pet and client-veterinarian bond on the care that pets receive. *J Am Vet Med Assoc*. 2008;232:531–540.

18. Rochlitz I. Housing and welfare. In: Rochlitz I, ed. *The welfare of cats*. Dordrecht, The Netherlands: Springer; 2007:177–203.

19. Ellis SL, Rodan I, Carney HC, et al. AAFP and ISFM feline environmental needs guidelines. *J Feline Med Surg*. 2013;15:219–230.

20. Griffin B, Hume KR. Recognition and management of stress in housed cats. In: August J, ed. *Consultations in feline internal medicine*. ed 5. St Louis: Elsevier; 2006:717–734.

21. Levine ED. Feline fear and anxiety. *Vet Clin North Am Small Anim Pract*. 2008;38:1065–1079.

22. Notari L. Stress in veterinary behavioural medicine. In: Horwitz DF, Mills D, eds. *BSAVA manual of canine and feline behavioural medicine*. ed 2. Gloucester, UK: British Small Animal Veterinary Association (BSAVA); 2009:136–145.

23. Milgram NW, de Rivera C, Landsberg GM. Development of a model to assess anxiety in cats. In: Mills D, da Graca Pereira G, Jacinto DM, eds. *Proceedings of the 9th International Veterinary Behaviour Meeting*. Lisbon, Portugal: PsiAnimal (Portuguese Association of Animal Behaviour Therapy and Welfare); 2013:46–47.

24. American Veterinary Medical Association's animal welfare principles. https://www.avma.org/KB/Policies/Pages/AVMA-Animal-Welfare-Principles.aspx. Accessed January 6, 2013.

25. Crowell-Davis S. Cat behaviour: social organization, communication and development. In: Rochlitz I, ed. *The welfare of cats*. Dordrecht, The Netherlands: Springer; 2005:1–22.

PART 2

Normal Feline Behavior

Feline Communication

Jacqueline M. Ley

INTRODUCTION

Communication between cats and humans is an important part of cat ownership, but a poorly researched area. The general view of the domestic cat is that they are enigmatic and solitary creatures.[1] Understanding the communication behaviors of cats is necessary to unravel feline behavior problems, as well as to help owners understand normal feline behavior. Understanding feline communication allows veterinarians and veterinary staff to better manage cats in their care. Shelters and catteries can reduce stress in the cats they house by understanding how fear and anxiety are communicated in the feline world. The aim of this chapter is to define communication and discuss its purpose before looking specifically at how domestic cats communicate.

DEFINITION OF COMMUNICATION

Communication can be defined as the process of sending messages from one individual to others with the purpose of modifying behaviors of the receiver(s) of that message.[2] The receiver interprets the signals to gain information about the physical characteristics and emotional state of the sender. This may include the size, sex, maturation, and sexual receptiveness of the sender. The signal may also inform the receiver about the sender's perception of and intentions to interact with the environment, both physical and social. This can be of particular benefit in a species that spends long periods of time avoiding social interaction, especially when resources are in short supply, and then needs to advertise its sexual status so that individuals can come together at the time of optimal fertility of the female. Information about the sender's use of the environment as territory or as a shared thoroughfare is particularly important in cats, where solitary surviving individuals live in overlapping territories and need to avoid unnecessary encounters.

For communication to be of value, it must be effective. The receiver must accurately receive the message and be able to understand the information within it. A visual signal is of no value as an indicator of danger if all of the potential receivers of that signal are blind. Many important messages are sent using several modalities to increase the chances of the signal being received.[2] Important messages share characteristics between species, which is useful when species' habitats overlap. Messages of danger often have sharp, loud, high-pitched vocalizations or sounds, and the sender often orientates toward potential danger. There may also be release of odiferous secretions that invoke fear and arousal in the receivers. The loud, repeated calls of a bird spotting a stalking cat, for example, alert all birds in the area, regardless of their species, to danger.[3] Another example of when messages have similar characteristics across species is that of threat behavior. Threat displays involve the sender appearing as large and imposing as possible. Anyone observing a cat threaten a dog can relate to the dog's uncertainty as the cat, through piloerection, body posture, and deep-throated growls, appears to grow larger and more dangerous.

Why Communicate?

Social species need to quickly identify members of their social group and recognize their emotional states in order to avoid conflicts.[4,5] The social group defends resources for its own use and must identify strangers in order to maintain control of resources such as food, water access, or resting areas. Within the group, it is important to keep competition over these resources to a minimum because conflict between members is detrimental to survival.[6,7] Cats are not obligate social creatures, and individual survival is the prime concern. Communication allows social group members or animals living in close proximity to signal their intentions and avoid conflicts.

Communication is extremely important for the survival of the most vulnerable members of a species. Mothers send signals to aid the survival of their young. The nature of the signals changes as the young develop. Queens initially use purring to communicate with their kittens until the kittens' ear canals open. Then the queen begins to use a call.[8] The mother also responds to the signals the young send and thus meets their needs for warmth, food, and protection. It has been shown that the isolation calls of kittens trigger retrieval behavior by the queen.[9]

METHODS OF COMMUNICATION

The method of communication used is dependent upon the structure and functioning of the sensory organs of the sender and the receiver.[2] This varies between species. Cats have large eyes with a large area of binocular vision and good night vision, but they do not see fine details clearly.[10] They have large mobile ears and can hear sounds up to 60 kHz (Figure 3-1).[11] Their olfactory sense is much more sensitive than that of humans but less acute than that of dogs, probably because cats use their sense of smell less for tracking prey and more for communication.[12] Cats have several scent glands on their body that allow them to leave a variety of signals

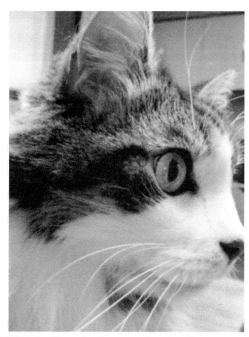

FIGURE 3-1 Portrait of a cat showing large, prominent eyes and large, mobile ears. These organs are used for hunting and for communication.

as they interact with their environment. They have a well-developed tactile sense, which is important in the affiliative behaviors of allorubbing and allogrooming. Cats mainly use visual signals and deposited odors to manage their territories. Vocal signaling is important in social interactions between cats and as an indicator of emotional state; however, because cats are ambush predators, they rarely use vocalizations during the hunting process so as to minimize their chances being located by either their prey or other predators.

The way a message is communicated varies with the type of message, the distance over which it is sent, and how long it needs to remain detectable to other animals. Some messages are immediate and fade quickly, whereas others last longer. Messages conveying danger need to be sent and received quickly, and they need to fade quickly once the danger has passed.[3] This is necessary for animals to avoid wasting valuable energy looking out for danger that has passed. Messages about sexual receptiveness need to remain in an area for longer periods to allow the message to reach as many potential mates as possible, but then needs to fade to prevent potential mates from wasting energy seeking an unreceptive female. Messages defining territorial boundaries need to be very long-lasting so that the claimant of a territory does not have to spend time better spent on other activities, such as feeding or raising young, renewing them.[2]

Signals can be sent using visual, olfactory, auditory, and tactile modalities. Cats make use of all of these and often use combinations to reduce ambiguity and maximize the advantages of each modality. Some signaling methods are better for certain types of signals. For example, depositing secretions is useful for communicating while maintaining distance between cats because the sender and recipient do not need to be in the same location at the same time and the signal has a long duration, thus increasing the time available for detection. See Table 3-1 for strengths and weaknesses of feline communication methods.

TABLE 3-1	Strengths and Weaknesses of Communication Methods Used by Cats		
Signal Modality	**Strength**	**Weakness**	**Example**
Visual	Immediate; message can be altered quickly to respond to information as it is received.	Sender is vulnerable as must expose self to send the signal; barriers block; most visual signals do not remain	Body posture, position
Auditory	Immediate; can be sent over distance while the sender remains hidden; can pass around or through some barriers	May be blocked by some barriers; does not last in the environment so receiver must be present; not able to be directed to only one individual	Kitten isolation cry; queen vocalizing during estrus
Olfaction	Long lasting signals; can diffuse around barriers	Slow transmission Lack of control of the spread of the message	Spraying Bunting/rub-marking
Tactile	Immediate, can alter as needed; can be directed at one individual	Must be close and in the same place, does not last	Allorubbing between conspecifics

Visual Signals

In general, visual signals are sent and received almost immediately. Changes in posture, piloerection, and position, for example, provide the receiver information about the sender's emotional state and behavioral intentions (Figure 3-2, *A–E*). Postural and facial visual signals require proximity between sender and receiver as well as visual access. In general, body postures give an overall impression of the emotional state and intention of the cat, whereas facial signals give more up-to-the-minute information and can be altered more rapidly in response to changing circumstances. For this reason, it is essential to read postural and facial expressions in combination, and where there is a discrepancy between the two, it is

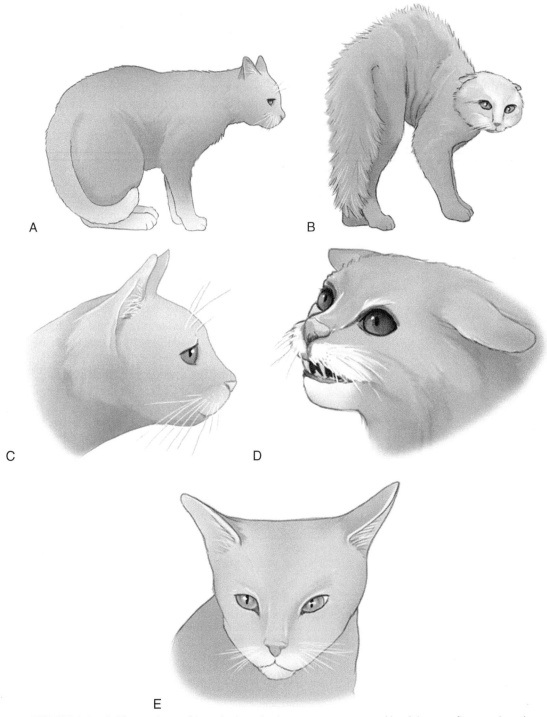

A

B

C

D

E

FIGURE 3-2 **A,** Uncertain cat. Note the hunched posture, ears rotated back but not flattened, and tail curled around feet. **B,** Defensive "Halloween" cat. The hunched posture with piloerection and ears flattened against the skull make the cat look larger and more threatening. **C,** Neutral, relaxed cat. **D,** Fearful cat with ears flattened against skull; mouth open; and threatening vocalization, hissing, and/or biting. **E,** Uncertain cat with ears semi-rotated and tight mouth.

important to pay attention to the more easily changeable facial expressions in order to obtain an accurate assessment of the message the cat is trying to convey.

Direct visual signals have the advantage of being rapidly delivered and can be altered quickly in response to new information (e.g., backing down from a threat when the other cat turns out to be much larger).[2] Sending visual signals can be dangerous for the senders, as they must expose themselves to being seen, allowing potential predators or rivals to identify their location. Visual signals are also easily blocked by physical barriers, lessening their usefulness in environments with heavy vegetation, hills, or other obstacles.[2]

There are some situations in which visual signaling could be described as indirect communication because it does not require the sender to be present to convey the message. For example, cats can leave visual messages by making scratch marks on trees (or furniture) or by leaving feces in prominent areas.[12,13] These visual signals attract receivers to investigate them and to find more information in the form of olfactory messages.

Auditory Signals

Cats have large, independently mobile ears. Being night hunters, their hearing is very sensitive. Attempts to quantify what cats can hear have suggested that ultrasound is within their range, with the upper limit of their hearing being measured at 60 kHz.[11] This makes evolutionary sense, as many prey species vocalize within the ultrasound range.[14] This would also explain why ultrasound devices designed to be deterrents to cats have been found to be less effective than expected.[15-17]

The vocalizations of domestic cats have been described by several authors. Moelk[18] described cat vocalization, identifying four categories of interaction in which cats may vocalize: antagonistic interactions, affiliative interactions, queen–kitten interactions, and cat–human interactions. In that study, vocalizations were grouped into murmur, vowel, and strained intensity patterns. Researchers in other studies have divided sounds cats make into closed-mouth, fixed open-mouth, and sounds produced while the open mouth is gradually closed. Many sounds associated with offensive and defensive aggression are made with the mouth held open.[18] Differences have been found between the vocalizations of domestic cats and those of feral cats, with domesticated cats making vocalizations of higher frequency and shorter duration in response to antagonistic interactions with people.[19] Many cats also have more interactive communication with people, and the role of conditioning needs to be considered.

The cries cats make vary with their sex, reproductive state, and time of the year. One study of feral cats identified three vocalizations: mew, yowl, and a rutting cry. The rutting cry was performed more frequently by male cats and only during the breeding season.[20] See Table 3-2 for more information.

TABLE 3-2 List of Vocalizations Made by Cats

Class	Vocalization	Situations Used
Closed mouth	Purr	Contact with familiar individuals—cat, human, dog
		Nursing kittens
		Pain/chronic illness
	Trill/chirrup	Greeting
		Contact with kittens
Fixed open mouth	Growl	Aggressive encounters
	Yowl	Aggressive encounters
	Snarl	Aggressive encounters
	Hiss	Defensive vocalization
	Spit	Defensive vocalization
	Shriek	Situations causing pain or fear
Gradually closing open mouth	Miaow	Greeting
		Interaction with people
	Female call	Advertising sexual receptiveness
	Male call/mowl	Courtship
	Howl	Aggressive encounters

Olfactory Signals

The advantages of many signals sent by odor are that they can diffuse around and through barriers which would obstruct visual and auditory signals and that they can be long-lasting, thus allowing the sender to have left the area before the recipient detects the message.[2] However, olfactory signals can also be sent quickly between individuals, such as when anal glands are expressed by a cat in a state of fear.

To detect olfactory signals, one needs suitable sensory abilities. The cat's olfactory skills are greater than humans', but they are less awe-inspiring than those of dogs and pigs. The ability to detect olfactory signals relies, in part, on the size of the nasal epithelium. The bigger the surface area, the more room there is for receptors to detect odors. The feline nasal epithelium is between 20 and 40 cm.[2,21]

Species	Size of Olfactory Epithelium	Number of Receptors	Sensitivity
Humans	2-5 cm^2	5 million	
Cats	20-40 cm^2	200 million	20 times better than humans
Dogs	Up to 170 cm^2	220 million	50-1000 times better than humans

Cats have several scent-producing glands on their bodies. They are located on the chin, around the mouth, at the base of tail, on the feet, and in the anus.[22] Scent from the facial glands is deposited on objects and individuals when the cat bunts or rubs its face against them.[21] It is understood that facial secretions have a number of roles to play in communication and are important in identification of territory, in transfer of information about the emotional state of individuals, and in the communication of information about sexual receptivity. Tomcats, for example, show more interest in the cheek secretions of queens when the queens are in estrus. Scent from the feet is deposited where cats walk, but also specifically when cats claw objects such as trees and furniture (Figure 3-3). Anal glands deposit scent on the feces and also are expressed when the cat is fearful. Cats have been found to spend differing amounts of time sniffing the feces of familiar and unfamiliar cats, with more time given to sniffing the feces of unfamiliar cats.[23,24]

Urine and feces also carry odors that convey information about the individual. For example, entire male cat urine has high levels of felinine compared with queens.[25] The amount of felinine in a male cat's urine varies with blood testosterone;[26] entire male cats have very high levels of this compound in their urine, neutered males have less, and females possess the least.[25] Where and how urine and feces are deposited varies with cats and their intentions. Small volumes of urine deposited on vertical surfaces (i.e., sprayed) let other cats know that the cat is claiming a territory or challenging for a territory. Marking is a normal behavior, but there is little information available about how often cats mark. Most work has been concentrated on problem marking.[27-30] Marking behavior appears to increase when cats are stressed, and marking in areas unacceptable to owners can become a reason for relinquishing cats.[31] When used to communicate between cats, urine spraying can be very effective in maintaining distance and avoiding conflict. The message is deposited by the sender and is persistent over time, thus enabling the receiver to read the information in the absence of the sender. Topping up urine marks on a regular basis enables cats to manage social encounters effectively, and cats are sensitive to the decaying of the signal for this reason.

In an indoor environment, this topping up mechanism may result in urine deposits' being renewed long after the original stressor has been removed (see Chapter 24).

Pheromones

Pheromones are chemicals that are released by the signaler and cause a change in the behavior and physiology of the recipient.[32] Pheromones are detected by specialized receptors in the nasal mucosa and the vomeronasal organ (VNO).[33] There are many different types of pheromones and many types of VNO receptors.[34] The feline VNO is similar to that of the dog, horse, pig, sheep, and goat in that it has only one connection to the accessory olfactory bulb.[35]

When a cat bunts against a surface, it leaves a complex chemical signal behind (Figure 3-4). As part of this signal, a pheromone complex identified as the feline facial pheromone is deposited.[36] Certain elements of this pheromone complex have been synthesized, and many cats show calmer behavior and stop unwanted behavior when exposed to it,[36-39] although not all researchers are in agreement with regard to its efficacy.[40] Feline facial pheromone is commercially available as Feliway (Ceva, Charlotte, NC) (see Chapter 18).

Fear pheromones tend to be released from the glands in the skin, and their presence is an indicator of the emotional state of the individual. Cats that are frightened may also empty their anal sacs and release fear-related pheromones in this way. This has a practical consequence in a veterinary context, when cats may be reluctant to be handled by personnel who have previously been interacting with a fearful feline.

Sex pheromones are released in urine and cheek gland secretion of the female cat and appear to inform the tomcat about her hormonal phase.[41] When he encounters the urine of female cats, the male cat sniffs and "gapes."[41] The gape or flehmen response forces pheromones into the VNO.

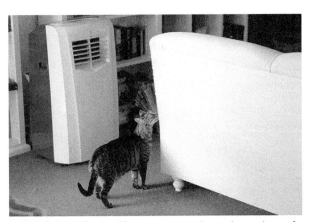

FIGURE 3-3   Cat sniffing at a scratch mark on the sofa. Cats may choose to mark with urine or by scratching items that are along thoroughfares or that are otherwise significant to cats.

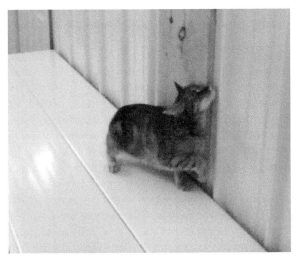

FIGURE 3-4   Laboratory cat bunting a scratching post in its run. (Courtesy J. Ley, CanCog Technologies)

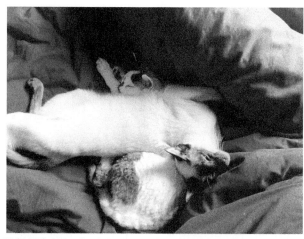

FIGURE 3-5 Socially bonded cats may be found in close physical contact. These cats could generally be found in close proximity wherever they were in the owner's apartment.

Tactile Signals

Tactile signals are very immediate and require the sender and receiver to be in close contact. Cats are very tactile and appear to enjoy interactions with individuals with which they have a social bond (Figure 3-5). Cats that are familiar and friendly with each other will rub heads and bodies after a period of separation and may twine their tails together.[42] The physical closeness displayed may be affected by the relatedness of the animals. Adult littermate cats that live together spend significantly more time in physical contact than unrelated adult cats who share a house, even those raised together from kittenhood.[43]

The evidence with regard to sex-related differences in allogrooming is not conclusive, and there is a lack of recent studies into this form of tactile interaction. Many owners report that male cats do allogroom other male cats, and it appears on the basis of other studies that the relatedness or social compatibility of the cats is an important predictor of allogrooming.[44] It may be that the relationship between the cats, their sex, and their sexual status (neutered or entire) all may play a role in allogrooming.

COMMUNICATING COMPLEX MESSAGES

Cats often use several communication modalities to build complex messages. Combining modalities such as visual signals, olfactory signals, and vocal signals increases the chances of a message being received and understood. This complexity can make it difficult for people with less experience in reading feline signals to interpret what is occurring between cats. However, most signals can be categorized as either distance-decreasing, distance-increasing, or neutral messages. Some of the combination signals that cats may use to send broad messages are described in the subsections that follow.

Distance-Decreasing Signals

Greeting

When cats recognize an approaching cat or person, they may give a greeting meow or trill. This is a closed-mouth sound. Often, they will raise their tail vertically, whereas at other times it may be held lower.[45] Kittens generally hold their tails vertically when approaching their mother. Olfactory exchange may occur through sniffing and bunting once the cat has come into proximity with a person or another cat, and tactile communication occurs through the process of allorubbing. One study of feral colony cats found that if both cats raised their tails, then mutual and simultaneous head-rubbing occurred.[46]

Sexual Receptivity

Vocalization is used to send an immediate message over longer distances and to a broader audience. Vocalizing by in-season queens is one way they advertise their availability, and entire tomcats also use vocalization to ensure that the queens are aware of their presence. Sexual receptivity can also be communicated indirectly through pheromones in urine and skin gland secretions. Tomcats spent more time investigating the urine and cheek secretions of queens in estrus.[41]

The queen may also roll on the ground and rub against objects in her environment in an obvious manner, perhaps to gain the attention of other cats in the vicinity and also to deposit important scent information.

Neutral Signals

The cat that is relaxed may look at another cat or a person and then squint its eyes shut in a blinking action. This action has also been reported to occur when a cat is seeking reassurance in a tense environment and does not appear to aim for either a reduction or an increase in distance. It has been suggested that humans can help to relax cats by blinking slowly or making "winky-eyes" (Figure 3-6) in the direction of the cat, and this has

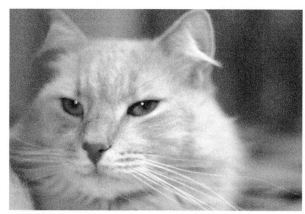

FIGURE 3-6 Cat showing "winky eyes" during his photo shoot. He was not interested in interacting with the photographer, but was signaling that her presence was of no bother to him.

been advocated as a means of making cats feel more comfortable in the veterinary consultation room (see Chapter 20). In contrast, turning the head away seems to signal that the cat does not want to be approached. In both cases, the cat does not approach the other party.

Distance-Increasing Behavior

Behaviors in this category have the intent of increasing distance between the cat and another individual. This may be a cat, a human, or another animal. The cat who feels threatened or unsafe may attempt to leave the area, especially if it is away from its home territory (Figure 3-7). Cats new to shelters hide and avoid other cats if given the opportunity.[47] If a cat is unable to leave or is in its home territory, then it may attempt to drive the other individual(s) away. This pattern of behavior in these situations tends to be delivery of threatening responses which are then followed either by a strategic retreat by the cat or by escalating aggression.[48] Anyone who has introduced a new cat to an incumbent cat will have witnessed this sort of interaction[49] (see Chapter 26).

The cat orientates toward the potential adversary. A cat that is unsure if it will leave or attempt to fight will often crouch with its feet tucked under its body (Figure 3-8, *A*). If the other cat continues to approach,

the cat may growl and rotate its ears backward. It may attempt to bluff the other party by assuming a "Halloween cat" posture. The hunched back, extended legs, and piloerected hair of this posture all serve to make the cat look larger.

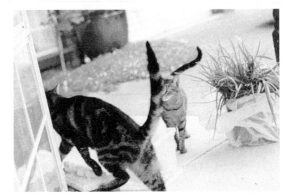

FIGURE 3-7 Nonaggressive communication between cats. Cheetah (facing) has approached the area Tommy (cat facing away) occupies. She stared at him, and he elected to leave the area. His tail is up, although his ears are rotated a little, indicating that he is not completely comfortable. Cheetah and Tommy cohabitate but do not have a social bond. Tommy tends to move away when Cheetah approaches.

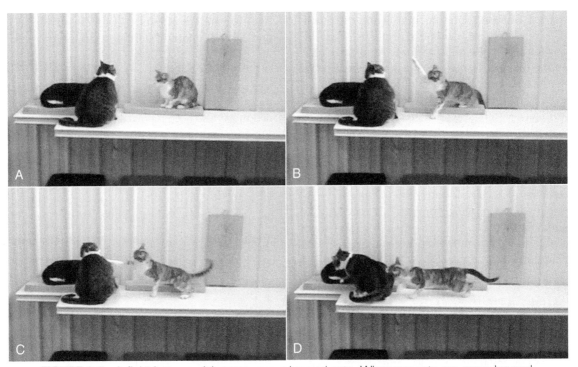

FIGURE 3-8 A fight between laboratory group-housed cats. Wherever cats are group-housed, aggressive interactions will occur; however, if there are enough resources (e.g., food, water, resting places, toilets), the cats will settle in a stable group with only minor altercations happening. **A,** Threat behavior in the form of staring between tabby and white cat with back to us and tortoiseshell and white cat. **B,** Tortoiseshell cat raises forepaw to strike as tabby and white pulls back. **C,** The tortoiseshell cat makes repeated strikes with her forepaw. **D,** The tortoiseshell cat sees the tabby and white cat off with a bite to its rump. The tabby and white cat moved to the end of the bench behind the black and white cat in the picture, which was sufficient to stop the aggressive behavior by the tortoiseshell cat. (Courtesy J. Ley, CanCog Technologies)

If the encounter progresses to a fight, the forefeet are used to strike (Figure 3-8, *B* and *C*), and there may be wrestling using a combination of the forefeet to grapple, the hindfeet to scratch, and the teeth to bite (Figure 3-8, *D*). The cats may give a very loud vocalization, referred to as a shriek or give a pain cry.[18] If one cat breaks away, the other may continue to pursue it or may remain in the area of the fight and spend time bunting objects and leaving important scent signals should the other cat return.

CAT–HUMAN COMMUNICATION

Cats are often perceived as unfriendly, lazy, and arrogant because they tend not to show the emotional responses that dogs do after absences from the people with whom they have a bond. Cats are a cautious species whose evolutionary history with people lacks the intense selection applied to dogs and agricultural animals.[1] However, scientists interested in cognition and communication are starting to look at how cats and people communicate.[50]

Preliminary research comparing communication with people by domestic dogs and cats shows that cats can follow human pointing gestures (as dogs do), but that they lack some of the behaviors, such as repeated gazing at the human and then at unobtainable food, that attract human attention to their needs.[51] Purring is used by some cats to solicit attention, food, and other needs from people.[52] The purring seems more intense than ordinary purring, because the cat appears to be vocalizing simultaneously while purring.[52] Cats reliably respond to their owners' calling their name, but they do not respond to strangers who mimic their owner's call.[53] People are able to identify differences between vocalizations by domestic cats and African wild cats[54] and rate domestic cat vocalizations as more pleasant.[55]

The Value of Understanding Cats

Understanding the communication behavior of cats makes it easier for people to respond appropriately to their cats and meet their needs for companionship; time alone; and food, water, rest, and toilet facilities. It also allows assessment of how well cats are living together and helps owners to accurately assess feline stress in multicat households (Figure 3-9). Similarly, understanding feline communication can reduce some cat–human conflict.[48]

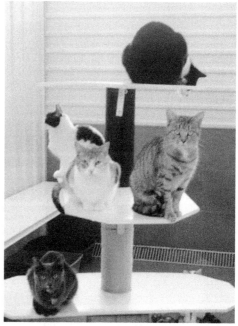

FIGURE 3-9 Managing a group of housed cats requires understanding of how cats interact socially and how they show they are comfortable and uncomfortable. These laboratory cats are not showing socially bonded behaviors, but are comfortable in close proximity on the multilevel platform. Supplying adequate amounts of resources in different areas of the space allows the cats to find a spot where they can rest and also guarantees them access to other resources when they need them. (Courtesy J. Ley, CanCog Technologies)

Understanding feline communication signals helps to manage cats in situations such as catteries, animal shelters, and veterinary practices. Recognizing signs of stress and signals indicating that cats need to be left alone or given time to settle makes it safer to handle them.[56] When there is successful communication, there is relief of some stress on the cat, which can make them easier to handle, more adoptable,[47] and less prone to outbreaks of stress-related disease.

The most important concept for owners, veterinarians, and people who work with cats to understand is that feline communication differs from human communication and that humans need to take some time to study feline signaling in order to avoid common misunderstandings that can detrimentally affect the cat–owner relationship.

REFERENCES

1. Budiansky S. *The character of cats: the origins, intelligence, behavior, and stratagems of Felis silvestris catus.* New York: Viking; 2002.
2. Price EO. *Principles & applications of domestic animal behaviour: an introductory text.* Wallingford, UK: CAB International; 2008.
3. Leavesley AJ, Magrath RD. Communicating about danger: urgency alarm calling in a bird. *Anim Behav.* 2005;70:365–373.
4. Bonnie KE, Earley RL. Expanding the scope for social information use. *Anim Behav.* 2007;74:171–181.
5. Broom DM, Fraser AF. *Domestic animal behaviour and welfare.* ed 4 Wallingford, UK: CAB International; 2007.
6. Christian JJ. Social subordination, population density, and mammalian evolution. *Science.* 1970;168:84–90.
7. Young AJ, Spong G, Clutton-Brock T. Subordinate male meerkats prospect for extra-group paternity: alternative

reproductive tactics in a cooperative mammal. *Proc Biol Sci.* 2007;274:1603–1609.

8. Luschekin VS, Shuleikina KV. Some sensory determinants of home orientation in kittens. *Dev Psychobiol.* 1989;22:601–616.

9. Buchwald JS, Shipley C, Altafullah I, Hinman C, Harrison J, Dickerson L. The feline isolation call. In: Newman JD, ed. *The physiological control of mammalian vocalization.* New York: Plenum; 1988:119–135.

10. Jacobson SG, Franklin KBJ, McDonald WI. Visual acuity of the cat. *Vision Res.* 1976;16:1141–1143.

11. Neff WD, Hind JE. Auditory thresholds of the cat. *J Acoust Soc Am.* 1955;27:480–483.

12. Beaver BV. *Feline behavior: a guide for veterinarians.* ed 2. St Louis: Saunders; 2003.

13. Ishida Y, Shimuzu M. Influence of social rank on defecating behaviors in feral cats. *J Ethol.* 1998;16:15–21.

14. Burgdorf J, Kroes RA, Moskal JR, Pfaus JG, Brudzynski SM, Panksepp J. Ultrasonic vocalizations of rats (*Rattus norvegicus*) during mating, play, and aggression: behavioral concomitants, relationship to reward, and self-administration of playback. *J Comp Psychol.* 2008;122:357–367.

15. Nelson SH, Evans AD, Bradbury RB. The efficacy of collar-mounted devices in reducing the rate of predation of wildlife by domestic cats. *Appl Anim Behav Sci.* 2005;94:273–285.

16. Mills DS, Bailey SL, Thurstans RE. Evaluation of the welfare implications and efficacy of an ultrasonic 'deterrent' for cats. *Vet Rec.* 2000;147:678–680.

17. Nelson SH, Evans AD, Bradbury RB. The efficacy of an ultrasonic cat deterrent. *Appl Anim Behav Sci.* 2006;96:83–91.

18. Moelk M. Vocalizing in the house-cat: a phonetic and functional study. *Am J Psychol.* 1944;57:184–205.

19. Yeon SC, Kim YK, Park SJ, et al. Differences between vocalization evoked by social stimuli in feral cats and house cats. *Behav Processes.* 2011;87:183–189.

20. Shimizu M. Vocalizations of feral cats: sexual differences in the breeding season. *Mammal Study.* 2001;26:85–92.

21. Houpt KA. *Domestic animal behavior for veterinarians and animal scientists.* ed 3. Ames, IA: Iowa State University Press; 1998.

22. Meyer W, Bartels T. Histochemical study on the eccrine glands in the foot pad of the cat. *Basic Appl Histochem.* 1989;33:219–238.

23. Nakabayashi M, Yamaoka R, Nakashima Y. Do faecal odours enable domestic cats (*Felis catus*) to distinguish familiarity of the donors? *J Ethol.* 2012;30:325–329.

24. Fogle B. *The cat's mind: understanding your cat's behavior.* New York: Penguin; 1991.

25. Hendriks WH, Rutherfurd-Markwick KJ, Weidgraaf K, Ugarte C, Rogers QR. Testosterone increases urinary free felinine, N-acetylfelinine and methylbutanolglutathione excretion in cats (*Felis catus*). *J Anim Physiol Anim Nutr.* 2008;92:53–62.

26. Tarttelin MF, Hendriks WH, Moughan PJ. Relationship between plasma testosterone and urinary felinine in the growing kitten. *Physiol Behav.* 1998;65:83–87.

27. Dehasse J. Feline urine spraying. *Appl Anim Behav Sci.* 1997;52:365–371.

28. Frank DF, Erb HN, Houpt KA. Urine spraying in cats: presence of concurrent disease and effects of a pheromone treatment. *Appl Anim Behav Sci.* 1999;61:263–272.

29. Horwitz DF. Behavioral and environmental factors associated with elimination behaviour problems in cats: a retrospective study. *Appl Anim Behav Sci.* 1997;52:129–137.

30. Olm DD, Houpt KA. Feline house-soiling problems. *Appl Anim Behav Sci.* 1988;20:335–345.

31. Patronek GJ, Glickman LT, Beck AM, McCabe GP, Ecker C. Risk factors for relinquishment of cats to an animal shelter. *J Am Vet Med Assoc.* 1996;209:582–588.

32. Sommerville BA, Broom DM. Olfactory awareness. *Appl Anim Behav Sci.* 1998;57:269–286.

33. Ma M. Odor and pheromone sensing via chemoreceptors. *Adv Exp Med Biol.* 2012;739:93–106.

34. Koh TW, Carlson JR. Chemoreception: identifying friends and foes. *Curr Biol.* 2011;21:R998–R999.

35. Salazar I, Sánchez-Quinteiro P. A detailed morphological study of the vomeronasal organ and the accessory olfactory bulb of cats. *Microsc Res Tech.* 2011;74:1109–1120.

36. Pageat P. Functions and use of the facial pheromones in the treatment of urine marking in the cat: interest of a structural analogue. In: Johnston D, Waner T, eds. *XXIst Congress of the World Small Animal Veterinary Association*; October 20th-23rd, 1996, Jerusalem, Israel.

37. Kronen PW, Ludders JW, Erb HN, Moon PF, Gleed RD, Koski S. A synthetic fraction of feline facial pheromones calms but does not reduce struggling in cats before venous catheterization. *Vet Anaesth Analg.* 2006;33:258–265.

38. Ogata N, Takeuchi Y. Clinical trial of a feline pheromone analogue for feline urine marking. *J Vet Med Sci.* 2001;63:157–161.

39. Griffith CA, Steigerwald ES, Buffington CA. Effects of a synthetic facial pheromone on behavior of cats. *J Am Vet Med Assoc.* 2000;217:1154–1156.

40. Frank D, Beauchamp G, Palestrini C. Systematic review of the use of pheromones for treatment of undesirable behavior in cats and dogs. *J Am Vet Med Assoc.* 2010;236:1308–1316.

41. Verberne G, de Boer J. Chemocommunication among domestic cats, mediated by the olfactory and vomeronasal senses. I. Chemocommunication. *Z Tierpsychol.* 1976;42:86–109.

42. Crowell-Davis SL, Curtis TM, Knowles RJ. Social organization in the cat: a modern understanding. *J Feline Med Surg.* 2004;6:19–28.

43. Bradshaw JWS, Hall SL. Affiliative behaviour of related and unrelated pairs of cats in catteries: a preliminary report. *Appl Anim Behav Sci.* 1999;63:251–255.

44. Curtis TM, Knowles RJ, Crowell-Davis SL. Influence of familiarity and relatedness on proximity and allogrooming in domestic cats (*Felis catus*). *Am J Vet Res.* 2003;64:1151–1154.

45. Cafazzo S, Natoli E. The social function of tail up in the domestic cat (Felis silvestris catus). *Behav Processes.* 2009;80:60–66.

46. Brown SL, Bradshaw JWS. Classification of social behaviour patterns in feral domestic cats. *Appl Anim Behav Sci.* 1993;35:294.

47. Kry K, Casey R. The effect of hiding enrichment on stress levels and behaviour of domestic cats (*Felis sylvestris catus*) in a shelter setting and the implications for adoption potential. *Anim Welf.* 2007;16:375–383.

48. Virga V. *Hissing, scratching, biting, & marking: how can we work with aggressive cats? Small Animal and Exotics Proceedings.* Orlando, FL, USA: North American Veterinary Conference; January 19-23, 2013.

49. Levine E, Perry P, Scarlett J, Houpt KA. Intercat aggression in households following the introduction of a new cat. *Appl Anim Behav Sci.* 2005;90:325–336.

50. Saito A, Shinozuka K. How should we study social intelligence in cats? *Jpn J Anim Psychol.* 2010;59:187–197.

51. Miklosi A, Pongracz P, Lakatos G, Topal J, Csanyi V. A comparative study of the use of visual communicative signals in

interactions between dogs (*Canis familiaris*) and humans and cats (*Felis catus*) and humans. *J Comp Psychol.* 2005;119:179–186.

52. McComb K, Taylor AM, Wilson C, Charlton BD. The cry embedded within the purr. *Curr Biol.* 2009;19:R507–R508.

53. Saito A, Shinozuka K. Vocal recognition of owners by domestic cats (Felis catus). *Anim Cogn.* 2013;16(4):685–690.

54. Nicastro N. Perceptual and acoustic evidence for species-level differences in meow vocalizations by domestic cats (*Felis catus*) and African wild cats (*Felis silvestris lybica*). *J Comp Psychol.* 2004;118:287–296.

55. Nicastro NS. Evolution of a domestic cat vocalization under anthropogenic selection. *Diss Abstr Int.* 2004;64:6317.

56. Sparkes A. Developing cat-friendly clinics. *In Pract.* 2013;35:212–215.

CHAPTER 4

Normal Social Behavior

Jacqueline M. Ley

INTRODUCTION

Cats have been thought of as solitary animals. They are often seen alone, and they are less gregarious than dogs and many domestic species. Incumbent cats drive new cats away if they enter claimed territories. But cats can and do live in groups with all the stresses and benefits that these involve. What makes cats really interesting is that they have a flexible social system, and can live solitarily or form social groups when conditions allow.

Living in a social group does have its benefits, but there can be drawbacks, especially for less confident individuals. Being part of a social group means conflicts must be managed and affiliations made and maintained to maximize the benefits of social living for every member. Ritualized social behavior allows animals to inform other animals of their intentions and to avoid conflicts.

In this section, social behavior and how cats organize themselves are considered. Feline affiliative and antagonistic behaviors are discussed. Development of social behavior is explored and related to how new cats can potentially integrate into an existing feline group and how social behavior allows cats to live with humans.

LIVING TOGETHER

Many animals live in close contact with others. Some species form tight-knit social groups where members support and defend each other. The group offers a survival advantage to the individual, to the group itself, and to the species as a whole. In other species, the individuals live in close contact but form less close-knit social relationships. The individuals may recognize each other and have organized contact but do not defend each other from outside threats. Before it is possible to understand how cats organize themselves socially, an understanding of the value of social behavior and how it can be described is necessary.

What is Social Behavior?

Social behavior describes the behavior that affects conspecifics.[1] Social behavior usually involves direct interaction with conspecifics or communication with them.

So, social behaviors, at least in mammals, encompass those behaviors such as finding a mate, raising young, marking territory, and fending off rivals (Figure 4-1). Of particular interest here is the formation of social groups. The size, composition, cohesiveness, and genetic makeup of a social group varies with the species and, in some flexible species, such as domestic cats, the environment they inhabit and mating strategies they employ.[1]

Some animals form transient social groups; they come together at particular times in their lives or at particular times of the year for mating and raising of young. This system is utilized by some felid species such as the jaguar *(Panthera onca)*.[2] Other species form more permanent social groups, with individuals of different generations present within the group. Often there is cooperation within the group on tasks such as raising young or finding food. Within the larger cat family, this is seen in the lion *(Panthera leo;* Figure 4-2).[3] Other species appear to be more flexible in the nature of the social groups they form. This appears to be the type of organization that is utilized by the cat. Social groups form in cats only if there are sufficient resources, such as food and space in the area to support the cats. Cats are interesting, as they are capable of living and thriving in a variety of systems ranging from high-density colonies to solitary animals.[4,5]

Living in a social group or in close contact has several benefits for individuals. Members of the group can access food sources, water, and resting places and control the ability of others of different social groups or species to access these resources. Cats that live in a group have more eyes and ears available to keep a lookout for predators and other dangers.[6] The concentration of animals enhances the chances of finding a mate when a female is receptive and increases her choice of mates. There are more animals available to help with raising young (in species that do this), and the young also benefit from increased vigilance made possible by the increased numbers of eyes and ears provided by the group.[6]

For the individuals of a social species or a species comfortable with close-contact living, group living benefits the species. But some individuals benefit more than

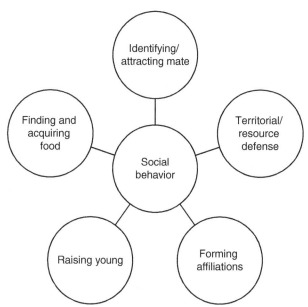

FIGURE 4-1 Social behavior encompasses many complex behaviors directed towards adult conspecifics. The exact nature of the behaviors varies with the species being examined.

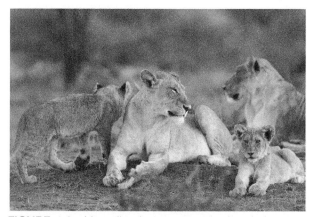

FIGURE 4-2 Lions live in groups and raise their young cooperatively. (Copyright © iStock.com)

others.[7] Some animals will find it easier to access food, water, desirable resting places, and mates than others. They will do this by virtue of their size, age, sex, personality, and level of confidence.[8,9] Thus, in colonies and multicat households, some cats will have it all, and others will struggle for access to resources unless these are spread throughout the area inhabited by the cats. Because of this unevenness in access to resources, conflict is a common occurrence within a social group. Managing it is important for the benefit of individuals.

Managing Conflict

Living together is stressful. Although research measuring stress parameters in indoor cats living in multicat households has not demonstrated changes in urinary cortisol,[10] research in other highly social species shows that maintaining social systems is stressful.[7,11,12]

Where individuals are living in close contact, conflict is inevitable and carries the risk of injury to both parties. Injury can lead to a reduction of fitness if the individual is weakened and cannot hunt, forage for food, or claim mates. Therefore, conflict must be avoided where possible. If conflict cannot be avoided, the risks of injury must be minimized for the best survival of the individuals and the group. Conflict is managed using ritualized behavior that demonstrates the confidence of the animal and its willingness to fight or its willingness to avoid conflict. Within a cat colony, threat behavior, including controlling access to resources, is used by cats to manage conflict. Some cats choose to avoid other cats that they have had conflicts with in the past or that are sending signals of agitation and a willingness to fight.[13] Other cats may stay in the area but send signals that say they are not willing to interact. They may avoid eye contact or pointedly look away. If a conflict escalates, then ritualized or passive aggression is used to minimize injury to either party. This usually involves many threat postures and vocalizations to attempt to bluff the other party.

Another method for managing conflict is to create a system for organizing the priority of access to resources. In cats, it is thought that priority of access is negotiated between the animals involved on the basis of their size, weight, age, experience, and motivation as well as the outcome of previous interactions.[9] In this system, the animal that appears to be the "winner" may change at every interaction, and this is explained in terms of the relative value of the resource to the individual at that time as well as the perceived cost of hostile confrontation. For a list of benefits and costs of living in a feline social group, see Table 4-1.

CATS: KIND OF SOCIAL ANIMALS

As has been discussed, social systems are varied and range from living closely together to living in a complex group with affiliations and ritualized behavior.

TABLE 4-1	The Benefits and Costs of Living in a Social Group
Benefits of Social Living	**Costs of Social Living**
The group can control resources such as food, water, and resting places	Some members of the group do not have equal access to resources
Safety is increased because more animals are looking out for danger	Some members will be less protected, owing to their location in the group
	Lookouts may be in places of increased danger
Greater chance of finding a mate when fertile	Unequal access to mates
More individuals to look after young	May not have the opportunity to reproduce
More individuals to locate and acquire food	Unequal access to food between group members

Domestic cats defy easy classification into one style of social organization, as the form of their social group may vary depending upon the amount and spread of resources within the environment. This is partly because of the biology of cats and the fact that they are small hunters that prey upon small animals—meals for one, in effect. Thus, domestic cats do not form close-knit groups that rely on each other to procure food as lions[14] and wolves do.[15] They also do not form the complex social relationships and affiliations that characterize social groups in some species, such as baboons,[16] chimpanzees,[17] and elephants.[18] Cats lack dominance hierarchies that prevent repeated conflicts and behaviors that allow the repair of social bonds after conflicts.[13] The success of the domestic cat as a pet and a feral animal is due, in part, to the ability of cats to form some types of social bonds and also to be able to live without them.

Cats are a territorial species. Male territories are larger and overlap female territories,[19] whereas queens have smaller territories, perhaps due to their need to remain close to their kittens while raising them.[20] External factors, such as the amount and dispersal of food and resting places in an area, play an important role in how closely together cats live, how much territorial overlap there is between neighboring cats, and how much interaction individuals have.

Where food is abundant but clumped, cats tend to live closely together. Where it is scarce and widely spread, cats disperse and have large territories.[19] Within cats' territories, there are differences as to how the sexes and individuals behave socially. Male cats tend to be solitary or to move around, visiting females. If resources can support them, many female kittens stay with or close to their dams and sisters. Some females even share kitten-raising duties.[5]

In cat social groups, the female animals tend to be related.[21,22] The group is friendly or at least tolerant of group members and often aggressive toward unfamiliar animals.[21,22] Affiliative or friendly behavior builds bonds between group members, whereas agonistic behavior protects the group from intruders.

SOCIAL BEHAVIOR OF CATS

As discussed earlier, social behaviors are those directed towards conspecifics and include affiliative and antagonistic behaviors as well as behaviors related to reproduction and care of young. Cats are highly flexible in their behavior due to inhabiting environments where resources may be unpredictably dispersed. In this section, the social behaviors of cats are examined in detail.

Feline Antagonistic Behavior

There will be conflicts within any social group, and this is true for feline groups. Conflicts arise over scarce resources such as food, water, resting places, and mates.

To minimize the risk of a conflict resulting in debilitating injury to one or both parties, cats have developed strategies to manage these interactions. Each cat acts as an independent unit in terms of its survival, with the aim of maximizing access to resources while minimizing the risk of confrontation and injury. Distribution of resources is therefore an important factor in feline harmony, and the ability to manage access to resources, both in terms of physical location and the times when the resources are available, is beneficial in terms of avoiding confrontation.

Feline threat behavior shares many characteristics with threat behavior of other animals. The goal of threat behavior is to make the other animal move away or to maintain the threat sender's access to a resource.[23] Threat behavior may involve the animal increasing its apparent size and aggressiveness by changing body posture and using vocalizations and aggressive behaviors. A cat conveys a message of confidence by showing upright body posture, staring at the other cat, moving with little or no hesitation towards the other animal, and possibly exhibiting bunting or even urine-marking behavior. If this behavior does not cause the other cat or cats to give way or move out of the area, the cat may increase the aggressiveness of its behavior. It may stand taller and position itself laterally to the other animal so that it looks as big as possible. By raising the hair on its tail and body, it increases its appearance of size and bulk, and dilation of the pupils means big, black eyes are staring at the other cat. It may growl, lash its tail, and raise a paw to strike. All of these behaviors send the message that the cat is big, strong, and willing to be aggressive to achieve its aims.

When faced with this threatening behavior, a cat may do one of the following:
1. Make itself scarce: It moves away from the threatening cat.
2. Seek to avoid conflict: It may do this by lowering its body, avoiding eye contact, and freezing until the other cat moves away.
3. Meet the threat with one of its own: Depending on factors such as the cat's personality, previous experience, and location of the conflict, the cat may meet the other cat's aggression with upright body language. If it is on neutral or claimed territory or is younger or less experienced, it may take a more defensive, lower position while remaining aggressive (Figure 4-3).

If a threat is met with a threat, then a fight may ensue, with the victor chasing the loser away.[24] Similar behavior is directed towards cats that are not recognized as part of the social group.

Feline Affiliative Behavior

The opposite of conflict behavior is affiliative behavior. These behaviors encourage contact and decrease distance

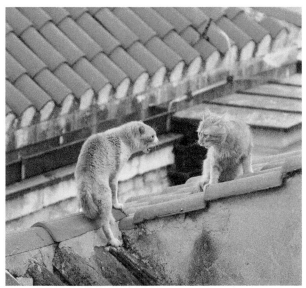

FIGURE 4-3 The cat on the left is threatening the cat on the right. The cat on the left has raised body posture, piloerection, and flattened ears. The cat on the right is not sure if it will move away or respond aggressively to the threat. Its body is lowered, but not completely, and its ears are rotated out to the side, but not completely to the back. (Copyright © iStock.com)

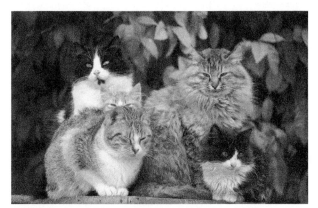

FIGURE 4-4 Bonded cats can often be found in close proximity to each other. (Copyright © iStock.com)

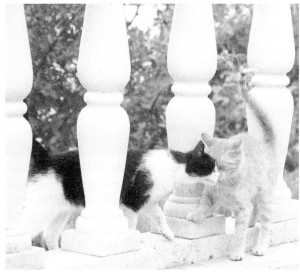

FIGURE 4-5 Bunting is an affiliative behavior. (Copyright © iStock.com)

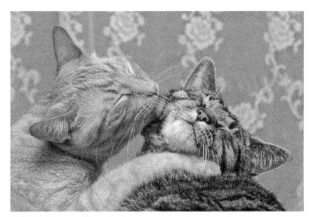

FIGURE 4-6 Bonded cats may show mutual grooming. (Copyright © iStock.com)

between members of a socially compatible group. Cats that are affiliated are said to have bonded (Figure 4-4). They can be recognized by being in close proximity to each other,[24] touching each other, bunting (Figure 4-5), allorubbing, twining their tails, and exhibiting mutual grooming (Figure 4-6). Allorubbing describes the way cats rub against each other.[5] They may share food or eat close together, especially if they are related; however, cats are naturally independent feeders, and this may be related to a higher level of tolerance of being fed in proximity rather than an actual desire to feed in this way.[25] If separated, cats exhibit behavior such as greeting vocalizations, allorubbing, and bunting when reunited. Many affiliative behaviors are also directed towards people with whom the cat has bonded.

Group scent is very important for feline group identity and affiliation. It is achieved by group members' mingling their scents by allorubbing and bunting each other as well as objects and surfaces in their environment. This behavior is not driven by dominance. All cats within a group display these marking behaviors.[26] Any cat that does not share this group odor may be driven off.

Understanding the importance of odor can help cat owners introduce a new cat into homes with existing cats or minimize the disruption if a cat from a multicat household is removed and then reintroduced. Rubbing all the cats with one towel (toweling) can artificially create a group smell and help with the integration of new cats and returning cats.[27] For more information on this topic, see Chapters 6 and 26.

Social Behavior of Kittens

Kittens are social from a very early age. They rely on interaction with the queen for survival and to learn important life skills such as grooming, hunting, feeding, and

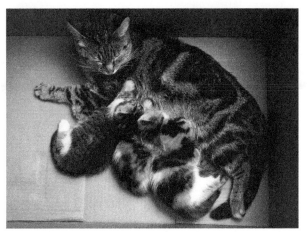

FIGURE 4-7 Kittens are social from an early age, as they must rely upon their mother not only for survival but to learn important skills. (Copyright © iStock.com)

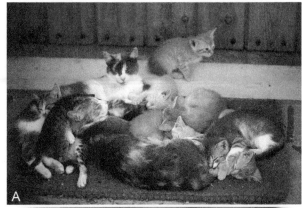

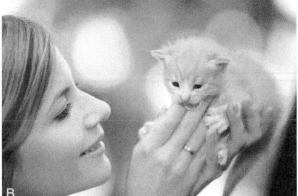

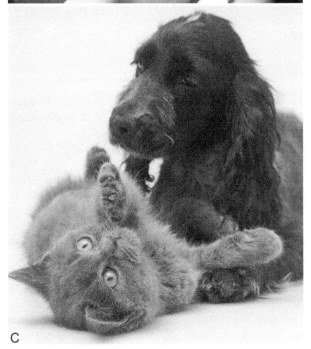

FIGURE 4-8 Kittens develop social relationships with other animals and display affiliative behavior towards cats **(A)**, people **(B)**, and dogs **(C)**. (Copyright © iStock.com)

agonistic and affiliative behaviors (Figure 4-7). They also rely on interaction with littermates to learn social skills such as threat behaviors and affiliative behaviors. Kittens begin to show social behaviors as their eyes and ears open and their nerves and muscles develop enough that they can change the position of the ears, tail, body, and hair. This begins to occur from 7 days of age onward.

During the first 2 months of their lives, kittens form social relationships. These include relationships with other cats, with people, and with other animals (Figure 4-8, *A–C*). The kittens prefer their mother over other adult cats but will accept care from familiar adult female cats. This is seen when related queens cross foster their kittens.[28] The developmental stages of the kitten and socialization with people have not been studied as thoroughly as in dogs.[29] It has been suggested that kittens pass through their major developmental stages at earlier ages than dogs do,[30] although more recent research into dog development has suggested that the important phase in terms of dogs' social development may be earlier than first thought. Certainly, kittens need socialization opportunities at a very young age if they are to accept other cats, people, and other animals as part of their milieu, and research has suggested the period from 2 to 7 weeks of age is of particular importance. When kittens were raised with rats of different strains, in general they did not prey on the strain of rat with which they were raised but would attack rats of different strains,[31] which illustrates how important early exposure is to the kittens' perception of other species later in life.

There are lifelong consequences for a kitten whose social environment is impoverished. Kittens isolated starting from a young age were found to develop behavioral, emotional, and physical problems. They were fearful and aggressive, had difficulty learning, and exhibited random, undirected locomotor activity.[32] They also did not play when exposed to other kittens.[33] This has important implications for hand-rearing single kittens. Whereas a queen with a single kitten socializes her kitten by playing with it,[34] a solo hand-reared kitten does not experience this important interaction. Where possible, single orphan kittens should be fostered onto a queen or raised with

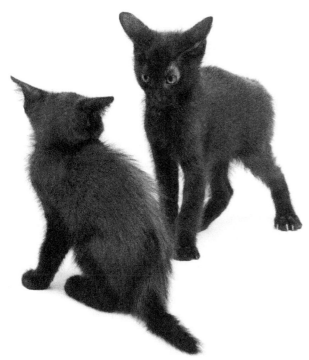

FIGURE 4-9 Kittens practice all behaviors, even antagonistic ones. (Copyright © iStock.com)

other kittens or cats that are friendly towards kittens. If these options are not available, some have suggested that euthanizing the kitten may be better than raising an animal likely to develop behavior problems.

Young kittens also practice hunting behavior in a social setting. The presence of the mother and littermates increases their interest in prey animals.[35,36] Kittens learn how to deal with different species of prey from watching their mother dispatch and dismantle them. This social learning continues into adult life as they learn how to deal with novel prey species by watching other cats kill them.[31] Kittens also learn a novel operant-conditioning activity faster when they watch their mother learn it and perform it.[37]

Play is used to practice behaviors needed for adult life. The play behaviors kittens show changes with their age and development. Social play is seen before approximately 8 weeks of age, but it gradually is replaced with play directed at inanimate objects after 8 weeks.[38]

After weaning, when play is directed towards littermates, it includes predatory and agonistic behaviors[30] (Figure 4-9). Play bouts may end in a fight, with the fighting part of the bout becoming more prevalent.[30] As kittens reach the age of dispersal, social play and interactions begin to decline.[39]

SOCIAL BEHAVIOR AND THE OWNED CAT

In communities and within individual homes, problems arising between owned cats are not uncommon. In a feral colony, a new cat stays at the periphery of the social group, attempting to avoid being attacked until it is accepted. If it is not accepted or if there is a lack of resources available for it (and it cannot displace an incumbent cat), it moves on. New animals entering existing colonies are disruptive.[24]

The owned cat often has no choice in where it lives, how many cats live in adjoining homes, how many cats share the home of the owned cat, and how many resources there are available to it. If the density of cats is too high for the level of resources available, there is a potential for problems of chronic stress, which can lead to both behavioral and physical health consequences. Young cats may also be driven off by bigger, older, incumbent cats, which may be a factor in cases where young cats are lost.

The individual differences of cats are often not considered when cat owners add cats to the household. Feral cats tend to form groups with related animals, usually female littermates and their dam.[5] Male cats may or may not belong to these groups. Therefore, expecting unrelated cats to form social bonds does not take the biology of the cat into consideration. Many cats form social bonds with other cats with which they share a household, but many more simply learn to tolerate the other cats. The cats appear to use a "time-share" routine for managing access to resources, with one cat using an area and then giving way to the next cat coming into the area.

Multicat households are often affected by soiling issues within the house. It is important to use extensive behavior history-taking to ascertain whether this is caused by one or more cats' experiencing anxiety disorders, whether it is a result of inadequate toilet facilities or management, or whether it is due to one or more cats' controlling resources. Management may involve separating some cats and providing more toilet facilities, resting places, water sources, and feeding places to prevent resources from being monopolized by a few cats (see Chapter 24).

A survey of cat owners who introduced new cats found that over half of the multicat households surveyed introduced the cats by just putting them together. The study authors also found that fighting between cats occurred in half of the multicat households.[40] Understanding what cats need and the time it takes for cats to adjust to the addition of new cats can help reduce conflict and stress within multicat households. Separation of cats, provision of plenty of resources, and toweling all cats can help integrate new cats into the household (see Chapter 26).

CONCLUSION

Cats are complex creatures capable of living alone or in high-density colonies. Groups maintain cohesiveness in part by creating a group odor by allorubbing and allogrooming. The stresses and benefits of living in social groups are managed by using agonistic and affiliative behaviors. These minimize within-group conflict and also prevent outsiders from entering the group and utilizing group resources.

Kittens need a positive social environment for proper development. They practice social behaviors with littermates and their dam. Social facilitation helps attract their attention to stimuli, such as prey, that are important for future survival.

Owned cats live in environments where they have very little control over the density of cats. Although many cats form social bonds with other household cats, better understanding of what cats need and how they form social bonds improves their welfare significantly.

REFERENCES

1. Kappeler PM, Barrett L, Blumstein DT, Clutton-Brock TH. Constraints and flexibility in mammalian social behaviour: introduction and synthesis. *Philos Trans R Soc Lond B Biol Sci.* 2013;368:20120337.
2. Rabinowitz AR, Nottingham Jr BG. Ecology and behaviour of the Jaguar (*Panthera onca*) in Belize, Central America. *J Zool.* 1986;210:149–159.
3. Kleiman DG, Eisenberg JF. Comparisons of canid and felid social systems from an evolutionary perspective. *Anim Behav.* 1973;21:637–659.
4. Izawa M, Doi T. Flexibility of the social system of the feral cat, Felis catus. *Physiol Ecol Jpn.* 1993;29:237–247.
5. Crowell-Davis SL, Curtis TM, Knowles RJ. Social organization in the cat: a modern understanding. *J Feline Med Surg.* 2004;6:19–28.
6. Petracca MM, Caine NG. Alarm calls of marmosets (*Callithrix geoffroyi*) to snakes and perched raptors. *Int J Primatol.* 2013;34:337–348.
7. Archie EA, Altmann J, Alberts SC. Social status predicts wound healing in wild baboons. *Proc Natl Acad Sci USA.* 2012;109:9017–9022.
8. Bonanni R, Cafazzo S, Fantini C, Pontier D, Natoli E. Feeding-order in an urban feral domestic cat colony: relationship to dominance rank, sex and age. *Anim Behav.* 2007;74:1369–1379.
9. Price EO. *Principles and applications of domestic animal behavior.* Cambridge, UK: CAB International; 2008.
10. Lichtsteiner M, Turne D. Influence of indoor-cat group size and dominance rank on urinary cortisol levels. *Anim Welf.* 2008;17:215–237.
11. Moosa MM, Ud-Dean S. The role of dominance hierarchy in the evolution of social species. *J Theory Soc Behav.* 2011;41:203–208.
12. Morrison KE, Swallows CL, Cooper MA. Effects of dominance status on conditioned defeat and expression of 5-HT1A and 5-HT2A receptors. *Physiol Behav.* 2011;104:283–290.
13. van den Bos R. Post-conflict stress-response in confined group-living cats (*Felis silvestris catus*). *Appl Anim Behav Sci.* 1998;59:323–330.
14. Stander PE. Cooperative hunting in lions: the role of the individual. *Behav Ecol Sociobiol.* 1992;29:445–454.
15. Moehlman P. Intraspecific variation in canid social systems. In: Gittleman J, ed. *Carnivore behavior, ecology, and evolution.* New York: Springer; 1989:143–163.
16. Buirski P, Kellerman H, Plutchik R, Weininger R. A field study of emotions, dominance, and social behaviour in a group of baboons (*Papio anubis*). *Primates.* 1973;14:67–78.
17. Chapman CA, Wrangham RW. Range use of the forest chimpanzees of Kibale: implications for the understanding of chimpanzee social organization. *Am J Primatol.* 1993;31:263–273.
18. Wittemyer G, Douglas-Hamilton I, Getz WM. The socioecology of elephants: analysis of the processes creating multitiered social structures. *Anim Behav.* 2005;69:1357–1371.
19. Kerby G, MacDonald DW. Cat society and the consequences of colony size. In: Turner DC, Bateson P, eds. *The domestic cat: the biology of its behaviour.* ed 1. Cambridge, UK: Cambridge University Press; 1988:67–81.
20. Fitzgerald BM, Karl BJ. Home range of feral house cats (*Felis catus*, L.) in forest of the Orongorongo Valley, Wellington, New Zealand. *N Z J Ecol.* 1986;9:71–81.
21. Dards JL. Home ranges of feral cats in Portsmouth dockyard. *Carnivore Genet Newsl.* 1978;253:357–370.
22. Izawa M, Doi T, Ono Y. Grouping patterns of feral cats living on a small island in Japan. *Jpn J Ecol.* 1982;32:373–382.
23. Barrow EM. *Animal behavior desk reference: a dictionary of animal behavior, ecology and evolution.* ed 2. Boca Raton, FL: CRC Press; 2001.
24. Wolfe RC. The social organization of the free ranging domestic cat (Felis catus). *Diss Abstr Int.* 2002;62(9-B):4265.
25. Bradshaw JW, Hall SL. Affiliative behaviour of related and unrelated pairs of cats in catteries: a preliminary report. *Appl Anim Behav Sci.* 1999;63:251–255.
26. Natoli E, Baggio A, Pontier D. Male and female agonistic and affiliative relationships in a social group of farm cats (*Felis catus* L.). *Behav Process.* 2001;53:137–143.
27. Landsberg G, Hunthausen W, Ackerman L. *Handbook of behaviour problems of the dog and cat.* ed 2. Edinburgh: Elsevier Saunders; 2004.
28. Feldman HN. Maternal care and differences in the use of nests in the domestic cat. *Anim Behav.* 1993;45:13–23.
29. Scott JP, Fuller JL. *Genetics and social behaviour of the dog: the classic study.* Chicago: The University of Chicago Press; 1965.
30. Bateson P. Behavioural development in the cat. In: Turner DC, Bateson P, eds. *The domestic cat: the biology of its behaviour.* ed 2. Cambridge, UK: Cambridge University Press; 2000:9–22.
31. Kuo ZY. The genesis of the cat's response to the rat. *J Comp Psychol.* 1930;11:1–35.
32. Seitz PFD. Infantile experience and adult behaviour in animal subjects: II. Age of separation from the mother and adult behaviour in the cat. *Psychosom Med.* 1959;21:353–378.
33. Guyot GW, Cross HA, Bennett TL. Early social isolation of the domestic cat: responses during mechanical toy testing. *Appl Anim Ethol.* 1983;10:109–116.
34. Mendl M. The effects of litter-size variation on the development of play behaviour in the domestic cat: litters of one and two. *Anim Behav.* 1988;36:20–34.
35. Caro TM. Effects of the mother, object play, and adult experience on predation in cats. *Behav Neural Biol.* 1980;29:29–51.
36. Caro TM. Predatory behaviour in domestic cat mothers. *Behaviour.* 1980;74:128–148.
37. Chesler P. Maternal influence in learning by observation in kittens. *Science.* 1969;166:901–903.
38. Barrett P, Bateson P. The development of play in cats. *Behaviour.* 1978;66:106–120.
39. West M. Social play in the domestic cat. *Am Zool.* 1974;14:427–436.
40. Levine E, Perry P, Scarlett J, Houpt KA. Intercat aggression in households following the introduction of a new cat. *Appl Anim Behav Sci.* 2005;90:325–336.

Feline Learning
Sophia Yin

INTRODUCTION: CAT STUCK IN A TREE SAVED BY A CAN OF CAT FOOD

When Brenda Farrow heard her stealthy Bengal cat meowing from high up in a tree, she wasn't concerned at first. "Punky's athletic, and the tree's in our front yard. I figured he'd come down when he was ready." But when she returned home from work and found that he was still meowing from the same spot, she became worried. "We tried to coax him down, and neighbors tried to help, but he wouldn't budge." Local firefighters even came to the rescue with their giant ladder. But upon seeing them approach, Punky climbed even higher! Then Brenda had a clever idea. She went into the house and came out armed with a secret weapon: a can of Punky's favorite cat food. "I didn't know if he could see the can, but he sure heard it!" Immediately upon hearing the familiar "schwack" of the can opening, he ran down the tree and followed Brenda and his meal into the house.

Punky's owner had spent hours in distress, and even called the fire department to help out, when the solution was so simple. Punky had been classically conditioned to associate the sound of the can of cat food being opened with the yummy taste of his favorite food. By consistently associating the sound of the can opening with food, Punky's reaction was strong—so strong that the positive emotions the sound triggered overcame his fear and prompted him to run down the tree. Furthermore, in the past he had been rewarded for running toward the sound, because as soon as he reached the source he'd been rewarded with a meal. So, two types of learning worked to rescue Punky, and, if the humans involved had known about these processes, they could have saved a lot of time and money.

We are very pleased to have two chapters in this book written by Sophia Yin and deeply saddened that she did not see her work published. In a multi-author book it is customary to edit chapters with a common writing style. Dr. Yin's other chapter has been edited as part of a series of chapters about handling, but we have intentionally left this chapter in its original form out of respect to Sophia Yin.

Likewise, in veterinary practice, shelter, and other feline-related settings, staff members deal with cat behavior issues on a daily basis. In order to find simple, time-saving solutions, it's essential to know about how cats learn and how human actions affect their behavior.

This chapter is focused on the two most important types of learning—classical conditioning and operant conditioning—that guide behaviors in cats as well as all other animals, ranging from rats and finches to horses, giraffes, and whales. Once you have a grasp of these guiding principles, your work and relationship with cats will be enriched.

CLASSICAL CONDITIONING

The young calico eyes the bowl as if savoring the sight. The scent of the warmed food drifts up. It's the same food she ate ravenously just one meal ago, but now she won't touch it, and it's the fourth type of food she's been offered today. She devours each type at one meal, then rejects it at the next.

What has happened? This cat has a liver shunt, so she often feels sick after she eats a meal. Therefore, she associates the feeling of sickness with the food she just ate and consequently learns to avoid that food in the future. She has learned through what's called classical conditioning to avoid new foods. Classical conditioning is one of the two major mechanisms of learning in animals. Through classical conditioning, animals learn on a daily basis. To understand what classical conditioning is, it's important first to know the history.

Pavlov's Dog

In the early 1900s, a Russian physician and researcher named Ivan Pavlov was studying digestion in dogs.[1] He fed meat powder to dogs and then measured their salivation. After several repetitions, he noted that the dogs frequently began salivating before food entered their mouths. This salivation response was triggered by the sight of food and upon hearing the sound of people approaching with their meals. After making this discovery, Pavlov changed the focus of his research and began investigating what he called "psychic secretions."

Pavlov took his dogs and paired feedings with the sound of a stimulus that previously had no meaning to them. He chose a bell because animals don't normally have any innate response to bells. He rang the bell and then immediately presented the food. After doing this many times, he found that when he tested the dogs by ringing the bell in the absence of food, the dogs salivated.

These results can be explained as follows. The food on its own elicits an involuntary physiologic (and emotional) response—one that occurs without conditioning or training. Consequently, this stimulus is called an *unconditioned stimulus,* and the salivation response is called an *unconditioned response.* After pairing the neutral stimulus bell with the food enough times, the bell elicits the salivation even in the absence of food. Thus, the bell starts off as a neutral stimulus, but, when paired enough times with food, it essentially takes on the same meaning as the food. It becomes a *conditioned stimulus* because it is one that was learned, and it elicits the salivation, which is now called a *conditioned response* because it was trained.

Physiologic Effects of Classical Conditioning

Since Pavlov's findings, this process of *associative learning* has been found to work across many different stimulus–response systems. In the 1950s, John Garcia and his colleagues at the Radiologic Defense Laboratory at Hunter's Point in San Francisco found that rats developed a taste aversion to solutions they were drinking while they were being irradiated.[2] This scenario is similar to the situation of the cat with the liver shunt and the food she was eating. Similarly, most humans have had an experience in which they have eaten a particular food while or immediately prior to becoming ill and subsequently have developed an aversion to the food.

Classical conditioning can have even more dramatic physiologic effects. For instance, even severe allergic responses can be classically conditioned. In one study of this phenomenon, researchers found that guinea pigs could be trained to exhibit a histamine release in response to a novel odor.[3] These guinea pigs were immunologically sensitized to bovine serum albumin (BSA) by injecting BSA into the foot pad, which led to histamine release. Then, during classical conditioning, each guinea pig received an injection of either saline as a control or BSA on five separate occasions spaced 1 week apart. The injections were paired with one of two odors: a sulfurous smell or a fishy smell. In half of the guinea pigs, the sulfurous odor was paired with BSA and the fishy odor was paired with saline. In the other guinea pigs, the pairing was reversed. After the training trials, each animal underwent test trials.

In the first test trial, the researchers presented the odor that had been paired with BSA (i.e., the sulfurous smell in half of the guinea pigs, and the fishy smell in the other half), but in the absence of a BSA injection. All eight guinea pigs showed a marked histamine response upon presentation of the odor that had been paired with BSA. Thus, the odor paired with BSA had become a conditioned stimulus. The histamine response level was comparable to the response that would be elicited by an allergen.

In the second trial, the odor that had been paired with saline was presented in the absence of a saline injection. The histamine release was minimal. Hence, the guinea pigs had been classically conditioned to have an allergic response to a previously neutral smell, whereas they had no response to the smell paired with saline.

Accidental Conditioning of Negative Associations

When does classical conditioning occur in real life? Not surprisingly, it occurs every day and in every interaction we have with animals, as well as in many other situations. For example, imagine that a newly adopted kitten is brought to a veterinary practice for the first time. The client puts the kitten into a travel carrier, which is a new experience for the kitten, and drives her to the practice in a car. Along the way, the kitten may salivate or vomit as a result of nausea induced by the ride. When the client and kitten arrive at the veterinary practice the kitten often encounters foreign scents and sounds, causing an additional fear response (Figure 5-1). Then, in the examination room, the kitten receives a painful vaccination. Although the examination may have seemed to go well because the kitten did not hiss or struggle, the visit 3 weeks later may reveal something different. This time, when the owner brings the carrier out, the kitten may hide. Whereas the owner may be surprised, the veterinarian should not be. The kitten has been accidentally classically conditioned to associate the carrier with the pain, fear, and nausea of her last trip to the veterinary practice and now she is having an involuntary fear response.

The situation continues to worsen once the now fearful kitten, which has been stuffed into the carrier she fears, arrives at the veterinary practice for a visit several months later to be spayed. Again the veterinary practice is scary and the kitten would like to hide, but the staff, oblivious to the kitten's condition, make no special effort

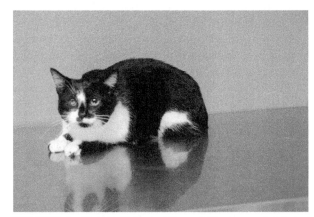

FIGURE 5-1   This cat's fear at the veterinary practice is not likely to decrease on its own. (Courtesy S. Yin)

to calm her down. Instead, they dump the kitten out of her carrier so that she's fully exposed to the environment, and then they scruff her in the hope that doing so will cause her to hold still, but this only serves to agitate her more. A towel over the kitten's head and a slight towel wrap or just a hand in front of her chest would have served to help her feel more comfortable and secure.

The kitten is then put into a cage to wait for surgery. With each human contact of naïve rough handling, the kitten continues to associate the veterinary practice with scary experiences. Then a dog walks by, throwing her into maximal high-alert mode. The next time a person enters to handle the kitten, rather than stiffly lying sternally with her ears back and head low, a posture indicating fear, she hisses and yowls. The kitten has been trained to associate the veterinary practice and veterinarian with aversive conditions, and now, when she can't escape the situation, she responds aggressively. In addition to developing a learned fear response to their handlers, animals can develop aggressive behaviors when techniques involving fear and pain are applied.[4] This finding has been demonstrated in many species, ranging from rats to humans.[5,6] The aggression can be directed toward the object causing the fear and pain, or it can be redirected toward humans, other animals, or inanimate objects. At this point, if the cat described here is restrained and receives an injection, her anxiety, fear, and aggression may remain at the same level, but they are likely to increase both in this visit and in future visits.

Using Classical Conditioning to Address Everyday Situations

We may unintentionally classically condition undesired associations in our pets, but these problems can be alleviated by classically conditioning a different association.[7,8] For instance, the fearful kitten can be trained to associate the carrier, car ride, and veterinary practice with food, thus eliciting all of the pleasurable physiologic changes associated with food. This is called *classical counterconditioning* because it involves countering the association that was previously classically conditioned.

Usually, counterconditioning the stimulus is started at low intensity because the animal will be too fearful of the normal-intensity stimulus to eat the food. Then the intensity is increased in small increments. This process is termed *systematic desensitization*. For instance, to countercondition a cat to the carrier, one would start by feeding the cat her meal outside the carrier at whatever distance she will approach and eat the food without hesitation (Figure 5-2, A and B). When she has comfortably eaten at least one meal in the new location, the food can be moved closer for the next few meals and then into the carrier until the kitten will comfortably eat the food while in the carrier. When the kitten will walk into the carrier and lie down in anticipation of food or in the absence of food, she has been counterconditioned successfully. This training usually takes less than 1 week in both dogs and cats and requires little extra time because it occurs for the duration of the meal. In general, with desensitization and counterconditioning, progress is quickest if the association is made clear by presenting the food immediately when the aversive situation or stimulus is present and by taking away the food when the aversive stimulus is removed. Furthermore, the desensitization steps should be incremental so that the animal experiences little or no fear response during the sessions.

This pattern of desensitization and counterconditioning is the same, regardless of the situation. For instance, with regard to the car-ride aversion, the cat would be fed

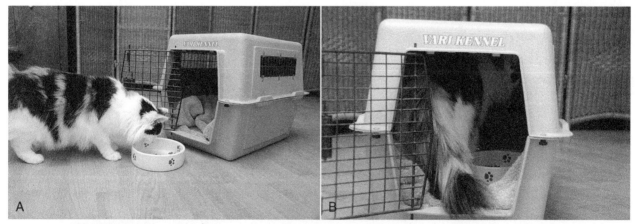

FIGURE 5-2 Desensitization and classical counterconditioning a cat to a carrier. **A,** To train a cat to be comfortable in a travel carrier, start by feeding the cat its meals just outside the carrier. **B,** Systematically move the food further into the carrier until the cat readily goes inside it to eat. The goal at each stage is for the cat to show little to no hesitation and to immediately walk over to the bowl and eat. (Used with permission from Yin S: Low stress handling, restraint, and behavior modification of dogs & cats: techniques for developing patients who love their visits. Davis, CA: CattleDog Publishing; 2009)

her daily meal in her carrier within the stationary car. When the cat comfortably eats her food at this level of stimulus several days in a row, the car engine could be turned on for a short period during the feeding. The next step would be to take the cat on a short car ride around the block. If the ride triggers a salivation or vomiting response due to earlier classical conditioning, an antiemetic may be needed for the first several sessions.

Next, the cat should be counterconditioned to the aspects of a veterinary practice that cause fear, such as encounters with unfamiliar people, receiving injections, and toenail trimming. Some of the behavior modification can be done by the owners at home and can be performed preventatively. For instance, kittens can easily be trained to lie on their backs for toenail trims (Figure 5-3) if they are first given treats continuously while they are on their backs in their owner's lap. Then add increasing intervals between treats until the kitten needs very few treats to remain lying in its owner's

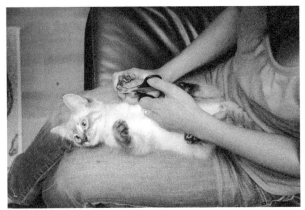

FIGURE 5-3 Desensitization and counterconditioning a kitten to toenail trims. Holding a kitten on its back does not always work well for nail trimming. If the kitten is not adapting to this position in a relaxed way, the training should not continue and another method should be tried when the kitten is calm. (Courtesy S. Yin)

lap. Next, pair treats with gentle foot handling and then systematically more rigorous foot and toenail handling, followed by actual clipping of the nails. For kittens, this process is very quick!

Owners can also easily help desensitize and counter-condition their cats to other procedures, such as injections (Figure 5-4, A and B). For injections, one could start by giving a treat and simultaneously rubbing the cat at the injection site. This contact should cease immediately as the cat finishes the treat. Additional steps include grasping the fur for a second, grasping it for longer periods of time, shaking the skin, pinching the skin softly, poking the tented skin with a capped needle, and, last, injecting the needle.

In general, cats should be counterconditioned to any procedure they may need to endure now or later in life so that they learn to like it. As always, the goal is to stay below the threshold where the animal responds negatively to the handling. During the process, the cat should remain stationary, relaxed, and focused on the food.

It's also important to know that cats can even be counterconditioned by using petting, generally by scratching around the head and ears, but one must focus carefully on making sessions short enough that the cat has a positive experience and no negative or neutral experiences.

These procedures may sound time-consuming, given the number of steps, but they can take just minutes when performed correctly, thus saving time during future visits. Additionally, when performed preventatively, they take only a fraction of the time required later. In either case, the pleasant results should also classically condition the veterinary staff, the cat, and the cat's owner to enjoy the veterinary visits.

OPERANT CONDITIONING

It's evening and you're home from work, but you still have some paperwork to complete. Fluffy, your cat, has just finished her dinner and is making attention-seeking rounds.

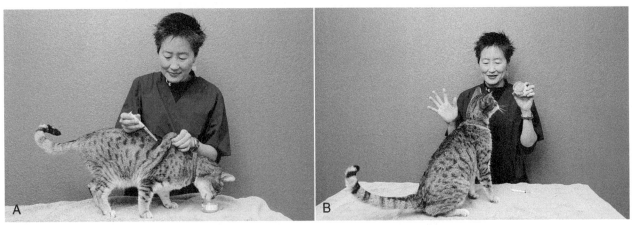

FIGURE 5-4 Desensitization **(A)** and counterconditioning **(B)** to injections. (Courtesy S. Yin)

She first walks up to your husband, who's watching television, and stops to look for a second. Your husband ignores Fluffy, so she moves on. She then walks up to your daughter, who's sitting on the couch, and sits politely. Your daughter scratches Fluffy on the chin on and off for a minute and then gets up to head out to meet her friends. Next, Fluffy gets to you and shows completely different behavior. She meows, not once, but over and over while rubbing against your legs. When you push her, she walks away a few steps and then comes right back and meows even more.

Why is Fluffy so polite with your daughter and your husband but so rude and demanding with you? She's learned through operant conditioning, or trial-and-

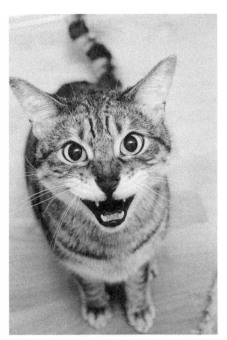

FIGURE 5-5 Cats commonly vocalize excessively because the meowing behavior has been reinforced by their human family. (Courtesy of S. Yin)

error learning. With operant conditioning, the animal repeats behaviors that have desired consequences and avoids behaviors that lead to undesirable consequences (Figure 5-5).

For instance, Fluffy has learned that no matter how much she meows at your husband, the meows fall on deaf ears. Nothing will work to get his attention when he's watching sports. With your daughter, Fluffy has learned that meowing won't work, but sitting quietly will. With you, the loud strategy is the best. You're so busy that you notice her only if she's wailing. Sometimes you give in and pet her. At other times, you push her away. In either case, she's gotten your attention, which reinforces her noisy behavior. Luckily, even if you've accidentally trained an unwanted behavior, you can easily change it once you know the rules of operant conditioning. How? Read on.

The Four Categories of Operant Conditioning

In order to understand operant conditioning, it's important to know some terminology. A good understanding of these terms will allow you to evaluate the knowledge of trainers and behavior consultants with whom you will be dealing, as well as that of companies designing products for behavior modification (Figure 5-6).

The first two terms are *reinforcement* and *punishment*. Reinforcement is anything that increases the likelihood that a behavior will occur again. For instance, if you give your cat a treat when she walks up to you and sits, she is more likely to sit the next time she walks up to you. Punishment is anything that decreases the likelihood that a behavior will occur. For instance, if your cat walks up to you and you pet her roughly in a manner she dislikes, she'll be less likely to walk up to you.

The second pair of terms is *positive* and *negative*. *Positive* and *negative* do not mean good and bad; rather, one should think of them as a plus sign or a minus sign. *Positive* means something is added, and *negative* means something is subtracted.

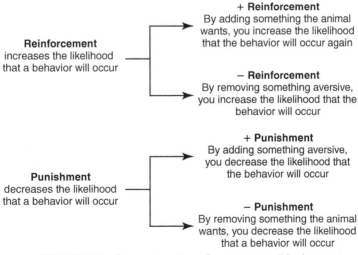

FIGURE 5-6 Four categories of operant conditioning.

These terms can be combined to create four categories of operant conditioning: positive reinforcement, negative reinforcement, positive punishment, and negative punishment.

With positive reinforcement, by adding something the animal desires, the likelihood that the behavior will occur again is increased. For instance, cats can be trained to come to you by rewarding them with a treat when they walk over and sit in front of you (Box 5-1). By rewarding the kitten for walking over and sitting with treats she likes, the likelihood that she will repeat this behavior is increased (Figure 5-7, *A* and *B*).

With *negative reinforcement*, by removing something aversive, the likelihood that the behavior will occur again is increased. An example of negative reinforcement is teaching a dog to come when called, or a horse to follow, by hooking the animal up to a leash or lead rope and pulling with constant pressure and then releasing pressure as soon as the animal takes a step toward you. The dog and the horse will eventually learn to come to you or follow your lead in order to avoid being pulled. Note that it is imperative that the pressure stops as soon as the animal starts performing the correct behavior, otherwise, it will not know that the behavior turns the pressure off.

Punishment can also be positive or negative. The term people are most familiar with is *positive punishment,* the punishment category people most commonly use. With *positive punishment*, by adding something aversive, the likelihood that the behavior will occur again is decreased. It could be physical punishment, such as whacking a cat with a newspaper (not recommended), verbal punishment, or something else that is seemingly benign, such as a squirt of water, if it causes

---

BOX 5-1   Training a Cat to Sit

To train a cat to sit, start in a distraction-free environment with a cat or kitten that is hungry. Be sure to have food rewards that the cat likes. The food can be treats, canned cat food, or the cat's regular food. Use whichever type of reward the cat is motivated for at the time. Method 1 for training a cat to sit is to show the cat the food, but out of the cat's grabbing range, and, when the cat sits, deliver the treat right to her face. Make sure you deliver it in such a manner and to such a location where the cat can eat it while remaining seated instead of accidentally placing the treat in a location that will lure the cat to stand up. Give one treat for sitting. Then remove your hand far enough away so that the cat knows that it shouldn't get up to try to get to the food. Next, before the cat gets up, give it a second treat as a reward for remaining seated.

Continue giving the cat a few more sequential treats. Increase the interval between treats as quickly as you can, but before the cat has a chance to stand up. To repeat the entire exercise, just walk away a few steps so that the cat follows you. Then, when you stop and she catches up, wait for her to sit, or, if need be, lure her. You should need to lure her for only one or two 5- to 10-minute sessions at most. Later, if you want to add a cue word, *sit*, just say "sit" once, right before you know the cat will sit. If the word is always paired with the action of sitting and stated only one time, the cat will learn to associate the word with the action of sitting. Ideally, the cat learns to sit automatically whenever she comes up to you and wants food or something else, but it's good to also be able to have the cat perform the behavior on cue (see Figure 5-7, *A* and *B*).

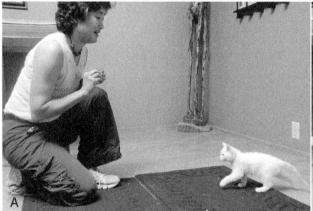 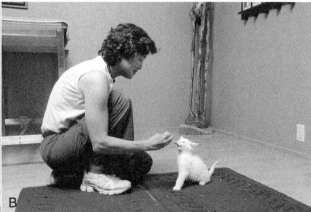

FIGURE 5-7   Training a cat to sit. **A,** Show the cat the food, but keep it out of grabbing range. **B,** When the cat sits, deliver the treat right to its face. Before the cat stands up, give a second treat to reward it for remaining seated. Continue giving the cat a few more sequential treats, increasing the interval between them before the cat has a chance to stand up. Ideally, the cat learns to sit automatically whenever it comes up to you (see Box 5-1). (Used with permission from Yin S: Low stress handling, restraint, and behavior modification of dogs & cats: techniques for developing patients who love their visits. Davis, CA: CattleDog Publishing; 2009)

the cat to run away. If it is aversive to the animal and discourages the behavior, it is a punishment. If it seems aversive to you but is not aversive to the animal, then it is not an effective punishment. In fact, technically, it's not even a punishment.

With **negative punishment**, by removing something the animal desires, we decrease the behavior. For instance, when you are feeding them, kittens as well as adult cats often climb on or claw you to try to grab the treat more quickly. If you remove the treat as soon as the cat starts to raise its paw, you will decrease the pawing and climbing behaviors (Figure 5-8, *A* and *B*).

Classification of Training Techniques Used in Operant Conditioning

The different training techniques used in operant conditioning may seem straightforward at first, but they often become confusing when one starts to classify them. The reason for this is that some techniques may fall into more than one category, depending on how the behavior and the technique are described. In order to avoid confusion, classification should be approached methodically. One such approach is outlined below:

1. **Define the behavior to be modified and decide whether you want to increase or decrease that behavior.** If the goal is to increase the behavior, you will, by definition, use reinforcement. If the goal is to decrease the behavior, you will, by definition, use punishment. For example, say your cat likes to run up to you and grab your leg like it's an interactive squeaky toy and you want to change that behavior. You can define two goal behaviors. You can either decide to train the cat to stop grabbing you or train him to greet you in a more acceptable manner, such as by sitting calmly. If your goal is to train the cat to stop grabbing, by definition you will be using

punishment. If your goal is to train a more appropriate behavior such as to sit upon greeting, you will be using reinforcement.

2. **Decide whether you're adding something or subtracting something in order to determine whether the operant category will be negative or positive.** If you squirt a cat with water to stop it from grabbing (not a recommended technique), you are adding something the cat finds aversive or undesirable in order to decrease the behavior. Consequently, you are using positive punishment. Alternatively, you may opt to remove the interactive attention that your cat wants by standing completely motionless and silent in order to make it clear to your cat that you are not an interactive squeaky toy. By doing so, you will decrease the grabbing behavior, so you are still using punishment. In this case, though, you are using negative punishment. You are removing something the cat wants in order to decrease the grabbing behavior.

3. Conversely, if your goal is to train the cat to greet by sitting, you will be using positive reinforcement or negative reinforcement. If you wait until the cat sits and then give it a treat for sitting, you are using **positive reinforcement**. If you hook the cat to a leash and collar and step on it so that it causes pressure when he tries to grab (not a recommended technique) and then release the pressure immediately when he sits, you're using **negative reinforcement**.

Which Categories of Operant Conditioning to Use: A General Approach to Solving Behavior Problems

Although animals learn in ways that fall under all four categories of operant conditioning in the wild, at home, and in specific training sessions, the categories that by

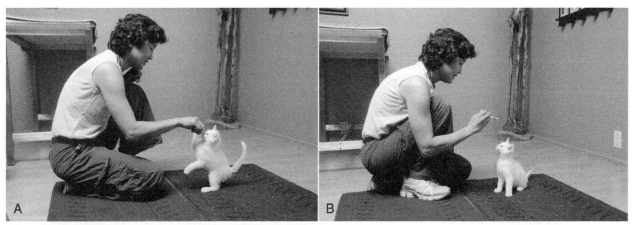

FIGURE 5-8 A, This kitten is excited to get the treat, so she tries to grab it with her paws. If she gets the treat while she's pawing, she will learn to paw or claw to get treats. **B,** The treat must be pulled away and out of the kitten's reach so she learns that pawing does not work. As a result, she exhibits the other behavior she has learned for getting treats; that is, she sits. (Used with permission from Yin S: Low stress handling, restraint, and behavior modification of dogs & cats: techniques for developing patients who love their visits. Davis, CA: CattleDog Publishing; 2009)

far work the best for our interactions with animals are positive reinforcement and negative punishment (i.e., rewarding behaviors we want and removing rewards for unwanted behaviors). Consequently, whereas we tend to solve behavior problems by asking how we can stop or punish an undesirable behavior, we should focus instead on how to reinforce a more appropriate behavior and how to avoid reinforcing the inappropriate behavior. Thus, step 1 in solving common behavior problems is to identify possible reinforcers of the undesirable behavior to avoid reinforcing it. The second step is to decide on a behavior you would rather have the animal perform. Note that in many cases you don't actually have to identify the reinforcer for the undesirable behavior; you can just focus on training the behavior you would rather have.

Example 1: The Cat That Bothers You When You are Working on the Computer

Your friend complains that her cat bothers her by pawing at her when she's working on the computer. How can we fix this problem?

First, identify the reinforcer of the unwanted behavior (that is, the positive reinforcement for the behavior). In this case, the cat paws its owner because the owner pets or talks to it when he does so (Figure 5-9, *A* and *B*). To fix the problem, the human must remove the reinforcer (negative punishment). If the human moves away when the cat starts to paw and remains quiet and avoids touching and/or petting the cat, then the cat can understand that that pawing leads to removal of attention (Figure 5-10, *A* and *B*).

Next, the human must reinforce the behavior she wants (positive reinforcement). In this case, once the cat sits quietly, the human should make sure to pet the cat for short periods, but at frequent intervals at first, so that the cat is rewarded for sitting and remaining

seated. Then the human should increase the interval between petting quickly, but systematically, so that the cat learns to remain quiet and seated for long periods of time (Figure 5-11, *A* and *B*).

Example 2: The Cat That Wakes You up Early in the Morning

Every morning your cat wakes you up at 5:00 AM. He cries and cries and even climbs all over you when you're lying in bed. Sometimes you push him off the bed, but he continues anyway until you feed him. Why does the cat wake you up every morning?

The cat wakes you up because you are reinforcing his behavior by getting up to feed him, and you're interacting with him when he jumps on the bed. If you can clearly remove your attention from him and feed him only after he's quiet, preferably at the time at which you want to feed him, then he will understand that the meowing doesn't work. For instance, you could lock him outside your room and start the training on days when you can wear earplugs and sleep until after he's quiet. Another technique is to get a remote-controlled, automated treat dispenser such as the Treat&Train[9] and train the cat that waiting calmly and quietly earns rewards (Figure 5-12). Start by rewarding the cat at frequent intervals, but quickly increase to longer intervals between treats, being careful to still reward frequently enough so that the cat stays quiet and stationary. Next, early in the morning when the cat starts to meow, wait for him to be quiet, then as soon he's quiet hit the Treat&Train remote control so that treats are dispensed at a rate that will keep him quiet. Alternatively, you can train him with a cue that tells him to perform a behavior, such as go to the rug where the Treat&Train resides, and if he sits there he will get treats. That way, if he's meowing and you give him that cue, he will run to the rug and

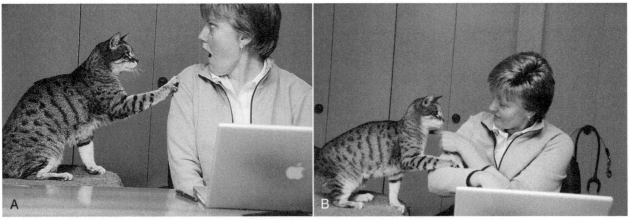

FIGURE 5-9   Identify the reinforcer for the unwanted behavior (the positive reinforcement). This cat paws because the person sometimes responds by petting or talking to it, thereby reinforcing the behavior. (Courtesy S. Yin)

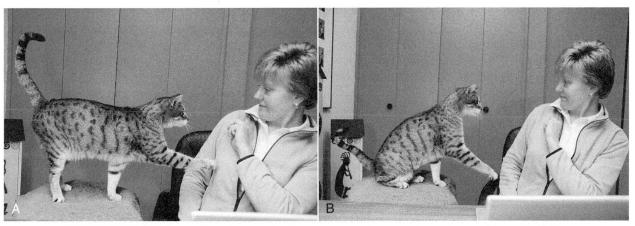

FIGURE 5-10 Remove the reinforcer for the unwanted behavior (negative punishment). If the human moves away when the cat starts to paw and remains quiet and avoids touching and/or petting the cat, then the cat can understand that pawing leads to removal of attention. (Courtesy S. Yin)

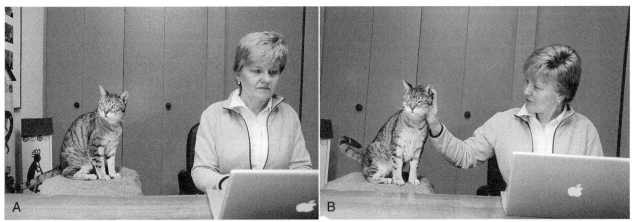

FIGURE 5-11 Reinforce the correct behavior instead (positive reinforcement). **A,** Once the cat is sitting quietly, make sure to pet it for short periods but at frequent intervals at first so that it gets rewarded for sitting and remaining seated. **B,** Increase the interval between petting quickly but systematically so that the cat learns to remain quiet and seated for long periods of time. (Courtesy S. Yin)

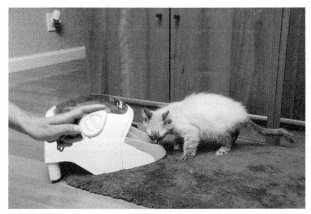

FIGURE 5-12 The Treat&Train can be used to reinforce quiet behavior even when your cat is in a different room. Start with frequent treats, and systematically and rapidly increase the interval between treats. (Courtesy S. Yin)

sit quietly. Then you can start rewarding quiet, calm behavior instead of waiting for the cat to be quiet on his own.

Example 3: The Outgoing Cat That Pesters a Shy or Fearful Feline Housemate

Your cat Lincoln loves to play with other cats, but you've introduced a new cat, Merlin, into the household. Merlin is fearful of other cats. What do you do when Lincoln walks up to Merlin and wants to interact?

In this case, interacting with Merlin would be a reward for Lincoln, and it is difficult to make this potential reward disappear. So, you could preemptively reward Lincoln for more appropriate behavior before he gets to Merlin. For instance, you could have him come when called and then reward him for performing this behavior quickly.

This two-step approach to modifying behavior in cats is fairly straightforward. However, people are sometimes unsure about which replacement behavior to use. Realistically, with cats, three replacement behaviors can be used to solve a huge number of problems. The first one, sit quietly, is covered in Box 5-1. The second two—come when called and targeting—are covered in the next section. For every unwanted behavior your cat performs, you can think of a way to use one, two, or a combination of all three replacement behaviors to solve your problem.

Reasons to Avoid Punishment and Aversive Stimuli

Although the most effective methods of modifying behavior are a combination of positive reinforcement and negative punishment, owners typically choose positive punishment and aversives (Figure 5-13). Whereas aversive stimuli can work under a very specific set of conditions, their use is also associated with many side effects, including fear of the human who delivers the aversive stimulus, aggression, and an actual strengthening of the unwanted behavior when the animal is punished inconsistently.[10,11]

Shaping Complex Behaviors

So far, we've covered the general approach to solving behavior problems; however, in some cases, it may seem impossible to just remove rewards for unwanted behavior and suddenly your cat will perform the desired behavior for a treat reward. For instance, it may seem impossible to train a cat to run to you for a food reward from across the room instead of running to play with another cat.

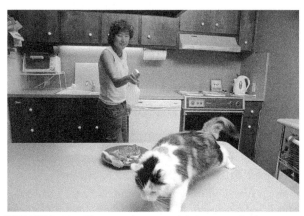

FIGURE 5-13 If you squirt a cat with water and this causes the cat to get off the counter, then by adding the aversive water you are using positive punishment to decrease the cat's behavior of jumping on the counter. Unfortunately, however, the cat may only learn that he should stay off or get off the counter if you are present and holding the squirt bottle. (Used with permission from Yin S: Low stress handling, restraint, and behavior modification of dogs & cats: techniques for developing patients who love their visits. Davis, CA: CattleDog Publishing; 2009)

In many cases, it *is* impossible to train cats toward the goal behavior, at least in one step. That's because we generally have to start with a behavior that we can train and systematically train behaviors that are closer to the goal behavior. In other words, we shape the behavior through incremental steps called *successive approximations*.

Example 1: Training a Cat to Stop Meowing

Say you have a cat that meows incessantly for your attention, a behavior that you want to stop.[12] The general approach is to reward for quiet behavior and remove your attention when the cat meows. But the problem is that you want the cat to be quiet for long periods of time. At first, you must reward for just an instant of quiet. Once you can capture that, continue rewarding for that instant of quiet before the cat has a chance to meow again. Then, once you can get that a few times, start rewarding increasing intervals of quiet. You'll be able to increase the interval quickly if you are systematic about the process. In fact, you can often fix this behavior altogether in just a couple of short training trials.

Example 2: Training a Cat to Come When Called

Remember the case of Lincoln, the cat that loves to play with other cats, and Merlin, the new household cat that's afraid of other cats? A good come-when-called will be important for keeping Lincoln away from Merlin when the two are out. But what if Lincoln is far away and you need to call him? Will his come-when-called be reliable enough? To train the cat to come when called, you can start with the sit exercise, in which you first give Lincoln a treat for sitting and then walk away a few steps. If he's hungry, he will follow and sit. Repeat this a few times, and, when he's consistently successful at immediately following you after he's finished with the first treat, systematically increase the distance you walk away until you can be sure he'll run to follow you even if you're 10 or more feet away. Note that if he's not following consistently or quickly, stop the session and try later when he's hungrier, or use a better food treat. If he's motivated to receive your reward and he's in a comfortable environment, it should take only a couple of short sessions to have him following you well.

When he consistently runs to you and sits, you can add the cue word *come*. Say, "Lincoln come" right after he finishes the treat from the previous repetition and is ready to follow you. In order for him to learn that he should come when called every time, the word must be followed by the behavior of come. So, only say "come" if you know he will come running within a second.

The next step is to increase the distance that Lincoln comes running. For instance, if you will need to have him come when called from the other side of the house, then you'll need to systematically increase your distance. You can also start practicing with mild distractions such as toys in the room or other people. Make sure your sessions are short so that your cat views it as play and wants more. Remember that cat at the beginning of the chapter that came running down the tree at the sound of the can opening? If you can be equally consistent about the meaning of the word *come* and the reward is equally valuable, then your cat's come-when-called behavior will be equally impressive.

Another technique that can be used to keep cats such as Lincoln engaged is **targeting,** an exercise in which the cat learns to touch a target with its nose (Figure 5-14). Most often with cats, the target is a ball on a stick. To teach this behavior, begin by holding the target out of view. Then place it in view about 1 cm from the cat's nose. When the cat investigates the object by sniffing it with its nose, remove the target and simultaneously place a treat where the target was to reward the target-touch. Repeat this training 5 to 10 times, and, as soon as the cat can touch the target five times in a row, increase the criteria by presenting the target far enough away so that it has to take one step. Once the cat can consistently walk one step, increase the criteria again to several steps until it can go to the target at whatever goal distance you decide you want it to be. Targeting can then be used as a way to get your cat to move to a location where you want it to be. Or it can just be used as a game to keep the cat engaged. In the case of Lincoln, it can be used to keep him engaged with something other than Merlin.

When Your Shaping Plan Stalls

Frequently, you devise a rough shaping plan that seems perfect, but it doesn't work when you go to apply it. When a shaping plan doesn't work, it's due to one of the following three problems.

1. **Going to step 2 before the animal has fully learned step 1.** Just because an animal can perform a behavior correctly a few times does not mean that it knows the behavior well. In general with animals, it should perform the behavior correctly 80% to 100% of the

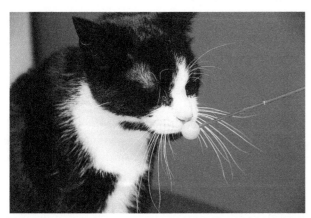

FIGURE 5-14 Targeting, an exercise in which the cat learns to touch a target with its nose, is a handy replacement behavior. (Courtesy S. Yin)

time before you go on. To make things simpler, you can choose a number such as 5 or 10 correct responses in a row and see if that criterion results in the pet performing well on new steps.

2. **Skipping steps.** The trainer may expect too much from the animal by accidentally skipping steps. For instance, just because a cat can touch a target in front of its nose does not mean it will be able to jump through a hoop to get to a target. In general, if the animal was doing well at one step and does poorly at the next step (40% or less often correct), then go back and add additional steps.

3. **Staying on the same step too long.** Trainers also err by staying on the same step too long. For instance, the goal when using food rewards is to use them only temporarily in the early-learning and habit-forming stages and then to wean the cat off the food rewards. So, in the case of the cat that meows incessantly, at first reward an instant of quiet, but start rewarding increased intervals of quiet as soon as possible. Where most people get stuck is that they may quickly increase the rewards to every 3 or 4 seconds, but then they stay at that interval instead. Their cat may bother them while they are studying, so they give the cat a few sequential treats or petting bouts for being quiet and then go back to working, but they fail to systematically pet or treat the cat at increasing intervals of quiet. As a result, the cat is only good for a few minutes and then bothers them again. If the humans were systematic for just a few sessions, the incessant meowing would be cured. A variation of this situation is one where the owner builds up a very high reinforcement rate at one step, such that the cat has learned the step so well that it has trouble learning the new criteria when the owner wants to increase the criteria. For instance, if the owner rewards the cat for 5 seconds of quiet 50 times a day for 10 days in a row, the cat should become highly consistent at being quiet for 5 seconds and may have a strong expectation that the treat will come at exactly 5 seconds of quiet. Subsequently, if the owner decides to increase the criterion to 7 seconds of quiet, he may sometimes encounter problems. The cat may be quiet for 7 seconds a few times, but other times may start pacing, become impatient, and start meowing when the reward does not come as expected at 5 seconds. In general, it's a good idea to know ahead of time what your shaping steps will be and try to get 80% to 100% correct trials during the shaping steps and repeat each step for only 5 to 10 trials in a row.

Training is a Technical Skill: Timing, Criteria, and Rate of Reinforcement

Now that you know the principles of operant conditioning, you can picture training an animal. Implementing these principles effectively requires practice, however, because, like playing tennis or a musical instrument, training animals is a technical skill. In this particular "sport," the keys to success are good timing, well-defined criteria, and the correct rate of reinforcement.

Timing

When training any animal, timing is critical. The reinforcement or punishment must occur as the behavior is occurring, within 1 second of the behavior, or at least well before the next significant behavior occurs. Take as an example teaching a chicken to peck a black dot on a target. What happens if he pecks the dot, you start to deliver the food reward, but he's moving so quickly that he pecks the yellow area and then grabs the food (Figure 5-15)? The chicken will learn that pecking the yellow area leads to food rewards. In other words, he'll think he's supposed to peck the yellow area. The take-home message here is that animals learn to perform the behaviors that are reinforced, not the behaviors you think you reinforced or meant to reinforce.

Well-Defined Criteria

To train a cat successfully, you have to firmly establish your criteria so that you can be clear and consistent. That means the picture of what you want should be so clear in your mind that if you describe the criteria to someone else, he or she will reward the exact behavior that you pictured. Using the chicken example above, what if the chicken sometimes hits the center of the dot, sometimes hits right at the border, and sometimes grabs at the dot and rips at it? You must decide exactly which behaviors to reinforce. If you want the chicken to peck only at the center, then you must provide reinforcement only when he pecks the center of the dot. Otherwise, you will get all of the above-mentioned pecking behaviors. In the photograph shown in Figure 5-15, the chicken pecked just outside the dot.

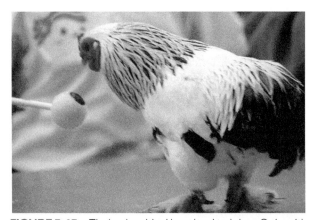

FIGURE 5-15 Timing is critical in animal training. Only with proper timing of the reinforcement can the desired behavior be trained. (Courtesy S. Yin)

Sometimes it is difficult to convey a correct behavior to the animal exactly when it is performed, because the animal is moving quickly and it is difficult to get the treat to the animal quickly enough or the animal is facing away from you while performing the correct behavior or is far away. In these cases, we can use what's called a *bridging stimulus* to tell the animal when it has done something right. First, train the animal that a novel, conspicuous sound, such as a clicking sound produced by a clicker, means food is coming. Do this by pairing the clicking sound with food. That is, every time you make the clicking sound, deliver food to the animal within one-half of a second. Once you've classically conditioned the association between the clicking sound and food, you can use the clicker to "mark" when the animal's done something right. Now, instead of getting the food to the animal immediately so that it knows when it has done something right, you can just use the clicker, which will cause it to stop what it is doing and orient it toward that direction to look for the treat reward. That is, as a bridging stimulus, the clicker bridges the time between the correct behavior and the food reinforcement. You should follow the click immediately with the reward every time in order to avoid diminishing the association. You should also still be ready to get the reward to the animal quickly, because a long or unpredictable delay will diminish the value of the reward.

Rate of Reinforcement

When working with chickens, exotics, cats, piglets, and other animals off-leash, you have to reinforce their behaviors enough to keep them interested in the game or else they will just wander away. With dogs and horses, we often force them to stay near us by using a leash or lead rope halter; however, they also need a high-enough reinforcement rate to stay focused on us and to do what we ask. The leash or halter is just a safety device to keep the dog out of trouble. We should rely on our good timing, well-defined criteria, and correct rate of reinforcement to keep the animal interested in sticking with us during training.

Continuous Reinforcement

When animals (and people) are first learning a behavior, reinforce the behavior on a **continuous basis**. That is, every time they perform the behavior correctly, reinforce the behavior until they know the behavior well. Make sure that the behavior is easy enough so they have many opportunities to earn rewards, or you will lose their attention. If the behavior you are teaching is one in a number of shaping steps, then, as soon as they perform the behavior to 80% to 100% proficiency, increase the criteria (shaping)! Otherwise, you'll stay on the same step forever. But continue reinforcing the correct behavior every single time, until you have reached the goal behavior. In the case of pecking a dot, the goal behavior is just pecking the dot. But for cases such as training your cat to sit and remain seated for long periods of time when greeting you, you'll first reinforce sitting for 1 or 2 seconds consistently and then rapidly increase the criteria to longer periods of sitting.

Variable Ratio of Reinforcement

Once the pet performs the goal behavior well enough to get it right close to 100% of the time and you can bet money the animal will perform the behavior on cue the next time, you may go to a **variable ratio** of reinforcement. With a variable ratio reinforcer, the animal doesn't know which time the correct behavior will earn the reward. That is, you can reinforce the behavior, on average, every two, three, four, five, or more times, depending on your goals and the animal's training level. This is how slot machines work: because you don't know, you try harder. Variable ratio reinforcement is the strongest schedule of reinforcement, which is why so many people are hooked on gambling! In the case of training your cat to sit quietly instead of meowing, a variable ratio of reinforcement might mean that you give him a treat or reward with petting, on average, every 5 minutes, but sometimes the reward comes at 1 minute and sometimes at 10 minutes. It's the average that is 5 minutes.

Motivation

Throughout this chapter, we've talked about removing reinforcers for unwanted behavior and reinforcing desired behaviors instead. In order to do this effectively, we need to know what is reinforcing or motivating to our pets. All animal species are motivated by three innate reinforcers: food, the need to avoid pain and danger, and the need to reproduce. For general training purposes, opportunities to engage in reproductive acts are not a practical reinforcer, and using aversives that generate fear is fraught with side effects.[7,11] That leaves food as one common motivator. All animals have to eat to survive. This means that if we alter the manner in which animals are fed, we can use food to our advantage for training purposes. However, we may need to adjust how they get their food. For instance, if they have food out all the time, they may not be motivated to work for it when we want them to. As a result, we may need to control access to the food source.

If we want to use food as the reward, we should make sure the cat is hungry by measuring his daily food allowance and subtracting his reward allotment from this. We can also plan to train him before he's received the rest of his meal, or we can train him using his total daily food allotment so that all of his food is being used for training purposes until he's well behaved. In general, for cats, it is a good idea to get them onto meal feeding if you want to train them in behaviors quickly and in a short period of time. If cats are used to free feeding, you can switch them to meal feeding in the following way. Measure a morning allotment and an evening allotment. Then put the morning allotment out in the morning. If the cat doesn't want to eat it or starts to eat but then walks away, remove that allotment and toss it out. If you want, instead of immediately tossing it out, you can offer it 15 minutes later so that your cat has a second chance. If he walks away again, however, then toss it out. His next opportunity to eat will be at the evening meal. Generally, within one or two meals, the cat starts to learn that the food is in limited supply. Once the cat is eating meals consistently, you can easily use his meal and mealtime for training, or you can use his meal for training throughout the day.

Another strategy for training cats using food without first having to switch his eating routine much is to use treats or canned cat food for training. If the cat likes canned food better than dry, you can try continuing to free feed it dry food and use the canned cat food for training. For ease of treat delivery, we often take a 3- or 5-mL syringe, cut off the tip, and fill the syringe with wet cat food. Alternatively, we put the cat food on a tongue depressor or a spoon. If canned cat food is not a good option, another option is to train your cat to enjoy treats; however, treats should make up a maximum of 10% or less of your cat's diet. So, your training session will be shorter if you're using treats instead of your cat's regular food. Cats are naturally afraid of trying new foods, and some may not know how to eat treats. To train a picky cat to enjoy treats, just sprinkle in the treats with the regular meal so that the cat tastes them on his own. Once he gets used to the taste, if the treat is tasty, he's likely to prefer them over his regular food, and then you can use them for training.

In addition to using food as a motivator, different species and individuals are motivated by different things. For instance, some cats love attention and petting, whereas for others petting may be considered aversive. It's important to evaluate your cat's response to potential motivators to see what he likes. It's also essential to recognize that motivators vary with context. For instance, some cats may enjoy petting when they are relaxed at home in a calm environment, but not when they are outside or when their level of activity in the room is high. Or they may enjoy short bouts of petting, but long bouts cause them to become agitated. When choosing a reward, it's essential that you choose something that is truly a motivator or reinforcer for your cat and that the cat finds reinforcement in that context and at that point in time.

Communication

It turns out that, as humans, we are at a disadvantage when communicating with animals. Whereas humans are used to communicating by talking and language, animals focus primarily on body language and whether it leads to a positive or negative consequence. For instance, even if you've taught your cat to sit upon hearing the cue word *sit,* if you say "sit" but accidentally wave your hand in a way that indicates to the cat that you are handing him the treat, you may be luring your cat to stand to get the treat. Or, if your cat tries to paw you to get your attention, you may say "stop," but the cat may continue pawing if you do not move away in a manner that clearly indicates you are removing your attention.

So, when training our pets, we have to be aware of our actions more than our words. We also need to watch the cat's body language to see what it is perceiving and how it is responding so that we can adapt what we do based on our cat's response. For instance, if you're rewarding your cat's calm sitting behavior with petting and every time you pet the cat he gets up, then you're actually rewarding standing. The cat learns he has to sit for only an instant and then can get up. If you then decide that you will remove your attention when he starts to stand and you remove your attention by pulling your hand back, if he sits pretty quickly, then it indicates you have removed your attention in a manner that is clear to him. If, however, he paws you or continues to stand, then perhaps you need to remove your attention in a different way, such as by removing your hand and moving a step away.

PUTTING IT ALL TOGETHER

Now you know about classical conditioning, operant conditioning, shaping, timing, criteria, rate of reinforcement, motivation, and communication. The following case is an example of how to integrate this information to solve common behavior problems.

Typhoon is an 8-week-old kitten that loves to play. She especially loves to play with human hands and legs, because her owners have rewarded her when she grabs their hands and legs by flailing them like toys. Whenever she's loose in the house and people walk across the living room, she rushes over and grabs them. Also, when they go to pet her, she sometimes starts to grab and bite their hands. She's also difficult to restrain for even simple handling, such as placing her collar on her, because for several weeks the owners mimicked an interaction they saw on a YouTube video. They would grab her, place her on her back in their laps, and then scratch her on her belly, which caused her to become overly aroused.

This case may seem complex, but it's relatively straightforward. The owners can easily teach Typhoon two or three of the main replacement behaviors—sit and come, for example—and use them to solve the overly aroused play issue. If they reward sit and remain seated with, for instance, 50 reinforcements per day, and control the environment so that Typhoon doesn't have the opportunity to race up to greet them when they are not training, they can quickly change her habit of greeting and playing. Once Typhoon knows how to sit

automatically for a treat, they can have a treat ready every time they enter the living room and reward her for sitting and remaining seated before she has a chance to grab their legs. Then they can redirect her attention to a more appropriate toy. The key factors here are that, for the fastest learning, Typhoon's owners should use the kitten's regular allotment of food and must make sure that the food they are using is of high-enough value to work as a motivator. Then they must practice the sit first until the kitten knows it well. Generally, 10-minute sessions while the kitten is hungry are enough to train this behavior. When Typhoon's owners are practicing the sit with her, they need to make sure to reward her while she is sitting and before she gets up. Then they need to reward longer intervals of sitting. They'll also need to reward Typhoon when she follows and then sits when she catches up to them. They'll need to do this every single time until the behavior is consistent. After that, they should go to a variable schedule of reinforcement. Now, once she has learned the sit as well as the follow and sit behaviors, they can practice in the impromptu sessions, in which they enter the living room and get up and walk around in her presence. They must be ready each time to reward Typhoon for sitting before she has a chance to grab them, and then they must be ready to either continue rewarding the follow-and-sit behavior or redirect her attention to a toy. If Typhoon can do this for many interactions in a row over sequential days, then her leg-grabbing behavior can be changed quickly.

For Typhoon's rough play with the hands, her owners should pet her slowly and gently, and, if she starts to become aroused, they should remove their hands within half a second. They must remove their hands far enough away so that it's clear that they are not interacting with her if she gets rough. They must do this every time until her new behavior of remaining calm during petting is a habit.

Another approach to training a cat to allow petting is to desensitize and countercondition the way that will be needed to train her to allow being restrained or having her collar put on. That is, feed the cat treats such as canned cat food and, while she's eating, pet the cat gently. Then, after about 5 to 10 seconds, stop petting and stop the food. Then wait another 5 to 10 seconds and repeat. The reason for waiting between food–handling pairings is to help make the association clear. Handling equals treats. No handling equals no treats. During this process, the goal is that the kitten be focused only on the food while being handled and that the petting always remain below the level of stimulus that causes the cat to react. In being systematic in petting and handling the cat only during the counterconditioning sessions, the owners can change the cat's attitude toward petting and handling as quickly as a few sessions to 1 week. Sessions should be short (5 to 10 minutes), and it's best if the cat has multiple sessions throughout the day as long as she's motivated to eat the food being used.

CONCLUSION

Overall, training cats to perform appropriate behaviors, as well as using classical counterconditioning and desensitization to change their emotional state, is fairly straightforward; however, it does require practice. For the quickest results, both behavior modification processes require good timing, an understanding of feline body language, and knowledge of the types of motivators that will work well for the cat. Furthermore, operant conditioning generally requires some simple shaping steps, and cat owners need to be aware of how they interact with their cats during every interaction in which the undesired behavior might accidentally be rewarded. Once cat owners can learn basic principles and develop basic skills, they can effect change within a surprisingly quick time frame and develop a better understanding of and stronger relationship with their cats.

ADDITIONAL RESOURCES

Videos

How to Train a Cat: http://drsophiayin.com/videos/entry/training_a_kitten_to_sit?/resources/video_full/training_a_kitten_to_sit

Teaching a Cat to Be Quiet: http://drsophiayin.com/videos/entry/teaching-a-cat-to-be-quiet
Target Training Kittens: http://drsophiayin.com/videos/entry/target_training_kittens

Blogs

The Case of Finn, the Cat Who's Afraid of Toenail Trims and the Vet: http://drsophiayin.com/blog/entry/the-case-of-finn-the-cat-whos-afraid-of-toenail-trims-and-the-vet
Cat Injections: Training Your Cat to Love Injections Without Ruining Your Relationship: http://drsophiayin.com/blog/entry/cat-injections-training-your-cat-to-love-injections-without-ruining-your-re
Training a Cat to Be Quiet: My Cat Meows Too Much, What Do I Do?: http://drsophiayin.com/blog/entry/training-a-cat-to-be-quiet-my-cat-meows-too-much-what-do-i-do
How to Teach a Cat to Use a Cat Door: http://drsophiayin.com/blog/entry/how-to-teach-a-cat-to-use-a-cat-door
A Super Simple Method for Training Cat Tricks: http://drsophiayin.com/blog/entry/a_super-simple_method_for_training_cat_tricks
Release Your Inner Kitty Through Tricks and Training http://drsophiayin.com/blog/entry/release_your_inner_kitty_through_tricks_and_training

REFERENCES

1. Hunt M. *The story of psychology*. New York: Anchor Books; 1993.
2. Garcia J, Koelling RA. Relation of cue to consequence in avoidance learning. *Psychon Sci*. 1966;4:123–124.
3. Russell M, Dark KA, Cummins RW, Ellman G, Callaway E, Peeke HV. Learned histamine release. *Science*. 1984;225:733–734.
4. Azrin NH, Rubin HB, Hutchinson RR. Biting attack by rats in response to aversive shock. *J Exp Anal Behav*. 1968;11:633–639.
5. Berkowitz L. The experience of anger as a parallel process in the display of impulsive, "angry" aggression. In: Geen RG, Donnerstein EI, eds. *Aggression: theoretical and empirical reviews: Vol. 1. Theoretical and methodological issues*. New York: Academic Press; 1983:103–133.
6. Overall KL. *Clinical behavioral medicine for small animals*. St Louis, MO: Mosby; 1997, p. 544.
7. Yin S. *How to behave so your dog behaves*. Neptune City, NJ: TFH Publications; 2004.
8. Wright JC, Reid PJ, Rozier Z. Treatment of emotional distress and disorders: non-pharmacologic methods. In: McMillan FD, ed. *Mental health and well-being in animals*. ed 1. Ames, IA: Blackwell Publishing; 2005:145–158.
9. Treat&Train. http://drsophiayin.com/treatntrain Accessed December 29, 2014.
10. American Veterinary Society of Animal Behavior (AVSAB): AVSAB position statement: The use of punishment for behavior modification in animals. 2007. http://avsabonline.org/uploads/position_statements/Punishment_Position_Statement-download_-_10-6-14.pdf Accessed December 29, 2014.
11. Yin S. *Low stress handling, restraint and behavior modification of dogs & cats: techniques for developing patients who love their visits*. Davis, CA: CattleDog Publishing; 2009.
12. Yin S: Teaching a cat to be quiet. http://www.youtube.com/watch?v=FSwUw9DiT6A Accessed June 2, 2014.

PART 3

Prevention of Behavior Problems: The Cat at Home

Pet Selection

Debra F. Horwitz and Amy L. Pike

INTRODUCTION

Choosing the right feline friends is the first step in a long line of decisions owners have to make in the lives of their companions. Although some owners set out to purchase a pedigree kitten and spend a long time looking into their breed selection, it is well recognized that the majority of new cat owners rarely put much effort into researching this major decision. Pet owners may obtain a cat as a stray that shows up on their doorstep, from a friend needing a home for a litter of kittens, from a shelter, or at an adoption event. Interestingly, more than 50% of clients report that they did not seek cat ownership; they say that their cats "found them." Also, 69% of cat owners did not pay anything for their cats. This method is very informal and usually results in little or no veterinary instruction on proper cat care or behavior.[1] Impulsivity may be the predominating factor when choosing a new feline companion, but it does not have to be.

Veterinarians need to be the gold standard source of information for their clients. Owners trust their veterinarians to guide them through the decisions they will need to make during their cat's lifetime. Questions owners should ask include the following:

- What annual vaccinations does my cat need?
- When my cat is ill, what diagnostics are the best choices based on the presenting symptoms?
- What treatments are appropriate for my cat?

As a reliable and trusted source of information, a veterinarian must take a proactive role in assisting clients in selecting their new feline companions. Many options are available: client handouts about pet selection, information about feline breeders in their area, and partnering with local rescues and shelters to assist these entities in their efforts to select and place up for adoption cats that are behaviorally and medically healthy (see handout titled **Did You Know? Fun Facts and Figures to Help Select a New Feline Family Member**). Assessing cats for behavioral health can be complex and may be outside the expertise of a general veterinary practice. The shelters may need to rely on expertise provided within their organization or on outside help, but practices that have the requisite knowledge or are willing to invest the time to acquire it to assist in this area can be hugely beneficial to shelters in this way. The practice's website or social media outlets can contain links to reputable breeders in the area, rescues, and shelters and can include a digital bulletin board on which current clients can post their own advertisements for cats needing a new home. Some practices may wish to take a more active role by creating a good working relationship with local area shelters and become a resource of cats up for adoption. However, if information is obtained from a veterinary practice, it will be seen as a form of endorsement, and therefore it is very important for a staff member to visit each of these premises to ensure that it is indeed reputable.

Without appropriate guidance, clients may obtain a kitten or a cat from an inappropriate source or perhaps make an impulsive selection of an animal with serious health problems requiring short- or long-term care. In other cases, a family may choose the wrong cat for their family situation, perhaps adding a cat to a household where the existing social dynamics cannot support it or choosing a cat with already established behavior problems that may require behavior management that the client may be unable to appropriately implement.

Of course, many clients arrive at a veterinary practice with a cat or kitten already in their arms, possibly with some of the issues mentioned above. At that time, veterinarians should help them to improve the possibility of success with their new feline friends. In some cases, the difficulties may be encountered that make keeping the cat in the home impossible, in which case providing the clients with professional and appropriate advice about how to rehome the cat may be in the best interests of all parties.

SOURCES

Clients have a variety of options available when they make the decision to add a feline companion to their family. Potential cat owners can obtain their new pet from a breeder if they are looking for a particular breed, from family or friends who have a litter of kittens to give away, or from a rescue or shelter organization, or they may get an abandoned or hand-raised individual.

Breeders of Pedigreed Cats

There can be significant differences in quality between breeders, as well as in the quality of their breeding stock. Unfortunately, most pet owners have limited education about cat breeders and the differences that may exist between them. Breeders of pedigreed cats can generally be classified into two categories: those who are considered highly involved breeders (HIBs) and those who are hobby breeders. HIBs often have larger facilities (catteries) with more breeding females and males on the premises. As a general rule, they are also highly invested in the future of the breed. They may show their cats for various titles, perform genetic testing on their breeding stock to minimize genetic disorders in their lines, and take great care to propagate breed-specific traits. HIBs are also extremely invested in who purchases their cats, often being very particular about to whom they will sell a kitten or adult cat. Because of the care and effort that has gone into the selection, testing, and breeding of the individuals, cats purchased from an HIB may be more costly, especially rare breeds or individuals with champion blood lines. Despite their undoubted investment in their cats, not all HIBs are aware of the behavioral needs of kittens or breed-specific medical and behavioral needs, and questions about these areas are appropriate to ask before taking home a kitten.

Hobby breeders, on the other hand, engage in breeding cats for a myriad of reasons, but often for the fun and experience of breeding a particular cat breed. Although hobbyists may place as much emphasis on the selection and quality of their breeding stock, they typically do not own a large number of breeding cats, attend cat shows, or have large cattery facilities. Often they may only have one or two litters of kittens available and may not have both the queen and the tomcat available in their home. It is equally important that hobby breeders pay attention to selection and rearing from a behavioral perspective.

When obtaining a purebred cat from either an HIB or a hobby breeder, pet owners should take certain factors into considerations. Potential families should research the breeding stock, the medical history of the lines, and the behavioral traits seen in previous litters of the breeding pairs. Unless the individual is too far away, most HIBs will allow you to visit their facility to meet not only the breeder but the cats as well. Owing to distance in some cases, an on-site visit may be impossible. In those situations, some targeted questions regarding health testing and genetic lines will be useful, and gathering information about socialization experiences, including handling and interaction with different people and animals, may provide useful behavioral information about the kitten to be adopted.

If a suitable breeder is nearby, every effort should be made to visit the breeder in person. A breeder who discourages the prospective pet owner from visiting the home or facility should raise concern. In-person visits allow a potential owner to assess the cleanliness and sanitation of the facility where the kitten was raised and the time kittens spend interacting with their mother, siblings, and human caregivers. The environment should be friendly, hospitable, enriched, and maintained for the behavioral and medical well-being of the cats that live there. Veterinarians are trained to recognize sanitary conditions and assess a facility for its ability to provide for the basic medical and nutritional needs of the animals housed there. It is also important to assess whether the social and behavioral needs of the cats are being met, which may be outside the expertise of the general practitioner. If this is the case, advice can be sought from colleagues and the literature, including the American Association of Feline Practitioners (AAFP)/International Society of Feline Medicine guidelines on the environmental needs of cats. To be comfortable with a breeder's recommendation, a hands-on assessment of the facility conditions and an on-site visit to the breeder's cattery or home are essential to providing recommendations with confidence. It is also important to carry out these visits on a frequent and regular basis, as situations can change over time.

To be considered sanitary, a facility's operators must properly dispose of waste and provide clean drinking water and housing for the animals. Litter boxes must be cleaned in a timely fashion, and the feces and urine clumps must be disposed of regularly (ideally by scooping daily and cleaning out the tray completely weekly). Any unacceptable elimination must be cleaned up at the time of discovery, which should not be less frequently than once per day, and ideally the reason for this behavior should be investigated. All the animals housed at the facility must be free of external and internal parasites and bathed when necessary. There should be no odors associated with excrement. In short, the facility should be kept as clean as a veterinary kennel area.

Caretakers also need to provide for the medical needs of the animals they house. Regular veterinary examinations with routine vaccinations and testing need to be provided based on the current recommended guidelines. In the United States, some breeders may choose to perform initial kitten vaccinations themselves; however, this is less than ideal and is not recommended. Vaccines must be handled in an appropriate fashion, including storing them in a refrigerator and mixing them correctly. Those vaccines should also be dispensed from a reputable source and manufactured by a trusted company. Ideally, breeders should rely on their veterinarians to perform necessary testing, vaccinations, and medical treatments. Veterinarians can also provide health certificates, like those used for airline travel, for the kittens and cats being adopted so that clients can be assured of the cats' health status.

Nutrition is a key component in the overall health of an animal. The cats being housed in the facility also need to be fed a complete diet that is compatible with their current life stage, such as a growth or kitten formulation for cats up to 6-12 months of age. Commercial brands of cat food can vary widely in their nutritional composition, and a veterinary nutritionist can provide additional guidance if there are questions or concerns about a particular diet's merits.

The social and environmental needs of the animals housed in the facility are also extremely important to their well-being. Enrichment opportunities for the cats must be made available, including a variety of different types of toys, vertical perching and climbing towers, time spent in positive interaction with other cats, and time interacting with human caregivers. It is important for kittens to have social contact with their own species through their littermates and mother, but it must be remembered that cats are not obligate social creatures and that social interaction with unfamiliar and unrelated cats can be a negative experience for them. Appropriate enrichment is imperative to alleviate stress, provide exercise, stimulate normal predatory behavior towards appropriate targets, and provide adequate early socialization for kittens.

Some breeders may sell kittens directly to pet stores, although this practice is becoming less common. In one study in 2009 by Amat *et al.*, the authors showed that cats obtained from pet stores were more likely to demonstrate problem behaviors,[2] providing evidence for veterinarians to discourage the practice of obtaining animals from this source.

Pet owners who would like to own a purebred cat, but are unwilling or unable financially to purchase from a breeder, may be able to locate a suitable pet through a breed-specific rescue organization. Unfortunately, unless the pet comes with papers, there is no guarantee that the cat is of the genetic line of the breed purported. However, the physical characteristics and coat colors and patterns should be closely aligned to the breed specifications. In certain breeds, behavioral traits may also be recognized and may provide a further indication of the authenticity of the breed description. These breed-specific rescue organizations obtain their cats from a number of different sources, including shelters that are low on space, directly by owner surrender, or as a result of hoarding situations, or they may actively seek out cats up for adoption through other venues to obtain individuals that share the breed's characteristics. Pet owners should be advised that breed-specific rescue organizations often take in any cat that meets the breed criteria, as long as space is available, and house them until a suitable adoptive home is found. In these situations, little or no information may be known about the previous home or the reason for pet surrender. Some breed rescue operations may have more stringent rules for adoption, requiring previous ownership of that particular breed or knowledge above a basic understanding of the unique characteristics and quirks of that breed.

Shelters and Strays

Humane shelters house numerous species up for adoption at any one time. These animals may arrive by direct owner relinquishment or court-ordered relinquishment from hoarders, as abused animals, or as neglect cases or strays. Behavior problems continue to be a common reason why owners relinquish their pets to shelters.[3] Although many shelters perform an intake interview upon relinquishment, owners may be reluctant to reveal all the reasons for the surrender out of concern that these may decrease the chances of adoption success for their pet. Therefore, potential behavior problems may not be revealed at intake and may reoccur in the new home.

Stray cats present another challenge because there may be no knowledge of the cat's prior life experiences. A cat may be found on the street for a variety of reasons; it may have been born and raised on the streets (possibly even as a feral), left outdoors at a previous home because of behavior problems, or simply wandered away and did not return home. In such situations, there will be no information about the past social history of the cat, raising questions such as to whether it was raised with other cats or was ever in a home with dogs or children and giving no indication as to how the cat fared in its previous environment.

The origin of the cat, whether it is owner-relinquished or a stray, can influence the behavior of the cat, not only while in the shelter but also in its subsequent adoptive home. Dybdall, Strasser, and Katz[4] examined behavior differences in shelter settings between owner-surrendered cats and those that were found as strays. These results indicated that cats relinquished by their owners were more stressed by being housed at the shelter, and also more likely to become ill sooner, than their stray counterparts, and both these factors had an impact on their chances for successful adoption. The amount of time the cat spends in the shelter can also affect its behavior while there, impact its adoptability, and possibly influence its post-adoption behavior. Gouveia, Magalhães, and de Sousa[5] looked at duration of stay within the shelter and its effect on cats. They found that, compared with cats housed for less than 1 year, cats housed in a shelter longer than 7 years showed greater inactivity, increased time spent in negative social encounters with conspecifics, decreased time eating, and a decrease in eating frequency. To the best of our knowledge, no additional studies have been done to ascertain whether these behaviors remain after adoption and persist in the new home.

Abandoned and Orphaned Kittens

Clients often obtain a new kitten that they believe has been orphaned or abandoned. Kittens that are emaciated or dehydrated are likely to have been abandoned, and their medical health needs must be addressed promptly. However, if the kitten appears in overall good condition, the client should attempt to reunite the kitten with its mother by canvassing the neighborhood for signs of a nest because queens may hide their kittens while they hunt, and thus some kittens are not truly abandoned. In addition, it can be helpful to ask others if they have seen either the queen or other kittens in the area. If these efforts are unsuccessful, the client can contact a nearby humane shelter that may have a lactating queen to foster the kitten, as this is the ideal choice.

Alternatively, the client can hand-raise the kitten by feeding it commercially available kitten formula via a gastric tube or bottle-feeding. Veterinary expertise is necessary in these situations, not only to help the client provide for the kitten nutritionally and medically but also to discuss the potential behavioral consequences of hand-raised, bottle-fed kittens. Despite best efforts to feed them frequently, these kittens lack the 24-hour constant care, attention, and presence of the queen, as well as important interaction with littermates. This lack of maternal interaction in a kitten can lead to increased fearfulness, aggression, and timidity when it reaches adulthood.[6] Limited research and anecdotal evidence indicate that hand-rearing of kittens is a potential risk factor for their development of future behavior problems.[7] However, in a 2005 study of 67 hand-reared kittens (all reared by veterinary students) and 58 control cats, researchers demonstrated that hand-reared kittens were no more likely than queen-reared kittens to become aggressive or fearful or to develop behavior problems.[8] Some behaviorists posit that kittens hand-reared by their human caregivers may not learn the boundaries of normal and appropriate play. They can often be too rough, using their claws and teeth, with a potentially detrimental effect on their owners.[9,10] One study demonstrated that kittens that are raised in the absence of feline maternal care tend not to readily socialize with humans.[11]

For all of the above-described reasons, whenever possible, a kitten should be placed with a nursing queen and her kittens to simulate the normal development of conspecific interaction. When this is not possible, clients must be aware of the need to introduce an element of frustration into the feeding process and to resist the temptation to always feed the kitten when it wants to eat while making sure to provide adequate nutrition for optimum development.[12]

Heritability of Behavioral Traits

Heritability of behavioral traits is another factor that must be considered when owners are picking their new feline companion. There is no way of knowing the genetic contributions derived from the mother and father when adopting an adult cat with no available history. Unless the cat is coming from a breeder, most information available is on the mother. Although the mother does contribute 50% of the genetic material to each kitten, numerous studies have established that heritability of certain behavioral traits appears to be linked to those of the father.[13] Turner and colleagues[14] showed that the friendliness rating of a kitten was directly influenced by the friendliness of its father. This correlation was evident even when the kitten had not actually interacted with its father, eliminating emulation as a possibility for their friendliness rating. Paternal influences are also evident in the amount of time a kitten is willing to spend with an unfamiliar person.[14] When interactional differences were examined between early socialized versus unsocialized kittens, and between kittens with friendly versus unfriendly fathers, paternity was found to be significantly responsible for these differences.[15] Socialized kittens with a friendly father were more likely to approach a person and did so more rapidly than those who were unsocialized or had unfriendly fathers. They physically interacted with people, showed relaxed body postures, and remained closer for longer periods of time than the other kittens. They were also less likely to hiss, demonstrate defensive or fearful body postures, or attempt to hide when in the presence of the unfamiliar person, whereas the unsocialized cats and those with unfriendly fathers were most likely to hiss. Although socialized and unsocialized cats were equivalent during the portion of the study during which the researchers examined responses to a novel object, the cats with friendly fathers were more likely than those with unfriendly fathers to approach a novel object and spend more time investigating that object. This effect on the kitten's ability to interact successfully with the environment as well as with people and with other cats has led to the use of the broader term *boldness* to describe the trait that has been found to be heritable. The characteristics of these cats with bold fathers include friendliness towards familiar and unfamiliar people and lack of fearful responses to novel objects, both of which are traits that owners desire in their feline companions. Veterinarians should therefore emphasize to potential owners the importance of knowing a kitten's genetic inheritance from both the mother and the father, as well as the importance of early socialization.

BREED SELECTION

Presently, there are two feline breed organizations in the United States: the Cat Fanciers Association, which currently recognizes 43 feline breeds,[16] and The International Cat Association (TICA),[17] which lists 70 breed categories, including the common household cat. In the United

Kingdom, the Governing Council of the Cat Fancy recognizes over 60 breeds. Contrast these breeds with the types of cats most familiar to potential owners and many veterinarians: the domestic shorthair, the domestic longhair, and perhaps a handful of easily recognizable breeds, such as the Persian, Siamese, and Abyssinian.

Behavior Specifics

Each registered cat breed has its unique visual characteristics, which often are compelling reasons for an owner to seek out an individual member of that breed. Information provided for potential owners considering a feline companion should go beyond the physical attributes of a breed and include the behavioral tendencies and medical disease predispositions. Armed with this information, pet owners can select traits that match not only their personal preferences for a cat but also their current household composition, their ability to provide the cat with care for potential medical diseases throughout its lifetime, and their ability to provide for the environment, enrichment, and activity needs of that particular breed.

Numerous written and electronic resources are available for behavioral and personality trait information about each breed, allowing owners to inform themselves of their available choices and considerations. The plethora of information from a variety of sources may either overwhelm or provide clarity as to which breed would be best for each individual's unique desires in a cat. To aid veterinarians in helping in this process, this information is consolidated in Table 6-1. The information on

TABLE 6-1   Feline Breeds and Their Behavioral Traits, Personality Descriptions, and Disease Predispositions

Feline Breed	Behavioral Traits and Personality Descriptions	Disease Predispositions
Abyssinian	Aggressive towards humans Aggressive towards other cats Highly intelligent Interactive with owners Loyal Not lap cats Playful Scratches furniture Songbird predation Urine marking Very active	Amyloidosis Blastomycosis Congenital hypothyroidism Cryptococcosis Dilated cardiomyopathy Griseofulvin sensitivity Hyperesthesia syndrome Increased osmotic fragility of erythrocytes Myasthenia gravis Nasopharyngeal polyps Psychogenic alopecia Pyruvate kinase deficiency Rod-cone retinal degeneration Rod-cone retinal dysplasia Shaft disorder
American shorthair	Adaptable Even-tempered Quiet Tolerant of children	Hypertrophic cardiomyopathy
Balinese	Active Affectionate Bonds closely with family Gregarious Mischievous Playful Vocal	Feline acromelanism
Bengal	Aggressive towards humans Aggressive towards other cats Confident Inquisitive Loves water Loving Not affectionate Rambunctious Scratches furniture Songbird predation Urine marking Very active Very playful	None known

Continued

Feline Breed	Behavioral Traits and Personality Descriptions	Disease Predispositions
Birman	Affectionate Sweet Vocal	Atypical granulation of neutrophils Birman cat distal polyneuropathy Congenital cataract Congenital hypotrichosis Corneal dermoid Corneal sequestration Hemophilia B Spongiform degeneration Tail tip necrosis Thymic aplasia
British shorthair	Affectionate, but not lap cats Calm Friendly towards humans Quiet	Hemophilia B Hypertrophic cardiomyopathy
Burmese	Affectionate towards humans Good litter box usage Playful Social Very little urine marking Very tolerant Vocal	Agenesis of the nares Burmese head defect Calcium oxalate urolithiasis Congenital deafness Congenital hypotrichosis Congenital vestibular disease Corneal and lateral limbal dermoid Corneal sequestration Dilated cardiomyopathy Endocardial fibroelastosis Feline acromelanism Generalized demodicosis Hyperesthesia syndrome Hypokalemic polymyopathy Meningoencephalocele Prolapsed gland of the nictitating membrane Psychogenic alopecia
Cornish Rex and Devon Rex	Active Affectionate Energetic Good litter box use Lively Love to climb and jump Very low urine marking	Anesthetic sensitivity Congenital hypotrichosis Hereditary myopathy of Devon Rex *Malassezia* dermatitis Patellar luxation Umbilical hernia Vitamin K–dependent coagulopathy
Domestic longhair	Good litter box use High urine marking Moderate affection Moderate aggression	Alpha-mannosidosis Basal cell tumor Congenital portosystemic shunt Cutaneous asthenia Hypertrophic cardiomyopathy Polycystic kidney disease
Domestic shorthair	Active Affectionate Aggressive Friendly towards unfamiliar people Good litter box use High urine marking Playful Songbird predation	Alpha-mannosidosis Coloboma Congenital cataract Congenital myasthenia gravis Congenital portosystemic shunt Corneal dermoid Cutaneous asthenia GM1 gangliosidosis Hemophilia A Hereditary porphyria Hyperoxaluria Hypertrophic cardiomyopathy Krabbe disease Lentigo simplex Methemoglobin reductase deficiency Microphakia

TABLE 6-1 Feline Breeds and Their Behavioral Traits, Personality Descriptions, and Disease Predispositions—cont'd

Feline Breed	Behavioral Traits and Personality Descriptions	Disease Predispositions
		Mucopolysaccharidosis
		Mucopolysaccharidosis type I
		Neuroaxonal dystrophy
		Niemann-Pick disease
		Pelger-Huet anomaly
		Psychogenic alopecia
		Pyruvate kinase deficiency
		Sebaceous gland tumors
		Solar dermatitis
Egyptian Mau	Active	Spongiform degeneration
	Aloof with unfamiliar people	
	Sensitive to loud noises	
	Shy	
Exotic	Affectionate	Epiphora
	Fearful towards unfamiliar people	Polycystic kidney disease
	Low affection towards humans	
	More active than the Persian	
	Quiet	
Havana Brown	Affectionate	Blastomycosis
	Attention seeker	
	Busy	
	Curious	
	Playful	
Himalayan	Affectionate	Basal cell tumor
	Playful with toys	Calcium oxalate urolithiasis
	Sedate	Congenital cataract
		Congenital portosystemic shunt
		Corneal sequestration
		Cutaneous asthenia
		Dermatophytosis
		Feline acromelanism
		Griseofulvin toxicity
		Hyperesthesia syndrome
		Idiopathic facial dermatitis
		Multiple epitrichial cysts
		Systemic lupus erythematosus
Korat	Active	GM1 gangliosidosis
	Affectionate	GM2 gangliosidosis
	Gentle	
	May not accept other cats	
Maine Coon	Affectionate towards humans	Hip dysplasia
	Good litter box use	Hypertrophic cardiomyopathy
	Not fearful towards unfamiliar people	
	Not very vocal	
	Relaxed and easygoing	
Manx	Even-tempered	Constipation
	Forms strong bonds with family	Corneal dystrophy
	Low level of affection towards family	Intertrigo
	Moderately fearful	Megacolon
	Not very vocal	Rectal prolapse
		Sacrocaudal dysgenesis
		Spina bifida
Norwegian Forest	Active	Glycogen storage disease type IV
	Interactive with family	
	May or may not be playful	
	Moderately fearful	
	Not very vocal	
	Sweet	

Continued

TABLE 6-1 **Feline Breeds and Their Behavioral Traits, Personality Descriptions, and Disease Predispositions—cont'd**

Feline Breed	Behavioral Traits and Personality Descriptions	Disease Predispositions
Oriental	Active Affectionate Good litter box use Less aggressive than Siamese Moderate urine marking Vocal	Psychogenic alopecia
Persian	Affectionate High urine marking Inactive Not playful Poor litter box usage Quiet Sweet Very fearful	Alpha-mannosidosis Basal cell tumors Calcium oxalate urolithiasis Chediak-Higashi syndrome (blue smoke Persians only) Coloboma Congenital cataract Congenital polycystic liver disease Congenital portosystemic shunts Corneal sequestration Cryptorchidism Dermatophytosis Entropion Griseofulvin toxicity Hypertrophic cardiomyopathy Idiopathic epiphora Idiopathic facial dermatitis Idiopathic periocular crusting Lacrimal punctal aplasia Lysosomal storage diseases Multiple epitrichial cysts Peritoneopericardial diaphragmatic hernia Polycystic kidney disease Primary seborrhea Prognathism Retinal degeneration Sebaceous gland tumors Systemic lupus erythematosus
Ragdoll	Affectionate Docile Friendly towards unfamiliar people Great with children Not aggressive	Hypertrophic cardiomyopathy
Russian Blue	Cautious with unfamiliar people Gets along well with children and with other pets Good litter box use Low urine marking Playful Quiet Shy	
Scottish Fold	Affectionate Inquisitive Intelligent Laid-back Loyal to family	Arthropathy
Siamese	Active Affectionate Aggressive towards other cats Demanding High urine marking Intelligent Lively Playful Scratches furniture Talkative Vocal	Aguirre syndrome Amyloidosis Basal cell tumors Blastomycosis Ceroid lipofuscinosis Chylothorax Cleft palate and/or lip Congenital cataract Congenital deafness Congenital hypotrichosis Congenital idiopathic megaesophagus

TABLE 6-1	Feline Breeds and Their Behavioral Traits, Personality Descriptions, and Disease Predispositions—cont'd	
Feline Breed	**Behavioral Traits and Personality Descriptions**	**Disease Predispositions**
		Congenital myasthenia gravis
		Congenital portosystemic shunt
		Congenital vestibular disease
		Convergent strabismus and nystagmus
		Corneal sequestration
		Cryptococcosis
		Cutaneous tuberculosis
		Dilated cardiomyopathy
		Endocardial fibroelastosis
		Eyelid coloboma
		Feline acromegalism
		Feline asthma
		Feline pinnal alopecia
		Food hypersensitivity
		Generalized demodicosis
		Glaucoma
		GM1 gangliosidosis
		Hemophilia B
		Hereditary porphyria
		Hip dysplasia
		Histoplasmosis
		Hydrocephalus
		Hyperesthesia syndrome
		Insulinoma
		Junctional epidermolysis bullosa
		Lipomas
		Mammary tumors
		Mast cell tumors
		Microphakia
		Mucopolysaccharidosis type VI
		Mycobacterium avium
		Nasal cavity tumors
		Niemann-Pick disease
		Patent ductus arteriosus
		Periocular leukotrichia
		Persistent atrial standstill
		Primary hyperparathyroidism (due to parathyroid tumors)
		Psychogenic alopecia
		Pyloric dysfunction
		Retinal degeneration
		Small intestine adenocarcinoma
		Sporotrichosis
		Sweat gland tumors
		Systemic lupus erythematosus
		Tail sucking
		Vitiligo
Somali	Active	Increased osmotic fragility of erythrocytes
	Affectionate	Myasthenia gravis
	High energy	Pyruvate kinase deficiency
	Interactive with owners	
	Not a lap cat	
	Not good in large cat populations	
	Very curious	
Sphynx	Active	Anesthetic sensitivity
	Affectionate	
	Extremely friendly	
	Good lap cats	
	Good litter box use	
	Inquisitive	
	Low urine marking	
	Playful	
	Unfriendly towards unfamiliar people	

Continued

TABLE 6-1	Feline Breeds and Their Behavioral Traits, Personality Descriptions, and Disease Predispositions—cont'd	
Feline Breed	**Behavioral Traits and Personality Descriptions**	**Disease Predispositions**
Tonkinese	Active Affectionate Friendly towards unfamiliar people Good lap cat Good litter box use Lively Low urine marking Playful Social Strong-willed Vocal	Congenital vestibular disease Gingivitis

Data from: Hart BL, Hart LA: Behavioral profiles of cat breeds. In: *Your ideal cat: insights into breed and gender differences in cat behavior*, West Lafayette, IN, 2013, Purdue University Press, pp. 68–120; http://www.cfa.org/FutureOwners/BreedPersonalityChart.aspx; and http://www.tica.org/public/breeds/to/intro.php

behavioral traits was compiled from three sources. The websites of the Cat Fanciers' Association[16] and The International Cat Association[17] provide detailed descriptions, pictures, and histories of each breed recognized by their respective associations. Breed enthusiasts predisposed to favor their breed, extolling good traits of the breed, and perhaps underestimating possible negative attributes generally compile these descriptions; thus, they may contain bias. Additional information gathered through a survey of 80 feline practitioners, all of whom are members of the AAFP, is now available. These individuals were asked to rank each breed on a variety of characteristics and common behavioral traits or problems.[18] None of these sources is a controlled scientific study of breed traits or behavior problems; yet, when evaluated in combination with one another, they allow a fairly accurate representation of the breed in question. However, there are several instances where two sources had a completely opposite description of the breed's characteristics, highlighting inconsistencies in the information available. Further information about breed types is also available on the International Cat Care website.[19]

Medical Issues

Information on the medical and disease predispositions was tabulated from information found in the book *Breed Predispositions to Disease in Dogs and Cats.*[20] The recent completion of both the canine and feline genome sequences has resulted in enormous amounts of information, and 230 hereditary disorders have already been documented in the cat.[21] The list of diseases, their screening tests, diagnostic procedures, preventive measures and subsequent treatments can be overwhelming to the veterinary practitioner. To help create some clarity, practitioners can avail themselves of the most comprehensive updated list of feline hereditary diseases by visiting the International Cat Care website.[22] Those clinicians wishing to learn about the clinical symptoms, diagnostics, and management of the various hereditary feline diseases should also visit the World Small Animal Veterinary Association global veterinary community websites for more comprehensive information.[23,24]

AGE AT ADOPTION

There are many factors to consider when choosing between a kitten and an adult cat as a new household pet. Both age groups come with their own challenges.

Kittens

Several factors must be considered and evaluated when choosing a kitten to bring into the home. One set of factors is related to the environment from which the kitten will be obtained (already covered in this chapter), and the other relates to the needs of the kitten once it arrives at its new home. The playfulness of a young kitten can be one of the behavioral attributes that owners enjoy most, but at the same time it is one of the main reasons to avoid adopting a young animal, as it can be frustrating, hazardous, and time-consuming. Owners need to be willing and able to meet the play and activity needs of a kitten and address a kitten's special physical and social needs. For this reason, kittens may not be suitable for frail individuals or older adults due to the potential hazards to their own safety from owning a young, active kitten. Similarly, very young children may find a playful and exuberant kitten overwhelming and frightening.

Kittens begin to develop play behaviors as early as 2 to 3 weeks of age.[25] Play behaviors of kittens include biting, batting with their paws, stalking, chasing, pouncing, wrestling, jumping, leaping, and climbing (Figure 6-1).

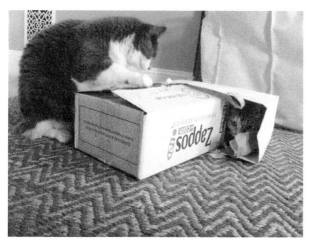

FIGURE 6-1 A kitten exhibiting play behavior.

Although these behaviors are entertaining, their timing and consequences may lead to frustration on the part of the owner and to concerns about the safety of people or other pets within the household. For example, kittens often play throughout the night, awakening their owners, and may attempt to leap onto and balance on high vertical perches, causing damage to personal property. Fast chase games through the home can also injure people if the kitten gets underfoot. This exuberant play needs plenty of outlets, including a plethora of toys, and, most importantly, structured owner initiated playtime to encourage appropriate object play. If suitable outlets are not provided, the kitten may become frustrated and begin to direct predatory play towards the owner or destroy the owner's personal belongings. Play behavior will diminish with increasing age,[25] as older cats tend to play during natural awake periods and their behavior is not as intense or as lively as a kitten's. The high requirement for play is one aspect of owning a kitten that must be taken into account when deciding whether to adopt a kitten or an adult cat.

Socialization

Providing for adequate and appropriate socialization is another time-consuming characteristic of owning a kitten. In the behavior literature, socialization is often thought of as a "window of opportunity" or the sensitive period of development. During this time, the animal is more receptive to meeting new people and other animals (including conspecifics), as well as to new experiences. Researchers have examined the effects of human interaction and early handling and have identified the sensitive period of socialization for cats as being from 2 to 7 weeks of age, perhaps extending to 9 weeks.[26] Because weaning does not usually occur before 7 weeks and kittens need time to interact with their mother and other kittens, this creates complications for adequate socialization to people unless it is provided in the natal environment. The endpoint of socialization is not

absolute, thus allowing a continued window of socialization that should be vigorously utilized to help kittens adjust to their new home environment. Although each kitten is an individual, clients should be counseled on appropriate socialization techniques for all new kittens. A more detailed discussion of socialization can be found in Chapter 4.

Litter Box Preferences and Food

Despite their young age, kittens may already have established preferences when they enter their new home. Litter substrate preferences will be influenced by the litter type provided to the mother and her kittens. Most research has indicated that cats seem to prefer clay clumping litter over other commercial litter materials,[27] and this is probably the best litter type to offer when bringing a kitten home. However, house-soiling problems may arise if the kitten was not exposed to this particular material or has not yet been litter box–trained because of having had an early outdoor environment, and the new owner may then need to try several different types of litter material (a "litter box cafeteria") to see which the kitten prefers. Anecdotally, some veterinarians recommend that clients bring home some of the used litter from the tray at the rearing establishment and place a small amount in their box at home so that the odor is familiar to the cat, which will help facilitate the use of the new box and litter substrate. It is vital that the kitten have easy access to the litter facilities provided, and, depending upon how small the kitten is, its owner may need to provide a litter box that has minimal height on the sides, such as a cookie or baking sheet, or cut out a deeper opening in a commercial plastic litter box. The location of the boxes may also need to be changed if the kitten is too small to access the current site, perhaps because it is up or down a flight of stairs.

By the time a kitten comes to its new home, it will have been weaned and had experience with certain food types in its previous environment. This can influence food preferences, and, if the new owners wish to alter the kitten's diet, the transition should be made gradually over a number of days.

Predatory Behavior

Some owners wish to obtain a cat not just for companionship purposes, but also to fulfill a need for pest control. In contrast, others find the predatory components of normal feline behavior abhorrent. Cats are naturally predatory, a behavior that develops during the weaning period as the kitten switches from nursing to eating prey that the mother brings back to the nest.[28] At this time, the kittens' play behaviors start to focus on capturing prey, and, even if the cat is domesticated and kept in a home, it will still display predatory play and may become an avid, successful hunter if allowed the opportunity. With recent concerns over the effect of domestic cat predation on urban bird and wildlife populations in some countries, cat owners in those countries are being urged to keep their felines indoors. Songbird predation is anecdotally highest in the most active breeds, including the Bengal, Abyssinian, domestic shorthair, and domestic longhair.[18] If the client wishes to have an indoor/outdoor cat, but also wishes to minimize its effect on local bird populations, avoiding one of these breeds and choosing a more inactive cat may be a consideration. Another option is to provide outdoor enclosures that prevent predation but still allow the cat access to an outdoor environment. Limited information is available on the efficacy of devices designed to prevent predation, such as large bells on the collar and "bibs." If cats with higher predatory drive are to be kept indoors, owners will need to provide them with more opportunities to "hunt" by appropriately using toys. Motion-activated toys and toys that look and move similarly to natural prey allow the cat to satisfy its need to forage, stalk, pounce, and kill. Food-dispensing foraging toys allow the cat to consume small meals throughout the day, which provides a more natural feeding pattern for a predatory cat while also fostering mental and physical enrichment. Allowing cats access to the outdoor environment and tolerating their natural hunting behavior is also an option and is commonly practiced in some countries.

Financial Considerations

If the kitten is adopted postweaning, the owner will need to bring it to a veterinarian for the necessary vaccination series, laboratory tests, and deworming based on the current preventive care and testing guidelines put out by the AAFP or another appropriate national veterinary organization, whereas adult cats may need only booster vaccinations. The owner will incur the cost of neutering, unless this has already been carried out, such as in the case of kittens adopted from shelters. In the United States, other surgical procedures, such as onychectomy, may be offered, although in other countries this would not be considered an acceptable practice, and it is declining in frequency in the United States. A more complete discussion of normal feline scratching behavior and appropriate methods for dealing with unwanted scratching can be found in Chapters 8 and 23. With the increased playfulness and exploration of kittens, the owner may also incur the cost of destroyed personal property. Although some may consider kittens easier to adopt than adult cats, it is clear that kittens have their own set of unique challenges, and the owner must be prepared to address their playfulness and need for adequate socialization, as well as to incur the financial costs of their care.

Adult Cats

When choosing an older cat, there are numerous behavioral factors to consider.

Food Preferences

Adult cats, and some older kittens, may have strong preferences for a certain food type at adoption.[29] These food types can comprise the brand and/or formulation (canned versus dry) that the breeder or original owner fed post weaning or the prey type that the queen brought home. Cats seem to show definite preferences for food type by 6 months of age,[30,31] despite any effort made by breeders or owners to feed them a variety of food types.[32] Veterinarians need to be proactive and warn new owners of adult cats that this preference can have serious detrimental health consequences upon adoption if the cat has an extremely strong preexisting preference. Cats with strong preferences that experience an abrupt change in diet upon rehoming may stop eating altogether,[29] potentially leading to life-threatening hepatic lipidosis. Knowledge of a cat's food preferences upon adoption can ease the adult cat's transition into the new home, minimize the risks of inappetance, and allow for slowly transitioning the cat to a new diet.

Preexisting Behavioral Tendencies

Potential owners may have reservations about adopting an older cat, thinking that problematic behaviors will be so ingrained as to be impossible to change. Behavioral maturity is thought to occur between 2 and 4 years of age, with many problem behaviors not manifesting or becoming firmly entrenched until that time. Urine marking, unacceptable elimination, and aggression are the most common behavior problems presented to behavioral referral practices.[2] Each of these behaviors is multifactorial, with genetics, gender, learning, and environment all playing a role in their manifestation. Amat *et al.* demonstrated that Persian cats were more likely than other breeds to eliminate unacceptably, with litter box aversion being the most common diagnosis.[2] Their study also revealed that cats without outdoor access exhibited more behavior problems than those with outdoor access, that aggression towards people was more common in single-cat than in multicat households, and that intact females were more likely than spayed females to be presented for aggression.[2] In each of these cases, if the new owners are able to provide a suitable environment, facilitate appropriate introductions into the new household, and responsibly neuter their new pet, many problem behaviors that were present in a previous home or facility may not manifest in an adopted adult individual.

When a prospective owner is evaluating whether to adopt a kitten or adult cat, veterinarians can facilitate the decision-making process by encouraging the prospective owner to make a list of which attributes they find most attractive in a cat. To help the prospective owner determine whether to adopt a young kitten or an older adult cat, this list can then be compared with the behavioral tendencies listed in Table 6-2.

TABLE 6-2 Behavioral Tendencies of Kittens versus Adult Cats

Behavioral Traits	Kittens	Adult Cats
Play and activity	Intensely playful Increased activity, even at night Multiple play sessions daily Increased destruction in the home due to exploring, biting, and scratching as well as energy expenditure needs	Less play, more time resting Less nighttime activity Need play and exercise, but exhibit less destructive energy More adaptable to being alone
Feeding behavior	Generally no strong food preferences before 6 months of age Can easily be trained into free-choice feeding pattern	May have strong food preferences Difficult to transition from meal to free-choice feeding or vice versa when the need arises
Litter box usage	May not be litter box–trained Need to ensure ease of access to litter boxes for small kittens May or may not have substrate preference	Likely to have substrate preference May already have unacceptable house-soiling behaviors such as nonuse of litter box or spraying and/or marking
Temperament and behavior	Current temperament may not be static Behavior problems are easier to prevent than to change	Temperament and personality are known qualities Behavior problems may be difficult to eliminate due to their learned component
Cost	Increased cost due to castration or spaying, preventive testing, and vaccinations	Increased expenses for older cats due to medical problems, including geriatric care issues

Note: These are only tendencies or trends and may not be true of the particular kitten or cat that is adopted.

SEXUAL CHARACTERISTICS AND NEUTERING STATUS

When deciding upon a male or female cat, owners have many factors to consider, and all desired behavior traits should be taken into account while making this complex decision.

Male versus Female

Some potential owners ask which sex cat to adopt, and others are unaware of any reasons to adopt one or the other. Research has identified some areas of cat behavior that are influenced by the sex and neutering status of the cat.[2,18,33–35] These include urine marking, aggression towards conspecifics, aggression towards family members, and friendliness towards strangers.

Neutered versus Unneutered

Veterinarians often emphasize the obvious health and population control benefits of neutering but may not draw attention to the behavioral traits that clients should consider when deciding to neuter their cat. Intact male kittens can potentially reproduce as early as 9 months of age, when the testes are mature enough to produce sperm and complete copulation can occur.[34] At that time, because of the male cat's testosterone surge, owners may begin to notice behaviors associated with sexual maturity, such as the desire to roam, presumably to find a receptive female.[34] This is also a time when evidence of territorial behaviors emerges, including intermale aggression and urine marking.[34] A study published by Hart and Barrett indicated that neutering status does not completely eliminate urine marking.

They reported that approximately 10% of castrated males and 5% of spayed females will urine-mark after surgical neutering.[33] The best age for neutering is a complex issue; however, only a 2.5% incidence of urine spraying was reported in one published study[36] in which researchers surveyed owners of kittens neutered by 2 months of age, suggesting that owners may wish to neuter their male cats significantly earlier than sexual maturity to maximize the likelihood of avoiding such behaviors. In a 2004 study, researchers examined early gonadectomized cats versus those neutered after 5.5 months of age. They determined that males neutered prior to 5.5 months of age were less likely to develop abscesses, show aggression towards veterinarians, demonstrate sexual behaviors, and urine-mark.[35] Although it is possible that territorial behaviors can be completely eliminated by castration, the neonatal masculinization due to testosterone may facilitate retention of such behaviors postcastration in some cats.[37] When an intact male cat is adopted and subsequently neutered, objectionable male behaviors may remain because of learning and the early effects of testosterone. See handout titled **Advantages and Risks of Spay or Castration Surgery** for advice on making informed decisions about neutering.

Intact females are seasonally polyestrous, often having multiple cycles throughout the year, typically occurring in the spring and fall months. These cycles are highly influenced by the presence of a receptive male or other estrous females, as well as by the female's breed, genetics, and climate of the environment in which it lives.[34] Behavioral traits seen in proestrus and estrous females can be quite distressing to owners, including the need to roam, physical affection demands, and characteristic vocalization by the female to attract a mate.

Inexperienced owners often mistake the highly distinctive yowling as a sign of pain or illness, leading them to bring the female cat to the veterinarian for this normal behavior of an intact estrous female. During pregnancy, females may be more aloof, seeking an isolated area in which to create their nest. They also may be more irritable, defensive, anxious, or frantic.[37] Maternal aggression postparturition is common when the queen feels her kittens are being threatened or moved, and this aggression may be directed at humans or other cats.[37] Aggression towards male cats by the queen is considered normal[37] in light of accidental kitten death by the tomcat and the male tendency to kill kittens not of its own genetic makeup. The intensity of maternal aggression, especially towards humans, often without any threat behavior prior to the act, can be high even in those female cats that are normally docile and friendly. Extreme caution and care must be taken when attempting to handle kittens in the presence of the queen to minimize danger to people. Owners who are incapable of or unwilling to cope with such behaviors should consider adopting an already spayed female and avoid taking in a pregnant or post parturient queen. In light of the problematic traits associated with intact males and females, it is important to emphasize to clients the behavioral benefits of neutering.

One recent study indicated that intact females were significantly more likely than spayed females to be presented to a behavioral referral practice for aggression problems.[2] According to an anecdotal survey of feline practitioners, spayed females, compared with their neutered male counterparts, tend to be more aggressive towards conspecifics.[18] This may seem counterintuitive to some because territorially motivated aggression seems to be more a male trait and because wild colonies of cats, living in group harmony and co-rearing their young, are matrilineal. Because these matrilineal colonies are groups of related females, evolutionarily it makes sense to help each other to perpetuate shared genes. However, in the typical multicat household, the humans have chosen the cats that live with one another and often are unrelated and therefore do not share that same evolutionary pull for cooperation and harmonious encounters. It is often suggested that owners desiring to get two cats at once choose two related kittens to perhaps decrease the likelihood of future intercat aggression (Figure 6-2). It has been suggested that the most successful combination of cats to adopt is female siblings and that different sex sibling pairs are the next most compatible combination; however, there is a lack of scientific evidence regarding the effect of sex on feline compatibility, and it can be very difficult to advise clients as to the best combinations. This is especially true when clients wish to introduce a new cat into an already established feline household. In view of the information that is available regarding feline social behavior, it is

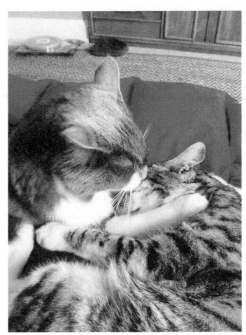

FIGURE 6-2 Two littermates grooming one another in their multicat household.

important to advise cat owners that social acceptance should not be expected in these situations and that the newcomer should be regarded as a separate social entity from the existing residents. This will lead to appropriate provisioning of separate key resources for the newcomer and prevent the client from having unrealistic expectations regarding establishment of feline friendships, although in many situations integration of a new cat may work out quite well (see Chapters 4 and 26, and Figure 2-3).

During feline behavior consultations, owners often state that they wanted to obtain a cat that is not only affectionate with its human family members but also friendly towards unfamiliar people and visitors. In a survey of feline practitioners by Ben and Lynette Hart,[18] respondents reported that they felt that males significantly outranked females on both accounts, with females scoring much higher on aggression towards family members. When friendly social interactions with humans are a priority for an owner, a male cat may be the better choice based on this information. However, there is a lack of scientifically robust evidence as to the effect of sex on behavior.

TEMPERAMENT

The terms *temperament* and *personality* are closely related and attempt to describe an animal's fixed behavioral attributes that define its individuality and sets it apart from others within its own species. Temperament testing is a method commonly used to determine an animal's particular behavioral strategy and suitability for adoption and to delineate which traits the animal may exhibit throughout adulthood. Although most often applied to dogs, temperament testing for cats appears to be gaining favor, especially in shelter settings, as it provides a quantifiable measure, especially in reference to interactions with unfamiliar people, reactions to novel stimuli, and general handling. Testing can provide a means by which to assess the cat's baseline personality, thus providing potential owners with a realistic framework for evaluating how the cat will meet their particular expectations and fit into their household.

Testing

There are many versions of temperament testing currently available for use with both dogs and cats. In the United States, Dr. Emily Weiss, CAAB is the Senior Director of Research and Development for the American Society for the Prevention of Cruelty to Animals (ASPCA). She has developed various tests for use in the shelter setting, including the Feline-ality Assessment.[38] The aim of this test is to match potential cat adopters with the cat personality best suited to their desired experience as an owner as well as to their household situation. Potential adopters take a 19-question quiz that identifies their lifestyle and needs for integrating a new cat into their lives. The adopter is then classified using a color schematic: green for those adopters best suited to adopting a cat that quickly and easily adapts to new situations, purple for those owners who are able to adopt a kitten or cat that needs both time and encouragement to appropriately adjust to new surroundings, and orange for owners who need to adopt what the ASPCA classifies as the "quintessential companion" cat. Shelter staff then use the feline-ality temperament testing developed by Dr. Weiss to classify the cats into the same three color categories, each of which is composed of three distinct personality subclassifications.[39] According to the ASPCA, shelters using Dr. Weiss's Meet-Your-Match program (of which feline-ality is a part) have seen a 40% to 45% increase in adoptions and a 45% to 50% decrease in euthanasia and returns.[38]

The Feline Temperament Profile (FTP) is a test originally developed in the United States by Lee et al.[40] to determine a cat's suitability for living in a nursing home. The FTP includes a number of testing situations used to assess the cat's response to a variety of interactive stimuli and challenging circumstances in a novel environment. The cat's response to each situation is classified as acceptable or questionable, with a maximum acceptable score being 38 and a maximum questionable score of 16. Testing includes having an unfamiliar person call the cat from across the room and evaluating how the cat responds and subsequently interacts, or does not, with the tester. Three "challenges" are then applied: pulling the cat's tail, attempting to engage the cat with a play toy, and assessing the cat's response to a dropped object.

In a recent study, researchers attempted to validate the FTP[41] and found that it not only was easy to use and score but also provided an objective measure of the cat's sociability, aggressiveness, and adaptability that appeared to be stable, even upon retesting 3 to 6 months after adoption.

In the United Kingdom, there is ongoing research into developing ways to assess aspects of temperament in shelter cats focused specifically on the reliability and validity of measures. A final test model has not yet been developed, but this is the end goal.[42] In addition, International Cat Care is supporting research to develop a protocol for assessing the emotional state of shelter cats in response to humans. Also taking into account the age and health of the individual cat, the aim of this protocol is to provide a structured system to help people manage cats on an individual level and to promote the best possible welfare outcomes for cats. This protocol is still under development and will be accessible in the public domain in the future.

Numerous studies have shown validity in using the tests in the United States with both cats and dogs,[41,43] but other studies have shown a lack of stability of the results between young kittens and adult cats,[14] and similar findings have been noted in puppies.[44] One particular study on temperament testing in dogs revealed deficiencies in predicting certain types of aggression post adoption, thereby effectively questioning their usefulness to determine true long-term behavioral stability.[45] Although temperament testing may not be the perfect tool, it can provide ease of use and wide-range applicability across a number of species, and help to promote more successful pet adoptions. With appropriate training, veterinarians may also be able to apply these temperament-testing procedures to litters of kittens presented to their practice to help breeders and owners determine which kitten may be best-suited for a particular environment as well as the needs of the family interested in owning one.

When asked by clients to assess a feline's personality, a veterinarian can employ the use of one of the feline temperament tests available or can simply rely on classifying the cat into one of the three commonly recognized personality types. In a study done by Feaver et al.,[46] cats were scored on a variety of different aspects, allowing the authors to determine three basic personality categories: active/aggressive, timid/nervous, and confident/easygoing. However, there were some cats that did not necessarily fit perfectly into one of these three categories, indicating the need for a broader range or continuum, which temperament testing can often provide. Researchers in other studies have also attempted to define the categories of cat personality types and found results similar to the study by Feaver and colleagues.[47] Based solely on a cat's interactions with unfamiliar people, one study determined three different behavioral classifications: initiative/friendly, reserved/friendly, and rebuffing/unfriendly.[48] The various personality types become important not only when attempting to match owner preferences and expectations but also when the composition of the cats currently in the household is taken into account to assess compatibility when adding a new feline member into the mix.

Household Composition of Current Cats

Introducing a new cat into the household can be a time-consuming task (see handout titled **Creating Successful Transitions to Your Home**), made especially difficult when the personalities of the felines are seemingly incompatible. Owners with timid/nervous cats or those classified as rebuffing/unfriendly may be disappointed in their cats' unwillingness to interact with them or visitors to their home and thus may seek to adopt a bolder cat to satisfy their needs in a feline companion. However, this bolder cat may prove to be a poor companion by chasing and actively challenging the nervous cat. An alternative scenario may also be true: Owners with an active/aggressive cat may be disappointed in the aggression shown towards them and wish to adopt a cat that is more people-friendly, not thinking of the possibility that the resident cat may become aggressive towards the new addition. The problems these combinations create are not necessarily insurmountable, but, when coupled with the fact that cats vary considerably in their adaptability to sharing their lives with unfamiliar cats, they can pose a real challenge and are best avoided when possible. Care must be exercised that introductions are made very slowly, by never forcing or actively encouraging social interaction between the cats, by separating the cats when owner supervision is not possible, and by ensuring that adequate resources are available for each cat, especially feeding stations, hiding places, and vertical perching. Veterinarians should help clients pay careful attention to the possible consequences of introducing another cat into the home and facilitate their decision based on the best interests of the cats and not just on their desire to add to another cat. If introductions are inappropriately handled or fail to result in compatibility, despite the client's best efforts to integrate the cats successfully, permanent separate territories will need to be created to allow for the safety of all the cats. However, it must be understood that isolation of cats in separate territories may compromise the welfare of the cats. In such cases, rehoming one of the cats should be discussed.

HOUSEHOLD CONSIDERATIONS

Creating a household that is welcoming to the new cat or kitten is a primary consideration. When other cats are already in the home, provisioning the space with necessary resources in adequate places and numbers should be a priority. It is essential to create a dedicated space for the new feline member containing food, water, a litter box, and hiding and resting places adequately separated from the resident cats (see handout titled **Creating Successful Transitions to Your Home**). The proper way to introduce a new cat into the home is covered in Chapter 26 and is briefly discussed here. The goal is to demonstrate the resource allocation necessary when deciding whether to add a new cat to the household.

Resource Allocation and Management

Feline resources include litter boxes, food, water, toys, readily accessible pathways through its territory, scratching posts, resting places and vertical perches, and social interactions with the people in the home. Appropriate and abundant availability of resources for each member of the household can minimize intercat aggression and perhaps avoid or minimize future behavior problems (see Chapters 8 and 26).

Food Resources

Although cats rarely fight over food, they are solitary feeders; therefore, providing separate food bowls, feeder toys, or feeding stations for each cat spread throughout the house can alleviate the potential stress associated with feeding near a housemate, particularly an antagonistic one. Owners often assume that if cats are not actively antagonistic toward each other when they are being fed, they are happy to be eating alongside each other; however, it must be remembered that the value of the food is likely to temporarily override the potential cost of tolerating the presence of another cat. This does not mean that the situation is desirable for the cats, and it should be remembered that cats prefer to eat alone. Behaviorists in some countries use tasty food treats during introductions of new cats, but having cats eat side by side for their daily food allotment is not suitable. If treats are used, the introductions are done at times other than mealtimes, and the treats are fed to individual cats while they are at a significant distance from the other cats. The food is used not to bring the cats closer together, but rather to foster positive emotions in association with the distant presence of another cat. In many cases, once initial introductions are over and the newcomer is integrated into the household, daily provisioning of food needs to be managed carefully in a multicat household, with all cats having access to food in a private location. This becomes especially important if there is one cat or more receiving a special or prescription diet. The inability of an individual cat to safely and privately access a food resource is speculated to lead to overeating, undereating, obesity, or poor body condition scores, and perhaps to vomiting due to rapid ingestion of food. Appropriate, safe, and easy access to food sources is important to maintain an amicable household and healthy cats.

Litter Boxes

House soiling continues to be one of the top behavioral complaints of cat owners and is an indication for a referral to a behaviorist.[3] Unacceptable elimination is a multifactorial problem, and how litter boxes are placed and accessible to the cats in the home may often be contributory. Veterinarians often cite the "$n+1$" rule of thumb of having one litter box more than the number of cats in the household, although this is not a scientifically validated number. One must also keep in mind that, though the number of litter boxes is relevant, if all boxes are within the same room or location, that place is actually only one toileting site, regardless of how many boxes are located there. Many other factors contribute to the usability of those boxes (see Table 6-3), and simply providing increased numbers of boxes may not always be enough. The actual size of the litter box may also play an important role in whether the cat will use it. A Maine Coon or other large-bodied cat may exceed the length of a commercially available, standard size litter box. Even some of the common domestic cats are so large that they may not fit inside an average size litter box. Clients may not even realize that there are alternative solutions, including low-sided plastic storage bins found in the home storage aisles of many major chain stores. Providing a litter substrate with which the new cat is familiar is also important, and the new owner should ask which litter brand the cat prefers and currently uses. Taking a sample of used litter may help encourage the new member of the house to use this new litter box in its new surroundings, because the odor remnants of its old litter box will be mixed in. Clients wishing to decrease the possibility of unacceptable elimination need to be aware of appropriate resource provisioning when it comes to the number and location of litter boxes, as well as the size and cleanliness of the litter boxes and the substrate used (see Chapter 24).

Space Allocation and Usage

Territorial disputes upon introduction of new cats are commonly seen in a multicat households because of the ways in which cats choose to share the space in which they live. In the wild, most feral cats have individual territories that are upwards of 150 acres (male territories are typically much larger than those of females), and they may roam up to one-half mile per day.[7] Because of the sheer size of their territory, it is possible for cats never to encounter another cat if they choose not to. Certainly, in the average suburban house, there is no possible way to provide that amount of individual territory for each cat, and even less so in a city apartment dwelling. Feral cat colonies are matrilineal, composed of related females that share responsibility for rearing their young. When the male kittens are mature, they often venture out to seek new territory and for mates. As cat owners, humans choose who the cat is forced to live with, whereas in the wild, if cats within a territory or colony do not get along, either the

TABLE 6-3 Increasing the Usability of the Litter Box

Usability Characteristics	Making the Ideal Litter Box
Number of boxes	• $n+1$ boxes (i.e., number of cats in the home plus one) placed in sufficient different locations to allow all cats in the household to access a box whenever they need to without encountering another cat • More boxes and locations may be needed if unacceptable elimination or agonistic encounters are present
Location of boxes	• At least one on each level of a multistory home • Spread throughout the home • Placed at the edges of the core areas where each cat spends the majority of its time • Not placed in high-traffic areas or remote locations • Not located near noisy electronic devices or household items (e.g., furnaces, washing machines) • Placed in an area that allows multiple entrances and exits to avoid bottlenecks
Size	• Must be at least 1.5 times the body length (tip of nose to base of tail) of the largest cat in the house • Under-the-bed sweater boxes or large plastic storage totes are ideal for larger cats
Litter substrate	• Most cats prefer fine-grained clay clumping litter • Fill the box to a depth of approximately 1 to 3 inches • More litter should be added as clumps are scooped out in order to maintain the 1- to 3-inch depth • A choice of litter boxes with varying litters can be provided to determine which type of litter each cat prefers • A rug box (i.e., a litter box lined with a towel or bathroom throw rug) can be used for cats that prefer to urinate on rugs, carpets, clothing, or bedding
Cleaning	• Each box should be scooped once or twice daily • The box should be completely emptied and cleaned out with mild soap and water every week or more often if needed • Self-cleaning litter boxes may be too noisy or frightening for some cats to use • Worn, scratched, or damaged boxes should be replaced • All boxes, regardless of wear, should be replaced annually

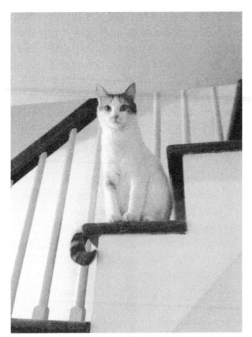

FIGURE 6-3 A cat perched in a high place, monitoring the room.

antagonist or victim cat will simply leave. This is not possible in the average household, unless sufficient territory is provided so that the cats are not forced to interact if they do not choose to do so. Vertical perching and resting places should be provided for each cat in its preferred core area. Vertical perching is important for cats to be able to survey their core area, monitor who enters, and seek refuge from enemies (Figure 6-3). Owners can be creative and provide additional climbing towers and vertical perches, such as wall-mounted shelving, and thus increase the amount of available territory within the limited confines of the home.

Clinicians need to take the time necessary to explain resource allocation to potential owners prior to the adoption of a new cat or, at the very least, at the new feline pet's first appointment. Clients may not be aware that such management is critical to the prevention of unwanted behaviors such as intercat aggression, anxiety, feline unacceptable elimination, and urine marking. If the clients are unable or unwilling to provide additional resources throughout the house, taking on another cat can be problematic and is not advisable. If the clients are insistent on doing so, they must carefully select the incoming cat with due consideration to the personality of the already resident feline(s) (as discussed above) to potentially prevent future behavior problems. For help with determining a client's ability or willingness to appropriately provision resources, see handout titled **Should I Adopt Another Cat?**

CONCLUSION

There are many facets that make up each cat's personality and behavior. Yet, pet owners know little about how to utilize these pieces of information in choosing their new feline companions. Karsh[26] studied cat placement and found that owners often chose their new feline companion based on looks alone, and in particular simply by coat color. This choice was driven by a similar look of the prospective cat to one that they once knew and liked, whether that was a childhood companion, a cat that they previously owned, or a cat owned by a friend. If owners are not armed with key information regarding the source of the cat and its sex, breed type, age at adoption, and temperament, they may choose a cat that does not fit their family and lifestyle and may not get along with the cats they already have. Poor decision-making in the beginning can lead to disastrous consequences in the end, including cat behavior problems, which may lead to relinquishment, abandonment, or euthanasia. Veterinary health care professionals need to educate clients about all the useful and credible scientific research available on the behavior of our feline friends and how that should play into their selection of a new companion.

REFERENCES

1. Bayer HealthCare Animal Health Division: Bayer veterinary care usage study III: feline findings. 2012. http://www.google.com/webhp?nord=1#nord=1&q=Bayer+Veterinary+Care+Usage+Study+III:+Feline+Findings Accessed December 29, 2014.
2. Amat M, Ruiz de la Torre JL, Fatjó J, Mariotti VM, Van Wijk S, Manteca X. Potential risk factors associated with feline behaviour problems. *Appl Anim Behav Sci.* 2009;121:134–139.
3. Salman MD, New JG Jr, Scarlett JM, Kass PH, Ruch-Gallie R, Hetts S. Human and animal factors related to the relinquishment of dogs and cats in 12 selected animal shelters in the United States. *J Appl Anim Welf Sci.* 1998;1:207–226.
4. Dybdall K, Strasser R, Katz T. Behavioral differences between owner surrender and stray domestic cats after entering an animal shelter. *Appl Anim Behav Sci.* 2007;104:85–94.
5. Gouveia K, Magalhães A, de Sousa L. The behaviour of domestic cats in a shelter: residence time, density and sex ratio. *Appl Anim Behav Sci.* 2011;130:53–59.
6. Mellen JD. Effects of early rearing experience in subsequent adult sexual behavior using domestic cats (*Felis catus*) as a model for exotic small felids. *Zoo Biol.* 2005;11:17–32.
7. Beaver BV. Feline social behavior. In: *Feline behavior: a guide for veterinarians.* ed 2. St Louis: Elsevier Science; 2003:127–163.
8. Chon E. The effects of queen (*Felis sylvestris*)-rearing versus hand-rearing on feline aggression and other problematic

behaviors. In: Mills D, Levine E, Landsberg G, et al., eds. *Current issues and research in veterinary behavioral medicine: papers presented at the Fifth International Veterinary Behavior Meeting.* West Lafayette, IN: Purdue University Press; 2005:201–202.

9. Overall KL. Management related problems in feline behavior. *Feline Pract.* 1994;22:13–15.

10. Overall KL. Feline aggression: part 1. *Feline Pract.* 1994;22:25–26.

11. Crowell-Davis SL, Curtis TM, Knowles RJ. Social organization in the cat: a modern understanding. *J Feline Med Surg.* 2004;6:19–28.

12. Neville P. The behavioural impact of weaning on cats and dogs. *Vet Annu.* 1996;36:98–108.

13. Reisner IR, Houpt KA, Erb HN, Quimby FW. Friendliness to humans and defensive aggression in cats: the influence of handling and paternity. *Physiol Behav.* 1994;55:1119–1124.

14. Turner DC, Feaver J, Mendl M, Bateson P. Variation in domestic cat behaviour towards humans: a paternal effect. *Anim Behav.* 1986;34:1890–1901.

15. McCune S. The impact of paternity and early socialisation on the development of cats' behaviour to people and novel objects. *Appl Anim Behav Sci.* 1995;45:109–124.

16. The Cat Fanciers' Association: CFA breed/color designation charts. http://www.cfa.org/Breeds/BreedColorPrefixChart.aspx Accessed December 29, 2014.

17. The International Cat Association (TICA): TICA-recognized cat breeds. http://www.tica.org/cat-breeds Accessed December 29, 2014.

18. Hart BL, Hart LA. Behavioral profiles of cat breeds. *Your ideal cat: insights into breed and gender differences in cat behavior.* West Lafayette, IN: Purdue University Press; 2013; pp. 65–120.

19. International Cat Care: Cat breeds. http://www.icatcare.org/advice/cat-breeds Accessed December 29, 2014.

20. Gough A, Thomas A. Cats. Breed predispositions to disease in dogs and cats. Oxford, UK: Blackwell Publishing; 2004, pp. 161–176.

21. Giger U: Feline hereditary diseases [abstract]. In: World Small Animal Veterinary Association (WSAVA) 38th Annual Congress Proceedings, Auckland, New Zealand, March 6–9, 2013. http://www.vin.com/Proceedings/Proceedings.plx?CID=WSAVA2013&Category=&PID=87406&O=Generic Accessed December 29, 2014.

22. International Cat Care: Inherited disorders in cats. http://www.icatcare.org/advice/cat-breeds/inherited-disorders-cats Accessed December 29, 2014.

23. PennGen, a project of the WSAVA Hereditary Disease Committee: Canine and feline hereditary disease (DNA) testing laboratories. http://research.vet.upenn.edu/Default.aspx?TabId=7620. Accessed December 29, 2014.

24. Veterinary Information Network homepage: http://www.vin.com/ Accessed December 29, 2014.

25. Beaver BV. Feline behavior of sensory and neural origins. *Feline behavior: a guide for veterinarians.* ed 2. St Louis: Elsevier Science; 2003, pp. 42–99.

26. Karsh EB, Turner DC. The human–cat relationship. In: Turner DC, Bateson P, eds. *The domestic cat: the biology of its behaviour.* ed 1. Cambridge, UK: Cambridge University Press; 1988:159–177.

27. Neilson JC. Pearl vs. clumping: litter preference in a population of shelter cats [abstract]. In: *Abstracts from the American Veterinary Society of Animal Behavior;* 2001:14, Boston.

28. Bateson P. Behavioural development in the cat. In: Turner DC, Bateson P, eds. *The domestic cat: the biology of its behaviour.* ed 2. Cambridge, UK: Cambridge University Press; 2000:10–19.

29. Kane E. Texture, odor, and flavor important in determining feline food preference. *DVM.* 1987;18:46–54.

30. Beaver BV. Feline ingestive behavior. *Feline behavior: a guide for veterinarians.* ed 2. St Louis: Elsevier Science; 2003, pp. 212–246.

31. Becques A, Larose C, Gouat P, Serra J. Effects of pre- and postnatal olfactogustatory experience on early preferences at birth and dietary selection at weaning in kittens. *Chem Senses.* 2010;35:41–45.

32. Hamper BA, Rohrbach B, Kirk CA, Lusby A, Bartges J. Effects of early experience on food acceptance in a colony of adult research cats: a preliminary study. *J Vet Behav.* 2012;7:27–32.

33. Hart BL, Barrett RE. Effects of castration on fighting, roaming, and urine spraying in adult male cats. *J Am Vet Med Assoc.* 1973;163:290–292.

34. Beaver BV. Male feline sexual behavior. *Feline behavior: a guide for veterinarians.* ed 2. St Louis: Elsevier Science; 2003, pp. 164–181.

35. Spain CV, Scarlett JM, Houpt KA. Long-term risks and benefits of early-age gonadectomy in cats. *J Am Vet Med Assoc.* 2004;224:372–379.

36. Lieberman LL. A case for neutering pups and kittens at two months of age. *J Am Vet Med Assoc.* 1987;191:518–521.

37. Beaver BV. Female feline sexual behavior. *Feline behavior: a guide for veterinarians.* ed 2. St Louis: Elsevier Science; 2003, pp. 182–211.

38. American Society for the Prevention of Cruelty to Animals (ASPCA): Feline-ality 101. https://www.aspca.org/adopt/meet-your-match/feline-ality-101 Accessed December 29, 2014.

39. American Society for the Prevention of Cruelty to Animals (ASPCA): Meet the feline-alities. https://www.aspca.org/adopt/meet-your-match/meet-feline-alities Accessed January 7, 2013.

40. Lee RL, Zeglen M, Ryan T, Hines L. Guidelines: animals in nursing homes. *Calif Vet Suppl.* 1983;3:22a–26a.

41. Siegford JM, Walshaw SO, Brunner P, Zanella AJ. Validation of a temperament test for domestic cats. *Anthrozoos.* 2003;16:332–351.

42. Finka L, Ellis SLH, Wilkinson A, Mills DS. Assessing cat sociability: effects of human familiarity and interaction style on the approach of cats in a rescue environment [abstract]. *Proceedings of the Ninth International Veterinary Behaviour Meeting, Lisbon, Portugal;* September 26–29, 2013, p. 144.

43. Dowling-Guyer S, Marder A, D'Arpino S. Behavioral traits detected in shelter dogs by a behavior evaluation. *Appl Anim Behav Sci.* 2011;130:107–114.

44. Wilsson E, Sundgren PE. Behaviour test for eight-week old puppies—heritabilities of tested behaviour traits and its correspondence to later behaviour. *Appl Anim Behav Sci.* 1998;58:151–162.

45. Christensen E, Scarlett J, Campagna M, Houpt KA. Aggressive behavior in adopted dogs that passed a temperament test. *Appl Anim Behav Sci.* 2007;106:85–95.

46. Feaver J, Mendl M, Bateson P. A method for rating the individual distinctiveness of domestic cats. *Anim Behav.* 1986;34:1016–1025.

47. Turner DC. The human–cat relationship. In: Turner DC, Bateson P, eds. *The domestic cat: the biology of its behaviour.* ed 2. Cambridge, UK: Cambridge University Press; 2000:193–206.

48. Mertens C, Turner DC. Experimental analysis of human–cat interactions during first encounters. *Anthrozoos.* 1988;2:83–97.

Providing Appropriate Healthcare

Susan Little

INTRODUCTION

Cats have now surpassed dogs as the most popular companion animal in many countries. In the United States, there are 74 million pet cats compared with 70 million pet dogs.[1] One-third of American households own at least one cat, and the average number of cats per household is 2.1. Canadians own 8.5 million cats compared with 6 million dogs.[2] About 35% of Canadian households own at least one cat and the average number of cats per household is 1.7. In the United Kingdom, there are about 10 million cats, with 26% of households owning a cat.[3]

However, some alarming statistics about feline veterinary care have been published in the United States, and other countries likely have similar findings.[1] For example, in 2011, spending on veterinary care for dogs increased almost 19%, whereas spending for cats increased only 4%. According to the Bayer Veterinary Care Usage Study, the number of feline veterinary visits declined by almost 15% between 2001 and 2011, despite an increase in the number of owned cats.[4] The reasons for the decline in feline veterinary care are multiple and complex.[5] They include issues such as the following:

- Difficulty getting the cat to the veterinary practice (Figure 7-1)
- A low level of owner awareness of basic medical needs of cats
- Difficulty recognizing subtle signs of illness in cats
- The perception that cats are able to take care of themselves
- The low perceived value of cats, since most cats are acquired for free
- Client discomfort and stress associated with experiences at the veterinary practice (Figure 7-2)

In contrast with some other companion animal species, cats are masters of disguise, and their signs of sickness are often subtle (Box 7-1).[4] Compounding this barrier is the attitude of many veterinarians, who believe that dogs are easier to work with than cats and that feline diseases are more challenging to diagnose and treat (Figure 7-3). In addition, a common misconception is that cats are independent and self-sufficient.

When cats lead primarily indoor lives, owners may falsely believe they are free from risk of disease. One result is that cats are often sicker than dogs by the time they are presented for evaluation of signs of illness. For example, in a study of 60 sick cats and 72 sick dogs over 6 months of age presented to an internal medicine service at a veterinary university, researchers evaluated body condition score (BCS), appetite, and changes in weight.[6] Cats had a lower median BCS than dogs (4/9 vs. 6.5/9) with 53% of cats having a BCS <5/9 (compared with 28% of dogs). Owners reported 57% of cats had recent weight loss (compared with 46% of dogs) and 53% had decreased food intake (compared with 35% of dogs).

Because cats are adept at hiding illness, clinicians must become expert at finding clues with a thorough medical history and feline-specific physical examination. Obtaining a medical history is easier than ever in today's electronic world. Clinicians can take advantage of multimedia tools to collect information, such as videos of a particular behavior that owners record at home. Questionnaires that are tailored to specific needs can be utilized, such as the Feline Musculoskeletal Pain Index.[7] The forms can be supplied to the client to fill out in advance of an appointment, thereby saving time and improving collection of detailed data.

Incorporating Behavioral Services into Healthcare

Behavior problems and problem behaviors are often overlooked in feline medicine and are a common reason for euthanasia or relinquishment to a shelter. Many cat owners do not realize that veterinarians can provide behavioral counseling or that many behavior problems have a medical basis. For example, in senior cats, many behavior changes are wrongly attributed to old age when the cause may be disease or pain. Conversely, sometimes signs of sickness (e.g., anorexia, vomiting, diarrhea) are caused by stressors in the cat's environment.[8] Instead of medications, these cats require a behavioral and environmental assessment with counseling for the clients on how to reduce stress and anxiety.

A behavior assessment should be conducted with every veterinary visit to help the client make changes necessary

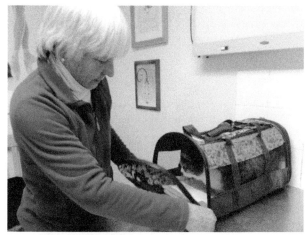

FIGURE 7-1 Providing clients with information on selecting an appropriate cat carrier and ways to reduce the stress of transporting the cat to the veterinary practice can help facilitate necessary veterinary visits.

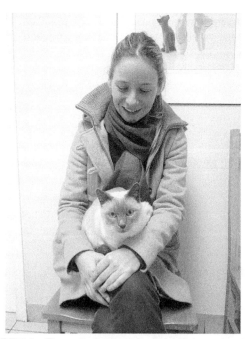

FIGURE 7-2 The veterinary visit should be as pleasant as possible for both cat and client.

BOX 7-1 **The 10 Subtle Signs of Sickness**

1. Inappropriate elimination
2. Changes in interaction
3. Changes in activity
4. Changes in sleeping habits
5. Changes in food and water consumption
6. Unexplained weight loss or gain
7. Changes in grooming
8. Signs of stress
9. Changes in vocalization
10. Bad breath

Adapted from: Have We Seen Your Cat Lately? Subtle Signs of Sickness. http://www.haveweseenyourcatlately.com/Health_and_Wellness.html

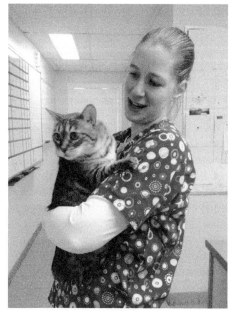

FIGURE 7-3 Veterinary staff who appreciate and understand cats help improve patient care.

BOX 7-2 **Examples of Behavior Questions to Ask at Every Veterinary Visit**

1. What changes in your cat's litter box have you noticed?
2. What problems with your cat hissing, biting, or scratching people have you noticed?
3. What problems with destructive behaviors, such as scratching or chewing objects, have you noticed?
4. What problems have you noticed with your cat's interactions with other pets in your home?
5. What changes in your cat's behavior or attitude have you noticed?

Adapted from: Overall KL, Rodan I, Beaver BV, et al.: Feline behavior guidelines from the American Association of Feline Practitioners. *J Am Vet Med Assoc.* 227:70–84, 2005.

to prevent behavior problems as well as for early detection of both behavior and medical problems. Cat owners may not provide information about potential behavior problems unless they are specifically questioned. Therefore, veterinary team members should be trained to ask screening questions about behavior at every visit (Box 7-2) and to use short behavior questionnaires. When screening identifies a behavior problem requiring more in-depth assessment, a follow up appointment specifically for that purpose can be scheduled or the patient can be referred to a board-certified veterinary behaviorist.

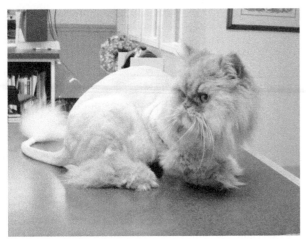

FIGURE 7-4 Clients should be counseled on the special needs of specific cat breeds. For example, longhair breeds such as the Persian require regular grooming to prevent matting of the hair coat.

Many veterinary practices are able to offer behavior services beyond assessment and treatment of common problems. Programs that help clients achieve success from the start of pet ownership may help reduce the risk of relinquishment. Prepurchase or preadoption counseling can help ensure that the pet is matched appropriately to the client and that the client's expectations are realistic. For example, adopting a cat of a very active breed (such as Siamese) or a breed requiring a commitment to grooming (such as the Persian, Figure 7-4) may not be appropriate for every family. Adopting a calmer adult cat may be better than adopting an active kitten in some cases. Adopting kittens in pairs is often recommended for healthy social development and prevention of unwanted behaviors (Figure 7-5).

Counseling should include information on how to handle cats safely, with special attention to handling by young children in the home. For example, hands and feet should never be used as toys to play with cats. Interactions with other pets in the home should also be discussed (Figure 7-6). For this type of counseling, veterinary team members should be familiar with different cat breeds and their characteristics, as well as with normal behaviors associated with life stages.

Kitten socialization classes have become very popular in recent years. The classes are usually small in size and often can be held in the veterinary practice waiting area. They can be conducted by a trained staff member, such as a veterinary technician. Benefits include exposing kittens and young cats to different stimuli and different people, and training clients how to handle cats properly and provide basic care (e.g., nail trimming, grooming, performing a basic physical examination). Clients can also be instructed how to select a cat carrier and accustom the cat to travel. These classes also provide an

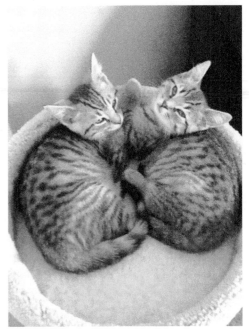

FIGURE 7-5 Adopting kittens in age-matched pairs is often recommended to improve bonding and prevent behavior problems. (Courtesy S. Butt)

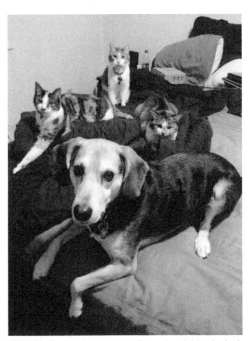

FIGURE 7-6 Behavior counseling should include interactions of cats with other pets in the home, such as dogs. (Courtesy K. Mantle)

opportunity to teach clients about a cat's basic environmental needs, such as the litter box, perching and resting places, and toys.

Life Stage Healthcare

A consistent approach to healthcare is necessary to prevent disease and for early detection of signs of illness.

Every visit should include a comprehensive medical history, a thorough physical examination, a nutritional assessment, a behavior assessment, and an environmental assessment. Veterinarians must educate cat owners about the importance of regular cat healthcare, including prevention and treatment of behavior problems. A life stage approach improves early recognition and treatment of problems, thereby improving feline health and welfare and preserving the human–animal bond. The American Association of Feline Practitioners (AAFP) and the American Animal Hospital Association (AAHA) have published guidelines defining six life stages with associated healthcare guidelines:[9]

1. Kitten: birth to 6 months
2. Junior: 7 months to 2 years
3. Prime/adult: 3 to 6 years
4. Mature: 7 to 10 years
5. Senior: 11 to 14 years
6. Geriatric: 15 years and older

Although assessment of healthcare needs varies by life stage (Table 7-1), it is important to remember that individual cats and body systems age at different rates. Some cats will develop an illness not typically associated with its life stage. In addition to the topics below, other topics that should be discussed at every preventive care visit include:

- Identification (e.g., microchip, collar and tag, tattoo)
- Pet health insurance
- Preparations for pet care in natural disaster response planning
- Benefits of oral healthcare
- Review of medications, supplements, nutraceuticals, botanicals, homeopathic remedies, and so on, that the cat is receiving

HEALTHCARE CONSIDERATIONS FOR ALL LIFE STAGES

Frequency of Examinations and Routine Health Screening

Annual health examinations are considered the minimum standard by organizations such as AAFP and AAHA. More frequent examinations are recommended for senior and geriatric cats as well as for those with chronic medical conditions (e.g., diabetes mellitus, chronic kidney disease). Changes in health can occur quickly in these patients, although the signs may not be readily apparent to owners. Educating clients about the subtle signs of sickness (see Box 7-1) can lead to more frequent visits, better communication, and more timely diagnosis and treatment.

Regular collection of a minimum database record based on life stage can allow early detection of disease and monitoring of trends in important laboratory parameters. An often overlooked benefit is the collection of baseline data that can be useful in interpreting data collected at future visits by providing context for the individual patient. Specific recommendations on which tests to perform and when to do them depend on many factors, such as the increase in incidence of many diseases with age. Recommendations for minimum database monitoring have been published in the AAFP senior care guidelines and the AAFP-AAHA feline life stage guidelines (see Resources, below). A summary by life stage is provided in Table 7-2.

Regular monitoring is especially important for older cats. In a study of 100 apparently healthy cats 6 years of age and older, routine health screening uncovered previously undetected problems such as hypertension, azotemia, diabetes mellitus, heart disease, hyperthyroidism, and proteinuria.[10]

Lifestyle and the Home Environment

The home environment is critically important in wellness, and veterinary staff should be trained to ask questions that uncover pertinent information and counsel clients about enriched environments. An indoor-only lifestyle decreases the risks of trauma and infectious diseases, but the cat's welfare may be compromised and illness induced by a stressful or sterile environment. A variety of conditions and diseases ("Pandora syndrome") may appear in susceptible cats placed into inadequate environments, so the patient's behaviors and its environment are key components of the medical history and assessment.[11]

Determining the adequacy (number and location) of key resources (e.g., hiding places, elevated resting places, food and water stations, scratching posts, litter boxes, and stimulating toys) is important for prevention of behavior problems. Asking the client to draw a floor plan showing the location of key resources can be very helpful. Veterinarians should be prepared to provide resources and guidance to help cat owners construct a suitable indoor environment to maximize health and well-being. Safe access to outdoor environments is also possible in a variety of ways and will be of interest to many cat owners (Figure 7-7).

Nutritional Assessment

Nutritional assessment is now referred to as the fifth vital assessment (after temperature, pulse, respiration, and pain). Nutritional needs must be assessed in order to maintain health and maximize quality of life, and as a component of therapy for many diseases, including behavior problems. Feeding management is not only important for health maintenance but also a key part of environmental enrichment and mental wellness. A nutritional assessment is therefore a critical part of every visit. The information gathered is used to determine

TABLE 7-1   Important Topics for Feline Preventive Care, by Life Stage

Life Stage	General	Behavior, Environment	Medical, Surgical	Elimination	Nutrition, Weight Management	Oral Health	Parasite Control	Vaccination
Kitten: birth to 6 months	Congenital and genetic diseases Breed predispositions to disease Claw care and grooming	Lifestyle choices Discuss resources and toys Teach simple commands Acclimate to car and pet carrier	Discuss sterilization, age to perform surgery	Litter box setup, cleaning Discuss normal elimination	Discuss growth requirements, healthy weight management Introduce to variety of foods, flavors	Acclimate to handling mouth Educate about dental care Start toothbrushing	Deworm every 2 weeks from 3 to 9 weeks of age, then monthly until age 6 months Fecal examination at least twice in first year of life	Administer core vaccines and other vaccines according to risk factors Vaccinate for rabies in accordance with local laws
Junior: 7 months to 2 years	Collect a thorough medical history Monitor for common health problems, such as asthma, intestinal disease, diabetes mellitus	Discuss social interactions with other pets, people, regular handling of mouth, ears, feet		Confirm litter box appropriate for growing cat Identify and correct litter box problems	Monitor for weight increase Adjust caloric intake after sterilization Feed to moderate body condition	Monitor, discuss ongoing needs	Fecal examination at least annually Ongoing parasite control based on lifestyle, risk factors	Ongoing management of vaccine needs according to lifestyle Continue core vaccines, others as indicated
Prime/adult: 3 to 6 years	Collect a thorough medical history Monitor for common health problems, such as asthma, intestinal disease, diabetes mellitus	Review environmental enrichment Discuss ways to keep active	Monitor for subtle changes Discuss mobility	Identify and correct litter box problems	Feed to moderate body condition Monitor for weight gain	Monitor, discuss ongoing needs	Fecal examination at least once annually Ongoing parasite control based on lifestyle, risk factors	Ongoing management of vaccine needs according to lifestyle Continue core vaccines, others as indicated
Mature: 7 to 10 years	Increase frequency of examinations Educate owner on changes associated with aging and common diseases in age group	Discuss access to litter box, bed, food, water	Discuss mobility Monitor for signs of illness	Ensure easy access to litter box with changes in mobility		Monitor, discuss ongoing needs	Fecal examination at least once annually Ongoing parasite control based on lifestyle, risk factors	Ongoing management of vaccine needs according to lifestyle Continue core vaccines, others as indicated

Senior: 11 to 14 years	Increase frequency of examinations Educate client on changes associated with aging and common diseases in age group	Discuss changing environmental needs Educate about changes in behavior and illness	Regular review of medications, diet, supplements	Adjust litter box size, height, location, cleaning, etc., as required to meet changing needs	Monitor for weight loss Adjust diet and feeding management as needed	Monitor for oral tumors, other sources of oral pain	Fecal examination at least once annually Ongoing parasite control based on lifestyle, risk factors	Ongoing management of vaccine needs according to lifestyle Continue core vaccines, others as indicated
Geriatric: 15 years and older	Increase frequency of examinations Educate client on changes associated with aging and common diseases in age group	Discuss access to litter box, bed, food, water, signs of cognitive dysfunction Discuss quality of life	Regular review of medications, diet, supplements	Adjust litter box size, height, location, cleaning, etc., as required to meet changing needs	Monitor for weight loss Adjust diet and feeding management as needed	Monitor for oral tumors, other sources of oral pain	Fecal examination at least once annually Ongoing parasite control based on lifestyle, risk factors	Ongoing management of vaccine needs according to lifestyle Continue core vaccines, others as indicated

From: Little S: Preventive healthcare: a life-stage approach. In: Harvey A, Tasker S, editors. *BSAVA manual of feline practice: a foundation manual*, Gloucester, UK, 2013, British Small Animal Veterinary Association (BSAVA), pp. 32–45.

TABLE 7-2   **Recommendations for Minimum Database Monitoring, by Life Stage**

	Kitten/Junior: <2 years	Adult: 2 to 7 years	Mature: 7 to 10 years	Senior/Geriatric: ≥11 years
Complete blood cell count with differential	O	O	R	R
Serum chemistry panels with electrolytes	O	O	R	R
Complete urinalysis	O	O	R	R
Total T4	NR	O	O	R
Blood pressure assessment	NR	O	O	R
FeLV/FIV testing	R	O	O	O
Fecal flotation	R	R	R	R

FeLV, Feline leukemia virus; *FIV,* feline immunodeficiency virus; *NR,* not recommended; *O,* optional; *R,* recommended.
Adapted from: Little S: Preventive healthcare: a life-stage approach. In: Harvey A, Tasker S, editors. *BSAVA manual of feline practice: a foundation manual,* Gloucester, UK, 2013, British Small Animal Veterinary Association (BSAVA), pp. 32–45.

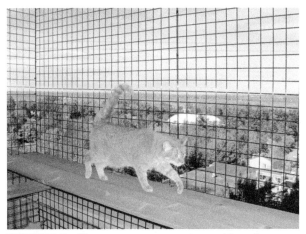

FIGURE 7-7   There are many ways to provide safe access to outdoor environments, such as this balcony enclosure, to provide stimulation and prevent boredom. (Courtesy W. Petrie)

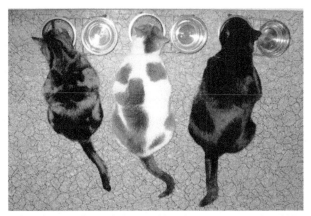

FIGURE 7-8   Part of the nutritional assessment should be collecting information on not only what cats are fed but also how and where they are fed. Although owners frequently place food bowls together, cats are solitary eaters and ideally would not be fed in close proximity to each other. (Courtesy W. Petrie)

whether the current nutritional plan is appropriate for the cat's life stage, health conditions, and body weight.

Information should be collected and recorded on the type of food fed (e.g., wet, dry, frozen, raw), the brands fed, the amount fed, how and where the food is provided (e.g., meal feeding, free choice feeding, food balls, or puzzles), and the frequency of feeding (Figure 7-8). Because many cat owners provide dry diets in a free choice manner, the amount actually eaten should be determined. As well, questions should be asked about the type and amounts of any supplements or treats provided. Questions about the provision of water and any changes in water intake are also part of the nutritional assessment. Reception staff can alert the client in advance to bring this information for the visit in order to provide a more accurate and efficient assessment. A follow-up phone call after the visit can help collect any missing details.

A nutritional assessment also includes monitoring weight, BCS, and muscle condition (Figure 7-9). Each cat's ideal body weight should be determined and recorded.

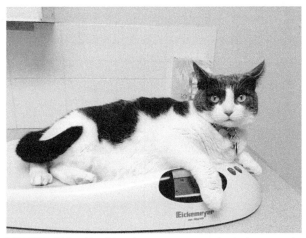

FIGURE 7-9   Nutritional assessment includes regular monitoring of weight, body condition, and muscle condition.

Ideal body weight can be determined by using several methods (e.g., five-point or nine-point BCS charts, morphometric measurements, body fat index). In addition to determining whether the cat's weight is stable or has changed, the percentage weight change may help detect insidious gains or losses over time, thereby allowing for early intervention. The percentage weight change is calculated as follows:

$$\% \text{ weight change} = ([\text{current weight} - \text{previous weight}]$$
$$/\text{previous weight}) \times 100$$

A simple muscle condition scoring system is currently undergoing development and validation; it is described in both the AAHA and World Small Animal Veterinary Association (WSAVA) nutritional assessment guidelines (see Resources, below). The patient's muscle condition is recorded as normal or wasted (scored as mild, moderate, or marked wasting). Muscle loss may be due to sarcopenia (age-associated) or cachexia (disease-associated), and some patients will have muscle loss of both types. A patient with muscle wasting may have a catabolic disease (e.g., neoplasia, hyperthyroidism), may be unable to absorb dietary protein efficiently (e.g., intestinal disease), or may require a diet with more protein. BCS and muscle condition scores are not related; for example, an overweight or obese cat may be muscle-wasted.

Nutritional requirements change with life stage and health status, so recommendations must be reviewed and updated accordingly. For example, maintenance energy requirements decrease by about 3% per year up to about 11 years of age.[12,13] After 11 years, energy requirements increase in many cats, leading some senior cats to be underweight if their energy needs are not met. As well, changes in digestive efficiency occur with age.[14] Older cats are less efficient at digesting fats and proteins, meaning that either daily food intake must be increased to compensate or a more appropriately formulated diet should be provided.

At every visit, the nutritional assessment should be reviewed and a recommendation made that includes a specific diet, the amount to be fed (preferably by weight), and the manner and frequency of feeding. The recommendation may be as simple as continuing with the current plan, or a revision in diet or feeding management may be required. When changes are made to the nutritional plan, appropriate follow-up should be planned.

Vaccinations

In many countries, vaccinations are no longer the main focus of regular veterinary visits. Reminders sent to cat owners for the annual visit are now often worded to reflect the need for a comprehensive physical examination and consultation rather than vaccination. This means it is important to ensure that cat owners understand that the veterinary visit is an opportunity to take measures that maintain good health (e.g., appropriate vaccinations and parasite control) and to detect and treat disease early. Prevention and treatment of behavior problems should also be emphasized.

Vaccination is a medical procedure and is not without risks. However, most adverse events associated with vaccination are mild and temporary and occur in less than 1% of vaccinated cats.[15] In general, vaccination decisions should be based on risk assessment and tailored to the individual patient. Information about the patient, the environment and lifestyle, and potential infectious agents are key components of risk assessment.

The Patient

Most infectious diseases are more prevalent in kittens, particularly those less than 6 months of age. Kittens, therefore, represent a principal target population for vaccination. Maternally derived antibodies (MDAs) provide important early protection against disease for kittens. However, MDAs may also interfere with the response to vaccination. The level of MDAs varies among individuals, so the age at which a kitten may be able to fully respond to vaccination also varies. In some cases, this may be 16 weeks of age or older, which is why most expert panels recommend that the last kitten vaccination be given no earlier than 16 weeks.

With aging, immunosenescence may blunt previously established immunity, so vaccinations should not be allowed to lapse in older cats. In fact, senior cats may have an increased need of protection against infectious disease compared with younger healthy adult cats.

The Environment and Lifestyle

Critical issues affecting risk of exposure to infectious diseases include population density and the opportunity for exposure to other cats. Patients in multicat households, those that may live in boarding facilities from time to time, and those with access to outdoors are likely to have a higher risk of infection than are cats in households with one or two indoor cats. However, indoor cats are not without risk of exposure to infectious disease during their lifetime and also require protection.

The Infectious Agent

Infectious diseases vary in geographic distribution, resulting in substantially different risks depending on where the cat lives. Determining a cat's risk for infectious disease should also include any plans for travel away from home. Variables associated with the infectious agent itself, such as severity of disease, will also influence vaccination decisions.

Vaccines are designated as core (where vaccination of all cats is justified), noncore (where vaccination is justified based on risk assessment), and not generally recommended. Several organizations have recently reviewed and updated vaccination guidelines for cats; these documents should be reviewed to help practitioners devise their own practice protocols (Box 7-3).

Table 7-3 contains a summary of the current feline vaccination recommendations for household pet cats.

Retrovirus Testing

Feline leukemia virus (FeLV) and feline immunodeficiency virus (FIV) are among the most common infectious diseases of cats, although their prevalence in the cat population varies by geographic location and risk factors. Comprehensive data on the seroprevalence of retroviral infections and risk factors for cats have been published for some countries (Table 7-4).

Guidelines for prevention and management of retroviral infections have been published (see Resources, below) and should be consulted. Ideally, the retroviral status of all cats should be known. Following are suggestions for determining which cats should be tested for FeLV and FIV:

- All cats at increased risk, including sick cats, cats with bite wounds or oral disease, cats with known exposure to a retrovirus-infected cat, and cats in multicat environments where the status of all cats is not known. A sick cat should be tested even if it had a negative test for FeLV or FIV in the past.
- Newly acquired cats and kittens, either before adoption or as soon after rehoming as possible.
- Cats about to be vaccinated for FeLV or FIV.

BOX 7-3   Published Vaccination Guidelines for Cats

American Association of Feline Practitioners

Scherk MA, Ford RB, Gaskell RM, et al.: 2013 AAFP Feline Vaccination Advisory Panel Report. *J Feline Med Surg* 15:785–808, 2013. http://www.catvets.com/guidelines/practice-guidelines/feline-vaccination-guidelines

European Advisory Board on Cat Diseases

Horzinek MC, Addie D, Belák S, et al.: ABCD: update of the 2009 guidelines on prevention and management of feline infectious diseases. *J Feline Med Surg* 15:530–539, 2013. http://www.abcd-vets.org/Pages/guidelines.aspx

Hosie MJ, Addie D, Belák S, et al.: Matrix Vaccination Guidelines: ABCD recommendations for indoor/outdoor cats, rescue shelter cats and breeding catteries. *J Feline Med Surg* 15:540–544, 2013.

Möstl K, Egberink H, Addie D, et al.: Prevention of infectious diseases in cat shelters: ABCD guidelines. *J Feline Med Surg* 15:546–554, 2013.

World Small Animal Veterinary Association

Day MJ, Horzinek MC, Schultz RD: WSAVA Guidelines for the Vaccination of Dogs and Cats. *J Small Anim Pract* 51:338–356, 2010. http://www.wsava.org/sites/default/files/VaccinationGuidelines2010.pdf

---

- Cats at ongoing risk of infection (e.g., cats with unconfined access to outdoors) should be tested annually for FeLV and for FIV (if not FIV-vaccinated).

Since most cats test positive for FIV antibody within 60 days of FIV exposure, testing should be repeated a minimum of 60 days after the last potential exposure. Positive FIV antibody tests in kittens younger than 6 months of age must be interpreted carefully. Kittens born to infected queens (or FIV-vaccinated queens) may acquire FIV antibodies in colostrum. Because it is uncommon for kittens to acquire infection from the queen, most kittens with a positive FIV antibody test are not truly infected and will have a negative test when reevaluated. Kittens with a positive test for FIV antibody at 4 to 6 months of age are most likely truly infected.

FIV-vaccinated cats produce antibodies that cannot be distinguished from antibodies due to natural infection using some currently available screening tests. Antibodies due to vaccination persist for several years. Validated polymerase chain reaction (PCR) tests may enable the clinician to determine a cat's true status.[16] Owing to its low sensitivity, PCR is not useful as a screening tool and cannot replace rapid in-practice assays or referral laboratory enzyme-linked immunosorbent assay tests. PCR testing should be used only in FIV antibody–positive cats that have an unknown vaccination history and in FIV antibody–positive cats that have been vaccinated against FIV but in which infection is still suspected. PCR cannot be used to determine a cat's vaccination status. PCR test results must be interpreted with caution. A positive PCR result for FIV confirms FIV infection and should not be affected by FIV vaccination. However, for several reasons, a negative PCR result for FIV does not rule out infection. The level of viral nucleic acid in the sample may be below the limit of detection, or the sample may contain a strain of FIV that cannot be detected with the test.

Since most cats will test positive for FeLV antigen within 30 days of exposure, testing should be repeated a minimum of 30 days after the last potential exposure. Kittens can be tested at any age, as MDA does not interfere with testing for viral antigen. Vaccination does not interfere with FeLV testing.

Because the consequences of a positive test result for FeLV or FIV are significant and currently available screening tests may have low positive predictive value (<90%), particularly in low-risk populations, confirmatory testing is recommended (Figures 7-10, 7-11, and 7-12).

Parasite Control

Effective control of external and internal parasites is essential to maintain patient health, enhance public safety, and preserve the bond between pets and people. Veterinarians often focus on the family dog for prevention of zoonotic disease, but the family cat should also be evaluated. Special care should be taken to give accurate information to immunocompromised pet owners or caregivers and

TABLE 7-3   Summary of Current Feline Vaccination Recommendations for Household Pet Cats from the American Association of Feline Practitioners, World Small Animal Veterinary Association, and European Advisory Board on Cat Diseases Vaccine Guideline Groups

Vaccine	Primary Series: Kittens <16 Weeks	Primary Series: Adults and Kittens >16 Weeks	Boosters
CORE VACCINES			
Feline panleukopenia	First dose as early as 6 weeks, then every 3–4 weeks until 16–20 weeks old	Two doses 3–4 weeks apart	1 year after primary series, then no more often than every 3 years
Feline herpesvirus and calicivirus	First dose as early as 6 weeks, then every 3–4 weeks until 16–20 weeks old	Two doses 3–4 weeks apart	1 year after primary series, then no more often than every 3 years unless high risk perceived (e.g., entry into boarding cattery)
Rabies (where legally mandated or in an endemic area)	Start as early as 12 weeks, then 1 year later	Two doses 1 year apart	Annually or less often, depending on local laws and product licensing
NONCORE VACCINES			
Feline leukemia virus (may be considered a core vaccine for kittens)	Start as early as 8 weeks, then 3–4 weeks later	Two doses 3–4 weeks apart	1 year after primary series, then annually for cats at ongoing risk. AAFP and ABCD recommend booster vaccines every 2–3 years after 3–4 years of age for cats at low risk
Feline immunodeficiency virus	Start as early as 8 weeks, then every 2–3 weeks for two additional doses (three doses required in total)	Three doses required, administered 2–3 weeks apart	1 year after last kitten vaccine, then annually for cats at ongoing risk
Chlamydophila felis	Start as early as 8–9 weeks, then 3–4 weeks later	Two doses 3–4 weeks apart	Annually for cats at ongoing risk
Bordetella bronchiseptica	Single dose as early as 4 weeks	Single dose	Annually for cats at ongoing risk
VACCINES NOT GENERALLY RECOMMENDED			
Feline infectious peritonitis	First dose at 16 weeks, then 3–4 weeks later	Two doses 3–4 weeks apart	Annual booster recommended by vaccine manufacturer

ABCD, European Advisory Board on Cat Diseases; *AAFP*, American Association of Feline Practitioners.

TABLE 7-4   Seroprevalence of Feline Leukemia Virus and Feline Immunodeficiency Virus in Selected Countries

Country	FIV Seroprevalence (%)	FeLV Seroprevalence (%)
Canada[*]	4.3	3.4
United States[†]	2.5	2.3
Germany[‡]	3.2	3.7
Japan[§]	9.8	2.9
Czech Republic[‖]	5.8	13.2

FeLV, feline leukemia virus; *FIV*, feline immunodeficiency virus.

[*]Little S, Sears W, Lachtara J, Bienzle D: Seroprevalence of feline leukemia virus and feline immunodeficiency virus infection among cats in Canada. *Can Vet J* 50:644–648, 2009.

[†]Levy JK, Scott HM, Lachtara JL, Crawford PC: Seroprevalence of feline leukemia virus and feline immunodeficiency virus infection among cats in North America and risk factors for seropositivity. *J Am Vet Med Assoc* 228:371–376, 2006.

[‡]Gleich S, Hartmann K: Feline immunodeficiency virus and feline leukemia virus: a retrospective study in 17462 cases [abstract]. *J Vet Intern Med* 21:578, 2007.

[§]Maruyama S, Kabeya H, Nakao R, et al.: Seroprevalence of *Bartonella henselae, Toxoplasma gondii*, FIV and FeLV infections in domestic cats in Japan. *Microbiol Immunol* 47:147–153, 2003.

[‖]Knotek Z, Hájková P, Svoboda M, Toman M, Raska V: Epidemiology of feline leukaemia and feline immunodeficiency virus infections in the Czech Republic. *Zentralbl Veterinarmed B* 46:665–671, 1999.

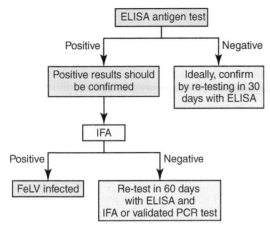

FIGURE 7-10 Algorithm for feline leukemia virus testing for kittens and cats of all ages.

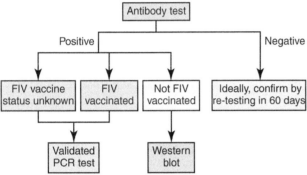

FIGURE 7-11 Algorithm for feline immunodeficiency virus for testing cats over 6 months of age.

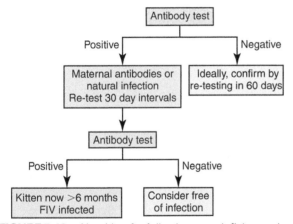

FIGURE 7-12 Algorithm for feline immunodeficiency virus testing for kittens less than 6 months of age.

where cats may be in contact with others with increased susceptibility to zoonotic disease, such as infants, young children, and the elderly.

A parasite control program is recommended for all cats and should be tailored to each patient's needs. Control programs should include evaluation of geographic, seasonal, and lifestyle factors that affect parasite prevalence and risk of exposure. Fecal testing is recommended as part of parasite control programs to monitor compliance with monthly preventive medication and to

diagnose internal parasites that may not be treated by broad-spectrum preventatives. However, veterinarians should be aware of the limitations of fecal testing, as false-negative results are common for many reasons. In kittens, fecal testing can be coordinated with vaccine administration so that two to four tests are performed during the first year of life.

KEY POINTS FOR DISCUSSION OF BEHAVIOR NEEDS DURING PREVENTIVE CARE VISITS, BY LIFE STAGE

Kittens (Birth to 6 Months)

Play

Kittens have strong play needs that must be met. Appropriate toys allow kittens to practice normal predatory behaviors. Clients should be advised to direct play toward toys and never use their own hands or feet.

Socialization

The primary socialization period is from about 2 to 7 weeks of age, so kittens should have positive experiences with people during this period. This is also the time to expose kittens in a positive way to a variety of situations and stimuli.

Training

Clients can be taught to trim their cat's claws at this time (Figure 7-13) and also basic physical examination skills such as inspecting the oral cavity. Selection of an appropriate cat carrier and training the cat to becoming accustomed to the carrier and car trips should begin as early as possible.

Lifestyle

Discussion about the cat's eventual lifestyle should encompass the risks and benefits of both indoor and

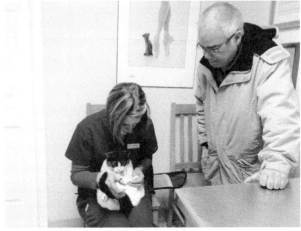

FIGURE 7-13 Clients should be taught how to trim their cat's claws as well as basic physical examination skills.

outdoor lifestyles. Clients should be introduced to the concept of environmental enrichment and resource management for cats that will live most or all of their lives indoors, especially in multicat households.

Junior (7 Months to 2 Years)

Training

Clients should be encouraged to continue efforts to acclimatize the cat to travel in a carrier and to accept handling for basic needs, such as nail trimming and grooming.

Intercat Relationships

In multicat households, intercat aggression may develop in this age group and can lead to problems with inappropriate elimination, urine spraying, and fighting. Clients must be educated on the need for adequate space and resources, and on the use of synthetic feline pheromones.

Adult/Prime (3 to 6 Years) and Mature (7 to 10 Years)

Play

In this age group, owners often find that cats are less playful. However, clients should be encouraged to provide stimulating environments (Figure 7-14) and regular play sessions (two or three sessions of 15 minutes each daily). Cats with access to outdoors may roam, hunt, and fight less in this life stage.

Senior (11 to 14 Years) and Geriatric (15 Years and Older)

Aging Changes

Older cats are often less active and spend more time sleeping (Figure 7-15). They are also less tolerant of change, whether it be changes in the environment or dietary change. Diminishing sensory abilities may contribute to a decreased appetite, reduced mobility, and changes in social interactions.

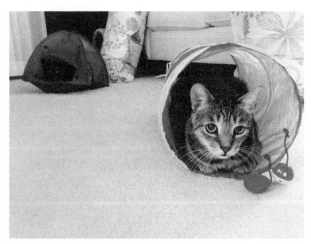

FIGURE 7-14 Cat tents and tubes can be used to provide a stimulating indoor environment as well as hiding places. (Courtesy K. Bailey)

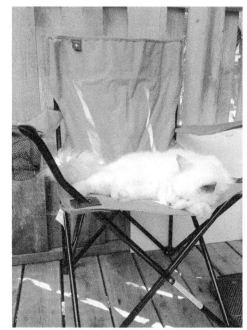

FIGURE 7-15 Many older cats spend more time sleeping and are less active than younger cats, even when outdoors. (Courtesy J. Lachapelle)

Behavior Changes

Behavior changes (e.g., inappropriate vocalization, change in litter box use) may be associated with underlying medical problems. Common diseases in this age group include chronic kidney disease, hyperthyroidism, dental disease, and neoplasia. It is important for clients to understand the difference between changes that occur naturally with aging and behaviors that are commonly associated with medical conditions. Painful conditions such as degenerative joint disease are common and may impair mobility, leading to inappropriate elimination and decreased social interactions with people and other pets.

Mobility

Because musculoskeletal disease is very common in older cats, attention must be paid to ensure litter box, food, water, and sleeping places are easily accessed. A night-light placed near the litter box may be helpful for cats with failing eyesight.

Cognitive Dysfunction

Changes associated with cognitive dysfunction include increased disorientation, vocalization, attention-seeking or reclusiveness, and altered sleep patterns.

Quality of Life

Aged cats may need palliative care for pain control as well as other types of assistance (e.g., help with grooming, provision of nightlights, moving key resources into a smaller area). Clients can be provided with questionnaires to assess quality of life and help with end-of-life planning (Box 7-4).

BOX 7-4   Quality of Life Scale

Each question is answered with a score from 1 (poor) to 10 (best). A total score of 35 to 70 represents acceptable quality of life.

Hurt: Is the cat's pain successfully managed? Are there any breathing problems? Is oxygen necessary?

Score: _____

Hunger: Is the cat eating enough? Does the cat require assisted feeding, such as hand or syringe feeding or a feeding tube?

Score: _____

Hydration: Is the cat well hydrated? Are subcutaneous fluids necessary to supplement voluntary fluid intake?

Score: _____

Hygiene: Does the cat require assistance with grooming and cleanliness?

Score: _____

Happiness: Does the cat express joy and interest? Is the cat responsive to family, toys, other pets? Is the cat depressed, lonely, anxious, or afraid?

Score: _____

Mobility: Can the cat move around without assistance? Are there any problems with seizures or stumbling? Can the cat access key resources such as food, water, and the litter box?

Score: _____

More good days than bad: When bad days outnumber good days, quality of life may be too compromised. When a healthy human–animal bond is no longer possible, the end of life is near. Decisions should be made to avoid suffering and provide a peaceful and painless death.

Score: _____

Adapted from: Villalobos A: Palliation and pawspice care. In: Villalobos A, Kaplan L, editors: *Canine and feline geriatric oncology: honoring the human-animal bond,* New York, 2007, Wiley, pp. 293–318.

ADDITIONAL RESOURCES

General

American Association of Feline Practitioners (AAFP): 2004 AAFP feline behavior guidelines. http://www.catvets.com/guidelines/practice-guidelines/behavior-guidelines

Feline Advisory Bureau: Essential cattitude: an insight into the feline world. http://www.icatcare.org/sites/default/files/PDF/essential_cattitude.pdf

Life Stage Healthcare

American Animal Hospital Association (AAHA)/American Veterinary Medical Association (AVMA): AAHA-AVMA feline preventive healthcare guidelines (2011). https://www.aahanet.org/PublicDocuments/FelinePreventiveGuidelines_PPPH.pdf

American Association of Feline Practitioners (AAFP)/ American Veterinary Medical Association (AVMA): 2010 AAFP-AAHA feline life stage guidelines. http://www.catvets.com/guidelines/practice-guidelines/life-stage-guidelines

American Association of Feline Practitioners (AAFP): 2008 AAFP senior care guidelines. http://www.catvets.com/guidelines/practice-guidelines/senior-care-guidelines

American Association of Feline Practitioners (AAFP): Ten solutions to increase cat visits (2013). http://www.catvets.com/public/PDFs/Education/Solutions/solutionsbrochure.pdf

Lifestyle and the Home Environment

American Association of Feline Practitioners (AAFP)/ International Society of Feline Medicine (ISFM): 2013 AAFP/ISFM environmental needs guidelines. http://www.catvets.com/guidelines/practice-guidelines/environmental-needs-guidelines

Nutritional Assessment

American Animal Hospital Association (AAHA): 2010 AAHA nutritional assessment guidelines for dogs and cats. https://www.aaha.org/professional/resources/nutritional_assessment.aspx#gsc.tab=0

Pet Nutrition Alliance: Tips for implementing nutrition as a vital assessment in your practice. http://www.petnutritionalliance.org/pdfs/pna_tipsguide_aahaproof2.pdf

World Small Animal Veterinary Association (WSAVA) Global Nutrition Committee Nutritional Toolkit. http://www.wsava.org/nutrition-toolkit

World Small Animal Veterinary Association (WSAVA): Nutritional assessment guidelines. http://www.wsava.org/sites/default/files/JSAP%20WSAVA%20Global%20Nutritional%20Assessment%20Guidelines%202011_0.pdf

Retrovirus Testing

American Association of Feline Practitioners: 2008 AAFP Feline retrovirus management guidelines. http://www.catvets.com/guidelines/practice-guidelines/retrovirus-management-guidelines

European Advisory Board on Cat Diseases: Guidelines. http://www.abcd-vets.org/Pages/guidelines.aspx

Little S, Bienzle D, Carioto L, et al.: Feline leukemia virus and feline immunodeficiency virus in Canada: recommendations for testing and management. *Can Vet J* 52:849–855, 2011. http://www.ncbi.nlm.nih.gov/pmc/articles/PMC3135027/

Parasite Control

Centers for Disease Control and Prevention (CDC): Healthy pets healthy people. http://www.cdc.gov/healthypets/

Companion Animal Parasite Council (CAPC): http://www.capcvet.org/

European Scientific Counsel Companion Animal Parasites (ESSCAP): http://www.esccap.org/

Worms & Germs Blog: Promoting safe pet ownership: http://www.wormsandgermsblog.com/

REFERENCES

1. American Veterinary Medical Association. *U.S. pet ownership & demographics sourcebook.* 2012 ed. Schaumberg, IL: American Veterinary Medical Association; 2012. https://www.avma.org/kb/resources/statistics/pages/market-research-statistics-us-pet-ownership-demographics-sourcebook.aspx.

2. Perrin T. The Business of Urban Animals Survey: the facts and statistics on companion animals in Canada. *Can Vet J.* 2009;50:48–52.

3. Murray JK, Browne WJ, Roberts MA, et al. Number and ownership profiles of cats and dogs in the UK. *Vet Rec.* 2010;166:163–168.

4. Bayer Healthcare/American Association of Feline Practitioners: Veterinary Care Usage Study III: feline findings. http://www.bayerdvm.com/show.aspx/resources/feline-practitioners-resource-center/bayer-veterinary-care-usage-study Accessed September 20, 2013.

5. Lue TW, Pantenburg DP, Crawford PM. Impact of the owner-pet and client-veterinarian bond on the care that pets receive. *J Am Vet Med Assoc.* 2008;232:531–540.

6. Chandler ML, Gunn-Moore DA. Nutritional status of canine and feline patients admitted to a referral veterinary internal medicine service. *J Nutr.* 2004;134(8 Suppl):2050S–2052S.

7. Comparative Pain Research Laboratory, Department of Clinical Sciences, North Carolina State University College of Veterinary Medicine: Feline Musculoskeletal Pain Index. http://www.cvm.ncsu.edu/docs/cprl/fmpi.html Accessed September 9, 2013.

8. Stella JL, Lord LK, Buffington CAT. Sickness behaviors in response to unusual external events in healthy cats and cats with feline interstitial cystitis. *J Am Vet Med Assoc.* 2011;238:67–73.

9. Vogt AH, Rodan I, Brown M, et al. AAFP-AAHA: feline life stage guidelines. *J Feline Med Surg.* 2010;12:43–54.

10. Paepe D, Verjans G, Duchateau L, et al. Routine health screening: findings in apparently healthy middle-aged and old cats. *J Feline Med Surg.* 2013;15:8–19.

11. Buffington CAT. Idiopathic cystitis in domestic cats—beyond the lower urinary tract. *J Vet Intern Med.* 2011;25:784–796.

12. Cupp C, Perez-Camargo G, Patil A, et al. Long-term food consumption and body weight changes in a controlled population of geriatric cats [abstract]. *Compend Contin Educ Pract Vet.* 2004;26(Suppl 2A):60.

13. Laflamme DP, Ballam JM. Effect of age on maintenance energy requirements of adult cats [abstract]. *Compend Contin Educ Pract Vet.* 2002;24(Suppl 9A):82.

14. Harper EJ. Changing perspectives on aging and energy requirements: aging, body weight and body composition in humans, dogs and cats. *J Nutr.* 1998;128(12 Suppl):2627S–2631S.

15. Moore GE, DeSantis-Kerr AC, Guptill LF, et al. Adverse events after vaccine administration in cats: 2,560 cases (2002–2005). *J Am Vet Med Assoc.* 2007;231:94–100.

16. Ammersbach M, Little S, Bienzle D. Preliminary evaluation of a quantitative polymerase chain reaction assay for diagnosis of feline immunodeficiency virus infection. *J Feline Med Surg.* 2013;15:725–729.

Providing Appropriate Behavioral Care

Kersti Seksel

INTRODUCTION

Providing appropriate behavioral care needs to be a priority for all feline patients, both new pets and those whose environmental needs have not been met. There are many things that veterinarians need to know in order to educate cat owners to address the environmental needs of both existing and potential new cats. These include the importance of the layout of the home environment to provide for feline environmental needs, the presence of other animals already in the household, and appropriate and adequate physical and mental stimulation.

Appropriate behavioral care may prevent behavior problems[1,2] and lower stress, which may, in turn, lessen the chances of stress-related diseases such as interstitial cystitis.[3–5] Enrichment can alleviate boredom[2] and may play a role in preventing obesity and associated medical problems, such as diabetes mellitus, hepatic lipidosis, and degenerative joint disease.[2] Stress has a negative role in the development of feline interstitial cystitis, skin conditions such as infections and pruritus, and conditions such as irritable bowel syndrome.[5–7]

Addressing the environment of affected cats may help in reducing the number and severity of outbreaks of chronic diseases such as feline interstitial cystitis (FIC).[8,9] Enrichment devices and activities need to address the biological needs of cats as well as their individual preferences to have a positive effect on feline welfare.

INCORPORATING BEHAVIORAL CARE INTO THE VETERINARY PRACTICE

Educating clients about appropriate behavioral care is important for cats during all life stages. This education is used for both prevention and treatment of behavior problems and to reduce feline stress within the household. Although the first appointment with the new cat or kitten is the ideal time to introduce this information, cats at all life stages need appropriate behavioral care, and modification of existing programs can assist in preventing stress and behavior problems. See the "Key Points for Discussion of Behavior Needs During Preventive Care Visits, by Life Stage" section in Chapter 7 for discussion of how to incorporate this information into preventive care appointments.

THE HOME ENVIRONMENT

In general, cats do not like change, so most cats are stressed by a change in the environment or if an unfamiliar animal is added to the home. New cats will also have some degree of stress when they arrive at their new home. Additionally, for a kitten, this will probably be the first time that it has been separated from its mother and littermates, so this separation will add to the stress of not only moving to a new house but also meeting new people. Therefore, there is a need to keep things relatively low-key initially to avoid overwhelming the cat. It will be important to explain to all family members, especially children, that the cat will need a calm environment and may not appreciate cuddles until it is more familiar with the new home and people.

It is important to have a designated area where the cat can stay until it is more settled. Having a room ready with bedding, resting places, a litter box, and access to food and water where the cat or kitten can adjust to the sounds and smells of the new household is an important part of the adjustment period. Using a Feliway diffuser can help the cat settle into the new home faster and decrease its stress. For more information on how to introduce a new cat to existing cats, see Chapter 26.

Resting Areas

During the day, cats will spend, on average, 2.8 hours resting and 7.8 hours sleeping.[10] Comfortable, protected areas for the cat to sleep and rest need to be provided. Every room that the cats visit frequently should offer them appropriate hiding and perching places, as these can reduce their stress.[11] As cats are both predators and prey, they often feel more secure when they have a place to watch activities without being watched.

Hiding is a coping behavior that cats may display in response to stimuli or changes in their environment.[12]

It is commonly seen in stressful situations and when cats want to avoid interactions with other cats or with people.[13] Cats are more likely to rest or sleep alone,[14] so multiple comfortable resting areas should be provided. Even affiliate cats need the option of separate resting areas; in a study of 60 pairs of neutered, indoor-only cats, researchers found that cats spent approximately 48% to 50% of their time out of each other's sight.[15]

Good options for resting areas are cat carriers, soft cat beds with high sides, and boxes with cutout holes (Figure 8-1). Some resting areas should be large enough for only one cat because many cats prefer to rest alone, and even affiliate cats do not spend all their time together.

A carrier with soft bedding, such as fleece, can be used to assist in the process of habituating the kitten. Initially the carrier should be left out in an area that is commonly used by the kitten and in which it feels safe and secure. Treats can be used to increase positive associations with the carrier, for example, by throwing treats inside it and leaving the kitten to enter at its own pace. The door or lid of the carrier should be left open until the kitten is comfortable with entering and hopefully sleeping in it. At this stage the door or lid can be closed very briefly; provided the kitten remains relaxed, the door can then be closed for increasing periods of time. (For more information on training a cat to enter the carrier, see Chapter 9.)

Perching Areas

Cats often prefer to rest on elevated surfaces. Having perches increases overall space and allows the cat to monitor the environment. Vertical or three-dimensional space provides a vantage point for the cat to observe its surroundings and the approach of people and other animals.[16] Having different locations and levels helps cats avoid conflict and competition for resources.[17] Cats are more secure in their environment if they have choices of elevated places to sit as well as to hide.

There are many great options for providing accessible three-dimensional space for cat use (Figure 8-2). The most common are cat trees, perches, or shelves. However, as cat lovers work hard to improve indoor life for cats, more elaborate options, such as stairs going up walls and beams or tunnels just below the level of the ceiling, are being offered as a source of environmental enrichment. The theory is that these features help to provide sufficient space for cats to move around the property while avoiding unnecessary contact with other cats. To achieve this goal the design is crucial, to ensure that there are no narrow passages or bottlenecks in the system that would lead to cats coming face to face with each other. Other, more cost-effective options include allowing cats to rest on top of bookcases or other pieces of free-standing furniture.

Arthritic cats still like to climb and get to high places. Providing ramps, steps such as pet steps, or other aids so that cats can reach their favorite perches or other bedding lets them continue to access favored places and be with other family members.

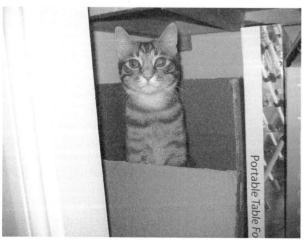

FIGURE 8-1 A cardboard box provides a favored resting place for this kitten. (Courtesy K. Lindsay)

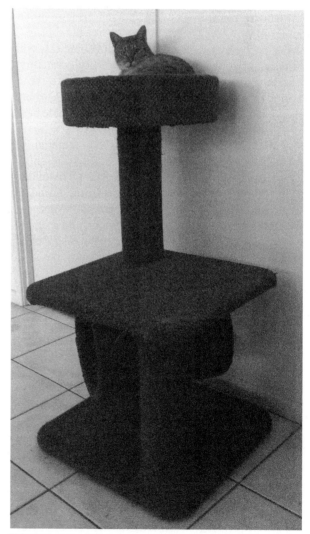

FIGURE 8-2 Cat towers provide multiple high resting places and opportunities to scratch. (Courtesy G. Perry)

Scratching Posts

Scratching is a normal feline behavior that is done to file or sharpen their claws, stretch their muscles, and leave their scent and visible markings. It is a form of communication with the deposition of an olfactory mark (pheromone) to convey temporal cues regarding its proximity or passage.[18] Cats often scratch when they are excited (such as when people come home or during play) and after sleeping.[18] Although both old and new objects will be scratched, many cats maintain interest in older scratching posts.[18]

Cats have individual preferences regarding the materials and orientation (vertical or horizontal) of the posts. Many cats prefer sisal rope or wood as scratching material. Every cat should have access to a scratching post that is attractive to it. If the cat does not like the material, it will scratch in other places, such as on the back of a couch with a material that may be more to the cat's liking. If the cat prefers to scratch on particular surfaces, it may help to provide a similar material on the scratching post. Owners should provide more than one scratching area and encourage the cat to use them by rewarding it with a food treat or quiet praise.

Most cats prefer vertical surfaces, but some cats will scratch at horizontal surfaces as well. Vertical scratching posts should ideally be tall enough for the cats to stand up on their back legs and reach up to scratch. Owners should ensure that posts are sturdy and on a stable base so that cats are not wary of using them.

Location is just as important as the material to scratch. It is advisable to have at least one scratching post in rooms most frequented by family members and in prominent well-traveled places in the home. If the cat is already scratching on furniture, the scratching post should be placed nearby and the furniture made less attractive by covering the areas the cat has scratched with plastic or double-sided tape. One study has also shown that spraying Feliway on scratched areas may decrease scratching.[19] More posts are needed in multicat homes, as not all cats share posts, depending on their relationship with each other.

Cats can be encouraged to scratch by using an interactive toy (such as a fishing pole–type toy with feathers) and waving it over the post or attaching a dangling toy to the post. Once a cat's scent is deposited on the post, the cat is more likely to return. Cats can also be clicker-trained to scratch at the posts as well.

Cat owners can use this information to both prevent and treat undesirable scratching, by providing scratching posts of a type and texture, as well as in a location, that would be most appealing to the cat.

When a cat's scratching appears to be excessive in frequency, locations, or duration, the possibility that the marking is related to stress or anxiety (as with urine marking) should be considered, and there may be a need for increased environmental enrichment (with care, as too many choices may increase anxiety and stress), identification and removal of potential stressors, and possibly pheromone therapy.

Litter Boxes

Cats that spend any time indoors need easy access to clean litter boxes. Litter boxes should be kept away from eating and sleeping areas. In multicat households, the rule of thumb is one litter box per cat "family", plus one extra, so that each cat in the family has suitable access to a toileting area. However, the positioning of the trays is as important as the number of them. For instance, in a two-cat household, three trays located side by side constitute just one toileting location, and, if the cats are not compatible, this provision may still be inadequate. The golden rule is that if all of the cats needed to eliminate at the same time, they should all be able to access a litter box without running the gauntlet of another cat. Ideally, all of the trays should be placed in separate locations.

Most cats prefer larger litter boxes over smaller ones.[20] It is often suggested that the litter box should be at least 1.5 times the length of the cat from the tip of its nose to the base of its tail, and therefore many commercially available litter boxes are not big enough. Good options are large plastic storage containers. For more information, see Chapter 24.

Many cats will toilet only in very clean trays, and cleaning regimes are therefore of particular importance from both a hygienic and a psychological perspective. All soiled material should be scooped from the trays as soon as it is noticed, and owners should completely change the litter at least once every week or two, depending on litter type. When the litter is completely changed, the tray should be cleaned with hot water and mild detergent; strong smelling detergents should be avoided. If possible, the tray should be left to air-dry, dried with a towel, or wiped out with an unscented cloth before refilling the tray with fresh litter. See Chapter 24 for more details on litter box care.

PLAY

Play is an important part of a cat's life. For animals that have all of their basic needs met, exploratory behavior becomes a greater priority in their time budget.[1] Most pet cats do not need to spend several hours each day hunting, so providing them with opportunities to play is an important part of enriching a well-fed and well-rested cat's time. Offering new toys or rotating toys every few days, as well as changing the location of toys, can create a "new" environment. Cats can habituate to hunt and chase toys within a few minutes, necessitating the introduction of a few different items within and between play sessions.[21]

Wild and feral cats spend a significant proportion of their waking time foraging and hunting for food. This behavior can be redirected to toys or feathers, for example, in domestic cats. Pet cats explore new objects in their environment and engage in play with small, prey-sized objects.[21] Toys that simulate prey are great outlets for predatory behaviors. Toys that dangle from a string or wire that can be made to "come alive" are excellent interactive toys and also allow "hunting."

During play sessions, owners should try to encourage appropriate games and interactions. Cats need to have clear rules about biting and clawing. Games should always be hands-off, and cats should not be allowed to play with human hands or feet, owing to the potential for injury from their claws or teeth. However, toys that encourage the behaviors of the hunting sequence, such as stalking, rushing, pouncing, and biting the toy are popular with cats and people and provide opportunities to engage in these normal behaviors. There are many suitable toy types available, including fishing rod–style toys.

Cats hunt in short bursts and owners can mimic this through interactive play with sudden changes in the toy's speed and direction.

Toys need to appeal to the cat in size and texture. Focusing on the cat's senses and its individual preferences will make the toy more appealing. However, many toys are designed to appeal to owners rather than their cats in terms of color, shape, size, and texture.

Visually, there are typically five ways for animals to differentiate between objects: luminance (or brightness), motion, texture, binocular disparity (depth), and color.

Perception of movement is a critical aspect of vision for catching prey. Rod photoreceptors are important for detecting motion and shapes, especially in dim light. Humans have a fovea, which is better equipped for detecting motion in bright light and in direct view, but cats do not have a fovea, so they appear to detect motion better peripherally, in dim light, and when the object is moving at a certain speed. This may explain why cats ignore static objects, but, once in motion, the objects elicit a chase response. Hence, toys that move are likely to be more appealing to the cat.

Whereas cats may quickly habituate and lose interest in one toy, play intensity actually may be heightened in the short term, so play should be repeated with up to three or four different toys with slightly different characteristics (e.g., interactive play with a toy on a wand, a ponytail holder on a string, self-play with a ball in a track, or chasing a milk ring). After play sessions, the cat's interest in further play may remain heightened for 15 minutes or more.

It is important that any toys or activities are suitable and safe for the cat (Figure 8-3). The fact that the toy is expensive does not necessarily mean that the cat will like

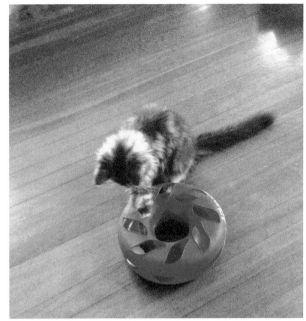

FIGURE 8-3 Cats often enjoy toys that allow movement and require manipulation. (Courtesy G. Perry)

the toy. Toys need to be carefully selected according to the cat's preferences and ability to destroy them. Owners need to be careful with parts that could snap or break off or that could be chewed off and potentially swallowed. Check toys regularly for damage, and always supervise the cat when introducing a new toy.

Cats can be taught to retrieve and often enjoy homemade toys, such as scrunched-up paper, or inexpensive jingle balls. Cats love tunnels (Figure 8-4) and cardboard boxes to hide in, but there is a need to be careful regarding where they are placed so that predatory behavior toward humans or between cats is not accidentally encouraged or stimulated.

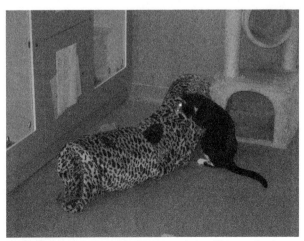

FIGURE 8-4 Cats love hiding, so many like to play in cat tunnels. (Courtesy G. Perry)

FEEDING

Normal Feeding Behavior

Cats are solitary hunters, eating 10 to 20 small meals per day, with repeated cycles of hunting to catch their small prey. Not all attempts to catch prey are successful. Some suggest that up to 50% of the feline hunt cycles are unsuccessful[12] and this results in cats expending a great deal of time and energy to survive.

Regardless of how much cats are fed, the hunting instinct still exists; cats often bring in unwanted "presents" to their people. Cats are also crepuscular animals, hunting primarily at dawn and dusk, when their prey is usually present.

Drinking Behavior

Cats in the wild drink water in locations separate from their food. Some cats prefer running water and enjoy drinking fountains (Figure 8-5), whereas others prefer still water. Water dishes should be provided in multiple locations and away from food.

Feeding Strategies

Many domestic cats tend to graze, so varying feeding strategies can encourage activity in sedentary individuals and provide a varied enrichment schedule for more active cats. Food can be placed inside toys (food puzzles) to provide additional stimulation. These can include simple toys that are nudged with a paw or nose to cause the cat kibble to fall out of specially made holes. There are also more complex toys that require more

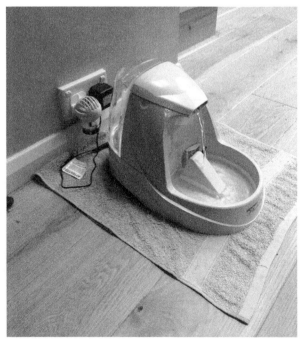

FIGURE 8-5   Some cats prefer running water and like to use drinking fountains. (Courtesy S. Heath)

sophisticated manipulation with the paws to get to the food. Food-dispensing toys can be homemade (yogurt containers with holes cut out are a good example) or purchased at the local pet store or online. Scatter feeding and hiding the food in various locations can also provide physical as well as mental stimulation for cats. Cats that hunt for food will chase, capture, and eat multiple small meals a day. Therefore, some cats may benefit from more play sessions and multiple, smaller, "prey-sized" meals. For more information, see Chapter 13.

Wild and feral cats frequently eat grass.[10] Cat grass offers a safe grazing choice for cats kept indoors. If the cat grass is periodically relocated, the cat will have to seek out the forage. This not only mimics a natural behavior but also provides physical and mental stimulation for the cat.

GROOMING

All cats need to engage in grooming behavior regardless of coat length, and for cats that enjoy physical contact and attention, brushing and hand grooming can be considered a form of enrichment. Grooming mitts are usually well tolerated but they are useful only for single-coated shorthair cats. Brushes and combs are good choices for grooming the top coat but when cats have a thick undercoat, a fine-toothed comb or deshedding tool (e.g., a "FURminator") is needed. Brushing and hand grooming can be considered a form of enrichment for cats that enjoy physical contact and attention.

Positive reinforcement training can be used to train a number of simple behaviors, such as "sit" and "come when called," so that the cat will come to be groomed and sit while the grooming occurs. With proper training, nail clipping and toothbrushing can be considered another positive form of human attention,[22] which highlights the overlap between providing appropriate behavioral care and appropriate healthcare for domestic cats.

CAT TRAINING

Visits to the veterinarian will be less frightening for the cat if it is trained to accept a health inspection, which involves being restrained and palpated thoroughly. Introduction to this sort of interaction should begin as early as possible, and acceptance of the handling can be enhanced by using well-timed rewards in the form of food or toys.

Cats respond really well to reward-based training using favored food treats, such as little pieces of chicken, meat, or fish. They can be taught to sit, come, "high-five," or anything you have the imagination to teach. Reward-based training provides mental stimulation for cats as well as owners. The reward must be highly desirable for the cat.

Positive reinforcement training can also be enriching to cats,[22] and training is another way to enhance the human–animal bond and improve the welfare of the cat.[23] (See Chapter 5 for more information about learning in cats.)

Kitten Kindy®

The idea of training cats, let alone the idea of holding kitten socialization and training classes, is a foreign concept to most people.[24] Kitten Kindy is an early socialization, training, and education program designed to help owners and kittens start off on the right track in life.

The classes socialize kittens at a young age so that they can adjust to going out into the world. The kittens are desensitized to the cat carrier and to car travel. Kittens in socialization classes are exposed to different people and other kittens, but the introductions are passive in nature and no kittens are forced to interact socially. Kitten class experiences may help make kittens more prepared to accept and enjoy more enriched lifestyles as they grow, as well as to become more malleable to change. These classes provide an opportunity to educate cat owners in appropriate handling and management and may help prevent behaviors that owners find unacceptable. The aim is also to establish close bonds between the cat, the owner, and the veterinary practice. Provided there is a suitable kitten-proof location within the practice, these classes represent another valuable service that veterinarians can offer their patients and clients. If an appropriate area is not available, the provision of kitten information evenings, where owners attend without their kittens, can be a more appropriate way to educate clients on the behavioral needs of their feline companion.

OTHER PETS IN THE HOME

Is There Already Another Cat in the Household?

Cats are social animals[2] and are often found in the vicinity of people with whom they have bonded. Being social animals, cats enjoy not only human companionship but also that of members of their own and other species. The most socially compatible groups of cats within households are those that are related to one another, and siblings from the same litter can make great housemates (Figure 8-6). However, there can be extensive individual variation in levels of sociability to other cats, depending on genetic predisposition, early experiences, and previous encounters with other cats. When owners are trying to introduce cats that are not genetically related to one another, it is important to take this variation into account. Even if the resident cat has lived amicably with a previous cat, it may not do so with a new cat. Owners who wish to add a second cat to their household need advice to maximize the likelihood the addition will be

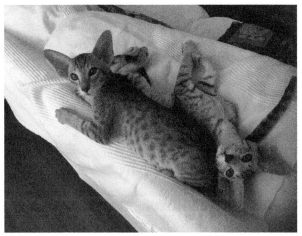

FIGURE 8-6 Two kittens from the same litter can provide great company for each other. (Courtesy G. Perry)

successful.[25] Separate areas for cats must be provided initially, and a plan must be developed for gradual introductions. It is not a good idea to bring the cat home, just place it in the same room with the other cat, and hope they get along or work it out.

Initial introductions should be gradual and positive to increase the chances of long-term success (Figure 8-7).[26] Introductions need to be handled with care, slowly and gradually, with supervision by owners. It is best to let the cats get used to the sounds and smells of the other cat for a few days (to weeks) and then, when they are both calm, allow a short period of time when they can see each other, perhaps through a glass or screen door. If there is no adverse response, such as hissing or spitting from either cat, then this step can be repeated on a daily basis, gradually increasing the periods of time that the cats can see each other. They should be rewarded for calm behavior with praise, gentle stroking, a game, or treats, depending on the cat's individual preference.

Over time, the cats can be allowed to come into contact with each other for longer periods of time. This may take several weeks, and progressing more slowly will pay dividends later. If the cats do hiss or spit at each other,

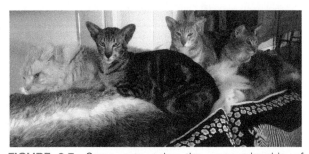

FIGURE 8-7 Some cats enjoy the companionship of other cats, whereas others are happier in a single-cat home. (Courtesy G. Perry)

then their owners will need to separate them for at least 48 hours before trying to introduce them again. For more information on introducing cats, see Chapter 26 and the handout titled **Creating Successful Transitions to Your Home**.

Is There Already a Dog in the Household?

For some cats, a dog may be easier to introduce as a companion. Exposure to dogs at an early age has been shown to be helpful in cats accepting dogs as adults (Figure 8-8).[27] Before introducing a new cat or kitten, the owner should consider whether the dog and cat will share the same living space or have separate areas. Will the cat live indoors or upstairs and the dog live outside or downstairs? Has the dog lived with cats before, or has the cat lived with dogs in its previous home? Is the dog a known cat chaser? These are all factors that need to be considered and addressed so that the introduction of the new cat is as smooth and stress-free as possible.

Gradual introductions should be done at times when both the cat and the dog are calm and relaxed. Ideally, the dog should reliably respond to verbal cues, such as sit, come, and stay, and should be able to settle on cue. These skills should be taught to the dog prior to any introduction of the cat.

Ideally, the introductions start with the cat in a cat carrier at a distance from the dog. The dog should be asked to adopt a relaxed, stationary position before the cat enters the room, and then it should be encouraged to remain in that position through appropriate use of positive reinforcement. If there is no adverse reaction from the cat or the dog to the sight, smell, and sound of each other for several short introduction periods, then the owner can progress to the next step. The dog should be asked to remain calm and relaxed on its mat, and the cat can be allowed to move freely around the room while the dog is rewarded for being relaxed in the presence of

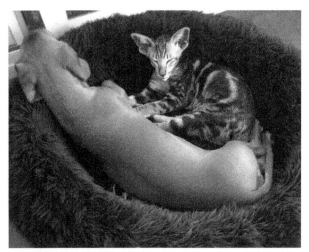

FIGURE 8-8 A dog and a cat can enjoy a harmonious relationship if introductions are made gradually. (Courtesy G. Perry)

the cat. If the sight of the moving cat is too salient for the dog at any stage and the dog is unable to maintain a relaxed posture, it may be necessary to confine the cat in a carrier again for shorter introduction periods. The cat could also be placed in a pen, which must be of appropriate size and should ideally include furniture that enables the cat to hide and/or elevate so that it can manage its own stress.

For welfare reasons, it is critical not to leave cat and dog together unsupervised until it can be established that there will not be an issue. Even when both seem relaxed in the presence of the other, the cat must be provided with safe places, or bolt holes, preferably up high where the dog cannot go.

INDOOR OR OUTDOOR CAT OR BOTH

These days many people, not only those who live in apartments, are choosing to keep their cats confined indoors for health and safety reasons. People who wish to prevent their cats from being hurt or killed on the roads, who do not want to have to deal with cat fights and the injuries and diseases associated with them, and those who do not want their cats to be responsible for hunting and killing wildlife are now choosing to keep their cats inside. Some jurisdictions have also introduced legislation to restrict the number of cats people can own, as well as cat curfews. This means that many more cats are living indoors 100% of the time.

Some authors feel that this is good news for cats, as it has been shown that the average life span of an indoor cat is much longer than that of an outdoor cat.[28] It also means cats are spending more time with their families. Many cats enjoy human companionship, and living indoors enables a cat to have this in abundance. Cats greet their owners when they come home, sleep in bed with them, sit on their laps, or beside them on the couch in the evening. They may not always want direct contact, but they often like being in the same room and follow their owners around the home. Special cuddle time, pats, and brushing are all activities many cats can enjoy with their owners.

If the cat is to be totally confined indoors, then the owner needs to appreciate that they will have to provide all the mental and physical stimulation necessary for the cat. Cats have a natural tendency to climb; therefore, access to vertical space (or three-dimensional space) is much more important than horizontal space. Cats tend to spend time in elevated locations and look down on the scene below. Many indoor cats climb up onto furniture or climb the curtains looking for an elevated resting space. If owners do not want the cat sitting on top of or in the wardrobe, then alternate (and more attractive for the cat) resting places will need to be provided. These may include scratching posts with raised platforms as well as shelves and cat towers. When making provision for resting places, it is important to use three-dimensional space to ensure that cats will not inadvertently contribute to the stress of other cats, especially in multicat households. Advising clients to invest in cat towers with hiding tunnels rather than boxes is a good example. If a cat in a hiding tunnel is approached by an incompatible feline, it can get out of the way by reversing or advancing, but if it is in a box with only one entrance and exit, it can become trapped. Similarly, it can help to ensure that some of the resting places in the house are big enough for only one cat, as this can avoid problems of incompatible cats attempting to share platforms. (See the Resources section at the end of this chapter for information on indoor cats.)

Other authors suggest that allowing cats some degree of free access to an outside environment is beneficial to allow them to fulfill natural behaviors such as exploring, hunting, and observing (Figure 8-9). It appears that there is a strong cultural influence on the decision whether to let cats have freedom to roam in the vicinity of their homes, with significant differences in the numbers of cats that are kept exclusively indoors in different countries.[29] In the United Kingdom, it is common for cats to be given freedom to roam and to have access to gardens adjoining their property in addition to that of their owners. In the United States and Australia, it is common for cats to be kept exclusively indoors.

Although life may be safer for indoor-only cats, and though being indoors has been shown to prolong a cat's life span,[28] it is acknowledged that cats do have a need for a wide range of visual and olfactory stimulation. Living inside does not mean that the cat's life has to be dull or that the cat never gets to enjoy the outside world. There are more and more options for people who want to keep

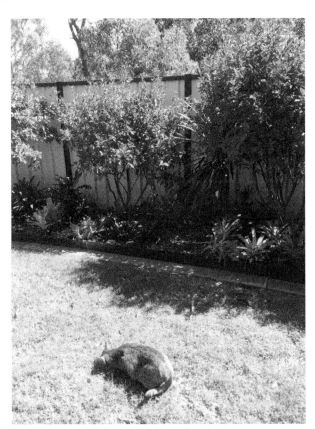

FIGURE 8-10 Access to this confined outdoor space provides a safe environment that allows for increased sensory stimulation and opportunities to perform normal feline behaviors. (Courtesy G. Perry)

their cats safe and sound, but also want to cater to their cat's physical and psychological needs (Figure 8-10).

Some owners may train their cats to wear a harness and walk on a lead. This allows the cat to have time outside in the sun, a walk around the garden, or a sniff of some grass and plants. Teaching a cat to wear a harness is not difficult, but it must be done gradually. Small pieces of tasty food can be used as rewards for the cat while the harness is slowly introduced. Once trained, many cats view the harness as a positive thing, as it means they will be able to explore the backyard. Some indoor cats can be a bit overwhelmed or frightened when first taken outside, so owners need to take things slowly and quickly return to the house if the cat seems concerned.

If the cat is to be let outside unsupervised but still kept within the confines of the yard, then the owner has to address ways to cat-proof the yard. These provisions may include high, solid fences, specifically designed cat-proof fencing, saggy wires that the cat is unable to climb over, or purpose-built outdoor cat enclosures (Figure 8-11).

There are many varieties of outdoor cat enclosures available, ranging from free-standing cat enclosures to complex modular systems that can be built onto the

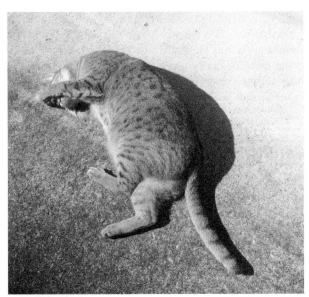

FIGURE 8-9 Cats enjoy spending time in the sunshine. (Courtesy G. Perry)

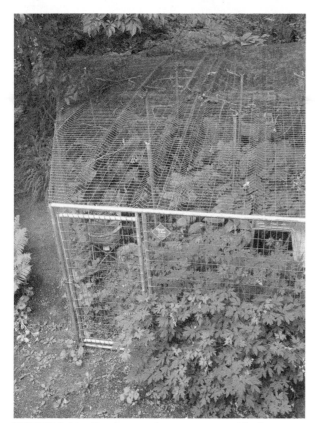

FIGURE 8-11   Outdoor enclosures can provide the opportunity for safe time outside the house. (Courtesy MA Test & I. Rodan)

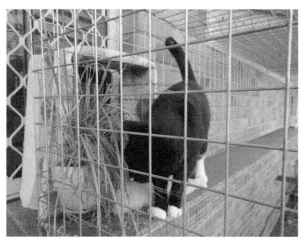

FIGURE 8-12   Cats with no access to a garden often enjoy grass in pots. (Courtesy K. Stevenson)

house. In most cases, a cat flap or open window allows the cat access to the enclosure (Figure 8-12). Another option is to cover an area of the yard with cat netting to make it escape proof. This is great for people who have a courtyard or similar area that can easily be made into a cat playground. Many apartments have a balcony or small courtyard. If the cat is to live in a high-rise

apartment with a balcony, then ways to keep the cat safe and prevent it from jumping or falling off the balcony will need to be addressed. Once cat-proofed, these areas enable the cat to sit in the sun or spend time outdoors. Many cats enjoy sniffing or chewing on cat grass or catnip, and these can be provided in pots indoors and on balconies, too.

Outdoor enclosures have many advantages, as they can provide the cat with safe outdoor access. However, there are also disadvantages, as the neighborhood cats may still threaten and even attack the cat through the enclosure walls, and, if access is through a tunnel, there may be social tension between household cats created by competition for access or by ambushing. The presence and view of other free roaming cats in the vicinity can be stressful to some cats, whether they are inside the house or in an outdoor enclosure, and can result in barrier frustration and redirected aggression towards other family members, both human and feline.[19]

In order to make access to an outdoor enclosure as beneficial as possible, there will need to be suitable furniture and resting places provided in the yard or enclosure. Cat ladders, cat trees, hammocks, igloos, shelves, and tops of furniture are often favorite places for cats to snooze. Inside the house, many cats like to be able to sit in the sun and look out of a window and watch the world go by, and an ability to engage in this sort of observational behavior from inside the enclosure will also be important.

Some owners prefer that their cat toilets outdoors, so allowing access to the outdoors is one of their primary objectives. However, this does not mean that litter boxes will not be needed at any stage, especially when the new cat first arrives in the household, as it will need time to settle in and become familiar with its surroundings. Ability to access outdoor toilets can be hampered by tensions with other cats in the neighborhood, and, in some cases, it may be necessary to provide purpose-built toilets close to the house to allow access (Box 8-1). If these toilets are designed to be used year-round, it is important to fill them with materials that will not freeze.[14]

CONCLUSION

Providing appropriate behavioral care takes effort, but it should be considered an important part of caring for companion cats (Figure 8-13). It strengthens the human–animal bond through interaction and play, and good environmental enrichment can also help reduce the incidence and severity of chronic diseases, such as feline idiopathic cystitis (FIC), chronic bowel conditions, and skin disease. More studies are required to investigate how best to enrich the environment of companion cats.

BOX 8-1 Providing Outdoor Toilets

House-soiling problems tend to be worse in the winter, which is probably because outdoor toilets become difficult or unappealing for the cat to use. Hard, frozen ground is difficult to dig and waterlogged, heavy soil is messy and unpleasant for the cat. Remember that cats are evolved from desert-living ancestors.

Outdoor toilets reduce your cat's need to have an indoor litter tray or can help to reduce the number of indoor litter trays needed in a multi-cat household. They can be constructed easily to make them low-maintenance and available for the cat to use all year round.

- Find a suitable location for the toilet at the edge of the garden, obscured by flowerbeds and bushes to give the cat some privacy.
- Dig a hole that is approximately 60–90 cm deep and 60–90 cm square.
- Fill the bottom two-thirds
- Top up the hole with soft, white sand. Use playground quality sand and not the orange type used for building (known as sharp sand).
- Once your cat is using the toilet regularly, you can scatter a little earth over the top to disguise it.
- Use a litter scoop to remove any feces, as you would with a conventional indoor tray.
- Dig out and replace the sand every few months to refresh the toilet.

Sand toilets get neither waterlogged nor frozen and they give the cat an easily accessible toilet close to the house. Some cats cannot find a proper toilet in their own garden and have to go several houses away to find a suitable location. Apart from increasing the probability of a house-soiling problem if that toilet ceases to be available, it also tends to annoy neighbors.

From Bowen J, Heath S: Improving the outdoor environment for cats: Appendix 3 In *Behaviour problems in small animals: practical advice for the veterinary team*, ed 1, St Louis, 2005, Saunders, pp. 265-266

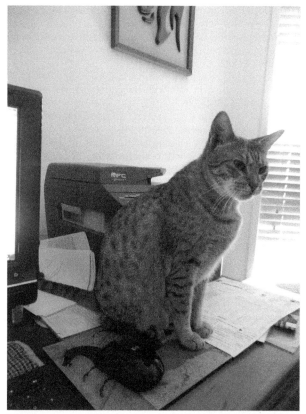

FIGURE 8-13 Well-socialized cats enjoy being with their owners while they go about their daily business. (Courtesy G. Perry)

Ellis S, Rodan I, Carney H, et al. AAFP and ISFM Feline Environmental Needs Guidelines. *J Fel Med & Surg*. 2013; 15:219-230. http://www.catvets.com/guidelines/practice-guidelines/environmental-needs-guidelines. Accessed September 2014.

Jackson V: Four legs // four walls design guidelines: a comprehensive guide to housing design with pets in mind. Camberwell, Australia, 2010, Petcare Information and Advisory Service Australia/Harlock Jackson. http://www.petsinthecity.net.au/sites/default/files/four_legs_four_walls.pdf

Your Cat's Environmental Needs: Practical Tips for Pet Owners. http://www.catvets.com/public/PDFs/ClientBrochures/Environmental%20GuidelinesEViewFinal.pdf. Accessed September 2014.

ADDITIONAL RESOURCES

College of Veterinary Medicine, The Ohio State University: The indoor pet initiative. http://indoorpet.osu.edu/cats/

REFERENCES

1. Young RJ. *Environmental Enrichment for Captive Animals*. New York: Wiley-Blackwell; 2003.
2. Overall K, Rodan I, Beaver B, et al. *American Association of Feline Practitioners (AAFP). Feline Behavior Guidelines from the American Association of Feline Practitioners*; 2004. http://www.catvets.com/public/PDFs/Practice Guidelines/FelineBehaviorGLS.pdf.
3. Buffington CA. External and internal influences on disease risk in cats. *J Am Vet Med Assoc*. 2002;220:994–1002.
4. Cameron ME, Casey RA, Bradshaw JW, et al. A study of environmental and behavioural factors that may be associated with feline idiopathic cystitis. *J Small Anim Pract*. 2004;45:144–147.
5. Buffington CA, Westropp JL, Chew DJ, Bolus RR. Clinical evaluation of multimodal environmental modification

(MEMO) in the management of cats with idiopathic cystitis. *J Feline Med Surg.* 2006;8:261–268.

6. Nagata M, Shibata K. Importance of psychogenic factors in canine recurrent pyoderma [P-5]. *Vet Dermatol.* 2004;15 (suppl S1):42.

7. Westropp JL, Kass PH, Buffington CAT. Evaluation of the effects of stress in cats with idiopathic cystitis. *Am J Vet Res.* 2006;67:731–736.

8. Bhatia V, Tandon RK. Stress and the gastrointestinal tract. *J Gastroenterol Hepatol.* 2005;20:332–339.

9. Ibáñez Talegón M, Dominguez Villalba C, Marin CY. Cats showing comfort or well-being behaviour in cages with an enriched and controlled environment. In: Overall KL, Mills DS, Heath SE, Horwitz D, eds. *Proceedings of Third International Congress on Veterinary Behavioural Medicine.* Wheathampstead, UK: Universities Federation for Animal Welfare; 2001:50–52.

10. Beaver BV. *Feline Behavior: A Guide for Veterinarians.* 2nd ed. St Louis: Saunders/Elsevier; 2003.

11. Kry K, Casey R. The effect of hiding enrichment on stress levels and behaviour of domestic cats (*Felis sylvestris catus*) in a shelter setting and the implications for adoption potential. *Anim Welf.* 2007;16:375–383.

12. Rochlitz I. Basic requirements for good behavioural health and welfare in cats. In: Horwitz D, Mills D, eds. *BSAVA Manual of Canine and Feline Behavioural Medicine.* 2nd ed. Gloucester, UK: British Small Animal Veterinary Association (BSAVA); 2009:35–48.

13. Carlstead K, Brown JL, Strawn W. Behavioral and physiological correlates of stress in laboratory cats. *Appl Anim Behav Sci.* 1993;38:143–158.

14. Bowen J, Heath S. An overview of feline social behaviour and communication. In: *Behaviour Problems in Small Animals: Practical Advice for the Veterinary Team.* 1st ed. St Louis: Saunders; 2005:29–36.

15. Rochlitz I. Housing and welfare. In: *The Welfare of Cats.* 3rd ed. New York: Springer; 2007:177–203.

16. Patronek G, Sperry E. Quality of life in long-term confinement. In: August J, ed. *Consultations in Feline Internal Medicine.* 4th ed. Philadelphia: Saunders; 2001:621–634.

17. Ellis SL, Rodan I, Carney HC, et al. AAFP and ISFM feline environmental needs guidelines. *J Feline Med Surg.* 2013;15:219–230.

18. Landsberg G. Feline behavior and welfare. *J Am Vet Med Assoc.* 1996;208:502–505.

19. Landsberg G, Hunthausen W, Ackerman L. *Handbook of Behavior Problems of the Dog and Cat.* New York: Saunders; 2004.

20. Guy NC, Hopson M, Vanderstichel R. Litterbox size preference in domestic cats (*Felis catus*). *J Vet Behav.* 2014;9:78–82.

21. Hall SL, Bradshaw JWS, Robinson IH. Object play in adult domestic cats: the roles of habituation and disinhibition. *Appl Anim Behav Sci.* 2002;79:263–271.

22. Yin S. *Low Stress Handling, Restraint and Behavior Modification of Dogs & Cats: Techniques for Developing Patients Who Love their Visits.* Davis, CA: CattleDog Publishing; 2009.

23. Bennett PC, Rohlf VI. Owner-companion dog interactions: relationships between demographic variables, potentially problematic behaviours, training engagement and shared activities. *Appl Anim Behav Sci.* 2007;102:65–84.

24. Seksel K. *Training Your Cat.* Carlton, Australia: Hyland House; 2001.

25. Casey RA, Bradshaw JWS. Evaluation of advice to owners on the introduction of an adult cat from a rescue shelter into a household with one or more adult cats. In: Heath SE, ed. *Proceedings of the 12th European Congress on Companion Animal Behavioural Medicine.* Lovendegem, Belgium: European Society of Veterinary Ethology (ESCVE); 2006.

26. Levine E, Perry P, Scarlett J, Houpt KA. Intercat aggression in households following the introduction of a new cat. *Appl Anim Behav Sci.* 2005;90:325–336.

27. Feuerstein N, Terkel J. Interrelationships of dogs (*Canis familiaris*) and cats (*Felis catus* L.) living under the same roof. *Appl Anim Behav Sci.* 2008;113:150–165.

28. Dodman N. *The Great Debate: Indoor vs. Outdoor Cats.* http://www.petplace.com/cats/the-great-debate-indoor-versus-outdoor-cats/page1.aspx.

29. Rochlitz I. A review of the housing requirements of domestic cats (*Felis silvestris catus*) kept in the home. *Appl Anim Behav Sci.* 2005;93:97–109.

PART 4

Prevention of Behavior Problems: The Cat at the Practice

CHAPTER

9

The Cat in the Veterinary Practice

Martha Cannon and Ilona Rodan

INTRODUCTION

A visit to the veterinary practice can be a highly stressful experience for a cat from start to finish. The experience is frightening for a species that needs a sense of control and familiarity to feel safe, and the distress this causes to both cat and client is a leading cause of cats not receiving the veterinary care they need and deserve.

From the moment that the carrier is brought out, the cat will be aware that its secure daily routine is about to be interrupted. It is then unwillingly loaded into that carrier, transported in a vehicle, carried into a veterinary waiting room from which there is no hope of escape, placed on an exposed and often slippery consulting room table, and then handled in unfamiliar and unpleasant ways by a stranger. Each of these stages runs contrary to the cat's natural inclination to be a solitary individual that exists within an established territory and uses avoidance and flight as its main means of dealing with conflict and fear. It is no wonder that cats may become frightened and then display fear-associated aggression at the veterinary practice (Figure 9-1); indeed, even those cats that appear to cope well with the experience are still exposed to a degree of stress and distress, which they may express in very subtle ways. To better understand the experience from the cat's perspective, encourage clients to watch the video "Scotty Goes to the Vet" by Dr. Sheilah Robertson produced on behalf of the CATalyst Council.[1] Clients may also gain some empathy from watching the video "Henri 3, Le Vet."[2]

By understanding the sources of stress and taking simple, inexpensive, but effective steps to reduce them, veterinarians can go a long way toward reducing the extent of the problem, allowing them to work more easily with feline patients and to do a better job for them and for their owners.

STRESS IN THE VETERINARY PRACTICE

The Impact on the Cat

For a cat, a trip to the veterinarian is unpleasant and frightening at the time it is happening, and the consequences of stress also have more far-reaching implications:

- The fearful state of the cat will be reflected in its behavior, often making it difficult to examine the cat and impossible to detect subtle changes in mobility and well-being.
- High sympathetic drive will affect parameters such as heart rate, respiratory rate, blood pressure, and blood glucose (Box 9-1). This has led to stress-associated findings being treated medically. For example, because stress hyperglycemia can be as high as 613 mg/dL,[3] some cats have been treated with insulin when not truly diabetic.
- A frightened, defensive cat will be more difficult to handle when more detailed examinations such as orthopedic, neurologic, or ophthalmologic examinations are required, and well-meaning but inappropriate methods of handling and restraint can rapidly make things worse.
- The inherent difficulty in handling such a cat often inhibits veterinarians from undertaking simple and essential procedures such as collection of blood and urine samples, so the cat receives a less than optimal level of veterinary care.
- Tight restraint (see Chapter 20 about appropriate handling) of the fearful, aggressive cat is likely to cause injury to staff and perhaps to clients. Situations resulting in legal liability to the veterinarian occur in litigious societies.

All of these inevitable consequences of a cat's fear and stress will contribute to a reduced ability to diagnose and manage its diseases.

The Impact on the Owner

Cat owners love their cats; in a U.S. survey,[4] 78% of cat owners considered their cats family members. Therefore, they want to do the best they can for their cats, and this is reflected in their spending in pet shops and online. However, this dedication to the cat's welfare and this willingness to spend money are often not reflected in the uptake of veterinary heath care for cats. The annually conducted Bayer Veterinary Care Usage studies indicate that, in the United States, cat owners visit veterinary practices less often than dog owners (an average of 1.7 visits per year compared to 2.8 visits

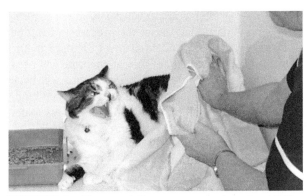

FIGURE 9-1   Characteristic appearance of a cat exhibiting fear-associated aggression.

per year).[5] Similarly, the American Veterinary Medical Association reported that cat owners spend less than half as much money at the veterinary practice than dog owners do (an average of $90 per year compared to $227 per year).[6]

Historically, this reluctance to come to the veterinary practice has been related to the perceived "low value" of a cat compared to a dog, leading to an unwillingness to spend money. In modern times, however, this is no longer the case—cat owners love their cats as much as dog owners love their dogs. It is important to recognize that a major factor in the reduced veterinary care received by cats compared to dogs relates to the stress and difficulty involved in bringing a cat to the veterinary practice as well as the fact that cats demonstrate only subtle signs of pain and illness. In a recent UK study,[7] 27% of cat owners said that stress to the cat during a veterinary visit was a very important factor when deciding whether to vaccinate their cat. The U.S. Bayer Veterinary Care Usage Study (2011)[8] demonstrated similar findings. In a survey of over 1000 cat owners, 58.2% said that their cat hates to go to the veterinarian, and, when asked about stress to the owners themselves, 37.6% said that "just thinking about taking their cat to the veterinarian is stressful." Furthermore, in a survey of 200 cat owners conducted jointly by International Society of Feline Medicine (ISFM) and a popular UK cat magazine (*Your Cat* magazine), 20% of the respondents said that their most recent visit to a veterinarian had been sufficiently stressful or unsatisfactory that they would either avoid going back or would change veterinarians.

The Impact on the Practice

Dealing with stressed cats and stressed clients is also stressful for veterinary staff.

- Fearful cats may rapidly become aggressive, and the need to handle them places veterinary personnel at risk of bites and scratches that would be avoided if the cat were calmer.
- Anxious and unhappy clients are less receptive to advice and less likely to return at recommended intervals for follow-up care for their cat. They may be more likely to find fault and be more aggressive in their communications simply because of the stress they are feeling while at the veterinary practice.

Keeping cats and their owners happy is clearly a worthwhile aim in itself, and it can also have positive benefits for the success of a veterinary practice.

Taking simple steps that will improve the experience of the cat and the owner when they visit the veterinary practice will improve cat welfare, bond cat-owning

---

BOX 9-1   Physiologic and Diagnostic Parameters That Are Affected by Stress

The following abnormalities are seen in healthy but stressed cats. It is important to assess the patient's fear prior to making a decision about illness or pain based on these examination or laboratory abnormalities.

Examination findings associated with fear
- Tachycardia
- Bradycardia (if long term)
- Increased respiratory rate
- Dilated pupils
- Hyperthermia
- Stress colitis, with soft stool, with blood, and/or with mucus on the surface of the stool

Diagnostic testing abnormalities that can be associated with fear
- Stress hyperglycemia* with or without glucosuria
- Hypokalemia due to epinephrine release‡
- Hypertension
  - Cats can have a systolic blood pressure over 200 mm Hg associated with stress†
- Platelet hypersensitivity‡
- Lymphocytosis‡
- Neutrophilia‡

*Rand JS, Kinnaird E, Baglioni A, et al: Acute stress hyperglycemia in cats is associated with struggling and increased concentrations of lactate and norepinephrine. J Vet Intern Med 16:123–132, 2002.
†DiBartola SP, de Morais HA: Disorders of potassium. In DiBartola SP, editor: *Fluid therapy in small animal practice*, ed 2. Philadelphia: Saunders; 2000:83–107.
‡Greco DS: The effect of stress on the evaluation of feline patients. In August JR, editor: *Consultations in feline internal medicine*, ed 1. Philadelphia: W.B. Saunders Company; 1991:13–17.

clients to the practice, and improve business. Furthermore, happier cat-owning clients will spread the word to their friends, improving the reputation of the practice and acting as the most effective marketing tool there is for growing the business.

Later chapters will provide more detailed advice on making all aspects of the veterinary practice more cat-friendly, but before this is discussed in detail, there are two guiding principles that should be kept in mind at all times: "cattitude" and species separation.

"Cattitude"

Cats and cat lovers sense when they are with those who understand and care about cats. One of the most important aspects of developing a cat-friendly clinic or practice involves the attitude of the staff, and that means all of the staff members who are involved with the healthcare of cats, including receptionists, technicians or nurses, veterinarians, and kennel assistants. It is essential that all staff members adopt a positive attitude toward cats and their owners—it is important to have "cattitude." For some people, this will come naturally; others may need to work at it, but learning more about cats and their behavior will help them to develop a genuine understanding of their needs and of their likely reactions to handling and stress, thus building confidence that will be reflected in a calm, professional, cat-friendly manner that cats and clients will recognize and respond to.

Promoting a cat-friendly attitude in all staff members involves good training and motivation and will be more challenging for some members of the staff than for others. Once the commitment has been made to drive forward with change, it can be helpful to appoint a "cat advocate" within the practice. This person will be a member of staff, whether a veterinarian or veterinary nurse or technician, who is passionate about the process and will be empowered to suggest and implement changes in the daily running of the practice. The cat advocate will need to be a diplomatic trainer and manager and will have a good understanding of how the entire practice functions in order to be able to identify and address issues that arise in all parts of the veterinary practice.

Species Separation

Cats tend to be solitary creatures; they do not appreciate the close company of other "unknown" cats, and they definitely do not like being in close proximity to unknown and excitable, scared, or aggressive dogs. Separating the species as far as possible and allowing cats their "personal space" will go a long way toward reducing their stress. Attempt to separate cats and dogs within the veterinary practice in every way possible. Consider the physical space the cats inhabit, but also try to separate cats from the sight, sound, and smell of dogs to the maximum degree possible within the confines of the building. Achieving separation of the species will have a huge impact on the cats treated by the veterinary practice. These actions can be simple and inexpensive and the long-term benefits to cats and cat owners will be rewarding.

To encourage and support veterinary practices in their efforts to reduce stress for feline patients and their owners, the American Association of Feline Practitioners (AAFP) and ISFM have each created the Cat Friendly Clinic/Cat Friendly Practice self-accreditation scheme[11,12] (Box 9-2, Figure 9-2). This scheme recognizes and applauds those practices that have embraced the challenge of thinking differently about cats as patients and allows clients to identify the cat-friendly veterinary practices in the area.

BOX 9-2   The AAFP/ISFM Cat Friendly Clinic or Practice Scheme

The ISFM Cat Friendly Clinic and the AAFP Cat Friendly Practice standards comprise a self-assessment accreditation scheme open to any veterinary practice that deals with cat patients. It lays out a set of requirements regarding the design, equipment, and facilities within the veterinary practice but, equally importantly, it also covers the quality of care provided to cats, the level of understanding of cats and their needs in the veterinary practice and interaction between the veterinary practice and cat owners.

On applying to AAFP or ISFM, veterinary practices will be provided with the comprehensive *A Guide to Creating a Cat Friendly Clinic*, which offers a step-by-step approach to understanding cats. It also lists the requirements for becoming an accredited veterinary practice at either the Silver (essential) or Gold (advanced) level of certification. The packet includes an application form that details the individual criteria and supporting materials that need to be included with the application. Successful applicants will be awarded the Cat Friendly Clinic or Practice standard (at the appropriate level) and given supporting materials to use within the veterinary practice along with the right to use the Cat Friendly Clinic or Practice logo (Figure 9-2) on their website and on their practice literature. Veterinary practices that have been successful in their application will also be listed on the relevant AAFP/ISFM websites so that cat owners can look for veterinary practices in their neighborhood that have the AAFP/ISFM Cat Friendly Clinic or Practice certification as a mark of the standard of care they can expect to receive. Veterinary practices need to reaccredit every 2 years to maintain their status. For more information, refer to the AAFP and ISFM websites.[11,12]

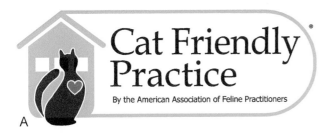

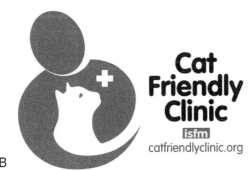

catfriendlyclinic.org

FIGURE 9-2   A practice that is accredited as an AAFP Cat Friendly Practice or an International Cat Care Cat Friendly Clinic can display the Cat Friendly Clinic or Practice Logo on its website, in the practice itself, and on all practice literature. (**A,** Courtesy American Association of Feline Practitioners. **B,** © International Cat Care)

GETTING OFF TO A GOOD START

For most clients, the visit to the practice will start with a telephone call to a receptionist. Receptionists are the first line of contact with the practice and are usually the first to meet and greet clients when they arrive in the building. Thus, receptionists have a key role in the relationship between the client and the practice, so they must have an understanding of the fears and needs of cats and their owners, as well as a willingness to accommodate their needs (Figure 9-3).

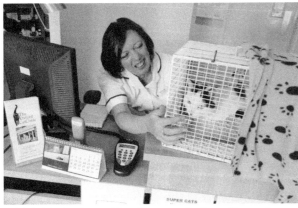

FIGURE 9-3   A cat-friendly receptionist will get the cat owner's visit off to a good start. (Courtesy International Cat Care, www.icatcare.org)

- In a multi-veterinarian practice, there will inevitably be differences between the veterinarians with regard to their attitude to cats. Some will be cat-lovers, but some may view treating cats as a challenge that cannot be avoided but is not necessarily to be welcomed. A survey of veterinarians in the United States conducted by Bayer and the AAFP[11] indicated that 48% of veterinarians prefer dogs, whereas only 17% prefer cats. Receptionists who know their veterinarians can diplomatically direct cat owners to those veterinarians for whom working with cats comes naturally and, in doing so, can avoid many stressful situations before they even arise.
- Designating a half-day or a surgery day as "cat-only" has been very beneficial in some practices. Cat owners recognize the knowledge and efforts of the practice to improve the environment for their cats. Even if they are unable to come during those times, or if a sick dog must be seen during that time, the awareness that an attempt has been made is important to them.
- Regardless of whether a veterinary practice chooses to have "cat-only" appointments, and surgery and dental days, it is important that the veterinary practice environment be "cat-friendly" at all times.
- Some cats do better with house calls, but some are more frightened by having an unfamiliar person(s) coming to the home and working with them in unfamiliar ways. In those situations where it is beneficial for the cat and cat owner, many clients are happy to pay the additional cost of a house visit to avoid the stress of a trip to the veterinary practice.
- A considerate conversation regarding the timing of the appointment will demonstrate to the client that the practice really cares about their cat and its well-being. Aspects to discuss include the following:
  - When is the best time to bring the cat to avoid unnecessary delays (e.g., avoiding rush hour to minimize journey time and offering appointments toward the beginning of consultation sessions to reduce the chance that the veterinarian will be running late)?
  - If the cat needs to be fasted prior to the appointment, when is the best time of day to schedule the appointment? Some clients will prefer to attend early in the day so that "breakfast" is only a little late and any other cats in the household can be fed once the target cat has been placed in its carrier. Others may prefer a late afternoon appointment so that 8 hours can have elapsed since the morning feed was given.
  - For cats with access to the outdoors, when is the cat most likely to be "available" for the client to catch it? Suitable times might be either early in the morning before the cat has been let out for the day or at feeding time, when the cat is likely to have returned home for food. Many cats are very predictable in

their habits, and the client may also know at which times of day the cat is typically active and outside and when it is likely to be resting indoors.

- If a urine sample is to be collected and the client is aware of the usual time of day that the cat urinates, the appointment can be scheduled for a time when the cat's bladder is most likely to be full or for a time when the client is likely to have been able to collect a fresh sample at home.

CAT CARRIERS

Once the veterinary appointment has been scheduled, the receptionist can help to educate the client about how to get the cat into the carrier and how to handle the transportation to the practice. All clients must be made aware that it is essential for the safety of both cat and client that cats be housed in secure traveling carriers at all times before leaving their home territory. Some clients will prefer to travel with their cat unrestrained (e.g., held on the lap of a passenger in the car) or restrained only by a harness and leash. This leads to a very high potential for distraction of the driver during the journey and is a hazard to the occupants of the car and to other road users. All clients must be made aware of this, and transport of cats not confined to a carrier must be strongly discouraged by all staff members. However, veterinarians must acknowledge that loading an uncooperative cat into an unsuitable cat carrier will cause problems for the client and stress for the cat long before the cat has even arrived at the practice. Receptionists, and indeed all other staff, can help to overcome this problem by advising clients as to which carriers are most suitable and by giving clients tips to assist them in getting the cat into the carrier. This may be done by telephone when the client first contacts the practice, and it can be supported by directing the client to a website or other source of more detailed information. A sample client handout and video options are provided in this chapter.

When buying a cat carrier, clients should be encouraged to spend their money wisely:

- The carrier must be sturdy, escape-proof, waterproof, and easily cleaned. Cardboard carriers are inexpensive and disposable, but they are easily damaged by a determined cat and may allow the cat to escape during the journey to the practice or while waiting to be seen (Figure 9-4).
- The carrier must be designed for easy loading and unloading: wide openings, top-loading carriers (Figure 9-5) and carriers with more than one opening present fewer problems than front-loading carriers (Figure 9-6).
- Plastic carriers that can be taken apart allow the top half of the carrier to be removed, leaving the cat in the bottom half for part or all of the examination (Figure 9-7).

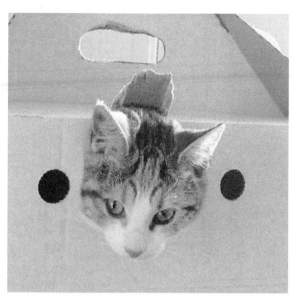

FIGURE 9-4 Cardboard carriers are not strong enough to safely contain a cat that is determined to escape.

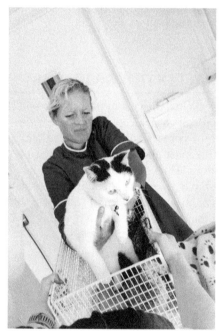

FIGURE 9-5 A top-loading carrier with a wide opening works well as long as no one looms over the cat. (Courtesy International Cat Care, www.icatcare.org)

- Hard-sided carriers, such as plastic carriers or those that are made from sturdy fabric stretched over a light metal frame can also be easily secured in the car by using the seat belt to prevent jostling and increase safety of the cat (Figure 9-8).
- Use a piece of the cat's bedding (Figure 9-9) or an old article of the owner's clothing to line the carrier so that it smells and feels familiar.

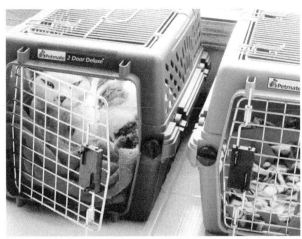

FIGURE 9-6 Carriers that can be taken apart in the middle are ideal so that the cat can remain in the bottom half during the veterinary visit. Having both a top and front opening allows the cat to go in and out on its own, and also makes it possible for the owner to place the cat into the carrier through the top. Owners should be instructed to leave the carrier out in the cat's favored location in the home.

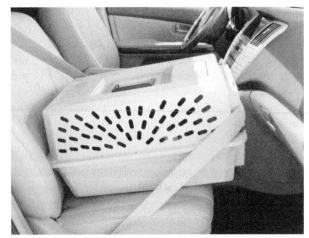

FIGURE 9-8 Clients must ensure that the carrier is stable and secure while transporting the cat in the car. (Courtesy E. Sundahl)

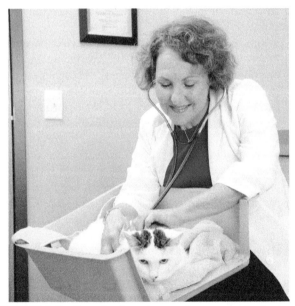

FIGURE 9-7 Examination of an anxious cat in the bottom half of its carrier.

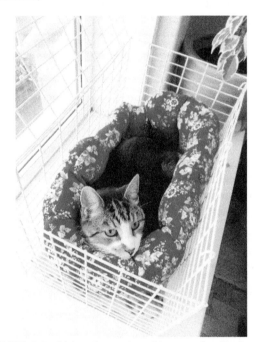

FIGURE 9-9 Lining the carrier with some familiar bedding helps the cat to feel more at home.

- Cover wire carriers with a towel or cloth to provide some cover for the cat (Figure 9-10).
- Spray the carrier with a feline pheromone product (e.g., Feliway Transport spray) at least 10 to 15 minutes before loading the cat into the carrier. In the United States, Feliway wipes are also available for use in carriers.
- If clients are bringing more than one cat to the practice, they should place each cat in a separate carrier—even cats that are usually friendly to each other may become highly stressed when forced to share a carrier, which may result in physical confrontation.

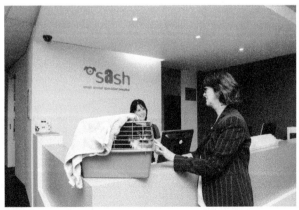

FIGURE 9-10 Cover wire or plastic carriers with a towel or cloth to provide some privacy for the cat. (Courtesy International Cat Care, www.icatcare.org)

Once the carrier has been acquired, the cat still needs to be placed into the carrier. Most clients have not been taught how to do this in a way that is comfortable for the cat. Again, client education prior to the veterinary visit can make all the difference. Staff members should be able to offer sensible advice, and client handouts can be useful too (see handout titled **Transporting Your Cat Made Easier**). Posting instructional videos (or links to videos) on your website can also be helpful (Table 9-1).

For a preventive care appointment that can be scheduled 1 to 2 weeks in advance, the client can be encouraged to acclimate the cat to the carrier in the home environment.

- Clients should be educated to keep the cat carrier in the house so that it becomes a familiar and non-threatening item. Easy access and leaving the carrier open and lined with comfortable bedding allows the cat a sense of control and choice to enter on its own terms. Playing games and/or feeding the cat in or near the carrier will increase the cat's familiarity and positive associations with the carrier. Clients should be made aware to never push the cat into the carrier, but rather entice it by calmly putting a treat in the carrier each day and providing a reward when the cat goes near or into the carrier.
- Cat owners who physically move the cat closer to the carrier or try to put them inside will frequently have negative experiences. In all their interactions with their cats, clients should be taught to reward or reinforce desired behavior and never to punish the cat, either verbally or physically.

TABLE 9-1	Cat Carrier Videos from the CATalyst Council*	
Title of Video	**Producer**	**Target Audience/ Purpose**
Cat Carriers: Friends, Not Foes	I. Rodan and Watson	Owners/carrier training and car trips
Tips for Taking Your Cat to the Veterinarian	I. Rodan	Owners/carrier training
Encourage Cat Vet Visits	I. Rodan	Veterinary teams/ education and handling
Cat Carrier Training	J. Neilson and Bug	Owners/carrier training using a clicker
Day 2 of Cat Carrier Training	J. Neilson and Bug	Owners/carrier training using a clicker

*The CATalyst Council website provides links to videos that help educate clients on how to transport their cats to the veterinary practice. These videos can be accessed from http://www.catalystcouncil.org/resources/video/ and from the CATalyst Council page on YouTube at https://www.youtube.com/user/catalystcouncil

For urgent appointments, clients may need to confine the cat to a small room with few hiding places before bringing the cat carrier out of storage. Ideally, the cat should still be given time to enter the carrier voluntarily, and owners can use food trails to encourage the cat to enter. However, if there is insufficient time for this passive approach, and if the carrier does not have a top-loading option, then it can be beneficial to turn the cat around and gently move it into the carrier backward to avoid causing the cat fear of being put into a dark place head first.

HELPING WITH THE JOURNEY

For many cats, the journey to and from the veterinary practice is the most unpleasant part of the whole process. Once it is in a carrier and leaving its familiar environment, the cat has no sense of control over its environment and will feel vulnerable. Exposure to unfamiliar sounds and sights will add to the cat's unease, and many will also experience nausea due to the combination of anxiety and motion. Clients need to be aware of this and should handle the carrier carefully and securely:

- When carrying the cat carrier, avoid swinging movements, do not bump the carrier against legs or doors, and try to keep most of the carrier covered to afford the cat security and comfort, but perhaps leave one side uncovered to allow communication with the cat if its nature is such that it will find this reassuring.
- When placing the carrier in the car, make sure it is level and secure so that it will not shift during the journey. Either place the carrier on the floor of the car where it cannot be jarred, or on a seat. Carriers on seats should be strapped in using a seat belt for safety and reduced motion of the carrier.
- Drive calmly; avoid rapid acceleration or deceleration; and take corners slowly and smoothly. Talk quietly and reassuringly to the cat and stay calm, as cats are very good at picking up tension in their owners. Providing some low-level background noise from the car's audio system may help to muffle other noises from outside, but avoid playing loud music that might distress the cat.
- Take spare bedding in case of accidents (i.e., urination or defecation in the carrier).
- Try to acclimate the cat to short car journeys that start and end at home so that the carrier and the car journey are not always associated with visits to the veterinary practice or to the boarding cattery.

Ideally, travel should occur when the cat has an empty stomach to reduce the likelihood of motion sickness and increase the cat's interest in treats at the veterinary practice, allowing for a more positive experience. Draping a blanket over the carrier can also help prevent fear and motion sickness. If the cat is still showing signs of nausea (e.g., lip-licking, drooling, or vomiting during transportation), maropitant (Cerenia) is effective against motion sickness[12] and may be prescribed for future journeys. The suggested dose is 1 mg/kg per os, dosed at between 1 and 24 hours in advance of travel. Note that maropitant is not currently licensed for oral use in cats, and it is the responsibility of the prescribing veterinarian to adhere to pertinent regulations in their country when prescribing medication for animals under their care.

THE WAITING ROOM

In an ideal world, there would be entirely separate waiting rooms for dogs and cats. Most practice buildings do not afford this luxury, but, if space allows, it may be possible to partition the waiting room into separate "zones." The cats and dogs will know that the other is present, but breaking up the direct sight line will provide some feeling of security for the nervous cat. The aim is to provide a waiting area that is as calm and quiet as possible. The following are simple steps that can help achieve this goal:

- Create a dedicated cat-only part of the waiting area, preferably located where there is the least human and animal traffic. Try to screen the area so that cats are not in direct visual contact with dogs. This may be achieved by building partitions (Figure 9-11), but it can also be done inexpensively by using a screen (Figure 9-12) or even by placing a line of chairs back to back.
- Make sure that the cat and dog areas are well signed and decorated (Figures 9-13) so that clients are immediately comfortable in knowing where they should take their pet.

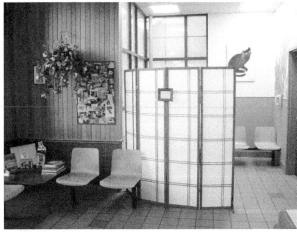

FIGURE 9-12 A screen can be used to prevent direct visual contact between cats and dogs. (Courtesy K. Wheel)

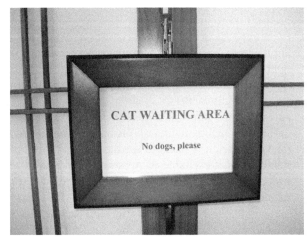

FIGURE 9-13 Clear signs indicate the cat-only section of the waiting area. (Courtesy K. Wheel)

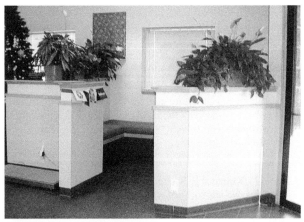

FIGURE 9-11 Physical partitions can be used to separate a dedicated cat-only waiting area. (From Bassert JM, McCurnin DM: McCurnin's Clinical Textbook for Veterinary Technicians, ed 7. Philadelphia, 2013, Saunders)

- When choosing where to situate the cat zone, consider the route the client will take from first entry into the waiting room, to the reception desk to check in, to the waiting zone, to the consulting room, and afterwards, back to the reception desk to pay. Look at how often the clients' route will take them through non-cat-only zones and identify any bottlenecks where cats and dogs may be in particularly close proximity to each other. The benefit of a cat-only waiting zone will be easily undone if the cat has been frightened by an encounter with a dog at the reception desk while its owner was checking in or was waiting to pay at the end of the previous visit.
- If possible, prevent noises from consultation rooms reaching the waiting area.
- Be aware of cats' exquisitely sensitive sense of smell. Clean up "accidents" quickly, and minimize artificial smells. Staff should not wear strong perfumes and should avoid excessive use of air fresheners or

strong-smelling floor polishes, for example. Wherever possible, use unscented disinfectants, make sure all rooms are well ventilated, and rinse disinfectants off surfaces thoroughly once the recommended contact time has passed. Consider designating one consulting room for cats so that lingering dog odors do not build up during the consulting session (and of course make sure the veterinarian working in that room is a cat-friendly veterinarian). Use Feliway diffusers in the reception area or in the cat-only section. The diffuser can be used at the same time as dog-appeasing pheromone (DAP) diffusers.

- Provide raised shelves or stools for clients to place cat carriers on, both by the reception desk and in the waiting area. Shelving systems can be made or bought (Figure 9-14), but, if space is limited, providing raised resting places may be no more complicated than encouraging clients to place the cat carrier on an empty chair (Figure 9-15) or on the reception desk itself rather than on the floor.
- Encourage clients to cover their cat's carrier with a familiar towel or piece of bedding to give the cat some shelter.
- Display notices asking clients with dogs to keep them away from cat carriers.
- At busy times, offer cat owners the option of waiting in their car, calling them into the building only when the veterinarian is ready to see them.
- Ask owners of excitable, aggressive, or noisy dogs to wait outside or in their car until they are called in for the appointment.

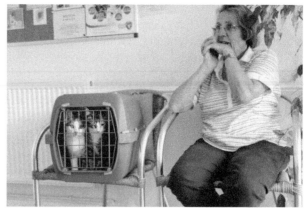

FIGURE 9-15 An empty chair provides an elevated resting point upon which to place the carrier.

The above recommendations are also important in a cat-only practice. Cats do not want to see, smell, or hear unfamiliar cats, and taking the steps outlined above can help to prevent fear associated with seeing other cats as well.

While the client is waiting to see the veterinarian, veterinary staff may use this opportunity to impress them with how cat-friendly the practice is. It will set the tone for the whole visit and create a positive impression from the outset. Here are some suggestions:

- Display evidence of feline-related continuing education that staff members have undertaken and certificates of membership of cat organizations, such as the ISFM or AAFP. Also, display awards and documentation of Cat Friendly Practice or Clinic status, and certificates of doctors with board certification in feline practice.
- Put up displays of cat breeds and photographs of clients' cats.
- Provide cat magazines and other information for clients to browse through.
- Display case histories of recently treated cats and design noticeboard displays to highlight cat-related health issues (e.g., lily toxicity, hepatic lipidosis, feline degenerative joint disease).

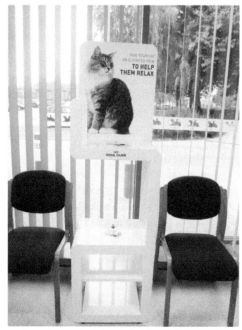

FIGURE 9-14 A portable shelving system provides secure elevated sites for cat carriers. (Courtesy Royal Canin)

REFERENCES

1. CATalyst Council: Scotty goes to the vet (video): http://www. youtube.com/watch?v=lubm_wHEegI (Part 1) and http:// www.youtube.com/watch?v=PH0ZXA6F3ZE (Part 2). Accessed May 14, 2013.
2. Henri 3, Le Vet (video). http://www.youtube.com/watch? v=IiYUzYozsAQ.
3. Rand JS, Kinnaird E, Baglioni A, et al. Acute stress hyperglycemia in cats is associated with struggling and increased concentrations of lactate and norepinephrine. *J Vet Intern Med.* 2002;16:123–132.
4. Taylor P, Funk C, Craighill P. *Gauging family intimacy: dogs edge cats (dads trail both).* Washington, DC: Pew Research Center; 2006. http://pewresearch.org/files/old-assets/social/ pdf/Pets.pdf.

5. Volk JO, Felsted KE, Thomas JG, Siren CW. Executive summary of the Bayer veterinary care usage study. *J Am Vet Med Assoc.* 2011;238:1275–1282.

6. American Veterinary Medical Association (AVMA). *US Pet Ownership & demographics source book.* 2012 ed. Schaumberg, IL: AVMA; 2012 [summarized at www.avma. org/news/javmanews/pages/130201a.aspx].

7. Habacher G, Gruffydd-Jones T, Murray J. Use of a web-based questionnaire to explore cat owners' attitudes towards vaccination in cats. *Vet Rec.* 2010;167:122–127.

8. Bayer HealthCare LLC, Animal Health Division: Bayer healthcare usage study [news release]. http://www.bayer-ah.com/images/AVMA%20-%20BVCUS%20Phase%20II%20Backgrounder.pdf. Accessed July 19, 2013.

9. International Cat Care/American Association of Feline Practitioners: The cat friendly practice program. http://catfriendlypractice.catvets.com. Accessed April 12, 2013.

10. ISFM: WellCat for life. http://www.isfm.net/wellcat.

11. Bayer HealthCare LLC, Animal Health Division: Bayer veterinary care usage study III: Feline findings. http://www.bayerdvm.com/show.aspx/news-release-bvcus-iii-feline-findings. Accessed May 23, 2014.

12. Hickman MA, Cox SR, Mahabir S, et al. Safety, pharmacokinetics and use of the novel NK-1 receptor antagonist maropitant (Cerenia) for the prevention of emesis and motion sickness in cats. *J Vet Pharmacol Ther.* 2008;31: 220–229.

The Cat in the Consulting Room

Martha Cannon and Ilona Rodan

INTRODUCTION

The veterinary consultation is one of the most important aspects of a veterinarian's job. Whether the animal presented is sick or well, the consultation is the only time during which veterinarian and clients are in direct face-to-face contact with each other; it is the most important opportunity to bond with the clients and gain their trust, and it is the time for them to express their concerns about their pet's health and behavior. During these critical minutes, veterinarians also need to assess the animal's well-being, perform a full physical examination, critically evaluate all findings, and produce a treatment or preventive healthcare plan that is suited to the individual animal and is acceptable to the clients. The challenge does not end there because one of the most important aspects of the veterinary consultation is the time spent explaining the findings and recommendations in such a way that the clients can understand them and believe in them, so that they will be motivated to follow the advice once they leave the consulting room. All of this has to be achieved in a very limited space of time, so every minute must be used effectively, and multitasking is often required. These considerations apply to every veterinary consultation, but when the animal presented is a cat, additional difficulties can arise from the essential nature of the cat: a solitary, self-sufficient animal that will feel threatened by the foreign environment in which it finds itself and may be unwilling to allow itself to be handled during the process of physical examination and/or diagnostic testing. Cats are also very subtle creatures and tend to hide signs of pain, weakness, and disease, so unraveling their problems can be more challenging than might be the case with some other species.

In Chapter 9, ways were presented to try to reduce the threat experienced by the cat during the process of being brought to the veterinary practice so that the cat is in a less stressed state when it arrives in the consulting room. This chapter will focus on how a veterinarian can approach the consultation process in a way that further reduces stress to the cat, the client, and the veterinary team, allowing maximum information to be gained and optimum benefit to be achieved during this vital but restricted period of time.

AN "EVERY CONSULTATION IS A BEHAVIOR CONSULTATION" APPROACH

When working with cats, every consultation is a behavior consultation because changes in the cat's behavior will have been noticed by the clients and raised their concern. Examples are a change in appetite, decline in grooming, or inability to get to its favorite spots or the litter box. Only by asking clients and encouraging them to describe these changes and exploring their underlying physical or behavioral causes will a true assessment of the cat's overall well-being be achieved. See Chapter 1 for more information.

Every veterinary consultation, regardless of the type of appointment, should follow a logical progression through a number of steps. This applies to preventive healthcare and "wellness" visits, as well as to consultations involving ill or injured animals, although clearly the emphasis will change according to the situation and to the needs of the pet and the client. Every consultation should include:

1. Greeting the client and gaining their confidence so that they are receptive to advice and recommendations and will also be willing to return in the future, thus becoming a "bonded" client for the veterinary practice
2. Finding out the client's concerns for their cat by asking open-ended questions that will encourage them to be forthcoming with regard to the cat's behavior and well-being
3. Identifying the veterinarian's concerns for the cat, which may not always be the same as the client's concerns, through careful history-taking, observation of the cat, and thorough physical examination
4. Developing a plan for investigation and management of any health or behavioral issues and for prevention of future problems
5. Communicating the plan to the client, ensuring that they will be both willing and able to apply it at home

6. Informing the client of the expected cost of the consultation and of any further investigations or recommended treatments, getting their agreement to the plan, or modifying it if it is not affordable

7. Advising the client when the cat should be seen next, either for a follow-up consultation or for the next planned preventive healthcare visit (preappointing or scheduling the appointment prior to the client's leaving reinforces the appointment's importance and has been shown to increase the client's return for future visits[1]).

By analyzing the consultation process in this way the importance of each step becomes evident, as well as the need for efficiency in this precious period of time. In the United Kingdom, the average time allocated to veterinary consultation is approximately 10 minutes. It is challenging to fit everything into that amount of time. Where possible, longer consultation times are the ideal, especially when working with cats that, by their nature, need more time to acclimate to the consulting room and with which the process of physical examination will need to be taken more gradually. When the consultation is well conducted, the additional time spent with the client will pay long-term dividends in terms of building a bonded and compliant client base and by allowing time to uncover and address issues that might otherwise be ignored, such as behavioral concerns, the need for routine dental care, implementation of dietary changes, and regular use of anthelmintics and ectoparasiticides.

GAINING THE CLIENT'S CONFIDENCE

When clients visit a veterinarian, they assume that he or she will have a high level of knowledge and technical skill. This may be a little unfair, but it is a fact of life. What clients are looking for, then, is more than just a competent veterinarian; they are looking for a kind, compassionate, empathetic veterinarian who understands how they feel about their pet, treats the pet as if it were a member of the family, and handles the pet in a gentle and compassionate way.

Taking the time for introductions with the client and the cat and complimenting the client on some noticeable aspect of the cat will start things off on a positive note; it will reassure the client and it will allow them to relax a little in the veterinary practice setting. For many clients, a trip to the veterinarian is an intimidating process. They expect their cat to be stressed by the visit; they are anxious about "what the veterinarian will find"; and, in many cases, they are worried about the potential costs of treatment. Establishing a friendly relationship will help to allay some of this anxiety, allowing the client to talk more freely about their concerns for their cat. It will also allow them to take in and remember professional advice more effectively.

Empathic listening with the goal of understanding and acknowledging the client's feelings will also increase the client's confidence and identify the client's concerns. Empathic listening involves attention to nonverbal cues such as body posture and facial expressions, asking open-ended questions, and using summary statements so that clients understand that their concerns have been heard.[2]

ESTABLISHING THE CLIENT'S CONCERNS

Most consultations will have been prompted by an immediate health problem, need for preventive care, or a requirement for a vaccination or repeat prescription of long-term medication. This primary purpose will be a natural focus for the consultation. In the majority of cases, however, there will also be other issues that the client might perceive to be less significant and therefore may not bring up without prompting from the veterinarian. These may include behavioral issues, chronic health issues that some clients may consider to be "normal" (e.g., vomiting of hair balls, halitosis, and reduced mobility), or difficulties that the client is experiencing in attempting successful application of preventive healthcare programs, such as in administering deworming or flea and tick preparations. The consultation period is the opportunity to uncover these concerns and to enlighten clients as to what can be done to alleviate them. Many clients will be unaware of the help that can be provided or will feel that these issues are an inevitable part of pet ownership and may not bring up these issues themselves. It is important to open the dialogue by establishing the primary reason that the client brought in the cat and to ensure that this concern is attended to, but it is also important to widen the discussion to all aspects of the cat's well-being.

Cats are very good at hiding the signs of disease, so their owners may be unaware when there is a problem. Conversely, clients may be aware of a behavior that is problematic, but they may not be aware of what it means or how to address it. Consider these two scenarios:

A 4-year-old cat is presented for an annual vaccination. It appears physically healthy, and there are no abnormal findings on examination. During your discussion with the client, however, you find that the cat is occasionally urinating outside the litter box. The client is frustrated by this but does not perceive it to be a health problem and would not have mentioned it if you had not asked. Now that you know about the problem, you can help the client to understand what the cat is trying to "say" (e.g., that it is suffering discomfort, stress, or aversion) and give advice about how to alleviate the problem. Thanking the client and reinforcing their input encourages them to continue to contact you with similar concerns in the future.

A 12-year-old cat is presented to you because it has been overgrooming. You immediately recognize that the cat has fleas and advise the client to treat the cat and the cat's environment with parasiticides. You know that this will resolve the overgrooming problem. You also identify that the cat has halitosis and significant periodontal disease, and you advise that the cat should be brought in for dental treatment under anesthesia. In view of the cat's age, you also recommend a preanesthesia blood test. This is good advice, but it does not relate to the problem that the client has identified. If you have not given sufficient time and attention to the client's primary concern, she will be left dissatisfied, and if the communication process has not been handled well, she may even perceive that you are recommending expensive and unnecessary treatment to deal with a problem that she did not know existed. The client leaves your consulting room feeling insecure and uncertain as to your motives and what is best for her cat. For these reasons, not only does the client not arrange for the necessary dental work, but she also feels unconvinced that the skin problem is due to fleas and thus does not follow the treatment plan you recommended either. Thus, the cat's overgrooming persists, the client feels that you were unable to "cure" the problem, and is unlikely to return to you in the future.

These contrasting examples illustrate the importance of both addressing the client's primary concern, however minor it may appear, and taking the opportunity to adopt a holistic view of the cat's physical and emotional well-being to identify currently "hidden" issues that are affecting its quality of life. Communication skills are essential. In addition to identifying the issues, it is important to take the time to explain and demonstrate to the client the reality of the findings. For example, in the second case above, showing the client the flea dirt that has been combed from the coat and teaching the client how to check for fleas at home will reinforce the diagnosis of flea-induced pruritus, and showing the client the affected teeth and gums while using photographs of a healthy cat's mouth will convince the client that the cat's dental disease is real and will become an even bigger problem if left untreated.

When taking a history, the veterinarian should ask the client open-ended questions that encourage dialogue rather than closed questions that can produce a "yes" or "no" response.

1. An excellent starting question is "What changes in behavior have you noticed since the last visit?" This question can be followed by "What else?" or a more specific question based on the client's answer. For example, if the client says that their cat is "slowing down," the veterinarian should ask a question such as "What are you noticing at home?"
2. Ask open-ended questions. Once the general information is provided, ask more specific open-ended questions, such as "What changes in eating are you seeing?" or "How is his appetite?" This encourages the client to consider and describe the cat's food intake and behavior at feeding time. Encourage the client to elaborate on the answer, which will often bring out related issues that the client might not otherwise have mentioned, such as "Oh, he eats really well. In fact, sometimes he eats his food so quickly that he vomits it up right away." This is a common issue that many clients consider to be normal. Now it is possible to open a discussion about eating too fast and regurgitation, food intolerance, or other potential causes of the cat's vomiting and give the client advice about what can be done to alleviate this issue.
3. Avoid asking closed questions. An example of a closed question might be "Is he off his food?" This prompts the client to reply simply "yes" or "no" without elaborating on the cat's feeding habits. In the example of a cat that is vomiting while eating, the answer "no" would be unlikely to uncover the presence of chronic vomiting.

ASSESSING THE CAT

As mentioned above, many cats in the veterinary practice may feel threatened and defensive, and they will not behave in the same way that they would at home. They are likely to be unwilling to walk freely around the floor. They tend not to flinch when mildly painful areas are manipulated or palpated. They may be very tense when handled, preventing good assessment of joints and limiting the ability to palpate the abdomen. A detailed neurological examination can be particularly challenging to interpret in a frightened, tense cat whose stress levels are overriding normal reflexes.

Distant Observation

Maintaining a low-stress experience for the cat is therefore crucial to allowing a timely and accurate health assessment. For most cats, the consulting table is one of the most frightening places in the veterinary practice. While on the table, they are exposed to "danger" and prevented from withdrawing to a safer place. On this table, the cat is intimately handled by a stranger during the physical examination, and if any areas of its body are painful, those areas will be focused on by the person who is forcing it to endure this ordeal. Many cats are reprimanded when they get onto a table at home, thus increasing their sense of anxiety when they are placed on the consulting room table. On the exam table, the cat may have its rectal temperature taken, its ears examined with a speculum or otoscope, and so forth. It may also associate this table with being restrained to receive injections or to be given oral medications. Placing and handling the cat on the consulting table therefore adds to its stress and further alters its behavior, reactions, and physiological parameters. The table can be made less threatening by placing a thick towel over its slippery, potentially cold surface; nevertheless, for the cat, the consulting room table is a high-stress zone. To get an accurate assessment of the cat, take every opportunity to observe the cat's demeanor, behavior, and gait from a distance, ideally without the cat knowing that it is being watched. This time can be spent greeting the client and taking the history to good effect by watching the cat carefully through these first minutes of the consultation.

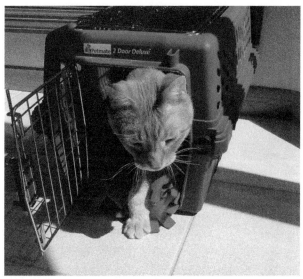

FIGURE 10-1 When the cat arrives in the examining room, allow it to step out of the carrier on its own.

- Getting the cat out of its carrier is the first challenge. If the cat is approached in a rushed or inappropriate manner, this simple first step can be damaging to a successful consultation. Reaching into the carrier, grabbing the cat by the scruff of the neck to drag him out, or tipping the carrier to shake the cat out onto the table will get the encounter off to the worst possible start, however good-natured the cat may otherwise be. Instead of using a direct and intimidating approach, start by asking the client not to place the carrier straight onto the consulting table and not to remove the cat from the carrier the moment they arrive in the room.

- Have the client place the carrier on the floor or, ideally, on a bench or low table, and have the client open the door of the carrier. Give the cat time to acclimate to the room and to your voice before approaching it. Many cats will naturally want to explore this new environment and will step out of the carrier, or at least step halfway out, to assess the room (Figure 10-1). This will allow you to greet the cat in a relaxed and nonthreatening manner while continuing to take the clinical history from the client. Talk to the cat in the tones that an client would use at home; extend a hand to allow the cat to sniff your fingers, and, if the cat remains confident, use this moment to stroke its head before withdrawing to allow the cat to continue to assess the environment for itself. This takes only a few seconds, but it allows the cat to feel more in control of its situation and establishes a level of friendly contact between the veterinarian and the cat.

- If the cat does not come out of the carrier of its own accord, have the client sit down on a chair next to the cat and encourage it to come out to interact. Do not

let the client dominate the cat, though. Some clients feel anxious, and they will transmit their anxiety to their cat. Sometimes you will need to gently educate the client that remaining calm and taking a slower approach is quicker in the end.

- If the cat is still not confident enough to come out of its carrier, place the carrier on a surface at a suitable height and, if possible, take the carrier apart (Figure 10-2, *A*) to allow you to start to examine the cat while it remains in the base of the carrier (Figure 10-2, *B*) (see Chapter 9 for advice about ideal carriers).

- If the carrier cannot be taken apart in the middle and you have no choice but to "encourage" the cat from the carrier, approach the cat gently and in a friendly way, talking to it in a reassuring tone before reaching into the carrier. Watch the body language of the cat carefully, and withdraw if the cat is becoming aggressive. Stroke the cat while it is still in the carrier and lift it out gently, handling it according to the principles of cat-friendly handling (see Chapter 20) and continuing to talk to it in reassuring tones as you do so. Never raise your voice to a cat, and never take the cat by the scruff of the neck and pull it from the carrier. Although many veterinary professionals have been taught to scruff, such an action is an aggressive way to handle a cat that will make it more likely to become aggressive. Even if the cat is not overtly aggressive, it will be less receptive to handling at that time as well as in the future, as it will associate the veterinary environment with its bad experience.

- Once the cat is out of the carrier, allow it to move around the consulting room or to interact with its

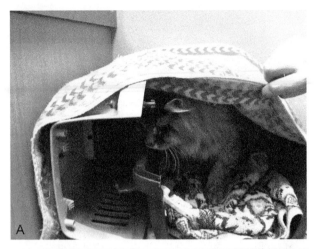

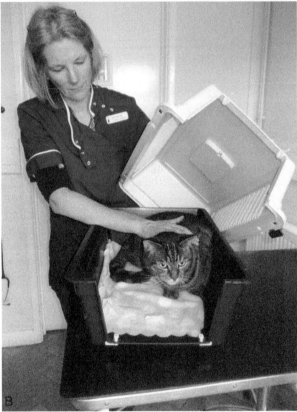

FIGURE 10-2 A, If necessary, the carrier can be taken apart to allow the cat to be examined. **B,** The cat can remain in the bottom half of the carrier for most of the examination.

the first encounter. Calmly and slowly reaching a hand out toward the cat may encourage it to rub against the hand. Cats prefer touch on the head and neck, the areas where cats that like each other groom. Approaching the cat from the side or behind avoids threatening the cat. Again, this process does not need to take long, a few minutes at most, and it happens while the relationship is being established with the client and the veterinarian is taking the history. It will also be time saved in the end, because the cat will be more receptive and cooperative during the physical examination.

- When the stage of the consultation that involves handling the cat is reached, consider how best to achieve this in light of the nature of the cat and the assessment to that point. When approaching a cat, always adopt a calm, soothing manner; move slowly; and never look directly into the cat's eyes. Talk to the cat throughout all interactions, maintaining a soothing tone at all times. However, remain quiet in the presence of the unusual cat that tenses, growls, or hisses each time it hears an unfamiliar voice and is calmer with quiet. "Shh-ing" or whispering can be confused with a hiss by a cat and should be avoided.

- Learn to read the cat's body language. For example, assess how the cat responds to an attempt to calmly stroke its head. Some cats will cower and adopt a defensive posture initially; if they are planning an attack, though, they will usually give due warning by hissing or growling. In the absence of an aggressive response, stroke the cat's head to reassure the cat that no harm is meant. With a bold and relaxed cat, a hand can be run along its back.

- The best experience for the cat is to be examined where it wants to be, which reduces its fear by allowing it to have a sense of control. Often this place is the floor or a bench or chair next to the client (Figure 10-3). Another option is on a window sill or perch if one is available (Figure 10-4). Many cats prefer to remain in the bottom half of the carrier, and the majority of the examination can be done there (Figure 10-5). Alternatively, the examination can be done with the cat directly in the lap of the veterinarian or client if socially appropriate and based on legal ordinances (Figure 10-6). This has an additional advantage in that the presence of an exam or consulting table or desk between the veterinary professional and the client is a barrier to empathic listening.[2]

- In some practices, the exam room may not have sufficient space and an exam table will be used. This can work for a bold, relaxed cat—one that approaches and rubs on you—if you can pick up the cat in a natural way, as you would your own pet cat, and place it on the consulting table. For a less confident but

client before you move in to handle it. Observing from a distance will allow you to assess the cat's general demeanor and behavior, including its level of fear, activity, gait, and mobility, as well as its body and coat condition. As the cat explores the room, it will most likely approach you as part of the exploration. It may rub against the veterinarian's or technician's legs. The cat should be allowed to continue to inspect the exam room so that it remains in control of

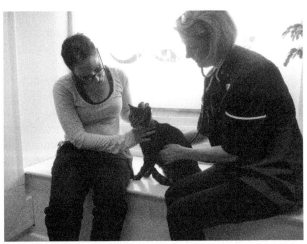

FIGURE 10-3   Ideally, the cat should be examined where it feels most at ease—for example, on a bench next to its owner.

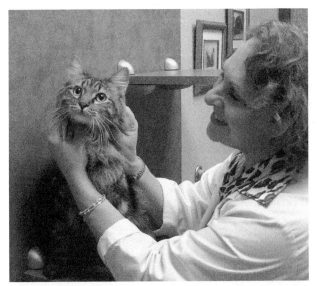

FIGURE 10-4   Cats often feel more comfortable being examined on an elevated surface or perch.

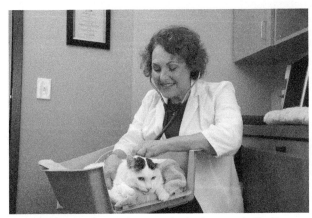

FIGURE 10-5   Examining a cat in the bottom half of its carrier often makes the cat feel more secure.

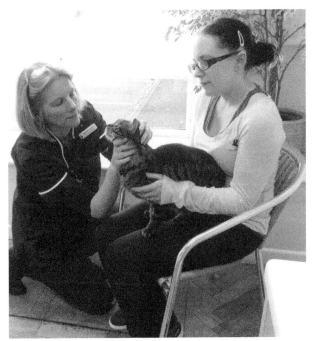

FIGURE 10-6   Examining a cat while it sits in its owner's lap is often the best option.

nonaggressive cat, you might ask the client to pick up the cat and bring it to the table, or you may consider starting the examination away from the table, as described above.

Physical Examination

All of your interactions with a cat should be conducted calmly and in a measured way, and this applies to the process of physical examination in the consulting room as much as anywhere else. Start the physical examination with the least invasive procedures, and leave less comfortable examinations until later (e.g., otoscopic exam, examining the mouth, and rectal temperature-taking). When handling the cat, also leave palpation of painful areas until last, but explain to the client that this is what you are doing. Otherwise, the client may become frustrated that you are "ignoring" the issue that they are most concerned about. The following are some other tips for feline-friendly consulting that might prove helpful.

- Maintain a constant level of background noise. Speaking in a soft and calm voice, conduct conversation and history-taking with the client, and during breaks in the interaction with the client, talk to the cat itself using the same tone of voice. You may feel self-conscious at first, but remember that all clients talk to their cats at home, so the cat expects this to happen when it is handled by a human, and silent handling may unnerve your feline patients. The client will also accept this as normal behavior, and if you are complimenting the cat on its charm and good behavior, the client will be charmed, too.

- Avoid direct eye contact with the cat as far as possible. In intercat interactions, "staring" is an aggressive action. Perform as much of the physical examination as possible with the cat looking away from you (Figure 10-7, *A* and *B*), and even when the cat is facing you, direct your gaze as far above, below, or beside its eyes as possible.

- When handling the cat's face, rub your hands over its pleasure centers: just below the zygomatic arches, the preauricular area, and the top of the bridge of the nose (Figure 10-8, *A* and *B*). This helps to calm the cat and often stimulates the cat to respond by nudging your hands with its head or stepping up to rub against your arms or body. When the client sees their cat befriending you in this way, you will have won them over forever!

- Once you have started your examination, keep a hand in contact with the cat at all times. The first touch is the most intimidating for the cat, and maintaining constant friendly contact is much better tolerated than repeatedly breaking and reestablishing physical contact.

- The same handling tips should be used for lab sample collections and treatments.

When you have finished working with the cat and while you discuss your findings with the client, allow the cat to return to the carrier or let it move freely around the consulting room or retire to a corner or other area where it feels safe (Figure 10-9, *A–D*). If you are dispensing any medication, take time to demonstrate to the client how to administer the medication before allowing the cat to return to its carrier. When it is time to leave, offer the cat the opportunity to go back into its carrier by itself (Figure 10-10). When you place the carrier onto the floor or a low surface with the door open, most cats will take the opportunity to move into what has now become a "safe haven," even though that same carrier may have been considered anything but a safe haven when the cat was introduced to it at home.

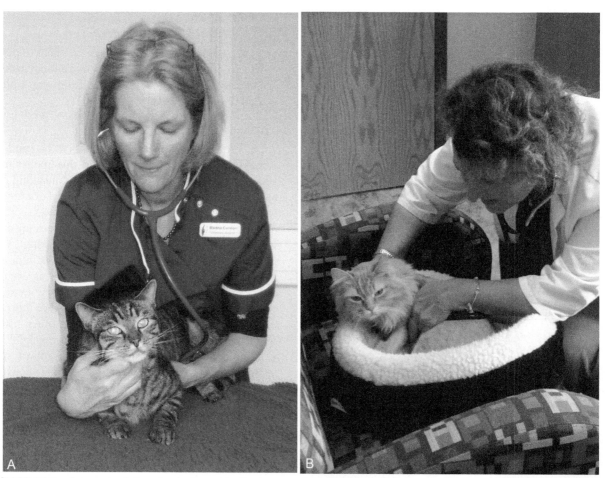

FIGURE 10-7 As much of the physical examination as possible should be performed with the cat facing away from the examiner. Eye contact should be avoided.

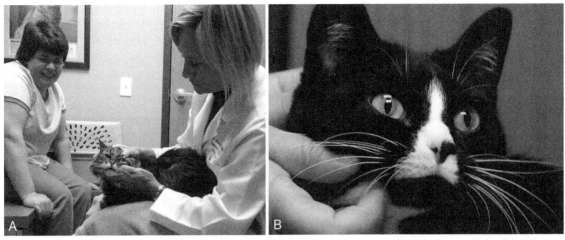

FIGURE 10-8   Rubbing the pleasure centers on the cat's face helps to calm the animal and may elicit a friendly response.

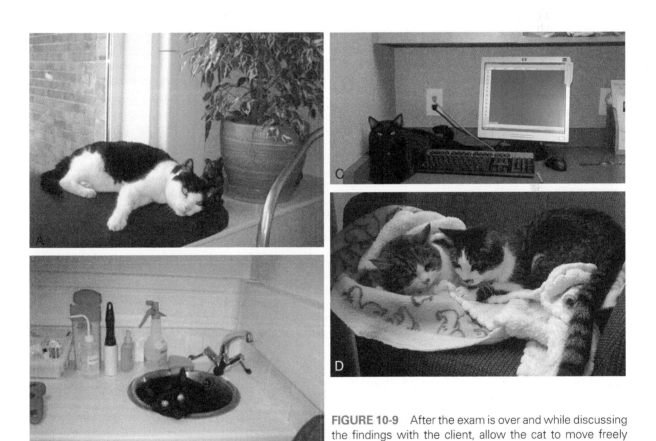

FIGURE 10-9   After the exam is over and while discussing the findings with the client, allow the cat to move freely around the consulting room and to retire to an area where it feels safe. This might be a corner in the room **(A** and **D)**, inside a sink **(B)**, or next to a computer **(C)**.

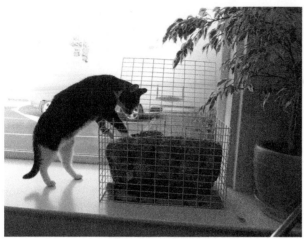

FIGURE 10-10   At the end of the examination, allow the cat to go back into the carrier on its own.

DEVELOP A PLAN, COMMUNICATE IT TO THE CLIENT, AND ENSURE THE CLIENT CAN COMPLY

To make the best use of time, use written advice sheets, handouts, or brochures as much as possible. Once you have established the client's concerns and your own regarding the cat's health and behavior and have physically examined the cat, you will develop a plan for future management, whether this involves further diagnostic investigations, a procedure within the veterinary practice, a course of medical treatment, a change of diet, or a plan for preventive healthcare measures that the client will implement at home between the current visit and the next scheduled visit. Whatever the plan involves, it will rely on the client to comply with your advice in order for the cat to benefit from it. Explaining the plan to the client so that she understands the recommendations and the reasons for them is therefore essential to the cat's future well-being. Teamwork and some forward planning will allow you to communicate more effectively with clients in a timely way.

- Use veterinary nurses or technicians to back up your recommendations and explain treatment options to clients in more detail and to demonstrate how to dose medications. This may be done in-person at the time of the initial visit or may be conveyed by telephone or e-mail in the days and weeks following the consultation to support the client at home as she implements a treatment plan or diet change. This follow-up support is valuable because it allows clients to ask questions and to talk about any difficulties they are having. It also provides an opportunity to remind the client of the importance of the treatment plan and of any follow-up visits that have been recommended. It can also be an opportunity to identify any problems or adverse effects that might arise.

- Use prewritten advice sheets or handouts that cover the common conditions that you deal with. Advice sheets can cover preventive healthcare issues, such as flea control, weight control, and dental care at home. They can also cover some of the common but often complex medical conditions that affect cats, such as chronic kidney disease, hyperthyroidism, diabetes, and degenerative joint disease. Many pharmaceutical and nutritional product companies and feline organizations publish product support literature that can be helpful (see Additional Resources for more information). However, to avoid confusion and to offer the full range of treatment choices available, develop your own independent advice sheets with your own practice branding guarantees that the written information given to the client exactly matches the verbal information they are given by you and all practice staff.

MEDICATING CATS

Medicating cats is not always easy, and the best drug in the world will not be useful if the client cannot get it into their cat. When planning a course of treatment, it is therefore important to think about the practical aspects of medicating cats and to discuss them with the client ahead of time, as well as to be aware of and discuss any potential adverse effects of the drugs themselves.

- Take the time to teach clients how to dose pills or liquids or how to apply spot-on preparations. Use your veterinary technicians to do this and provide links to videos that may be helpful (see Additional Resources).

- Use all the gadgets that you have available to help the client give tablets successfully:
  - Pill-givers or pill-poppers with a soft rubber end to reduce the risk of injury (Buster Pill Giver Soft Tip). Although some cats and people are better able to handle oral administration of pills without a gadget, others prefer pill-givers or pill-poppers.
  - Gelatin capsules: available from veterinary wholesalers, these are invaluable for dosing multiple medications at the same time or to mask the bitter flavor of unpalatable drugs, such as maropitant (Figure 10-11).
    - Make sure the capsule is washed down with water or food after dosing to avoid it sticking in the cat's esophagus, often most easily achieved by giving the cat some food or a treat immediately after administering the medication, unless instructions require medicating on an empty stomach.
  - Pill-crushers: crushing a tablet down to a powder allows it to be mixed with food or suspended in water to make a liquid formulation, which may be easier to administer.

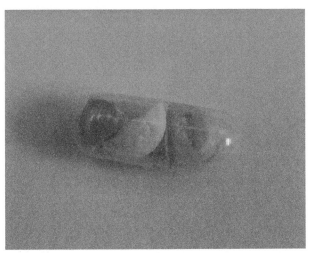

FIGURE 10-11 Mask bitter tablets in a gelatin capsule.

- Check that the tablet is suitable for crushing (e.g., not one with enteric coating).
- Crush finely enough not to affect the texture of the food.
- Check that the powder is tasteless and will not affect the flavor of the food.
- Wear gloves to crush tablets, and avoid breathing in the crushed powder.
- Pill pockets: use tasty treats that the tablet can be concealed inside, such as Greenies, Easytabs (Bayer); Vivitreats (Vétoquinol).
- Pill paste: wrap a palatable paste around a tablet, such as Pill Wrap Paste (Vétoquinol)
- Choose the medication carefully: consider the size, shape, and palatability of the product you prescribe.
  - If there is a safe and effective option that has an International Cat Care Easy to Give award, someone somewhere has road-tested it and found it to be reasonably cat-friendly for dosing.
  - Opt for smaller, oval tablets whenever possible.
  - Use "palatable" formulations whenever possible.
  - Consider the duration of action: fewer doses per day may improve compliance.
  - Discuss the alternative formulations that are available with the client, and let the client have a say in which formulation you prescribe.

- Chilling strongly flavored liquids or tablets prior to dosing may reduce their flavor, making them less bitter and potentially easier to hide in strong-tasting food.
- Tablets and capsules may lodge in the esophagus.
  - Some drugs are irritants and can cause esophagitis and esophageal strictures (e.g., doxycycline, clindamycin). These drugs must always be washed down with water or given with food.
  - Even if it is not inherently an irritant, a lodged tablet or capsule will be uncomfortable and may make the cat less amenable to dosing next time.
    - Lubricate capsules with oil or butter. Wash tablets or capsules down with food or water.
- Know what works: Ask for feedback from clients on how easy they find the medication to give. Remember the difficult ones and consider whether there is a more cat-friendly alternative.
- Ask clients to call you if they are having difficulty administering the medication.

ADDITIONAL RESOURCES

Product Support Information

American Association of Feline Practitioners: www.catvets.com. Accessed January 18, 2015.

International Cat Care: www.icatcare.org. Accessed January 18, 2015.

Winn Feline Foundation: http://www.winnfelinefoundation.org/. Accessed January 18, 2015.

Cornell Feline Health Center: www.vet.cornell.edu/FHC/health_resources/topics.cfm. Accessed January 18, 2015.

Medicating Cats

Cornell Feline Heath Center, www.vet.cornell.edu/FHC/health_resources/topics.cfm. Accessed January 18, 2015.

International Cat Care client instructional videos, Courtesy of Martha Cannon www.icatcare.org:8080/advice/videos. Accessed February 13, 2015.

REFERENCES

1. Bayer HealthCare LLC, Animal Health Division. *Bayer Veterinary Care Usage Study III: Feline Findings.* http://www.bayerdvm.com/show.aspx/news-release-bvcus-iii-feline-findings. Accessed January 18, 2015.

2. Osborne CA, Ulrich LK, Nwaokorie EE. Reactive versus empathic listening: what is the difference? *J Am Vet Med Assoc.* 2013;242:460–462.

Housing Cats in the Veterinary Practice

Ilona Rodan and Martha Cannon

INTRODUCTION

A period of hospitalization is essential at some point for many cats, but keeping cats in an unfamiliar environment and away from their families can negatively impact their welfare and recovery. A veterinary practice's goals for hygiene and patient monitoring often conflict with the hospitalized patient's ability to cope in an unfamiliar environment. Additionally, clients are often anxious about their cats and how they will do away from home. When these stressors are understood, steps can be taken to reduce both feline and client stress and ensure staff safety.

Most cages used to house cats do not meet essential feline needs; they are often too small for the cat to stretch, sleep in a comfortable position, and move around, and most caging setups do not allow cats to hide. Hiding is an important coping strategy for cats in an unfamiliar environment, and they also need a place to perch so they can "monitor" their environment. Consistency in routine, smells, sounds, and handlers is also important in the unfamiliar veterinary practice environment. This chapter provides practical advice for adapting cages and developing standard operating procedures for staff to address these important feline requirements.

Although caging for cats in shelters and catteries is beyond the scope of this chapter, the points discussed here will enhance cat care in those environments as well. These potentially long-term conditions make meeting the needs of cats even more important. For more information on enriching the shelter environment, see the link to the UC Davis Koret Shelter Medicine Program website provided in the Additional Resources section at the end of this chapter.

CHALLENGES ASSOCIATED WITH HOSPITALIZATION AND BOARDING

There are major challenges to hospitalizing cats and being able to provide optimal care for them in the veterinary practice environment. The most important problems are the cat's fear and stress due to disruption of the social bond, its lack of familiarity with the veterinary practice environment, and its inability to perform its normal behaviors.[1-3]

Cats are social animals, and studies indicate that the disruption of the social bond with their owners leads to stress in the hospitalized patient.[4-6] Ensuring provision of familiar bedding, toys, and food is helpful, but cats often do better when their owners also have regular visiting privileges in the veterinary practice.

As territorial animals, cats are most secure in the familiarity of their own territory. During hospitalization or boarding in the veterinary practice, the cat is confronted with unfamiliar smells, sounds, sights, people, and other animals. The unfamiliar schedules and handling can also be very frightening. Adjustment to the new environment can take anywhere from a couple of days to several weeks.[7-9] The outcome, despite the goal of providing the best care for the cat throughout hospitalization, is that the lack of familiarity and reduced sense of control can negatively impact the cat's health and welfare.[4,10]

A good example is seen in the veterinary practice goals of bringing the patient back to health and preventing the spread of contagious diseases, in that stress in a caged cat can increase the risk of upper respiratory infections[11] and stress-associated medical conditions can occur in hospitalized cats.[3,12] Inconsistencies in caregivers, feeding and cleaning schedules, and periods of light and dark can even lead to feline idiopathic cystitis (FIC) in healthy caged cats.[12] This information comes from studies of cats donated to The Ohio State University, some with FIC and some apparently healthy cats, both groups housed in veterinary practice cages. The FIC cats were exposed to a consistent schedule and caregivers, with consistent times to interact with people and have out-of-cage time. They also had places within the cages to hide and to perch, so that they had a sense of control. No medications or prescription diets were given; in fact, the diet provided was a commercial, nonprescription dry food. The option to control their environment, the predictability, and the familiar human interactions at consistent times resolved the signs of FIC.[3,12] Both the apparently healthy cats and the cats with resolved FIC were then exposed to cages without enrichment and to inconsistencies in schedules and caregivers, which did not provide the cats with predictability and familiarity, and both groups of cats developed signs of stress-related medical conditions such as FIC.[3]

Additionally, abnormal physical findings and diagnostic tests in hospitalized cats can occur secondary to fear and may erroneously be considered disease findings. These exam findings include hyperthermia and increased respiratory and heart rates.[13] The diagnostic findings include stress neutrophilia and lymphocytosis, as well as hyperglycemia. In one study, hyperglycemia was found in 64% of nondiabetic cats hospitalized at a primary referral veterinary practice, and cats with longer lengths of hospitalization had increased prevalence of hyperglycemia.[14]

Recognizing Stress in Hospitalized Cats

It can be difficult to recognize stress in a hospitalized cat as the signs of stress associated with lack of familiarity and reduced sense of control during caging are usually inhibited normal behaviors rather than more overt abnormal behaviors.[1,2,15] They include decreased activity, appetite, eliminations, grooming, play, and sleep, and the problem is even more complicated because these signs can also be seen in sick cats.[1,2,7] Cats that demonstrate these more subtle signs of fear and stress may suffer more than cats that demonstrate blatant signs of being upset.[2]

These inhibited signs pose a problem with regard to recovery, because veterinarians often think that a cat should not be sent home until it starts to eat again. However, because hospitalization inhibits eating and other normal behaviors, it is often in the cat's best interest to be sent home when other signs (e.g., hydration, vital signs, recovery from anesthesia) are back to normal. The client must be made aware of why a decision was made to send the cat home before it started to eat (i.e., because cats are often more willing to eat at home) and to contact the veterinary practice if there are any questions or concerns or if the cat does not eat within 24 hours (less for kittens) after getting home. It is important to follow up with the client and to schedule return visits to reassess the patient's progress.

Although inhibited behaviors are more common, some caged cats may become vigilant, watching every movement that occurs around them, and be alert to every sound. These cats cannot rest, because they must monitor the unfamiliar environment to protect themselves. Caged cats also often become fearfully aggressive as a protective mechanism. Although cats prefer not to fight, they will fight to protect themselves when their other defense responses—inhibition (freezing) and avoidance (fleeing) —are not possible or effective, such as when a person attempts to take them out of a cage. The cat usually bluffs, making itself bigger, with arched back and in a crouching position. If the person continues to remove such a cat from the cage, it will often react aggressively in an effort to protect itself.

Cats' positioning and posture in the cage can help to identify fearful cats in the veterinary practice. Compare the position and posture of the two cats in Figure 11-1,

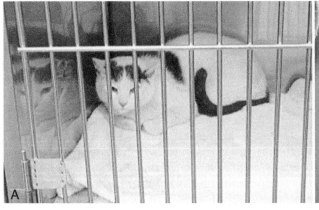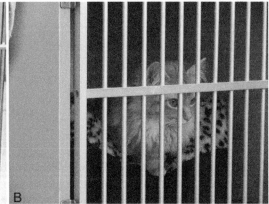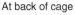

At back of cage
- Ears back
- Slightly arched back
- Vigilant
- Not able to rest
- Stainless steel shows cat's reflection
- Cat may think it's another cat

In front of cage, with hiding option
- Ears forward
- Relaxed body
- Curious
- Watching what is going on
- In Formica cage

FIGURE 11-1 Comparing the cats in A and B helps to differentiate between the fearful and non-fearful caged cat and highlights the importance of always reading facial signals. The cat in A has a body posture that could be mistaken for that of a relaxed cat, with the tail curled around the body and the front paws tucked in and the pads off the floor. Reading the cat's facial signals and considering its positioning at the back of the cage helps to accurately assess its emotional state.

BOX 11-1	How to Tell if a Cat is Fearful or Stressed

Inhibition of Behaviors: Most Common
- Feeding
- Grooming
- Toileting
- Play
- Sleep (may be difficult to recognize, because caged cats sometimes feign sleep)

Hiding
- Hiding in litter box
- Hiding under blanket, in newspapers
- Other attempts to hide (e.g., tearing up newspapers or blanket placed on cage floor to make a hiding place)

Position in Cage
- In back and huddled
- Up front and ready to attack when someone approaches

Posture
- Crouching as if pretending not to be there
- Back arched and appears larger than is (bluffing)
- Ears back
- Pupils dilated

Behavior That Indicates Illness (e.g., feline idiopathic cystitis)
Behaviors Considered Abnormal
- Overgrooming
- Soiling outside the litter box
- Fear-related aggression

A and *B*. For a summary of signs of fear and stress in caged cats, see Box 11-1.

Should the Cat be Hospitalized?

When making a decision to admit a cat to the veterinary practice, it is important to remember the degree of feline stress that can be induced by a period of hospitalization. Veterinarians should weigh the benefits and risks for the individual cat, the cat's condition, and the owner's ability to treat the cat at home. Most cats do better in their familiar home environment than in an unfamiliar veterinary practice, so the real question is what can be done for the cat at the practice that cannot be done at home. A number of questions need to be asked to ensure that the best decision is made for each feline patient.
- Does the cat require hospitalization to perform the needed observations, procedures, or treatments?
- How will this individual cat respond to hospitalization?

- Can the client medicate the cat as effectively at home, or is it possible to arrange for someone to go to the home to do so?
- Will the cat be better off receiving treatments today and returning after a certain period of time to be reassessed instead of being hospitalized?
- Will the client be willing to bring the cat back for recheck of its condition and to update the treatment plan?

Of course, there are several instances in which it is in the best interest of the patient to be hospitalized. These include anesthetic procedures, intravenous fluid administration, shock therapy, hypothermia, respiratory distress, monitoring of vital signs, and other critical treatments and procedures. When hospitalization is considered necessary, the following questions must be answered:
- How can feline fear and stress be prevented?
- How can staff safety be ensured?
- How can owner worries and stress be managed?

Another important consideration is when the patient should be discharged. A rule of thumb that is commonly used with dogs is to send the patient home after it starts eating or once it urinates or defecates, depending on the problem. However, cats often inhibit their normal behaviors, such as eating, due to the stress of hospitalization, and many of them do better if they are discharged as soon as is otherwise medically responsible. Therefore, it is important to consider whether it may be in the best interest of the patient and client if the cat is sent home overnight and then brought back to the veterinary practice for rechecking the next day. This is especially important in situations where there is no overnight care in the veterinary practice and no emergency facility to send the cat to overnight.

BUILDING DESIGN: HOSPITALIZATION AND BOARDING WARDS

Whenever possible, cat-only wards should be provided. Cats with high exposure to unfamiliar dogs have higher urinary cortisol levels than those with low exposure.[12] Providing separate cat and dog wards reduces cats' fear by eliminating or at least reducing the noise, scent, and visibility of dogs, all of which can be very frightening to cats. Dogs should not be walked or carried where cats can see them. Even cats that get along well with a familiar dog in their own household usually become frightened by unfamiliar dogs.

Cats are also more fearful if they see unfamiliar cats, so cats should be caged in a ward with a door closed to the rest of the veterinary practice. Within the ward, the visibility of other caged cats can be prevented by having one bank or row of cages per ward. When this is not possible, cages should be placed so that they are side-by-side or back-to-back instead of across from each other or at an angle to each other. Fear caused by visibility of unfamiliar animals and people can also be reduced by providing hiding places within the cage (see "A Place to Hide" below). Fear is increased in cats placed in bottom cages and therefore middle and upper cages should be used first, avoiding the use of bottom cages whenever possible. Many veterinary practices use the lower cages for storage or for resident cats that are already comfortable in the environment. Cats that are very anxious, displaying fear-associated aggression, or vocalizing excessively are best moved to an unused isolation area. If this is not possible, a towel should be placed over the front of the cage to screen out activity that may add to the cat's anxiety.

One study has shown increased stress levels in cats when they observed other cats being examined.[16] So, caging in treatment areas or leaving cats in carriers in the treatment area can be terrifying even in cat-only practices. Cats need to be examined out of sight of any other cats and resident cats should be kept away from hospitalized patients at all times. In particular, resident cats should not be allowed to play in front of caged cats or to stick their paws into another cat's cage.

It is not only unfamiliar dogs and cats that cause fear in caged cats. Unfamiliar people walking frequently in and out of wards and at inconsistent times also cause feline stress. Loud voices, machines beeping, and other sounds can further frighten feline patients. Having separate rooms for wards with closed doors helps minimize sound. Playing soft music or white noise in the ward helps prevent startling caused by other noises. Partial or full glass doors to patient wards allow monitoring and observation from a distance. Consistent times for hands-on patient monitoring by the same person—ideally a "cat-friendly" person—facilitate the ability to care for calmer feline patients.

Meeting the Needs of Caged Cats

Regardless of the length of stay (a few hours to several days or more), it is essential to provide for the cat's needs to support its well-being.[6] Both the size and complexity of the cage are important in meeting the needs of the caged cat.[6] Box 11-2 lists feline needs, which are also essential for caged cats.

BOX 11-2	**Meeting the Needs of the Caged Cat**

Ideally, caged cats need the following:
- Hiding place
- Vertical space
- Food*
- Water*
- Litter box*
- Human interaction if desired by the cat
- Predictability and consistency
- Gentle and respectful handling
- Ability to express normal behavior

*Note: Food, water, and litter box should not be next to each other.

Many cages made specifically for cats and other small patients are too small and do not allow sufficient space for the necessary resources to be provided. Even if a cage is of sufficient size, food is commonly placed near a litter box, which will be stress inducing for any cat. The largest cage size that can be accommodated within the veterinary practice should be used and the material that the cage is made from should be carefully selected.

Stainless steel cages are noisy and cold and can show the cat's reflection (see Figure 11-1, *A*). Cats are often frightened by the reflection in the cage, possibly thinking it is another cat, and have been observed to "attack" the reflection. Formica or polypropylene cages are quieter, warmer, nonreflective, and as easy to disinfect, making them preferable to stainless steel cages.

If the veterinary practice has stainless steel cages and they cannot be replaced in the near term, use cat beds with high sides and toweling to keep the cat warm and to prevent reflections of the cat from appearing or being noticed by the cat. Placing padding on the cage bottom, such as rubber matting, a blanket, or warmed thick towels, also helps keep feline patients warm.

Traditional cages usually lack a place to hide and a place to perch.

A Place to Hide

Hiding is an important coping mechanism for the cat in an unfamiliar environment. It is the cat's attempt to avoid interactions with others, especially in a potentially stressful situation.[17] The option to hide gives the cat a sense of control, allowing it to rest more comfortably. Not having a place to hide often results in fear, vigilance, lack of rest, and fear-associated aggression.[1] In feline terms, hiding occurs when the cat cannot see anything or anyone, and this is helpful information as it means that it is possible to provide cats with a place to hide and still be able to monitor them effectively.

Even if the cat is not allowed space to hide, it will try to do so, whether in the back of the cage, behind the box, or within or under papers or blankets, and it will often "trash" or disrupt things in the cage in an attempt to make a hiding place (Figure 11-2, *A* and *B*). Cats may shred newspaper placed in cages, or hide inside the litter box if there is no other place to hide (Figure 11-2, *C*).

Adding a place to hide, such as a cardboard box or a bed with high sides, reduces stress in caged cats.[5] The added benefit of a hiding place is that there is less potential for fear-associated aggression when a cat is removed from the cage, which greatly reduces one of the common causes of human injury in veterinary practices. The handler should pick up the box or bed while the cat is still within it. A towel covering the door of the cage can protect the cat from the sight of unfamiliar individuals and reduce any anxiety about being removed from the cage.

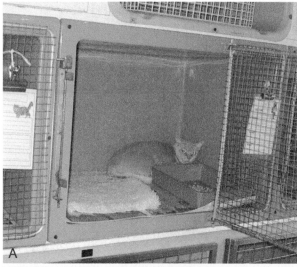

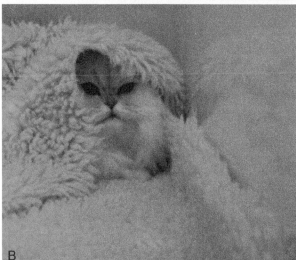

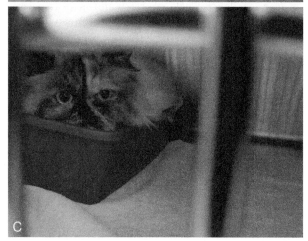

FIGURE 11-2 Cats that are not provided with a hiding place will make their own place to hide.

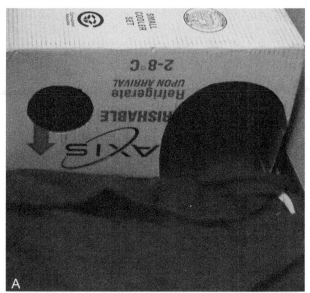

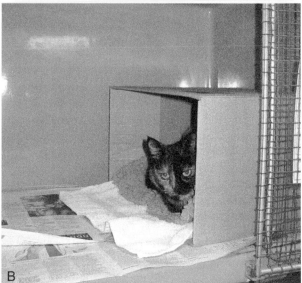

FIGURE 11-3 A cardboard box is easy to find in any veterinary practice and can be used as a hiding spot that allows the cat to see out and come out if desired. The box should be lined with fleece or a towel, preferably one from the cat's home that carries its scent.

Hiding places can be as simple as a sturdy cardboard box, a cat bed with high sides, an igloo-shaped cat bed, or the cat's carrier.

- Cardboard boxes are a great hiding place for a cat, which is proven by their desire to climb into any open boxes around the home (Figure 11-3, *A* and *B*). When used as hiding places in the veterinary practice, they should be lined with a towel or fleece bedding, preferably one that came with the cat and thus carries its scent (see Figure 11-3, *B*).
- Cat beds with high sides or igloo-shaped cat beds also make good hiding spots (Figure 11-4, *A–C*). They can be inexpensive and may last a long time, even when put into the washing machine, with diluted bleach added to the laundry soap, and then dried in the dryer. The beauty of these beds is that the cat is able to hide in a warm and comfortable place, and, when there is a need to remove the cat from the cage, this

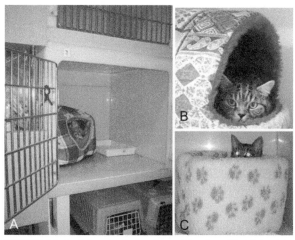

FIGURE 11-4 Igloo-style beds and beds with high sides make excellent places for cats to hide. Another advantage of this type of bed is that the cat can be moved from one place to another while inside the bed.

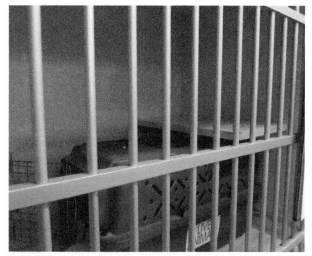

FIGURE 11-6 Placing the cat's own carrier inside the cage provides a familiar hiding space.

can be done by moving the bed with the cat still inside it.

- A litter box with high sides and soft bedding also makes a good place to hide (Figure 11-5)
- The cat's own carrier can also be placed in the cage and used as a hiding spot. Even cats that have not been carrier-trained tend to prefer their carrier at the veterinary practice to an unfamiliar space (Figure 11-6).

When the cat is fearful, the hiding place and bedding should be placed on a side of the cage that will allow the cat to look away from people who are walking by or looking into the cage. If the cat is comfortable and interested in the surroundings, the hiding place can be turned around so that the cat can see out. In a hiding place with multiple entrances, the cat can reorient itself and look out when it feels ready to observe. When a hiding place is provided, many cats will feel comfortable enough to leave the hiding spot and approach the front of the cage with curiosity.

Custom-made structures such as the Feline Fort (Cats Protection, Haywards Heath, UK) or the Hide, Perch, & Go box (British Columbia Society for the Prevention of Cruelty to Animals, Vancouver, BC, Canada) are also available (see Additional Resources for more information; also see section on vertical space).

In cages with internal shelves, a blanket or towel can be suspended from the shelf to give the cat the option of spending time behind the blanket in the back of the cage, or in the front of the blanket, where it can view its surroundings (Figure 11-7). If no internal shelf is available, then a blanket or towel can be placed over half of the cage door, thus providing additional privacy but allowing the cat to choose to look out through the open portion of the door when it is less fearful (Figure 11-8).

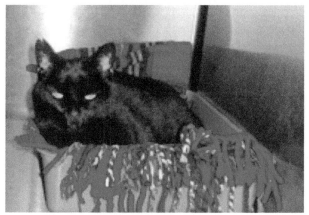

FIGURE 11-5 A litter box with high edges and soft bedding also makes a good hiding place.

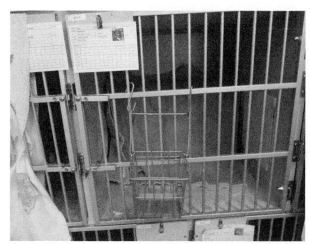

FIGURE 11-7 In cages with internal shelves, a towel or blanket can be suspended from the shelves to allow the cat to hide or look out as it wishes.

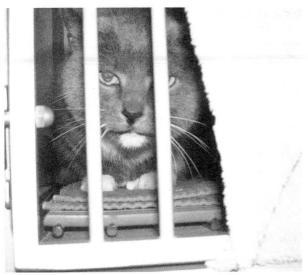

FIGURE 11-8   A towel partially covering a cage door provides additional security for the cat. The towel should be placed over half the cage door so the cat can choose to either hide or look out.

Vertical Space

Another important feline need is vertical space or a perch. There are two main benefits to having three-dimensional space in a veterinary practice cage. Cats use raised structures to monitor their environment and to anticipate the approach of others, which is especially important for a caged cat in an unfamiliar environment.[2] The vertical space also increases the overall usable space in the cage (Figure 11-9).

Most veterinary practice cages are not made with a shelf or other raised area, but excellent commercial options are now available. "Kitty condominiums" or "condos" are

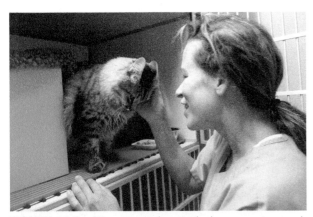

FIGURE 11-9   All cats need a vertical space or a perch from which they can monitor their environment. This is especially important for cats in an unfamiliar environment. Cages with raised shelves are ideal for this purpose. However, commercial cage inserts such as the one in this photo can increase both vertical and overall space.

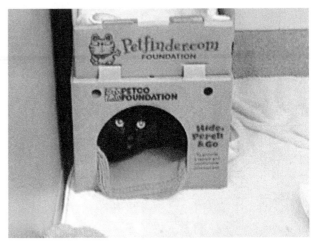

FIGURE 11-10   The Hide, Perch, & Go box, developed by the British Columbia Society for the Prevention of Cruelty to Animals, is a popular structure because it gives the cat the option to either hide or perch.

excellent for boarding cats in the veterinary practice, but they are more challenging to use for hospitalized patients.

Some commercial cages for cats are now built with a shelf; placing a towel or blanket over the shelf provides a hiding place for the cat (see Figure 11-7). For veterinary practices that have cages without shelves, there are other inexpensive solutions that will provide both a hiding place and a perch.

- A hard sided, flat-topped carrier can be used as a hiding spot and can also serve as a perch site on top. The carrier ideally stays with the cat throughout its stay, and it can be used to remove the cat from the cage, keep the cat within for treatments to be done in the bottom half, and carry the cat from one area to another.
- The Hide, Perch & Go box developed by the British Columbia SPCA is an excellent option that allows cats to hide or perch. It can be folded up into a carrier for them to go home (Figure 11-10).
- The Feline Fort developed by Cats Protection in the UK is a three-piece unit consisting of a cat step, table, and hiding spot. It provides the cat with the opportunity to hide or perch, thus helping the cat to feel safer. The Feline Fort can be purchased as a unit, or each element of it can be bought individually (Figure 11-11).
- A sturdy cardboard box turned with the opening on the side or with a door cut into the side can also be used to create vertical space.

Food and Water

Feeding the cat its regular diet during hospitalization or boarding helps with familiarity, as well as with prevention of food aversion by not introducing a new diet in a stressful environment. The client can be asked to bring the cat's favorite food and treats to help entice the cat to eat. If a

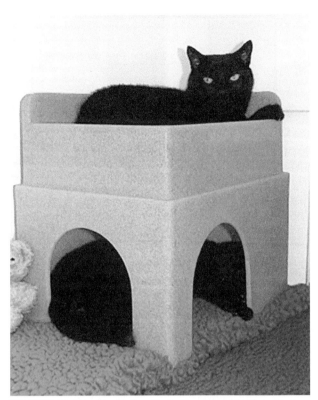

FIGURE 11-11 The Feline Fort, developed by Cats Protection in the United Kingdom, is a three-piece unit consisting of a cat step, a table, and a hiding spot. It provides the cat with a sense of security by giving it a place to either hide or perch.

dietary change is needed, it is ideal to start introducing it gradually once the cat has gone home. It is rare for a cat to need an immediate dietary change; it can usually wait until discharge. However, there are certain situations when a dietary change should be made during hospitalization, such as if the cat's normal diet has made it sick or if the cat has developed a food aversion because it became nauseous or sick when it ate that food.

In order to find out what food the cat is most likely to accept, questions should be asked about the cat's preferred diets, brands, and flavors, as well as its preference for dry and/or canned food. Providing frequent, small offerings of food allows for more normal feeding behavior and also prevents the food from becoming stale or dried. Flat food dishes with low sides are often easier for caged cats to eat from. If dry food is fed, it can be placed in feeding balls or toys to increase the cat's normal hunting behavior.

Many cats prefer warmed canned food. Microwaving the food for a few seconds on high can increase its palatability, but care must be taken to stir the food after heating in this way to avoid hot spots. This is especially true if the food was refrigerated. As cats are individuals, some do not prefer warmed food but do like food from a newly opened can, and some even want refrigerated

food. This is often seen in nauseous cats or in cats whose nausea has not been effectively controlled; the intense smell of warmed canned food makes these cats more nauseous.

If the cat has always eaten dry food, it is unlikely that its diet can be changed to canned food. Adding tepid water to dry food may be more acceptable to the cat if it needs increased liquids.

If the cat displays signs of possible food aversion (e.g., getting as far away as possible from the food, attempting to bury it, lip smacking or drooling), the food should be removed immediately. It is important to then wait before adding a different food.

If the cat is not nauseous, or if the nausea has been controlled but the cat is still inappetant, appetite stimulants can be helpful. Mirtazapine is an excellent appetite stimulant in cats. It is also an antiemetic, so it can be particularly helpful in these cats.

Toileting Area

The litter box or tray should be large enough for the cat to be able to get into it and move around without difficulty. In small cages, there is often insufficient space to provide an appropriate size litter box. When possible, the owner should be asked to bring in the litter that is used at home, but if this is not available or not considered appropriate, it is preferable to use a soft sand litter, which is comfortable underfoot and unscented.

Other Resources

Human attention is important for cats that want it. It should be given on a consistent schedule and preferably by the same caregiver so that the cat can adapt easily (see Figure 11-9). If the cat is being boarded or hospitalized on a more long-term basis, some time spent outside the cage is desirable if the cat's disease is not contagious. Long-term patients or boarders also need a place to scratch.

Spatial Arrangement of Resources

Each resource should be placed in a different area so that the cat's food, water, and litter box are separated.[6] Some shelters and veterinary practices modify their existing cages to create cages with two compartments. This is done by creating an opening, or "pass-through," between two adjacent cages (Figure 11-12, *A* and *B*). A litter box can be placed in one compartment and food and water in the other. These double-compartment cages give cats more space and more options, and ideally the cat can remain in one half of the cage while the other half is being cleaned. For more information on how to make these double-compartment cages, see the Additional Resources section.

In a small cage, the easiest way to separate the food, litter box, and resting area is by using three points as in a triangle (Figure 11-13).

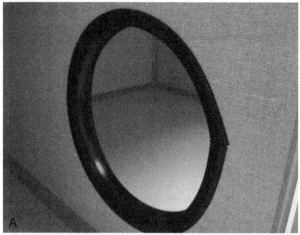

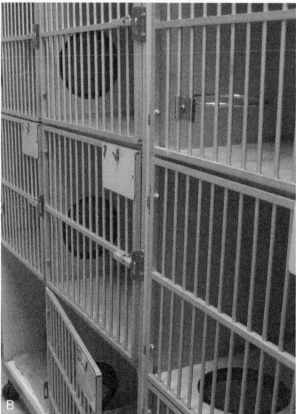

FIGURE 11-12 Some shelters and veterinary practices modify their cage banks by having a carpenter make an opening, or "pass-through," between two smaller cages to create larger spaces with two separate compartments. One compartment can be used for feeding and the other for toileting. (Courtesy E. Sundahl)

Isolation Areas and Their Additional Uses

The primary function of isolation rooms is to house cats with contagious or potentially contagious diseases. These cats should be housed in easily cleanable cages inside the isolation area. Formica or polypropylene cages are readily cleanable with bleach and other cleaning supplies and are warmer than stainless steel ones.

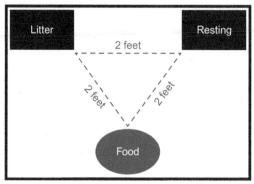

FIGURE 11-13 The easiest way to separate food, litter box, and resting areas is by using three points as in a triangle. (From Newbury S, et al: Guidelines for Standards of Care in Animal Shelters, The Association of Shelter Veterinarians, 2010)

The cage must meet the needs of the cat as described above. Provide a surface within the isolation room for examination and treatment so that the cat is not removed from the isolation area. Cats in isolation wards should always be treated last, and their cages should be cleaned last to prevent disease contagion to other cats.

In many of today's veterinary practices, isolation areas are needed only infrequently for contagious diseases; at other times they can be used to provide a nice, quiet space to house cats that are shy or displaying fear aggression. Removing these cats from the main wards reduces the stress of both these cats and other cats in the ward.

When using an isolation area for the fearful or shy cat with noncontagious disease, more creative alternatives are possible. If the cages in the isolation room are easily movable (e.g., on casters) and can be taken out of the room, these cats can have the entire room to roam, allowing them more space and capacity for enrichment (Figure 11-14, A and B). Provide warm blankets, especially on the floor, to ensure that the cat is warm enough. Even if the cages cannot be removed and there is only the one cat in the isolation ward, the cage door can remain open so that the cat can jump in and out.

HOSPITALIZATION PROCEDURES

Following certain procedures when hospitalizing a cat can make the process go more smoothly and the hospitalization experience less stressful for the patient, the client, and the veterinary staff.

Admitting Cats for Hospitalization or Boarding

In very busy veterinary practices, it is not uncommon to see several cats being brought in by their owners for admission during a relatively short time period. This can result in cats being left in carriers stacked upon one another or next to each other on the floor of the

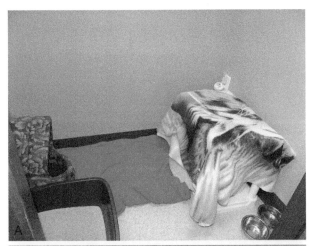
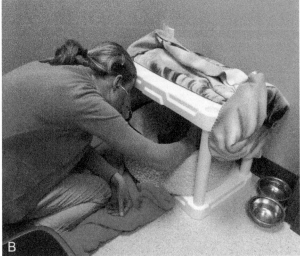

FIGURE 11-14   This shy cat did very well with the inexpensive hiding place. The cat could also choose to perch if desired.

treatment area until there is time to move the cats to the hospitalization cages. The result is increased fear and fear-associated aggression and the rest of the day going badly for both cats and staff.

It is ideal to have the ward prepared early in the morning, so that cats that are admitted can be moved to the cages without any delay. To help to create a positive and relaxed association with the enclosure, it is advisable to spray or wipe the cage and bedding with synthetic feline pheromone analog (Feliway; Ceva Animal Health, USA) a minimum of 10 to 15 minutes before it is needed. The spray version of this product has an alcohol carrier, and it is important to ensure that this has evaporated before the cat is put into the cage. Add water, litter, food if appropriate, and whatever other accessories the cat can have, prior to placing the cat inside. Preferably, move the cat while in its carrier and with bedding or something else with familiar scent. Ask clients to bring items that their cat favors, such as a piece of a favored person's clothing, toys, or anything else with a familiar scent that can be kept with the cat in the cage.

Even if there is not enough time to remove the cat from the carrier, it is important to take the cat to the ward as soon as possible and to avoid bringing it into a busy treatment area. The cat can be left in its carrier within the cage, and the carrier door can be left open so that the cat can leave the carrier if it so chooses and explore. If the ward is not prepared or there is not enough time to move the cat to the ward, then another option is to place each cat within its carrier in an unused room, such as an empty exam room or isolation area. If there is no space other than the treatment room for cats to be kept during the admission process, then place the carriers on counters instead of floors and ensure that the cats are facing away from other animals. It can be helpful to cover the carriers with towels sprayed or wiped with synthetic feline pheromone analog. The aim should always be to move the carrier to a cage as soon as possible.

Getting the Cat Out of the Cage

Removing a fearful cat from a cage can be especially challenging. Human injury frequently occurs if the cat's fear is not appreciated and the cat's sense of control is not respected during the process of removing it from what is now the safest space. Fearful cats hide, and if a hiding place is not provided, the cat often cringes in the back of the cage. When a person approaches or reaches into the cage, the cat's fear may increase rapidly, which it demonstrates by hissing, screaming, and/or lunging in the direction of the person. This is a common cause of injury to people who work with cats.

There are multiple reasons why the cat is fearful and trying to protect itself, and it is important to understand these reasons so that they can be addressed.

- Cats are often frightened because they have no place to hide, and the back of the cage is as far away as they can get from the fear-inducing situation.
- They can become more fearful if they see or hear unfamiliar cats and dogs or other animals when in the cage or while being taken out of the cage.
- When people stand in front of the cage, it is as if they are looming over the cat and blocking its only possible escape route. This will increase the cat's fear and make it more likely to display defensive aggressive behaviors.
- If a person tries to reach into the cage and grab the cat to get it out, whether with hands, towel, or gloves, the cat's fear will be exacerbated because other defense strategies—inhibition (freezing) or avoidance (fleeing)—are prevented from being successful. As a result, the cat is forced to use repulsion (fighting) as a defense and injuries to people are very common. (For more information on how to prevent this problem, see Chapters 20 and 22.)

The cat is vigilant from the start of this process and loses its sense of control rapidly as the scenario develops. The cumulative effect of each attempted interaction with the cat exacerbates its fear and increases the likelihood of fear-associated aggression being displayed.

Fortunately, several steps can be taken to make the task of getting the cat out of a cage easier for both the cat and caregiver. Safety for personnel and reduction of stress for the cat are the primary concerns. As with all interactions with cats, it is beneficial to engage in some forward planning and to make sure that all possible eventualities have been considered. The aim is for the cat to leave the cage as calmly as possible and for it to be at a low level of emotional arousal throughout the process.

In order to reduce feline stress and emotional arousal, it is beneficial to prevent them from seeing other animals, either from within the cage or when they are taken out of the cage. It is also important to prepare the room to which the cat is to be taken so that the room is safe. It would be preferable to use a small exam room rather than a large treatment room to decrease the potential for the cat to get trapped in inaccessible places if it escapes. Doors and windows should be shut and any potential escape routes blocked in case the cat gets away. This helps to reduce the temptation to use overly restrictive handling techniques. It is also necessary to ensure that the room is quiet and calm and that there are no loud or startling noises in the environment.

When approaching the cage to remove a cat, it is advisable to stand to the side and to avoid making eye contact with or staring at the cat. From the side, the door can be opened calmly, allowing the cat to choose whether to stay in its hiding place or approach. If the cat does not hiss or show other signs of aggression, the handler can put a hand into the cage so that the cat can sniff it and decide whether it wants to approach. (Figure 11-15). If there is a hiding place, such as a cat carrier, within the cage and the cat will not voluntarily come out of that area, then it would be beneficial to keep the cat within the carrier and remove it from the cage while still inside. This is particularly sensible if the cat needs to be transported over a distance, such as into an adjacent room. If there is no hiding place within the cage, it may be necessary to quietly encourage the cat to walk into a carrier that can be used to transport it to the intended destination.

If the cat is curious and approaches the front of the cage, the handler should stand to the side of the cage in order to avoid direct face-to-face contact. A hand should be moved slowly to gently touch the caudal part of the cat's abdomen to persuade it to move forward into a waiting carrier. No contact should be made with the head and neck region as this will encourage the cat to move backward and to be more resistant to the process of leaving the cage.

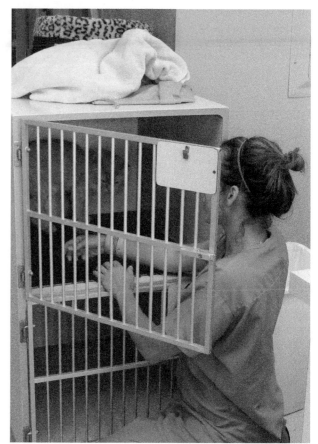

FIGURE 11-15 A calm approach is needed when taking a cat out of a veterinary practice cage.

In the majority of cases, by approaching the process of removal from the cage in this calm manner, the cat will remain in a low state of emotional arousal and the potential for fear-related aggression can be minimized. However, in some cases, cats can remain excessively aroused and the caregiver is faced with displays of overt, fear-related aggression, such as lunging and swiping. This is more likely in cats that have learned from previous negative experiences of being handled in a cage or carrier context and are therefore anxious as well as fearful. The anticipatory nature of the anxiety response leads to the cat preparing itself for a negative encounter and results in an elevated level of emotional arousal. It is ideal, if possible, to allow the cat time to relax before attempting handling, and it may help to cover the front of the pen or carrier with a towel to minimize sensory input. However, in cases where time is limited or where the cat's fear and anxiety are particularly high, it may be necessary to consider the use of chemical restraint or antianxiety medication to facilitate the handling. More information on potential approaches can be found in Chapter 20 (also see Additional Resources for a link to an online video produced by the CATalyst Council demonstrating how to remove a cat from a cage safely).

Cage Cleaning

Cats mark their territory with facial pheromones and will exhibit this behavior in a veterinary practice cage. They may display facial rubbing of bedding, boxes, cage walls, and doors. These marks are reassuring for the cat; therefore, it is important to avoid cleaning these marked areas while the cat is resident in the cage.

Most veterinary professionals have been taught to clean patient cages on a daily basis, with the cat moved from one cage to another to accomplish the thorough cleaning. However, complete cleaning of a cage during a cat's stay conflicts with the need to maintain its scent profile and familiarity. Additionally, the act of moving a cat from one cage to another can arouse and frighten both that cat as well as other cats that may hear, see, or smell the cat being moved. Often this leads to more fear and potential fear-associated aggression toward handlers. Despite these issues, it is possible to meet the hygienic requirements as well as the emotional and stress-related needs of caged cats.

If the cage is not soiled, the cat should be kept in the same cage throughout its stay. This allows the scent profile to remain familiar. The preferred method is to spot clean the cage if it is not soiled.[18] Instructions for spot cleaning are given in Box 11-3. The aim is to clean the cage with minimal disruption of the patient and areas should be wiped clean rather than sprayed. It is important to avoid wiping areas that are not soiled. The towels and blankets should not be changed unless they are soiled in order to avoid removal of familiar scents and introduction of unfamiliar ones. A similar approach is needed with litter boxes. The same litter box should be retained during the cat's stay and the litter should be scooped two or more times daily. A complete change of the litter box contents should take place only when necessary.

If the cage is soiled with urine, feces, vomit, or other deposits, the cat should be moved to a clean cage that has been prepared in advance of moving the cat. If something from the previous cage is still clean, it should be moved to the new cage to increase the cat's sense of familiarity. Arousal and fear should be prevented among all of the cats by using a visual barrier to prevent them from seeing each other. This can be achieved by moving the cat into its hiding area or to a new and clean hiding area (e.g., carrier, box, or tall cat bed). The cat should be moved directly to a newly prepared cage nearby that has been sprayed or wiped with a synthetic feline pheromone analog at least 10-15 minutes before the cat is placed into it and stocked with food, water, litter, and anything else the cat may need.

Cages, including the cage doors, should be cleaned thoroughly once a cat is discharged. All cages in one ward should be cleaned before moving on to the next ward, and isolation cages and all cages that have housed cats with contagious diseases should be cleaned last.

BOX 11-3 Techniques for Spot Cleaning

- Keep the cat in the same cage throughout the stay if possible.
- If the cage is clean, do not eliminate the smells that are now familiar to the cat.
- Keep the same bedding or towels if clean.
- Keep the same litter box and scoop a minimum of twice daily if it is easy to get to the box to do so. If not, replace the box with a clean box with minimal disruption to the caged cat.
- Cleaning should be done at a consistent time and by the same person so that the cat can anticipate this procedure.
- Prepare new food and water dishes and/or litter box, as well as anything else that may need to be replaced prior to opening the cage.
- Open the cage door quietly.
- If the cat is shy or fearful, stand to one side and allow the cat to run to or remain in its hiding area. Gently place a towel over the hiding area so that the cat can remain hidden. Tidy and remove old food and water dishes calmly and without making eye contact with the cat, but talk to the cat in a low and reassuring voice. Place prepared dishes inside the cage.
- If the cat is seeking attention, offer social interaction while tidying the cage. This can also occur at other times when the cat shows a desire for human attention.
- If the cage has a double compartment, first clean the compartment that does not contain the cat, then hopefully the cat will move to that section of the cage so that the second compartment can be cleaned.
- Close the cage door quietly.

Note: This procedure is a modified version of the spot-cleaning method recommended by the UC Davis Koret Shelter Medicine Program (Cat cage cleaning protocols for single compartment housing. Available at http://www.sheltermedicine.com/node/338. Accessed January 20, 2015).

Consistency in times for routine ward procedures, such as cleaning and feeding, is important so that the cats can be habituated to the schedule. Cage checks should be done twice daily or more frequently if the cage is being soiled. It is beneficial to have the same person—a person who enjoys working with cats—to clean the cages and interact with the cats, which will help to make the veterinary practice setting more familiar to the cat.

Considerations for "Out-of-Cage" Time

Even if the cage environment meets the cat's needs, an enriched area outside the cage is important for cats that are hospitalized or boarding for 1 week or longer. This allows them room to stretch, scratch, play, and interact with people. This is even more critical when cages are small. Options are an exam room when it is not in use or an isolation area that is not needed. Make sure the cat is provided with a hiding area and that the room provides opportunities for elevation (Figure 11-16, *A* and *B*). The hiding area can be the cat's own carrier, which can also be used to transport the cat from the cage to the "exercise/play" area.

Decisions regarding provision of "out-of-cage" time must be made on an individual basis because some cats become more fearful when taken away from the familiarity of the cage and do not benefit from having "out-of-cage" time. If the cat is hiding and stressed while in the cage, it is unlikely that taking it to another location will be beneficial, and thus it would be better to provide enrichment within the cage in the form of toys or catnip in addition to the cat's safe hiding place and perch. It is important to observe all cats that have been moved out of cages to make sure that they are doing well during the time out of the cage, and if there are signs of fear or distress, it would be advisable to return them to their more familiar environment.

Boarding Cats in the Veterinary Practice

The focus of this chapter is on caging for hospitalized patients, but many veterinary practices choose to board cats or at least to provide medical boarding for cats that need medication while owners are away from home. Cats that are boarded for several days or longer need larger spaces. "Kitty condos" are excellent options for boarding cats (Figure 11-17, *A* and *B*). However, many veterinary practices do not have these multitiered

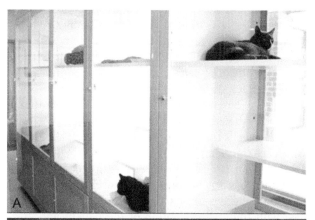

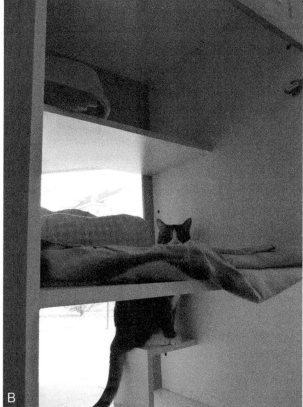

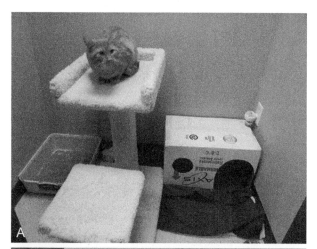

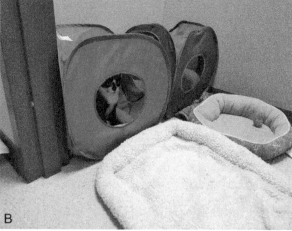

FIGURE 11-16 Having an enriched area outside the cage is important for cats that are hospitalized or boarded for 1 week or longer. Make sure that the cat is provided with opportunities for elevation, such as an elevated perch. Some fearful cats do much better in a quiet and isolated area.

FIGURE 11-17 Cats are more relaxed during boarding if they have large condominium-style accommodations with vertical spaces and familiar scents. Owners should be encouraged to bring items from home, such as beds, toys, and food.

arrangements, and other options also work well. For example, allowing the cat time out of the cage during quiet times of the day, perhaps in an exam room or in a place where they can look out a window and climb and scratch. When cats from multicat households are boarded together, it is important to remember that even cats that are bonded to another cat prefer to rest alone at least 50% of the time, and each of the cats should have its own resting area or cat bed.[10] It is also important to assess multicat interactions because those cats that are socially incompatible with their housemates may be able to manage the social tension between them when they have a whole house to occupy, but they may find being confined in a small boarding cage for 1 week or more highly stressful. Clients often want their cats to be housed together, but the decision has to be made with the best interests of the cats in mind, and, in some cases, being separated from each other is preferable from a feline perspective.

Decreasing Client Stress

Stress surrounding hospitalization is experienced not only by feline patients but also by their owners. Cat owners have multiple concerns when they leave their cat at the veterinary practice. In addition to dealing with their own worry about being separated from their feline friend, clients are also concerned about whether their cat will be scared or misbehave. They may also worry about their pet suffering alone and being ill, or even dying, away from home. In such situations, owners need reassurance that their cat will be handled lovingly and cared for in a friendly environment.

Addressing client concerns and fears about their hospitalized cat is essential to make the experience positive. There are several simple things that can be done to help the client. Most clients have never seen the hospitalization area of the veterinary practice, and the fear of the unknown can lead to a vivid imagination. Once the cage has been suitably prepared for the cat, the clients can come through to the ward to see where their cat will be staying. If it is feasible for the practice, it can also help to let the clients know that they are welcome to visit. The vast majority of clients will not abuse their visiting rights, and in fact many never visit, but the permission to do so can be reassuring.

Clients should be informed that their cat will be comforted by familiarity and that it is therefore helpful if they can supply a bed, a carrier, a toy, and some favorite food for their cat during its stay. The most important thing for clients to know is that their cat will receive the best possible care in as comfortable and respectful an environment as possible.

Clients also desperately want updates when their cat is away from them. Modern technology can be helpful in this regard, and owners of boarders can be sent short e-mails or text messages with information about how their pet is doing. Pictures can also be attached if veterinary practice staff have the time to take these. For hospitalized patients, it is important to set realistic expectations of when information, such as results of tests, will be available. It is best to set a time when a member of the practice staff will contact clients, but make it known that they can also call the veterinary practice whenever they want to, provided that they realize that it may not always be possible for them to speak to a specific member of staff and that additional information may not always be available if they initiate the call.

CONCLUSION

Because of the challenges of hospitalization for feline patients and the stress that results for their owners, it is advisable to admit cats into veterinary practices only when absolutely necessary. When the cat must be hospitalized, it is important to provide an environment that respects natural feline behavior and aims to meet the behavioral needs of feline patients. Simple steps based on an understanding of the cat's needs can help to reduce the stress of hospitalization or boarding. This not only benefits the welfare of the cat but also improves the veterinary practice's ability to treat and evaluate the cat and will result in an increase in safety and job satisfaction among staff members.

ADDITIONAL RESOURCES

British Columbia Society for the Prevention of Cruelty to Animals. CatSense: Hide, Perch, & Go Box. http://www.spca.bc.ca/welfare/professional-resources/catsense/CatSense-Hide-Perch-Go-Box.html. Accessed January 20, 2015.

Cats Protection. The Feline Fort–A Defence Against Stress. http://www.cats.org.uk/uploads/documents/feline_fort_-_info_for_vets_updated_vr3.1.pdf. Accessed January 20, 2015.

The CATalyst Council. Getting a Cat Out of a Cage (video). https://www.youtube.com/watch?v=Xr5W91nFK4M. Accessed January 20, 2015.

UC Davis Koret Shelter Medicine Program. Enriching the Shelter Environment. http://www.sheltermedicine.com. Accessed January 20, 2015.

UC Davis Koret Shelter Medicine Program. Cat Cage Modifications: Making Double Compartment Cat Cages Using a PVC Portal. http://www.sheltermedicine.com/shelter-health-portal/information-sheets/cat-cage-modifications-making-double-compartment-cat-cages-. Accessed January 20, 2015.

REFERENCES

1. Griffin B, Hume KR. Recognition and management of stress in housed cats. In: August JR, ed. *Consultations in Feline Internal Medicine*. 5th ed. St Louis: Saunders Elsevier; 2006:717–734.

2. Patronek GJ, Sperry E. Quality of life in long-term confinement. In: August JR, ed. *Consultations in Feline Internal Medicine*. 4th ed. St Louis: Saunders Elsevier; 2001:621–633.

3. Stella JL, Lord LK, Buffington CAT. Sickness behaviors in response to unusual external events in healthy cats and cats with feline interstitial cystitis. *J Am Vet Med Assoc*. 2011;238:67–73.

4. Gourkow N, Fraser D. The effect of housing and handling practices on the welfare, behaviour and selection of domestic cats (*Felis sylvestris catus*) by adopters in an animal shelter. *Anim Welf*. 2006;15:371–377.

5. Kry K, Casey R. The effect of hiding enrichment on stress levels and behaviour of domestic cats *Felis sylvestris catus* in a shelter setting and the implications for adoption potential. *Anim Welf*. 2007;16(3):375–383.

6. Rochlitz I. Recommendations for the housing of cats in the home, in catteries and animal shelters, in laboratories and in veterinary surgeries. *J Feline Med Surg*. 1999;1:181–191.

7. Zeiler GE, Fosgate GT, van Vollenhoven E, Rioja E. Assessment of behavioural changes in domestic cats during short-term hospitalisation. *J Feline Med Surg*. 2014;16:499–503.

8. McCobb EC, Patronek GJ, Marder A, et al. Assessment of stress levels among cats in four animal shelters. *J Am Vet Med Assoc*. 2005;226:548–555.

9. Rochlitz I, Podberscek AL, Broom DM. Welfare of cats in a quarantine cattery. *Vet Rec*. 1998;143:35–39.

10. Rochlitz I. Recommendations for the housing and care of domestic cats in laboratories. *Lab Anim*. 2000;34:1–9.

11. Tanaka A, Wagner DC, Kass PH, Hurley KF. Associations among weight loss, stress, and upper respiratory tract infection in shelter cats. *J Am Vet Med Assoc*. 2012;240:570–576.

12. Stella J, Croney C, Buffington T. Effects of stressors on the behavior and physiology of domestic cats. *Appl Anim Behav Sci*. 2013;143:157–163.

13. Quimby JM, Smith ML, Lunn KF. Evaluation of the effects of hospital visit stress on physiologic parameters in the cat. *J Feline Med Surg*. 2011;13:733–737.

14. Ray CC, Callahan-Clark J, Beckel NF, Walters PC. The prevalence and significance of hyperglycemia in hospitalized cats. *J Vet Emerg Crit Care*. 2009;19:347–351.

15. Buffington CA, Westropp JL, Chew DJ, Bolus RR. Clinical evaluation of multimodal environmental modification (MEMO) in the management of cats with idiopathic cystitis. *J Feline Med Surg*. 2006;8:261–268.

16. Wallinder E, et al. Are hospitalised cats stressed by observing another cat undergoing routine clinical examination? International Society of Feline Medicine 2012 Proceedings.

17. Rochlitz I. Basic requirements for good behavioural health and welfare in cats. In: Horowitz DF, Mills DS, eds. *BSAVA Manual of Canine and Feline Behavioural Medicine*. 2nd ed. Gloucester, UK: British Small Animal Veterinary Association (BSAVA); 2009:35–48.

18. Newbury S, Blinn MK, Bushby PA, et al. *Guidelines for Standards of Care in Animal Shelters*. Corning, NY: Association of Shelter Veterinarians; 2010. http://oacu.od.nih.gov/disaster/ShelterGuide.pdf, Accessed January 20, 2015.

Interplay between Behavior and Disease

CHAPTER
12

Stress as a Risk Factor for Disease

Christos Karagiannis

INTRODUCTION

In recent decades, many studies in medicine have emphasized the impact of stress on human health. In the field of feline medicine, the role of stress in a cat's health has started to be recognized as well. To address this, the field of veterinary behavioral medicine has developed paradigms to appraise the impact of stress on physical, mental, and social health.[1] Overall health is derived from these three dimensions (Figure 12-1), and disruptions to any one of them can affect a cat's well-being and may raise concerns for cat owners. Consequently, it is important for veterinary practitioners to identify the link between stress and feline health and be prepared to develop a treatment plan to target stress-related health issues. In order to do this, it is necessary to identify any factors—environmental or social—that can escalate the risk of a stress response and understand how they can affect the physical, mental, or social health of the cat.[2] Only then can the success rate of diagnosing, preventing, and managing stress-related problems be increased.

Stress can be defined as a condition in which predictability and controllability are compromised, restricted to conditions in which an environmental demand exceeds the natural regulatory capacity of an organism.[3] A stressor is a stimulus that can induce that state.[3] A stress response consists of the physiological, behavioral, and psychological alterations that occur when an individual's well-being is compromised.[4] However, measuring the level of stress in veterinary medicine can be challenging, and there is no single accepted method of doing so. Contrary to the initial theories regarding the stress response (e.g., general adaptation syndrome),[5] responses are in fact determined not only by the nature of the stressor but also by the perception of the stressor by the individual. Consequently, different types of stressors should be clinically individualized and managed, taking into account their quality and intensity. The quality and intensity of a stressor's characteristics—namely, predictability and controllability—are defined in this chapter as the emotional processes that a stressor triggers in the cat.

ASSESING A CAT'S STRESS RESPONSES

Unpredictability is characterized by the absence of an anticipatory response, and the consequent loss of control is reflected by a delayed recovery response and the presence of an atypical neuroendocrine profile.[3] Historically, this neuroendocrine profile was represented mainly by cortisol levels, but in reality an increased level of cortisol depicts a state of arousal and is not always indicative of a stress response. To assess a stress response, the emotional and/or psychological impact of unpredictability should be systematically triangulated with a range of psychological and behavioral observations, as psychological aspects cannot be assessed directly. To evaluate the emotional and psychological impacts of a potential stressor on a cat (e.g., when a visitor is coming into the house), all available behavioral (e.g., cat freezes, runs away, hides itself, hisses at visitors, meows) (Figure 12-2) and physiological (e.g., piloerection, pupil dilation, tachypnea, tachycardia, drooling) (Figure 12-3) changes must be considered. The aim is not only to evaluate the psychological impact of the quality and intensity of the stimulus to the cat, but also to further evaluate how the cat perceives the stimulus, which can vary tremendously between different individuals. Experience plays a significant role in behavior, as specific responses through time and repetition teach the cat how to act in such a way that it can control the situation and predict the outcome of its actions. Thus, in a clinical setting, differentiating a learned behavior (i.e., conditioned response) from a purely emotional behavior can be challenging.[2]

In addition, it must be noted that a stressor is not always a one-time stimulus; it often has a continuous presentation, developing effects that escalate over time. In such a setting, not only the quality, but also the intensity of the stressor must be considered. For example, when encountering a unfamiliar cat, the cat's behavior may shift from a passive inhibitory state to a more active behavior, such as avoidance (running away) or repulsion (biting or scratching), which often highlights the necessity for different case by case management, even

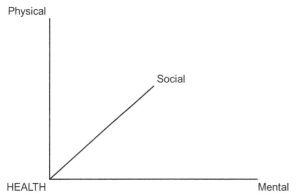

FIGURE 12-1 Health is derived from three dimensions, physical, social, and mental. Disruptions to any one of these dimensions can affect a cat's well-being and may raise concerns for cat owners.

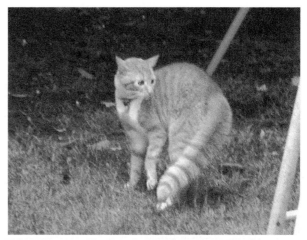

FIGURE 12-3 Physiological changes such as piloerection are indicators of the emotional impact of a stressful encounter. (Courtesy S. Heath)

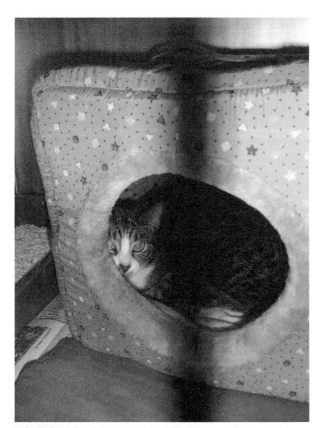

FIGURE 12-2 Behavioral manifestations of negative emotional states include hiding. (Courtesy S. Heath)

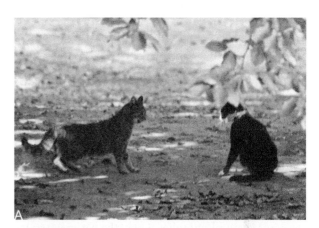

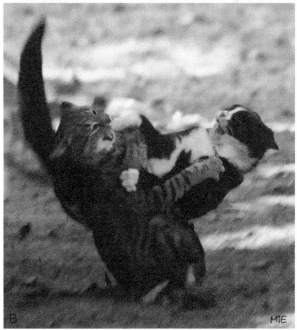

FIGURE 12-4 The cat's behavior may shift from passive inhibitory response to a more active repulsion behavior, sometimes referred to as a fight response. (Courtesy A. Dossche)

if the stress response is associated with the same emotional category (fear) (Figure 12-4, *A* and *B*).[2] For the same reason, acute and chronic stress should be managed differently.

From an affective neuroscience point of view,[6,7] emotional responses, whether induced by stress or not, are induced by triggers that can be broadly classified into the following categories:[2]

- Desirables (resources desired by the cat)
- Frustrations (denial or absence of things the cat wants)
- Fears (threats to the cat)
- Pain (bodily injury)
- Those with whom an affectionate bond is shared (social play and similar positive interactions)
- Attachment figures and objects (sources of safety and security)
- Potential sexual partners (courtship and reproductive activity)
- Offspring (parental activity)
- Undesirables (avoidance, including aggressive responses toward stimuli that do not pose an actual or perceived physical threat)

Different emotional responses can simultaneously coexist and are not mutually exclusive. For example, a cat that is uncomfortable during a clinical examination may be reacting for different reasons. A cat may be afraid of the veterinarian or may be in pain and not want to be manipulated. In both situations, the cat may express similar behaviors (e.g., avoidance of handling and manipulation), but fear will typically be triggered when the veterinarian approaches the cat, and be manifested through piloerection, retraction of the ears, arching of the back, marked pupillary dilatation, vocalization and/or hissing, and unsheathing of the claws,[8] whereas pain may be triggered when the veterinarian touches or examines the cat, resulting in hissing, snarling, growling, or biting.[9] If the cat, through experience, learns that the veterinarian's approach results in a painful experience, it may associate the veterinarian with an unpleasant, painful stimulus. Thus, the cat may try to avoid that interaction, not exclusively because it is painful, but because the cat is anxious or afraid of pain. With a repetition of this situation, the cat may learn to avoid the examination and display preemptive aggression without any signs of emotional involvement, through pain or fear, because it knows that this is the most successful strategy it can adopt in that context. Pain and fear of pain can be different emotions, and experience plays a significant role in the development of fear. Accordingly, the emotional response of the cat to different interventions must be followed and assessed.

It has been suggested that not all individuals with the same behavioral phenotype manifest improvements with the same treatment; for example, aggressive behavior in different cats may call for different intervention strategies. For this reason, an accurate diagnosis is a prerequisite.[10] However, apart from the emotional response of the animal, an additional important factor in assessing the stress response is the evaluation of the neuroendocrine profile of the underlying behavior.[2] Different neuroendocrine profiles and different neurotransmitters may be involved in the same behaviors. In dogs, different levels of stress are represented by the level of prolactin in blood plasma. Depending on the levels of prolactin, whether high or low, different psychopharmacologic agents have different efficacies.[11] Animals with lower levels of prolactinemia and signs of anxiety tend to improve after fluoxetine administration (a selective serotonin reuptake inhibitor), whereas animals with similar behavioral signs but high levels of prolactinemia show greater improvement with selegiline administration (a monoamine oxidase inhibitor). In cats, different neuroanatomical pathways are responsible for different forms of aggressive behavior (e.g., fear versus predatory attack)[8] and it is theoretically possible that this may hold true for the neuroendocrine system as well. As with the concept of personalized healthcare in humans, tailoring of medical management and patient care to the individual characteristics of each patient, beyond traditional disease-directed approaches,[12] allows the clinician to use more specific treatments. Targeted treatments for each feline patient and its owner also make compliance more likely,[2] because unnecessary measures can be identified and avoided. If the diagnosis is not accurate and the cat is not treated, or is treated inappropriately, the chronic high arousal associated with long-term stress can also elicit serious physical, mental, and social health problems (Table 12-1), emphasizing once more the significance of an accurate diagnosis and an appropriate, targeted intervention.

THE IMPACT OF STRESS ON A CAT'S PHYSICAL HEALTH

Stress in humans and animals is directly correlated with decreases in lifespan.[13,14] The mechanism behind this phenomenon, as it is found in humans, is based on DNA changes (shortened telomeres) that can accelerate aging.[13] Nevertheless, stress not only directly decreases lifespan, but can also affect the quality of life through various harmful changes in physical health, mainly though the impact of stress on the immune system. A wide range of well-documented associations in the feline veterinary literature are reviewed in this chapter, but it must be recognized that these associations do not automatically imply causality, because diseases *per se* can cause stress ("dis"-ease), and, in some situations, this bidirectional relationship is difficult to define.[2] For example, indoor cats have been reported to have a higher frequency of hyperthyroidism than outdoor cats.[15,16] Although an indoor environment may be stressful because it can be unchanging and nonstimulating,[17] recent data suggest that other indoor factors (e.g., fire retardants,[16] cat litter,[17] canned foods[18] that may be consumed in bigger proportions by indoor cats, tap water quality)[19,20] may act as thyroid disruptors or goitrogens, potentially leading to hyperthyroidism.[21]

TABLE 12-1	The Impact of Stress on Cats' Physical, Mental, and Social Health [22,23,25–31,33–35,40,42,44,47,50,52,53,55,56]

	Impact
PHYSICAL HEALTH	
Urinary system	Increased risk of interstitial cystitis
	Increased risk for cystitis
	Association between spraying and medical complications
Gastrointestinal system	Intermittent diarrhea, vomiting, or decreased appetite
	Decreased appetite and water intake, avoiding elimination for 24 hours, defecation outside the litter tray
Reproductive system	Kittens from stressed queens: lowered birth weight and slower weight gain
	Stressors can upset pituitary and ovarian functions or even terminate pregnancy
Immune system	Increased susceptibility to feline infectious peritonitis
	Increased risk of developing upper respiratory tract infection
Integument	Repetitive behaviors (e.g., overgrooming)
Genetics	Hyperactivity
MENTAL HEALTH	
	Chronic frustration
	Wool sucking in Oriental cat breeds
SOCIAL HEALTH	
	"Social phobias"
	Relinquishment
	May affect human–animal relationship

Urinary System

Stress has been reported to exacerbate clinical signs of feline idiopathic cystitis (FIC). Increased blood levels of catecholamines, which are released during stressful events, have been found in cats with severe FIC.[22,23] Catecholamine levels have been observed to return to baseline after periods of environmental enrichment.[22] For that reason, the latest treatment strategies for the management of FIC and the decline of stress levels call for environmental and behavioral measures in parallel with pharmacological intervention. This is referred to as multimodal environmental modification, or MEMO.[24]

In three different studies, researchers have reported that the risk for developing FIC is positively correlated with the amount of time that cats spend indoors.[25–27] Furthermore, specific stressors, such as moving to a new home, the presence of dogs or other cats in the house, and, especially, conflict between cats or difficulties accessing the litter tray are reportedly associated with increased risk of interstitial cystitis.[28,29] These studies suggest that the pathophysiology of FIC is related to changes in bladder permeability associated with stress.[22] In a study of healthy cats and cats with

FIC, researchers found that environmental stressors resulted in an increased number of sickness behaviors (e.g., vomiting, lethargy, anorexia) in cats with FIC.[30]

In another study, in which multicat households where a cat that sprayed or urine-marked were compared with multicat households where a cat failed to use the litter tray, researchers found that both behaviorally normal and problematic cats living with the urine-spraying cat had increased levels of fecal glucocorticoids compared with cats living without a urine-spraying cat in the household.[31] The elevated concentration of the fecal glucocorticoids is a possible biomarker of chronic arousal, suggesting that chronic stress more often drives cats to urine spraying than failure to use the litter tray. It is worth mentioning that in the Ramos et al. study,[31] 11 (48%) of 23 toileting cats and 7 (39%) of 18 spraying cats, which were described as otherwise physically normal by their owners, had signs of physical disease under clinical examination, suggesting that, regardless of chronic stress, urinating outside the litter tray or urine spraying may be associated with medical complications.

Gastrointestinal System

In humans, stress has been associated with different gastrointestinal disorders, including inflammatory bowel syndrome, peptic ulcers, and gastroesophageal reflux.[32] Similar associations have been reported in cats, and in one study, when a stressor was related to the cat's isolation or confinement, it was associated with behaviors such as vomiting, decreased appetite, or intermittent diarrhea.[33]

Reproductive System

In human medicine, stress and reproductive ability are closely related. However, in feline medicine, the association between the two has only been investigated in a few studies. For example, in one study,[34] researchers compared two groups of queens. One group remained in a location to which they had been accustomed for years (the non-stressed group) and the other was placed in a novel and stressful environment (the stressed group). The results were that the newborn kittens in the stressed group showed a significantly lower birth weight and slower weight gain after the third week of lactation compared with the nonstressed group. Furthermore, many environmental stressors can temporarily upset pituitary and ovarian functions, or even terminate a cat's pregnancy. These stressors can include shipping a queen by air or by land, moving a cat away from a familiar location, or adding new pets to a queen's environment.[35]

For pedigree cats in catteries, stressors can be more intense. They often include frequent exhibition and travel, overcrowding, extremes of temperature variation, and antagonistic social interactions.[36] Some cats can be so stressed by such factors that their ovarian functions are affected and their estrous cycles are interrupted.[37,38]

Immune System

The secretion of glucocorticoids is controlled by the brain (through corticotropin-releasing hormone), and stress can increase the secretion of these hormones, which suppress the activity of the immune system. However, in humans other mechanisms have also been described. For example, stress may lead to a rise in the likelihood of upper respiratory tract infection by suppressing the production of immunoglobulin A.[39] In general, stress can greatly impair the functionality of the immune system.

In highly stressful environments, such as catteries, it has been found that cats exhibiting high levels of stress are about five times more likely to develop upper respiratory tract infections compared with those in less stressful environments.[40] It has been described that feline viral rhinotracheitis virus (feline herpesvirus type 1) is shed at higher levels in cats who are exposed to stressful situations compared to those who live in non-stressful environments.[41] Another viral disease, feline infectious peritonitis, is also reported to be associated with stress, as stressful situations have been found to increase an animals' susceptibility to infection.[42]

The Integument

Self-grooming and scratching can be displacement behaviors and are often immediate reactions to conflicts with no apparent pathological impact.[43] Nevertheless, if the stressor is persistent, a cat may perceive a loss of control of the situation, and maladaptive overgrooming behaviors may develop.[44] This relationship between the skin and the nervous system is close, as they both are derived from the embryonic ectoderm during the developmental process[45] and share substantial numbers of hormones, neuropeptides, and receptors.[46]

Feline overgrooming is associated with a number of environmental and social stressors.[47] However, medical factors should be also considered, as it has been suggested that psychogenic alopecia is overdiagnosed, and, in most cases, the cause is primarily medical.[48] In reality, a multimodal approach similar to the one suggested for the treatment of FIC may be appropriate for the management of these cases, as medical causes may increase the risk for emotional overgrooming and vice versa (Figure 12-5).

Genetics

Epigenetics is a term that describes the mechanisms regulating how DNA is expressed and transcribed.[49] Studies in humans and rodents have shown that maternal stress can cause epigenetic changes that can lead to hyperactivity. This phenomenon not only affects the first generation offspring, but extends to the second generation as well.[50] In a study in cats, researchers found that stress can evoke changes in calcitonin gene-related peptide binding sites in the central nervous system.[51] It was suggested that cats raised in a stressful environment (e.g., strays; cats whose mothers were ill, malnourished, or undernourished), kittens experiencing dystocia, or those possibly experiencing

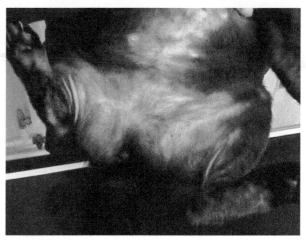

FIGURE 12-5 In cases of overgrooming, it is always important to consider medical differentials such as FIC before attributing alopecia to purely emotional triggers. (Courtesy S. Heath)

less than optimal social and/or nutritional environments may face a greater risk of becoming more hyperactive and should receive the appropriate multimodal management as soon as possible.[50]

THE IMPACT OF STRESS ON A CAT'S MENTAL HEALTH

Environmental or internal stressors, such as chronic pain, can elicit anxiety, which not only increases the risk of development of various physical health problems as already described but also increases the risk of psychological problems. In human medicine, anxiety in adults greatly increases the risk of social phobias, obsessive-compulsive behavior, and posttraumatic stress disorders, and in children it can increase the risk of separation anxiety, a psychological condition that may have comparable animal analogues.[47]

Environments that expose the animal to long-term, unpredictable, and unavoidable fear-related stressors may disturb its mental health due to a lack of perceived control. It has been described that unexpected stressful events lead to increases in elimination of both urine and feces outside the litter tray in a group of colony cats.[30] A pet cat that lives in a house with other unfamiliar cats, a situation where coping strategies are often restricted, may become more anxious during an especially stressful period, such as introduction of a new baby into the house, and may start to urinate outside the litter tray. This situation necessitates the use of multimodal treatment approaches to control both the emotional response to specific stressors (e.g., ensure appropriate distribution of essential resources) and a more general change in the mood of the environment (e.g., increase provision of hiding places, pheromone plug-in).

Chronic frustration may also elicit general behavioral changes, especially when a cat cannot have control of the situation.[6] Depending on the intensity, duration, and quality of the stressor, as well as the perception of each individual cat, the cat might respond passively or actively, with high arousal and possibly chronic displacement activities, such as overgrooming.[52] In Oriental cat breeds, genetic factors have been found to play a role in the expression of wool-sucking behavior.[53] Even if genetic predisposition increases the risk for the development of a certain behavior, environmental stressors should always be investigated, as they may catalyze the expression of the problem.

Mental health problems may develop not only from the chronic effects of a certain emotion but also from the emotional effects of motivational conflict as well. For example, a cat that is inconsistently treated by different members of a family may experience conflict anxiety. This form of anxiety is related to uncertainty about the present situation and is therefore different from anxiety associated with anticipation of aversive stimuli, which is related to concerns about the future. This is perhaps evident in a prevalence of ambivalent behaviors, such as approach-avoidance behavior and hesitancy.[2] The aim in management of these problems must be to resolve the conflict (i.e., a counterconditioning of the emotion) rather than focusing on desensitization,[2] as the goal is to encourage approach and make clear that interaction with the family has strong positive consequences for the cat.

Increased production of endogenous steroids as a result of environmental stress can have significant effects on cognitive processing, resulting in greater sensitivity to aversive stimuli. Increased aversive events in daily life can give rise to potentially negative psychological effects as well. This alteration in stimuli perception and sensitivity may impact the mental health of both normal and cognitively impaired senior animals. The pathophysiological mechanism underlying this alteration is that a stress response may increase cerebral metabolic needs and potentially result in the decline of cognitive function.[2] Veterinarians should consider the impact of exogenous steroids and critically evaluate their therapeutic benefits, since their chronic administration can also increase sensitivity to aversive events and result in behavior problems, a phenomenon well described in dogs.[54]

THE IMPACT OF STRESS ON A CAT'S SOCIAL HEALTH

The term *social health* encompasses a wide range of interactions between individuals and others, both conspecifics and heterospecifics.[2] In humans, if a person is exposed to someone who is in a stressful situation, stress responses can be triggered in their own bodies as well.[55] As cats are described by the majority of their owners as family members, their stress can affect their owners and consequently their relationship with them.

In animals, the most widely recognized problems in this domain are represented by social phobias.[9] When a stressed cat utilizes active strategies to cope with a stressful situation, including aggressive behavior toward household members or other cats, this can influence not only people and other cats, but also the stressed cat's welfare. Behavior problems are the most common reason for cat relinquishment, and house soiling is the most common cause of behavior problems, to which stress can act as a major contributor.[56] Accordingly, as the veterinary profession increasingly takes on a responsibility for the total healthcare of pets, it is essential that techniques aimed at managing and preventing these problems be embraced. These interventions form the focus of the next part of this chapter.

DIAGNOSIS AND MANAGEMENT OF STRESS-RELATED PROBLEMS

Stress Auditing

Rather than resulting from a single cause, behavior problems often stem from many different risk factors of varying importance and with an accumulating effect. Accordingly, any treatment should focus on the management of all the potential factors that can be stress-related, not just the obvious ones. The first step in developing a successful treatment plan for any behavioral problem is an accurate diagnosis of the underlying emotional motivation for the response. To this end, comprehensive history-taking is needed to identify not only the obvious triggers for the specific behavioral response, which are extensively described in other chapters, but also the more subtle background factors that can increase the risk of the problem behavior occurring (Figure 12-6). The focus here is on the diagnosis and management of all the risk factors that can alter the animal's perception of controllability and predictability of its environment and thereby trigger a stress response. In some cases, focusing on these stress factors may offer the solution to the behavior problem.[2]

As with all stress responses, background stress has a predominant quality and intensity that needs to be defined, as it affects the emotional response in a given situation. For example, in a relaxed environment, the animal may be less likely to express a fear response. However, if different stressors coexist on a frequent basis and result in a high level of background stress, a fear response may be more likely to be expressed. In cases where a cat acts aggressively toward humans, increased levels of background stress in the home have been described as one of the most pervasive risk factors.[57] Recognizing the background context of a problem and identifying non overt risk factors are essential steps in addressing this issue. This can be fulfilled through the stress audit, which provides a

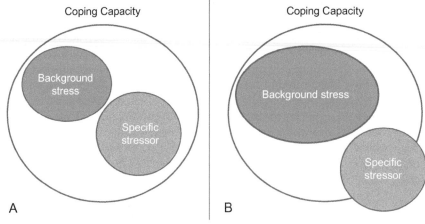

FIGURE 12-6 A cat may be able to cope with a specific stressor when the background stress is low **(A)**, but if the environmental stress is increased, the specific stressor may overwhelm the individual's coping capacity **(B)**.

framework for the systematic evaluation of possible stressors in a given situation (Box 12-1).[6] The elements of a stress audit are discussed in the next section. In practice, the stress audit can be done in the form of a written questionnaire, which can be part of the patient's history form, together with some verbal questions framed into the consultation, which would take no more than a few minutes.

Controllability and Predictability

The first step in stress auditing is to clarify the expectations placed on the cat—what role the caregivers expect

---

BOX 12-1 Stress Audit

- Husbandry
  - Daily management
  - Rules and regulations
    - Training given to enable the cat to understand them
    - Consistency of enforcement by everyone spending time with the cat
  - Level of routine
  - Quality of the general environment (physical and social)
- Expectations placed on the cat by its owner
  - Cat's role and is this the same for all family members
  - Clarity and consistency of expectations among all family members
  - Provision of resources needed by the cat to meet these expectations
- Ongoing change
  - Amount and type of change
  - Predictability within changing situations
  - Preparation for change and communication of ability to cope
  - Availability of coping strategies
- Specific stressors in the home affecting the client's family
  - Changes in behavior or circumstances that might impact the cat
- Associated changes in the expectations of a cat's behavior
- Associated changes in the cat's management
- Specific stressors in the home affecting the cat
- Physical characteristics of the stressors
  - Affective quality
  - Intensity
  - Magnitude
  - Duration
  - Predictability
- Expectation of a cat's behavior in relation to a stressor
  - Preparation given to enable coping
  - Appropriateness of the response to the cat's behavior
- Opportunities for the cat to control the stressor
- Supportive or conflicting social relationships in the home
- Support for the cat
  - Communication
    - Clarity of instruction provided to the cat expected to initiate appropriate behaviors
    - Provisions made for the cat to succeed in the appropriate behaviors
  - Feedback
  - Consistency

Adapted from Mills et al.[2]

the cat to fulfill, how these expectations are communicated, and how consistently the owners behave toward their pet.[6] For example, an owner may feed the cat when meowing, but ignore it when tired. This differential response may be detrimental to successful communication. If feeding is always associated with vocalization, the cat may start to meow excessively when food is not available. This, in turn, may irritate the owner. In this example, the expectation has not been communicated clearly to the cat and if the owner tries to use punishment to stop the unwanted vocalization, this will result in emotional conflict for the cat, who sees the owner as a positive caregiver. Such conflict is counterproductive in terms of resolving the behavioral issue.

The next step in stress auditing is to consider the physical characteristics of potential stressors and the preparation given and resources available to the cat to help it cope with the stressors.[2] A cat may be able to cope with a specific stressor, but if stressors are accumulated, especially those from the same emotional category, these triggers may overwhelm the cat's coping capacity (see Figure 12-6). Predictability may reduce the impact of the stressor, especially after repeated exposure. However, if the cat does not feel it can control the situation, any event, whether predictable or unpredictable, can lead to a stress response. If the cat learns through experience that it cannot control a specific condition, such as being manipulated by young children, predicting the situation may lead to anxiety. However, in the case of unpredictable stressors, the cat may generalize its state of anxiety to many new stimuli. For example, if the owner tries to cut the cat's nails when children are in the house, the cat may become anxious about children as well as the action of cutting nails.

Increasing a cat's controllability implies that the cat has an acceptable range of actions that it can perform to decrease the impact of the stressor. For example, if a cat that is afraid of children does not have an escape route or a safe place to go when children are around, it may feel that it has no control over the situation. Consequently, the cat may respond aggressively. The provision of hiding places or a defined safe haven is important (Figure 12-7). A safe haven can be extremely important in cases where the household stress level is high and exceeds a cat's coping ability. A carrier without a front door can be an ideal safe haven for a cat, and it can help if the carrier is not used for the sole purpose of visiting the veterinarian or the cattery in that context (Box 12-2).

Apart from the safe haven, owners actively need to be supportive and increase a cat's perception of control over a stressful situation. Many times owners feel the urge to punish their cat when the cat performs an unwanted behavior. Punishment not only increases anxiety, conflict, and frustration but also simultaneously affects human–animal relationships and compromises the owner's role as a trusted person. It has been described

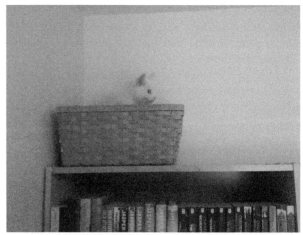

FIGURE 12-7   The provision of hiding places or a defined safe haven is important. (Courtesy S. Heath)

BOX 12-2   Train a Cat to Use the Carrier as its Safe Haven

A safe haven is a place where the animal is in control and one that has become a conditioned place of safety outside of times when there are significant stressors.[2] The aim is for the cat facing a stressor to be able to retreat to this place and feel that it has control of the situation. It is not the same as a "bolt-hole" where the animal goes when it is not confident, but just hopes that the threatening stimuli will pass. To establish a carrier as a cat's safe-haven, it is important that the cat not be anxious as a result of the presence of the carrier and that positive associations with the carrier be established through the use of food and toys. Pheromones may provide an additional positive, unconditioned, stimulus.[6] Using the carrier as a hiding place in the house can decrease the general household stress level for the cat.

In some cats, a strong negative association has already been established between the carrier and the veterinary visit and it can be difficult to override this. In these cases, placing the carrier in a small room where there are few hiding places may encourage the cat to enter it voluntarily. Removing the door of the carrier and using food and toys to create positive associations can help to teach the cat to consider the carrier a safe haven. This can decrease the cat's level of stress during veterinary visits. Further advice on how to teach a cat to use its carrier as a safe haven is given in the Feline-Friendly Handling Guidelines produced by AAFP and ISFM.

---

that punishment can alter a dog's perception of the owner as a consistently trustworthy person,[59] as well as its overall coping capabilities. Even though similar studies have not yet been carried out in cats, the presence of stressors in a cat's daily life should be identified and managed appropriately through owner education.

Management of Stress

As already described, specific stressors and problems may require specific management measures, but this falls outside the scope of this chapter, and the reader can refer to the other chapters of this book for advice on such matters. However, it should be emphasized that management measures must be tailored to the individual patient, its family, and the specific conditions where the problem developed.[6] If the veterinarian fails to understand the individual client's competence and resources, the potential to successfully support the client in resolving the cat's problems is low. Focusing on the diagnosis of the underlying motivation for the problem and developing the client's understanding of the situation from a feline perspective are vital for a successful outcome. Asking a client to change his whole lifestyle, or to spend hours of his day on the suggested treatment plan, is unreasonable for the majority of clients. Often, environmental modifications and simple management strategies, such as the avoidance of full-blown stressful circumstances and the use of pheromonotherapy, may be preferable as initial interventions, even if specific behavior modification management, and psychopharmacology in some cases, may be required as

the next stage of treatment.[2] Where possible, treatment suggestions should be framed within the context of normal daily interactions and routines because time can be a limited resource for many clients, drastically influencing their compliance with suggested behavioral modification procedures.[60]

Prevention of stress-related problems and minimizing the stress response in the first place are important aims in behavioral medicine. For this reason, the cat's early life experiences should be positive and structured in such a way that will help cats cope with environmental stressors that may evoke negative arousal and emotions. Assisting kittens in the development of a cat's life skills through the running of kitten parties has been suggested.[61] However, the aims of these classes are very different from the more familiar puppy party and not all practices are equipped with the necessary physical space or staff to run them successfully. Where a kitten party approach is not possible, the holding of kitten information evenings (where relevant information can be imparted to new kitten owners) can be extremely beneficial and can help the next generation of cat owners to be better informed about cats and their behavioral needs.

REFERENCES

1. World Health Organization. Preamble to the Constitution of the World Health Organization as adopted by the International Health Conference, New York, 19–22 June, 1946; signed on 22 July 1946 by the representatives of 61 States (Official Records of the World Health Organization, no. 2, p. 100) and entered into force on 7 April 1948.
2. Mills D, Karagiannis C, Zulch H. Stress—its effects on health and behavior: a guide for practitioners. *Vet Clin North Am Small Anim Pract.* 2014;44:525–541.
3. Koolhaas JM, Bartolomucci A, Buwalda B, et al. Stress revisited: a critical evaluation of the stress concept. *Neurosci Biobehav Rev.* 2011;35:1291–1301.
4. Carlstead K, Brown JL, Strawn W. Behavioral and physiological correlates of stress in laboratory cats. *Appl Anim Behav Sci.* 1993;38:143–158.
5. Selye H. Stress and the general adaptation syndrome. *Br Med J.* 1950;1(4667):1384–1392.
6. Mills D, Dube MB, Zulch H. Principles of pheromonatherapy. In: *Stress and pheromonatherapy in small animal clinical behaviour.* Chichester, UK: Wiley-Blackwell; 2012:127–145.
7. Panksepp J. *Affective neuroscience: the foundations of human and animal emotions.* New York: Oxford University Press; 1998.
8. Siegel A, Roeling TA, Gregg TR, Kruk MR. Neuropharmacology of brain-stimulation-evoked aggression. *Neurosci Biobehav Rev.* 1999;23:359–389.
9. Landsberg G, Hunthausen W, Ackerman L. *Behavioural problems of the dog and cat.* 3rd ed. Edinburgh, UK: Saunders; 2013, pp 76–112.
10. Heath S. Aggression in cats. In: Horwitz DF, Mills DS, eds. *BSAVA manual of canine and feline behavioural medicine.*

2nd ed. Gloucester, UK: British Small Animal Veterinary Association (BSAVA); 2009:223–235.
11. Pageat P, Lafont C, Falawée C, et al. An evaluation of serum prolactin in anxious dogs and response to treatment with selegiline or fluoxetine. *Appl Anim Behav Sci.* 2007;105:342–350.
12. Teng K, Eng C, Hess CA, et al. Building an innovative model for personalized healthcare. *Cleve Clin J Med.* 2012;79(Suppl 1):S1–S9.
13. Ahola K, Sirén I, Kivimäki M, et al. Work-related exhaustion and telomere length: a population-based study. *PLoS One.* 2012;7:e40186.
14. Dreschel NA. The effects of fear and anxiety on health and lifespan in pet dogs. *Appl Anim Behav Sci.* 2010;125:157–162.
15. Scarlett JM, Moise NS, Rayl J. Feline hyperthyroidism: A descriptive and case-control study. *Prev Vet Med.* 1998;6:295–309.
16. Kass PH, Peterson ME, Levy J, et al. Evaluation of environmental, nutritional, and host factors in cats with hyperthyroidism. *J Vet Intern Vet.* 1999;13:323–329.
17. van Rooijen J. Predictability and boredom. *Appl Anim Behav Sci.* 1991;31:283–287.
18. Edinboro CH, Scott-Moncrieff JC, Janovitz E, et al. Epidemiologic study of relationships between consumption of commercial canned food and risk of hyperthyroidism in cats. *J Am Vet Med Assoc.* 2004;224:879–886.
19. Gaitan E. Goitrogens in food and water. *Annu Rev Nutr.* 1990;10:21–39.
20. National Research Council. Effects on the endocrine system. In: *Fluoride in drinking water: a scientific review of EPA's standards.* Washington, DC: The National Academies Press; 2006:224–267.

21. Peterson M. Hyperthyroidism in cats: what's causing this epidemic of thyroid disease and can we prevent it? *J Feline Med Surg*. 2012;14:804–818.

22. Westropp JL, Kass PH, Buffington CA. Evaluation of the effects of stress in cats with idiopathic cystitis. *Am J Vet Res*. 2006;67:731–736.

23. Westropp JL, Kass PH, Buffington CA. In vivo evaluation of α_2-adrenoceptors in cats with idiopathic cystitis. *Am J Vet Res*. 2007;68:203–207.

24. Buffington CT, Westropp JL, Chew DJ, Bolus RR. Clinical evaluation of multimodal environmental modification (MEMO) in the management of cats with idiopathic cystitis. *J Feline Med Surg*. 2006;8:261–268.

25. Reif JS, Bovee KC, Gaskell CJ, et al. Feline urethral obstruction: a case-control study. *J Am Vet Med Assoc*. 1977;170:1320–1324.

26. Walker AD, Weaver AD, Anderson RS, et al. An epidemiological survey of the feline urological syndrome. *J Small Anim Pract*. 1977;18:282–301.

27. Willeberg P. Epidemiology of naturally-occurring feline urologic syndrome. *Vet Clin North Am Small Anim Pract*. 1984;14:455–469.

28. Cameron ME, Casey RA, Bradshaw JWS, et al. A study of environmental and behavioural factors that may be associated with feline idiopathic cystitis. *J Small Anim Pract*. 2004;45:144–147.

29. Pryor PA, Hart BL, Bain MJ, Cliff KD. Causes of urine marking in cats and effects of environmental management on frequency of marking. *J Am Vet Med Assoc*. 2001;219:1709–1713.

30. Stella JL, Lord LK, Buffington CAT. Sickness behaviors in response to unusual external events in healthy cats and cats with feline internal cystitis. *J Am Vet Med Assoc*. 2011;238:67–73.

31. Ramos D, Reche-Junior A, Mills D, et al. Are cats with house soiling problems stressed? A case-controlled comparison of faecal glucocorticoid levels in urine spraying and toileting cats [abstract]. In: Mills D, et al. ed. *Proceedings of the Ninth International Veterinary Behavioural Meeting Conference*; 26-28 September 2013:113–114, Lisbon Portugal.

32. Bhatia V, Tandon RK. Stress and the gastrointestinal tract. *J Gastroenterol Hepatol*. 2005;20:332–339.

33. Schwartz S. Separation anxiety syndrome in cats: 136 cases (1991-2000). *J Am Vet Med Assoc*. 2002;220:1028–1033.

34. Bilkei G. The effect of management and psychosocial stress on the fetal and postnatal development of the domestic cat [Article in German]. *Dtsch Tierarztl Wochenschr*. 1990;97:202–203.

35. Voith VL, Morrow DE. Female reproductive behavior. In: *Current therapy in theriogenology*. WB Saunders: Philadelphia; 1980:839.

36. Little S. Symposium on feline breeding and infertility. Uncovering the cause of infertility in queens: queens can have trouble producing litters for a variety of reasons, from inadequate daylight. *Vet Med*. 2001;96:557–569.

37. Feldman EC, Nelson RW. Feline reproduction. In: *Canine and feline endocrinology and reproduction*. 2nd ed. Philadelphia: Saunders; 1006:741–768.

38. Wolf AM. Infertility in the queen. In: Kirk RW, Bonagura JD, eds. *Current veterinary therapy, vol XI: small animal practice*. Philadelphia: WB Saunders; 1992:947–954.

39. Stone AA, Reed BR, Neale JM. Changes in daily event frequency precede episodes of physical symptoms. *J Human Stress*. 1987;13:70–74.

40. Tanaka A, Wagner DC, Kass PH, Hurley KF. Associations among weight loss, stress, and upper respiratory tract infection in shelter cats. *J Am Vet Med Assoc*. 2012;240:570–576.

41. Gaskell RM, Povey RC. Experimental induction of feline viral rhinotracheitis virus re-excretion in FVR-recovered cats. *Vet Rec*. 1977;100:128–133.

42. Peterson PK, Chao CC, Molitor T, et al. Stress and pathogenesis of infectious disease. *Rev Infect Dis*. 1991;13:710–720.

43. van den Bos R. Post-conflict stress-response in confined group-living cats (*Felis silvestris catus*). *Appl Anim Behav Sci*. 1998;59:323–330.

44. Willemse T, Mudde M, Josephy M, Spruijt BM. The effect of haloperidol and naloxone on excessive grooming behavior of cats. *Eur Neuropsychopharmacol*. 1994;4:39–45.

45. Fuchs E. Scratching the surface of skin development. *Nature*. 2007;445:834–842.

46. Panconesi E, Hautmann G. Psychophysiology of stress in dermatology: the psychobiologic pattern of psychosomatics. *Dermatol Clin*. 1996;14:399–421.

47. Overall K. Self-injurious behavior and obsessive-compulsive disorder in domestic animals. In: Dodman NH, Shuster L, eds. *Psychopharmacology of animal behavior disorders*. Malden, MA: Blackwell Science; 1998:222–252.

48. Waisglass SE, Landsberg GM, Yager JA, Hall JA. Underlying medical conditions in cats with presumptive psychogenic alopecia. *J Am Vet Med Assoc*. 2006;228:1705–1709.

49. Jensen P. Behaviour epigenetics–the connection between environment, stress and welfare. *Appl Anim Behav Sci*. 2014;157:1–7.

50. Overall KL, Tiira K, Broach D, Bryant D. Genetics and behavior: a guide for practitioners. *Vet Clin North Am Small Anim Pract*. 2014;44:483–505.

51. Guidobono F, Netti C, Pecile A, et al. Stress-related changes in calcitonin gene-related peptide binding sites in the cat central nervous system. *Neuropeptides*. 1991;19:57–63.

52. Mills D, Luescher A. Veterinary and pharmacological approaches to abnormal behaviour. In: Mason G, Rushen J, eds. *Stereotypic animal behaviour: fundamentals and applications to welfare*. Wallingford, UK: CABI; 2008:286–324.

53. Bradshaw JW, Neville PF, Sawyer D. Factors affecting pica in the domestic cat. *Appl Anim Behav Sci*. 1997;52:373–379.

54. Notari L, Mills D. Possible behavioral effects of exogenous corticosteroids on dog behavior: a preliminary investigation. *J Vet Behav*. 2011;6:321–327.

55. Engert V, Plessow F, Miller R, et al. Cortisol increase in empathic stress is modulated by emotional closeness and observation modality. *Psychoneuroendocrinology*. 2014;45:192–201.

56. Casey R, Vandenbussche S, Bradshaw J, Roberts M. Reasons for relinquishment and return of domestic cats (*Felis silvestris catus*) to rescue shelters in the UK. *Anthrozoos*. 2009;22:347–358.

57. Ramos D, Mills DS. Human directed aggression in Brazilian domestic cats: owner reported prevalence, contexts and risk factors. *J Feline Med Surg*. 2009;11:835–841.

58. Rodan I, Sundahl E, Carney H, et al. AAFP and ISFM feline-friendly handling guidelines. *J Feline Med Surg*. 2011;13:364–375.

59. Gácsi M, Maros K, Sernkvist S, et al. Human analogue safe haven effect of the owner: behavioural and heart rate response to stressful social stimuli in dogs. *PLoS One*. 2013;8:e58475.

60. Corridan CL, Mills DS, Pfeffer K. Comparison of factors limiting acquisition versus retention of companion dogs. *J Vet Behav*. 2010;5:22.

61. Seksel K. *Training your cat*. Melbourne, Australia: Hyland House; 2001.

Feline Obesity
A Medical Disease with Behavioral Influences
Alexander German and Sarah Heath

DEFINITION AND PREVALENCE OF OBESITY

Obesity is a disease in which excess body fat has accumulated to the point where there are adverse effects on health.[1] Cats whose weight exceeds an optimal level by >15% are said to be overweight, and those >30% above an optimal weight are considered obese.[2] As in humans, there is now irrefutable evidence that adverse consequences develop when cats are not maintained in optimal body condition.[3,4]

A number of epidemiological studies have estimated the prevalence of overweight and obese cats in the pet population to be between 34% and 41%.[5,6] Alarmingly, evidence suggests that the prevalence is increasing, with figures in North America suggesting a 90% increase in prevalence since 2007.[7]

RISK FACTORS FOR THE DEVELOPMENT OF OBESITY

Obesity arises from a positive mismatch between energy intake and energy expenditure. Intriguingly, research has demonstrated that some cats can maintain a stable weight, despite *ad libitum* feeding, while others cannot; the cats that cannot regulate gain weight gradually over time, and, if their weight gain is unchecked, they usually become obese by middle age.[8] A number of risk factors for the development of obesity have been identified, all of which alter energy balance and predispose individuals to unwanted weight gain.

Coexisting Health Problems

Concurrent disease affects overall energy balance, either through greater food consumption or because of reduced physical activity. A common example that is frequently neglected in cats is the concurrence of lameness.[3] For example, degenerative joint disease is now recognized as an important disease of aging cats and, in contrast to dogs, its clinical signs are more subtle,[9] meaning that it is frequently not recognized. The decreased activity resulting from degenerative joint disease can predispose individuals to weight gain. Another issue is use of a medical intervention that might predispose a cat to weight gain (e.g., drug therapy with glucocorticoids), although effects on appetite are less pronounced in cats than in dogs. Endocrine causes of obesity (e.g., hypothyroidism and hyperadrenocorticism) are rare in cats.

Rapid Early-Life Weight Gain

In humans, rapid early-life weight gain is a key predictor of obesity in later life,[10,11] and a similar phenomenon has been identified in cats.[8] Although the basis for this phenomenon is not yet known, a simple comparison of the ratio of weight at 2 months (i.e., second vaccination) and 12 months (first annual booster) could identify cats at risk of developing obesity in later years.[8]

Signalment

The prevalence of obesity in cats increases after 2 years of age and becomes most prevalent in middle age, then declines through the senior years.[4] Neutering is an important risk factor, mainly by impacting behavior through increasing food intake and decreasing physical activity.[12,13] Domestic shorthair cats are the most commonly affected breed, although obesity has the potential to manifest in any breed. Sex is also a predisposing factor, with a feline study suggesting that males might be overrepresented.[5]

Household Factors

Cats living with dogs or in houses with up to two other cats may be at greater risk of obesity.[14,15] The role of social stress needs further investigation, but the potential for compromising natural feline feeding behavior in multicat households due to poor distribution of feeding stations and the tendency to encourage proximity between cats during food preparation needs to be considered. Further, some, though not all, studies have suggested living exclusively indoors or apartment dwelling to be risk factors.[14,15] Possible factors include restriction of adequate physical exercise and mental stimulation due to a restricted environment. It may also be necessary to consider the potential for human nurturing behavior to be a factor in these situations where cats are living in more constant contact with their human caregivers.

Dietary Factors

Neither the use of commercial pet food nor home cooking predisposes cats to obesity, but offering cats food on an *ad libitum* basis might.[14,15] Further, some[4,16] but not all[14] studies have suggested an association with food cost, with cats consuming premium foods being more at risk of becoming overweight, possibly because such diets contain more fat and, therefore, energy. Many people believe that feeding a cat a diet with increased carbohydrate content can predispose it to obesity, as this is not typically the food consumed by cats in the wild. However, this supposition is not supported by the literature in that it is increased dietary fat, rather than carbohydrates, that predisposes cats to weight gain.[17]

Owner Influences on Weight Status

In humans, the weight status of the parents exerts a strong influence on the weight status of their children, with overweight adults typically having overweight offspring.[10] Although partly related to genetic predisposition (nature), there is also a significant effect of nurture, including parental guidance regarding food and exercise. The term *family food environment* has been coined to describe this association.[18,19]

There are a number of similarities between human and feline obesity, which is not surprising, given that both humans and felines are outbred species and have a shared environment. Furthermore, the care that owners provide for their cats mirrors that which parents provide for their children,[20] and can therefore influence the prevalence of obesity. The owners of obese cats tend to overhumanize them and use their cats as a substitute for human companionship.[21] They also play less with their cats and instead use food as a reward. Compared with the owners of cats in optimal condition, those who own overweight cats watch their cats more closely during eating, engage less with preventive veterinary care, and are more likely to be overweight themselves.[21] However, no associations with household income or owner age have yet been identified for cat owners compared with the owners of overweight dogs.[16,21,22] Further, although studies have suggested that owners of overweight dogs are more likely to be overweight themselves,[23,24] this has not yet been convincingly demonstrated in cat owners.[25]

Understanding of the parental influences on childhood obesity has improved as a result of mapping parenting styles. Four main styles are recognized, namely, authoritative, authoritarian, indulgent, and uninvolved.[26]

Not surprisingly, the indulgent style can have negative consequences, because the poor control of food intake leads to development of a poor relationship with food, predisposing to weight gain.[27] However, unexpectedly, too much parental control, as occurs with the authoritarian style, is also associated with greater body weight in the child,[28] suggesting that food restriction or pressuring children to eat certain foods can be counterproductive.[29]

In light of the similarities recognized between childhood obesity and feline obesity, an obvious question to consider is whether styles of cat ownership exist and what part they may play in the development of obesity in this species. To our knowledge, no studies have yet examined the concept of pet ownership style or the extent to which these mirror parenting styles.

The human–animal relationship is of importance and appears to be more intense in owners of obese cats,[30] and a lack of understanding of normal feeding behavior has also been identified as an important factor in feline obesity. In households where owners are more indulgent in their attitude toward their cats, it is likely that this will be manifested in more human involvement in the feeding process.

The fact that cats are solitary feeders and are by nature inclined to consume multiple small meals per day makes it difficult for owners to exercise their natural nurturing instincts, and many domestic cats find themselves being fed according to a schedule that is customary for humans. The need to be dependent on owners for the delivery of food at set times of day has the potential to be stressful for a species that is naturally in control of its own access to food sources. This can be exacerbated by the tendency for owners to use feeding time as one of the primary periods of social interaction with their pet. In multicat households, the potential for social stress is amplified by bringing multiple cats into close proximity during food preparation and delivering food in bowls that are positioned in close proximity to one another.

Lack of Knowledge of Normal Feline Feeding Behavior

Most knowledge regarding the feeding behavior of domesticated cats is derived both from observing wild felids and from observations made in laboratory animals.

Feeding Behavior in Wild Felids

Besides the lion, wild felids are solitary hunters and are considered to be strict carnivores because neither feral cats nor domesticated cats, when outside, demonstrate omnivorous feeding behavior.[31] When domesticated cats hunt, they typically seek small-sized prey, such as rodents, birds, lizards, and insects.[32–36] Interestingly, pet cats hunt more often when meat is not a component of their diet.[36] If a domesticated cat were to attempt to support its daily energy requirement solely from hunting, it would need to catch 8–12 prey animals every 24 hours, assuming that a mouse or small bird provides approximately 30 kcal of energy.

Voluntary Water Intake

The amount of water consumed varies depending on the type of diet, with no additional water consumed when eating some foods (e.g., canned food with approximately 70% water content).[37–39] However, because cats have a weak thirst drive, they do not compensate by drinking more when consuming dry food; their physiological response is thus increased urine concentration.

Diurnal and Seasonal Patterns

Cats do not have a clear circadian rhythm,[40] as demonstrated by the fact that, unlike most mammalian species, feline body temperature does not follow a circadian pattern.[41] With regard to feeding behavior, cats are both diurnal and nocturnal (e.g., sleeping and hunting both at night and during the day). Further, when cats' free-feeding patterns have been studied in laboratory conditions in which food was continuously available, they have been observed to consume between 12 and 20 meals per day that were evenly spread between light and dark periods.[42,43] Under such conditions, consumption of food was marginally greater during the light period.[43] However, farm cats can demonstrate nocturnal patterns by sleeping during the day and then traveling great distances during the night.[44] Nonetheless, such a pattern can easily be disrupted by minor disturbances (e.g., noise made by humans), suggesting that such patterns would be less likely in pet cats.

In a 4-year-long study of food intake in cats, a seasonal effect on food intake was identified, with approximately 15% less consumption during summer months than in winter.[45] Food consumption in the spring and autumn were intermediate between summer and winter intakes. Such changes in voluntary food intake were thought to be the result of changes in ambient temperature, daylight length, or both.[45] The fact that differences in food intake did not cause seasonal changes in body weight suggested that they occurred in response to changes in energy requirements.

Social Factors and Feeding Behavior

Early feeding experiences can influence feline dietary choices later in life. In this respect, when exposed to specific flavors and textures, preferences can be enhanced, with adults preferentially selecting these flavors at a later stage. On occasion, cats can become fixated on food of a single flavor and exclusively consume that food. However, once well-adjusted to a food, the adult cat will often select a new diet in preference to the existing one,[42,46–48] referred to as flavor fatigue. Although in the short term, change to a novel diet may lead to increased food consumption, once adapted to the diet, adult cats consume the same average meal size (e.g., 15 to 30 kcal), irrespective of the type of food provided (dry or wet food). In contrast to this preference for new foods (neophilia), when cats are in a strange environment, they become neophobic and avoid new flavors.[49]

Cats' preference for wet or dry food can vary. Although most cats prefer wet food, if they have had dry food for a prolonged period, they often select it in preference. Further, most cats prefer the food to be warm rather than hot or cold.[49] Thus, food kept in a refrigerator should first be warmed, and, when switching diets, it is best to do so gradually by increasing the proportion of the novel food in the existing diet.

The presence of certain amino acids (e.g., alanine, proline, lysine, histidine, and leucine) and peptides in food are important in driving food intake,[50,51] which may explain why cats especially enjoy meat flavors. Texture of food is also important. However, unlike dogs, which attempt to consume 25% to 30% of their energy intake as protein,[52,53] cats do not specifically select for protein and, indeed, may consume a protein-free diet in preference to diets with greater protein content.[54,55] These findings have been confirmed with the discovery that when offered diets with differing macronutrient content, cats attempt to balance their macronutrient intake.[56] Cats have a ceiling for carbohydrate intake, which limits ingestion when fed high-carbohydrate foods, possibly to the detriment of protein and fat intake. Thus, nutritional adequacy plays less of a part in dietary choice for cats.

Aside from proteins, certain other nutrients are known to influence food intake. Although sugar can increase the acceptance of food for a dog,[53] the same is not the case for cats.[57] Further, even small amounts (approximately 5%) of medium-chain triglycerides have a negative effect on palatability in cats.[58]

Taste

Given the presence of a genetic mutation, most cat species lack the T1R2 protein, which is required to enable the sweetness sensory receptor to function.[59] This suggests that the mutation arose in an early ancestor. Some scientists have speculated that the specialized evolutionary niche of cats (namely, being a carnivore and a hunter) perhaps, explains the observation that cats typically ignore plants, whose taste appeal often results from high sugar content.

Cat Behavioral Factors

Behavioral factors also play a part in the development of obesity, especially in cats. The factors implicated include anxiety, depression, failure to establish normal feeding behavior, and failure to develop control of satiety.[30]

Both anxiety and depression can affect appetite. If there is any suspicion of involvement of these behavioral disorders, it is advisable to refer the cat to a veterinary behaviorist for full investigation. The potential for chronic stress to play a role in obesity issues needs to be investigated through specific behavioral history-taking, and particular attention should be paid to the potential for social stress in multicat households and neighborhoods. Information about resource distribution and the potential for visual as well as physical intimidation should be gathered by questioning owners. Important additional information can be obtained through observation of the owner's property, either directly during a home visit or indirectly through the use of house layout plans or technologies such as FaceTime or Skype. Feeding cats in close proximity can be a significant source of stress (Figure 13-1) but it is beneficial to ask owners to submit video footage of their cats during food preparation as well as during food delivery, because it is not uncommon for cats that are fed in separate locations to be encouraged into proximity of one another during the preparation of their meals, resulting in significant levels of social stress. Video footage of households where food is left out on an *ad libitum* basis can be useful to gain information about feeding behavior of the resident cat in terms of how often the cat consumes food during the day. It also can uncover the involvement of neighborhood cats that are "breaking and entering" through cat flaps or open windows during the owner's absence.

The influence of feeding routines in terms of the potential for associated stress due to proximity of other cats and the potential to influence the cat's ability to control its food intake and consequently their body weight should be considered. Some reports suggest that cats do not regulate their body weight, such as by failing to maintain weight when consuming a diet diluted with cellflour and kaolin[60,61] or by failing to reduce intake when additional energy is provided with a liquid diet.[62]

However, one study suggested that two different feeding phenotypes may exist in domesticated cats.[8] In an 8-year feeding study in which cats were fed *ad libitum* for 8 years, some cats regulated their food intake and their body weight remained stable during adulthood. In other cats, their weight increased gradually after skeletal maturity, such that these cats had become overweight by 8 years of age. Although the mechanisms underlying this effect need clarification, awareness of phenotypic differences suggests that different approaches should be adopted for different cats. Cats that maintain their weight can feasibly be fed *ad libitum*, whereas some form of portion control is required for those that do not. Interestingly, there is some suggestion that these different phenotypes can be predicted early in life, before cats are overweight.[8] In this respect, and similarly to children, rapid weight gain during growth appears to be a key predictor of a cat becoming overweight later in life.[8] Thus, regular weight monitoring before 12 months of age has the potential to identify cats that may require external regulation to maintain weight. Clients can then be advised to feed their pet accordingly.

PATHOLOGICAL CONSEQUENCES OF OBESITY

Obesity increases the risk of mortality in humans, as well as increasing risk of various diseases, not least of which is metabolic syndrome. This syndrome comprises a group of metabolic and vascular disorders, which together increase the risk of an individual developing type 2 diabetes mellitus and cardiovascular disease (especially coronary artery disease, arthrosclerosis, hypertension, and dyslipidemias).[63–65] Other comorbidities in people include renal disease (e.g., diabetic nephropathy), osteoarthritis, respiratory disease (e.g., sleep apnea and asthma), hepatopathies (e.g., steatosis, cirrhosis, and hepatocellular carcinoma),[66] and various types of neoplasia (e.g., postmenopausal breast, prostatic, ovarian, colonic/rectal, renal cell, and esophageal cancers).[67]

Obesity-Associated Disorders in Cats

Table 13-1 gives details on obesity-associated disorders in cats.[68]

Longevity

Although studies have suggested a shortened lifespan in dogs that are overweight or obese,[69,70] no such studies have yet been conducted in cats. Further work is needed to determine whether cats of optimal weight have a similar lifespan advantage.

Endocrine and Metabolic Diseases

Cats usually develop an insulin-resistant form of diabetes mellitus akin to type 2 diabetes in humans, and obese

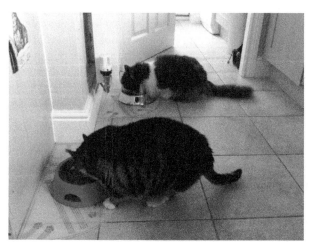

FIGURE 13-1   Cats that are fed in close proximity to one another may experience significant levels of social stress.

TABLE 13-1	Diseases Associated with Overweight and Obesity in Humans, Dogs, and Cats		
		SPECIES	
Disease Category	**Human**	**Dog**	**Cat**
Endocrine and lipid	Type 2 diabetes Metabolic syndrome Dyslipidemias	Hypothyroidism Hyperadrenocorticism Diabetes mellitus; insulin resistance Metabolic syndrome (experimental)	Diabetes mellitus Hepatic lipidosis

Cardiorespiratory	Coronary heart disease
	Atherosclerosis
	Hypertension
	Obstructive sleep apnea
	Asthma
		Tracheal collapse
		Expiratory airway dysfunction
		  (experimental)
		Hypertension (of doubtful clinical
		  significance)
		Portal vein thrombosis
		Myocardial hypoxia	

Orthopedic and impaired mobility	Osteoarthritis Musculoskeletal pain Gout	Osteoarthritis Cruciate ligament disease Humeral condylar fractures Intervertebral disc disease Hip dysplasia	Increased lameness

Oncological	Various cancers including breast
	  (postmenopausal), renal,
	  endometrial, prostatic,
	  esophageal, colon/rectal
	  hepatocellular carcinoma
		Variable neoplasia risk
		Transitional cell carcinoma
		Mammary carcinoma (some but not
		  all studies)
			Increased neoplasia
			  risk

Urogenital	(Diabetic) nephropathy	Urinary tract disease
		Urethral sphincter mechanism
		  incompetence
		Calcium oxalate urolithiasis[37]
		Transitional cell carcinoma
		Glomerular disease (experimental)
		Dystocia
			Increased risk of
			  urinary tract
			  disease

Alimentary	Pancreatitis
	Hepatic steatosis
	Cirrhosis
		Pancreatitis	Increased oral cavity
			  disease and
			  gastrointestinal
			  disease

Other	Depression Postoperative complication Various dermatological diseases	Immune function	Increased risk of dermatoses

Reprinted with permission from Elsevier. German AJ, Ryan VH, German AC, et al: Obesity, its associated disorders and the role of inflammatory adipokines in companion animals. Vet J 185:4–9, 2010.

cats develop insulin resistance,[71] which predisposes them to the development of clinical diabetes mellitus.[4] Successful weight loss in obese cats improves their insulin sensitivity, and,[72] in cats with diabetes, it can decrease the need for exogenous insulin therapy, sometimes eliminating it altogether.[73] Although the pathogenesis remains unclear, an association between feline obesity and hepatic lipidosis has long been known.[4]

Orthopedic Disorders

Obesity is a major risk factor for orthopedic disease in dogs, with associations identified for osteoarthritis, hip dysplasia, humeral condylar fractures, cranial cruciate ligament rupture, and intervertebral disc disease.[74-76] As mentioned above, obesity is a potential risk factor for orthopedic disease in cats, with one study suggesting that

obese cats are five times more likely to limp than cats of normal body condition.[3] However, not all reports have confirmed this association.[4] The lack of association in this later study[4] may relate to the fact that orthopedic disease is underrecognized, given that signs are subtle in this species.

Other Disorders

Obesity can negatively impact cardiorespiratory function in both humans[77] and dogs.[78-80] Unfortunately, given the absence of equivalent feline data, the extent to which the cardiorespiratory system is compromised in cats is not known. In epidemiological studies, researchers have reported an increased risk of neoplasia in cats that are obese.[4]

In experimental dogs, the onset of obesity is associated with glomerular pathology and changes in function, including increases in plasma renin and insulin concentrations, mean arterial pressure, and plasma renal flow.[81] However, no such association has yet been demonstrated in cats. In contrast, although the reasons for an association are unclear, obese cats are at increased risk of oral cavity disease, dermatological disorders, and diarrhea.[4]

Pathogenesis of Obesity-Associated Diseases

Excessive amounts of white adipose tissue (WAT) increase the risk of disease through both mechanical and endocrine etiologies. Mechanical causes include excessive loading of weight-bearing structures (exacerbating orthopedic diseases), constriction of collapsible structures (increasing risk of upper respiratory tract and urinary system disorders), inability to groom, and reduced heat dissipation due to the insulating effect of fat. However, there is now recognition that WAT is an important endocrine organ, synthesizing a range of cytokines, chemokines, and other inflammation-related proteins, collectively termed *adipokines*.[68] Thus, in addition to mechanical causes, WAT can predispose individuals to diseases via derangements in endocrine function. In humans, increases in the production of certain inflammatory adipokines (e.g., leptin, tumor necrosis factor α, IL-6, plasminogen activator inhibitor-1, and haptoglobin) have been directly linked to the development of the metabolic syndrome and other disorders linked to the obese state.[82] Although information is more limited, inflammatory adipokine gene expression in feline WAT has been documented.[81] Plasma leptin concentrations have been shown to be independently associated with insulin sensitivity in lean and overweight cats.[83] This suggests that pathogenetic mechanisms similar to those seen in human obesity may exist in companion animals.

CLINICAL INVESTIGATIONS

At first presentation, an overweight cat should be examined thoroughly to determine the severity of obesity, possible predisposing factors for weight gain, and whether there are any concurrent diseases that may be associated with obesity. The exact tests required to evaluate overall health status depend upon the individual patient, most notably the presence of other signs. This baseline information allows the clinician to determine the cat's ideal weight, choose the safest and most effective approach for weight loss, and determine a suitable target for weight loss.

History and Physical Examination

The history will have both medical and behavioral components and should include details of the cat's environment, lifestyle, diet, and exercise regimes, as well as a complete medical history, including previous or current therapy.

Assessing Body Weight and Composition

Body composition can be assessed in various ways. First, dual-energy x-ray absorptiometry (DXA) is known to be precise and reliable and can be used in a referral setting[84,85]; however, it is not widely available in first opinion veterinary practice. Instead, noninvasive methods are preferred, most notably using a combination of body weight and body condition scoring (BCS). Body weight is best measured using the same set of electronic weigh scales, and it is important to calibrate these regularly. The most reliable calibration method is to use test weights, although, given the expense, any object of known mass could instead be used (e.g., a bag of food).

Although body weight is a poor measure of body composition, since it does not enable fat mass to be differentiated from lean tissue or bone mineral, it is the most precise means of monitoring a weight loss plan. Therefore, body weight should be measured at the outset and regularly thereafter. A variety of systems for assessing body condition are available, all of which use both visual assessment and palpation to determine body fat mass subjectively.[86,87] However, the 9-integer-unit system is preferred. With appropriate training, the technique correlates well with body fat mass determined by other methods, such as DXA.[86] At the outset, BCS can be used to establish the degree of obesity and predict the likely ideal weight of a particular animal (see below).[86,87] BCS should also be used periodically during the weight program to check on progress, and target weight should be adjusted if required.

Further Investigations

Although it is not always essential, routine hematological examination, clinical chemistry, and urinalysis can be useful when determining the cat's overall state of health and to identify concurrent disease. In some cases, such as when the clinician is concerned about a specific associated disease, further tests may also be necessary. Examples include measurement of blood pressure, fasting blood glucose, and fructosamine concentrations (e.g., if diabetes is suspected), as well as diagnostic imaging, such as survey radiography (for possible orthopedic and respiratory disease) and abdominal ultrasonography (e.g., hepatic ultrasonography with fine-needle aspiration cytology or liver biopsy for suspected hepatic lipidosis). Targeted assessment of the urinary system (e.g., bacterial culture of urine, bladder ultrasonography, and radiographic contrast studies) might be necessary if there are concurrent lower urinary tract signs.

Ideal Weight Versus Target Weight

In setting a weight loss plan, it is essential to know the ideal weight because this target will be used to set the initial caloric intake (see below). The ideal weight is the estimated optimal weight for the particular cat, which is the weight at which fat mass is optimal. In reality, there will be a range of weights deemed to be ideal, which, when determined by DXA, is less than 20% for domestic cats.[87] For most weight loss plans, a simple way to determine ideal weight is based on the current weight and BCS. In this regard, each unit on the scale between 5/9 and 9/9 corresponds to approximately 10% to 15% excess weight.[86,87] Therefore, with a simple calculation, the ideal weight can be determined.[55] An alternative approach to determining ideal weight is to refer to historical records of body weight in the individual cat. For instance, if the veterinary practice has a record of an early-adulthood body weight (i.e., 12 to 18 months of age) with a concurrent normal BCS (4/9 or 5/9), this is arguably a more accurate indicator of optimal weight.

Although the terms *target weight* and *ideal weight* are commonly used interchangeably, they mean different things. The target weight is the final weight that the clinician determines to be appropriate for the individual cat. For some cats, the target weight and ideal weight may be the same, but that might not be appropriate for all. The main benefits of returning an animal to its optimal weight will be in disease prevention and extending lifespan.[69,70,73] Therefore, such an approach is most beneficial for a young cat that has not yet developed any associated diseases. However, those benefits would be less for an older cat and/or one with preexisting disease. Instead, in those cats, weight management should focus on improving quality of life, and it may not be necessary to return them to ideal weight for such benefits to be seen. In fact, a study in dogs has revealed that reductions in severity of disease typically occur with modest (i.e., greater than 5%) reductions in weight.[88] A partial weight loss protocol would also be most appropriate for an older cat with another chronic disease likely to cause chronic wasting. In humans, an obesity paradox has been identified:[89] Although being overweight often increases the risk of developing the disease, when present, survival is longer in overweight rather than ideal weight patients. Examples of the obesity paradox in cats include chronic kidney disease[90] and cardiac disease,[91] with a study demonstrating longer survival times in overweight cats. In such cases, a modest weight reduction (of 5% to 10%) to a target in the overweight range will not lead to significant loss of lean tissue,[85] but can improve quality of life, as seen in a recent canine study.[92]

TREATMENT AND PROGNOSIS

Weight management in cats can be immensely challenging. Many cats do not successfully reach their target weight, and about half of those that do subsequently rebound.[93] Therefore, for cats' weight management to be successful, owners must be extremely dedicated and veterinary professionals must closely support and encourage them. Successful weight management is not simply about reducing body fat; what is more important is improving quality of life, decreasing severity of associated diseases, and reducing the risk of developing another disease. It is also important to change clients' behavior, most notably regarding feeding habits. To ensure long-term success, it is essential that a healthier relationship between the cat and its owner be established. Cats should lose weight at a steady rate during their weight loss program; overly rapid weight loss should be avoided, given concerns over inducing hepatic lipidosis or causing excessive lean tissue loss. A study of pet cats suggested that approximately 1% weight loss per week represents a realistic goal and seems to be safe.[94]

It is important to consider two phases in any weight loss program: weight loss and weight maintenance. Weight loss can take a variable amount of time, depending upon how overweight the cat is and how fast the weight is lost; although most weight loss programs are completed within 1 year, occasionally longer periods are required. The main aim of the maintenance phase is to ensure that body weight is first stabilized at the chosen target weight and then maintained over the long term to prevent rebound. Because younger cats are more likely than older cats to rebound,[93] they require especially close monitoring during the maintenance phase.

Although microsomal membrane transfer protein inhibitor drugs are licensed for weight loss in obese dogs, they are neither licensed nor safe for use in cats.[95] Instead, dietary therapy in conjunction with increased activity is the most common approach to obesity management in felines. In cases where emotional disorders such as anxiety are involved, these will also need to be treated and referral to a specialist in veterinary behavioral medicine is appropriate.

Dietary Management

Diet Choice

Purpose-formulated weight loss diets are recommended because they are restricted in energy content while providing supplemental protein and micronutrients to avoid malnutrition. A high-protein (relative to energy) formulation does not speed up the rate of weight loss, but it ensures that lean tissue loss is minimized. Supplementing the diet with L-carnitine can also maintain lean tissue mass during weight loss. Altering the macronutrient content of a weight management diet can also improve satiety. For instance, increasing both protein and fiber content relative to energy provides the greatest benefit for satiety in dogs,[96,97] but this is less successful in cats.[25] This is because increased dietary protein content can increase voluntary food intake in cats, and too much fiber is unpalatable.[98] Instead, the best effect on satiety occurs with modest fiber and protein supplementation.[25] Studies have also suggested that increasing water content may be beneficial. Not only will this lead to caloric dilution, but there is also some evidence that activity levels will increase.[99,100]

Energy Intake During Weight Loss

When calculating energy allocation for weight loss, it is essential to base the calculations on the ideal body weight and not on the current weight. The rate of weight loss depends mainly upon energy intake, with greater restriction leading to more rapid weight loss but also to greater potential to lose lean tissue.[101] The exact energy intake needed to induce weight loss can vary between cats, and adjustments (typically reductions) in energy are often needed during a weight loss plan to maintain weight loss. One study suggested that pet cats with naturally occurring obesity lose weight at a mean rate of 0.8% body weight per week when mean energy intake over the whole course of weight loss was 32 kcal/kg ideal weight.[85]

Method of Feeding

Use of measuring cups should be avoided because such measurements are imprecise, especially with the small portions typically given to cats. In a study, there was marked intra- and inter-individual variability in the actual amount of food measured, with overestimates being most common.[102] Further, many cups were found to be incorrectly calibrated, such that the printed scale did not reflect actual portion size. Electronic kitchen scales are preferred as an alternative to using measuring cups. Clients can be instructed to weigh daily portions and partition them into bags. The food in each portion can then be readily divided across the required number of meals and/or be reserved for use as treats or in puzzle feeders.

If possible, no additional food should be given by the owners or scavenged by the cat. It is common for owners to underestimate the energy contribution of many such foods. In some cases, functional treats can be recommended (e.g., a treat to support oral cavity health), but the caloric content must be included in calculating the overall allocation and provide less than 5% of total daily requirements. Liquids (e.g., milk), and food used to facilitate oral administration of medications can also be a source of significant caloric intake.

From the perspective of feeding behavior, a range of strategies can be considered for cats. As mentioned above, some cats can safely be fed a free-choice diet, yet still maintain body weight.[8] Such a strategy is not suitable for others that overeat. Because cats will typically consume many meals daily, strategies involving a single large meal (or even two) daily are best avoided.[103] An alternative approach is to place the correct daily ration in a bowl and make the food available for as long as is required for the cat to consume it during the day. However, such a strategy does not always work, nor does the practice of feeding a cat a diet of lesser energy density. Further, it can sometimes be a challenge to control the energy intake of an outdoor cat if the cat is able to consume food elsewhere in the neighborhood (e.g., at a neighbor's house). Multicat households can also be a challenge, not least when the cats' feeding requirements vary (e.g., different feeding phenotype or requirement of a different diet). In such cases, individualized strategies that make use of spatial separation (feeding in different rooms) or supervised feeding must be considered. Where owners are unable to supervise feeding or are trying to offer a more self-service form of feeding, various forms of creep feeding have been tried, ranging from the use of cardboard boxes with cutouts that allow only the slimmer household cats to gain access to food to arrangements where food is placed in elevated locations that the obese cat is unable to access. If owners are willing to install microchip-operated cat flaps in internal doors within the house, this method can be used to create selective access to feeding bowls. An electronic feeding bowl has been developed that opens only when triggered by a registered microchip (Figure 13-2). Such devices, if used correctly, have the potential to maximize individual feeding and minimize risk of weight gain.

Changes in lifestyle to encourage increased expenditure of energy are described in the next subsection, and it is possible to combine these aims with the delivery of food through the provision of so-called puzzle feeders. These can take various forms, but the idea is that the cat gains mental and physical stimulation while gaining access to the daily food ration. Owners can make their own feeders by using plastic drink containers (Figure 13-3, *A*) or toilet paper tubes (Figure 13-3, *B*), or they can purchase more complex feeding devices (Figure 13-4, *A–D*).

Lifestyle Management

Increasing physical activity is recommended for most obese cats on a weight loss program, because it promotes fat loss, assists in lean tissue preservation, and aids with owner compliance. The activity program should be tailored to the individual cat and take account of any concurrent medical concerns. Cats can be encouraged to increase their activity through regular

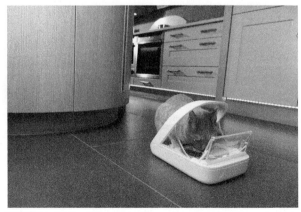

FIGURE 13-2 The use of a microchip feeder can help ensure that each cat in a multicat household has access to the correct diet. (Courtesy SureFlap)

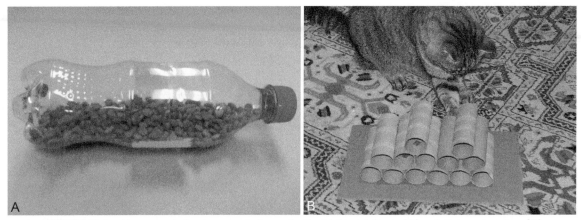

FIGURE 13-3 Homemade feeders made from plastic drink containers **(A)** or toilet-paper tubes **(B)** can provide both physical and mental stimulation for the overweight cat. **(B,** Courtesy I. Rodan)

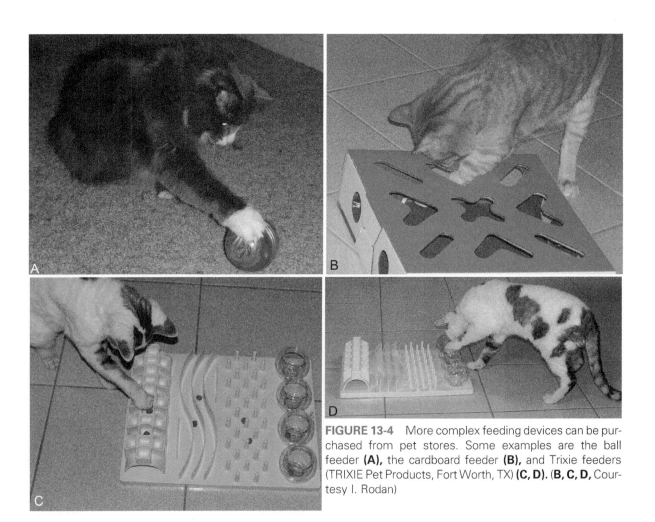

FIGURE 13-4 More complex feeding devices can be purchased from pet stores. Some examples are the ball feeder **(A)**, the cardboard feeder **(B)**, and Trixie feeders (TRIXIE Pet Products, Fort Worth, TX) **(C, D)**. **(B, C, D,** Courtesy I. Rodan)

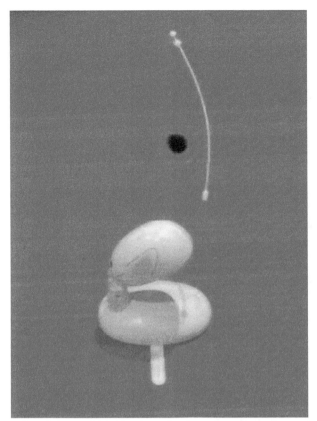

FIGURE 13-5   Motorized toy feeders encourage play and stimulate activity.

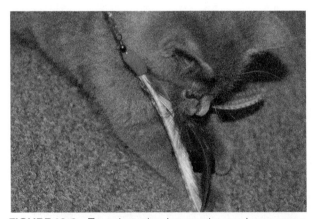

FIGURE 13-6   Toys that stimulate predatory play are especially useful in encouraging the cat to expend energy. (Courtesy I. Rodan)

play sessions with cat toys (e.g., fishing rod toys), motorized units (Figure 13-5), and puzzle feeders (see Figure 13-4, *A–D*). Toys that stimulate predatory play can be particularly beneficial (Figure 13-6). Energy expenditure can also be increased by providing access to high resting locations (Figure 13-7, *A* and *B*), which has the added benefit of giving cats the opportunity to moderate stress levels by allowing them access to elevated perches. In multicat households, the incorporation of feeding locations into cat trees can be beneficial by allowing better distribution of feeding stations and giving the cat the opportunity to eat in a quiet, protected, and elevated location (Figure 13-8, *A* and *B*).

Monitoring of Weight Loss

Regular weight checks should be scheduled during weight loss, and a 2-week interval is initially recommended because adjustments are often required shortly after starting a new program. It is then acceptable to extend the interval between checks if weight loss is consistent, but an interval longer than 4 weeks should be avoided because compliance may be lost. It is usually best if a single, dedicated member of staff be responsible for weight management in a particular cat. That way, a rapport can be established with the cat owner, and this can improve success. Given that some clients require intensive support throughout the program, training in client counseling is recommended. It is essential to continue to monitor a cat's body weight after ideal weight has been achieved to ensure that weight that was lost is not regained. As with humans, a rebound effect has been demonstrated after weight loss in cats.[93]

Prognosis

When a cat is predisposed to obesity due to both individual and environmental factors, many of these predispositions will remain after weight loss, and risk of rebound is therefore greater. Professional experience suggests that approximately one-half to two-thirds of dogs and cats successfully reach their ideal weight. That said, 90% of cats do lose more than 5% of weight, an amount that is known to improve disease status in both dogs and humans (AJG, unpublished observations). For unknown reasons, some cats fail to lose significant weight or are lost to follow-up. This might be related to the perception of poor quality of life[101] or may be due to metabolic disturbances. In this respect, one study has demonstrated that the adipokine adiponectin might be a key player in weight loss.[72] As in humans and other species, adiponectin concentration is lower in obese cats. Intriguingly, adiponectin concentrations are lowest in cats that fail to lose weight. Further, even when weight loss is successful, cats with the lowest pre–weight loss adiponectin concentrations lose more lean tissue during the process. Clearly, therefore, adiponectin status is a critical factor in the success of weight management, although currently it is unclear whether this is directly associated with treatment failure or represents an innocent bystander.

In addition to the fact that many cats fail to reach their target weight, approximately 50% of cats that successfully reach their ideal weight rebound, although most regain less than half their initial loss. Therefore, as mentioned above, continued monitoring of body weight during maintenance is recommended. Further, continuing to feed cats a purpose-formulated diet (i.e., the one used for weight loss)

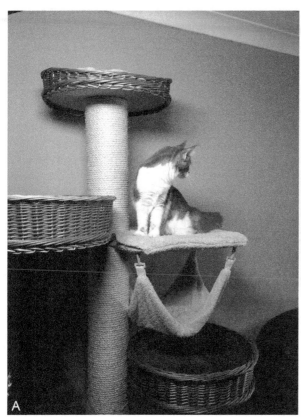

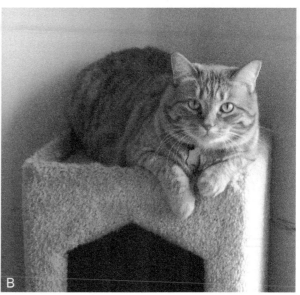

FIGURE 13-7 Cat trees and other elevated resting spots encourage the cat to jump and climb and also provide a stress-free place for the animal to rest. (**B,** Courtesy I. Rodan)

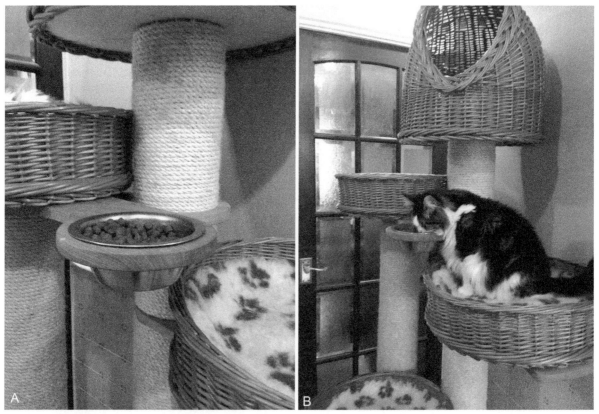

FIGURE 13-8 In multicat households, elevated feeding stations provide a place for the cat to eat in a quiet, protected, and elevated location.

can help to prevent rebound. Such diets have been shown to be appropriate for the low weight maintenance energy requirements of dogs after weight loss.[104]

Prevention

Given the variable outcome of weight management diets, prevention of obesity would appear to be a preferable strategy to weight management after obesity has developed and would appear likely to have a more significant beneficial effect on the health and welfare of cats. Advice on optimal nutrition and exercise should be included in all kitten consultations and continued for all cats throughout their lives. Ideally, body weight should be recorded at every visit, and BCS should be considered at least annually. Regularly monitoring body weight and BCS throughout a cat's life can enable subtle changes (e.g., ±5%) to be identified and rectified before they worsen (e.g., with subtle changes in routine). Veterinarians should be alert to the weight gain that can occur as a consequence of neutering. It is advisable to schedule two or three checks for weight and BCS in the first 6 to 12 months after neutering to identify those cats that gain excessive amounts of weight during that time.

Finally, knowledge of pet ownership styles could ultimately be used to help in obesity prevention. If certain styles are known to predispose to obesity, then targeted client education can be applied to those clients with ownership styles likely to predispose their cat to weight gain. A study has identified that different populations of cats exist that respond differently to long-term *ad libitum* feeding.[8] Some cats are unable to regulate their food intake, leading to gradual lifelong weight gain, whereas others maintain stable weight and optimal body condition throughout their lives, presumably by regulating intake. Therefore, this suggests that different groups of cats have different feeding styles, some of which are regulators, whereas others tend to overeat. When it comes to preventing weight gain, attention should be paid to the match of pet ownership style to feeding style. For example, owners with an indulgent feeding style might not be a good match for a cat that overeats, but might be fine for one that self-regulates. Such owners could be free to feed a cat that self-regulates as they wish, without the risk of inducing undesirable weight gain in their cat. A better match for an overeating cat would be an owner with an authoritative style.

REFERENCES

1. Kopelman PG. Obesity as a medical problem. *Nature.* 2000;404:635–643.
2. German AJ. The growing problem of obesity in dogs and cats. *J Nutr.* 2006;136(suppl 7):1940S–1946S.
3. Scarlett JM, Donoghue S. Associations between body condition and disease in cats. *J Am Vet Med Assoc.* 1998;212:1725–1731.
4. Lund EM, Armstrong PJ, Kirk CA, Klausner JS. Prevalence and risk factors for obesity in adult cats from private US veterinary practices. *Int J Appl Res Vet Med.* 2005;3:88–96.
5. Colliard L, Paragon BM, Lemeuet B, et al. Prevalence and risk factors of obesity in an urban population of healthy cats. *J Feline Med Surg.* 2009;11:135–140.
6. Courcier EA, O'Higgins R, Mellor DJ, Yam PS. Prevalence and risk factors for feline obesity in a first opinion practice in Glasgow, Scotland. *J Feline Med Surg.* 2010;12:746–753.
7. Banfield Pet Hospital: Banfield Pet Hospital state of pet health 2012 report. http://www.stateofpethealth.com/Content/pdf/State_of_Pet_Health_2012.pdf Accessed January 23, 2015.
8. Serisier S, Feugier A, Venet C, et al. Faster growth rate in *ad libitum*-fed cats: a risk factor predicting the likelihood of becoming overweight during adulthood. *J Nutr Sci.* 2013;2:e11.
9. Clarke SP, Bennett D. Feline osteoarthritis: a prospective study of 28 cases. *J Small Anim Pract.* 2006;47:439–445.
10. Danielzik S, Czerwinski-Mast M, Langnäse K, et al. Parental overweight, socioeconomic status and high birth weight are the major determinants of overweight and obesity in 5-7 y-old children: baseline data of the Kiel Obesity Prevention Study (KOPS). *Int J Obes Relat Metab Disord.* 2004;28:1494–1502.
11. Reilly JJ, Armstrong J, Dorosty AR, et al. Avon Longitudinal Study of Parents and Children Study Team: Early life risk factors for obesity in childhood: cohort study. *BMJ.* 2005;330:1357.
12. Flynn MF, Hardie EM, Armstrong PJ. Effect of ovariohysterectomy on maintenance energy requirements in cats. *J Am Vet Med Assoc.* 1996;9:1572–1581.
13. Harper EJ, Stack DM, Watson TD, Moxham G. Effect of feeding regimens on bodyweight, composition and condition score in cats following ovariohysterectomy. *J Small Anim Pract.* 2001;42:433–438.
14. Robertson ID. The influence of diet and other factors on owner-perceived obesity in privately owned cats from metropolitan Perth, Western Australia. *Prev Vet Med.* 1999;40:75–85.
15. Allan FJ, Pfeiffer DU, Jones BR, et al. A cross-sectional study of risk factors for obesity in cats in New Zealand. *Prev Vet Med.* 2000;46:183–196.
16. Kienzle E, Bergler R, Mandernach A. Comparison of the feeding behavior of the human–animal relationship in owners of normal and obese dogs. *J Nutr.* 1998;128(suppl 12):2779S–2782S.
17. Backus RC, Cave NJ, Keisler DH. Gonadectomy and high dietary fat but not high dietary carbohydrate induce gains in body weight and fat of domestic cats. *Br J Nutr.* 2007;98:641–650.
18. Birch LL, Davison KK. Family environmental factors influencing the developing behavioral controls of food intake and childhood overweight. *Pediatr Clin North Am.* 2001;48:893–907.
19. Campbell KJ, Crawford DA, Ball K. Family food environment and dietary behaviors likely to promote fatness in 5–6 year-old children. *Int J Obes (Lond).* 2006;30:1272–1280.
20. Archer J. Why do people love their pets? *Evol Hum Behav.* 1997;18:237–259.
21. Kienzle E, Bergler R. Human-animal relationship of owners of normal and overweight cats. *J Nutr.* 2006;136(suppl 7):1947S–1950S.
22. Courcier EC, Thompson RM, Mellor DJ. An epidemiological study of environmental factors associated with canine obesity. *J Small Anim Pract.* 2010;51:362–367.

23. Holmes KL, Morris PJ, Abdulla Z, et al. Risk factors associated with excess body weight in dogs in the UK. *J Anim Physiol Anim Nutr.* 2007;91:166–167.

24. Nijland ML, Stam F, Seidell JC. Overweight in dogs, but not in cats, is related to overweight in their owners. *Public Health Nutr.* 2010;13:102–106.

25. Bissot T, Servet E, Vidal S, et al. Novel dietary strategies can improve the outcome of weight loss programmes in obese client-owned cats. *J Feline Med Surg.* 2010;12:104–112.

26. Maccoby EE, Martin J. Socialization in the context of the family: parent–child interaction. In: Mussen PH, ed. *Handbook of child psychology: socialization, personality, and social development.* New York: Wiley; 1983:1–101, vol. 4.

27. Hughes SO, Power TG, Orlet Fisher J, et al. Revisiting a neglected construct: parenting styles in a child-feeding context. *Appetite.* 2005;44:83–92.

28. Faith MS, Scanlon KS, Birch LL, et al. Parent-child feeding strategies and their relationships to child eating and weight status. *Obes Res.* 2004;12:1711–1722.

29. Ventura AK, Birch LL. Does parenting affect children's eating and weight status? *Int J Behav Nutr Phys Act.* 2008;5:15.

30. Heath S. Behaviour problems and welfare. In: Rochlitz I, ed. *The welfare of cats.* London: Springer; 2005:91–118.

31. Ewer RF. Felidae. In: *The carnivores.* New York: Cornell University Press; 1973:205–230.

32. McMurry FB, Sperry CC. Food of feral house cats in Oklahoma. *J Mammal.* 1941;22:185–190.

33. Eberhard T. Food habits of Pennsylvania house cats. *J Wildl Manag.* 1954;18:2284–2286.

34. Coman B, Brunner H. Food habits of the feral cat in Victoria. *J Wildl Manag.* 1972;36:848–852.

35. Fitzgerald BM. Diet of domestic cats and their impact on prey populations. In: Turner DC, Bateson P, eds. *The domestic cat: the biology.* Cambridge, UK: Cambridge University Press; 1988:123–146.

36. Robertson ID. Survey of predation by domestic cats. *Aust Vet J.* 1998;76:551–554.

37. Caldwell GT. Studies in water metabolism of the cat. *Physiol Zool.* 1931;4:324–355.

38. Danowski TS, Elkinton JR, Winkler AW. The deleterious effect in dogs of a dry protein ration. *J Clin Invest.* 1944;23:816–823.

39. Prentiss PGA, Wolf AV, Eddy HE. Hydropenia in cat and dog: ability of the cat to meet its water requirements solely from a diet of fish or meat. *Am J Physiol.* 1959;196:625–632.

40. Hawking F, Lobban MC, Gamage K, Worms MJ. Circadian rhythms (activity, temperature, urine and microfilariae) in dog, cat, hen, duck, Thamnomys and Gerbillus. *J Interdiscipl Cycle Res.* 1971;2:455–473.

41. Sterman MB, Knauss T, Lehmann D, Clemente CD. Circadian sleep and waking patterns in the laboratory cat. *Electroencephalogr Clin Neurophysiol.* 1965;19:509–517.

42. Mugford RA. External influences on feeding of carnivores. In: Kare MR, Maller O, eds. *The chemical senses and nutrition.* New York: Academic Press; 1977:25–50.

43. Kane EJG, Morris JG, Rogers QR, Leung PMB. Feeding behaviour of the cat fed laboratory and commercial diets. *Nutr Res.* 1981;1:499–507.

44. MacDonald E, Apps P. The social behaviour of a group of semi-dependent farm cats, *Felis catus*: a progress report. *Carnivore Genet Newsl.* 1978;3:256–268.

45. Serisier S, Feugier A, Delmotte S, et al. Seasonal variation in the voluntary food intake of domesticated cats (*Felis catus*). *PLoS One.* 2014;9:e96071.

46. Kuo ZY. The dynamics of behavior development: an epigenetic view. New York: Random House; 1967.

47. Mugford RA, Thorne C. Comparative studies of meal patterns in pet and laboratory housed dogs and cats. In: Anderson RS, ed. *Nutrition of the dog and cat.* Oxford, UK: Pergamon Press; 1980:3–14.

48. Kane EJG. Feeding behaviour of the cat. In: Burger IH, Rivers JPW, eds. Nutrition of the dog and cat, *Waltham symposium 7.* Cambridge, UK: Cambridge University Press; 1989:147–158.

49. Bradshaw J, Thorne C. Feeding behaviour. In: Thorne C, ed. *Waltham book of dog and cat behaviour.* New York: Pergamon Press; 1992:115–129.

50. White TD, Boudreau JC. Taste preferences of the cat for neurophysiologically active compounds. *Physiol Psychol.* 1975;3:405–410.

51. Hargrove DM, Morris JG, Rogers QR. Kittens choose a high-leucine diet even when isoleucine and valine are the limiting amino acids. *J Nutr.* 1994;124:689–693.

52. Romsos DR, Ferguson D. Regulation of protein intake in adult dogs. *J Am Vet Med Assoc.* 1983;182:41–43.

53. Hickenbottom SJ, Torres CL, Rogers QR. Adult purified diets. *Fed Proc.* 2001;15:A981.

54. Cook NE, Kane E, Rogers QR, Morris JG. Self-selection of dietary casein and soy-protein by the cat. *Physiol Behav.* 1985;34:593–594.

55. Cook NE, Rogers QR, Morris JG. Acid-base balance affect dietary choice in cats. *Appetite.* 1996;26:175–192.

56. Hewson-Hughes AK, Hewson-Hughes VL, Miller AT, et al. Geometric analysis of macronutrient selection in the adult domestic cat, Felis catus. *J Exp Biol.* 2011;214:1039–1051.

57. Beauchamp GK, Maller O, Rogers JG. Flavor preferences in cats (*Felis catus* and *Panthera* sp.). *J Comp Physiol Psychol.* 1977;91:1118–1127.

58. MacDonald ML, Rogers QR, Morris JG. Aversion of the cat to dietary medium-chain triglycerides and caprylic acid. *Physiol Behav.* 1985;35:371–375.

59. Li X, Li W, Wang H, et al. Pseudogenization of a sweet-receptor gene accounts for cats' indifference toward sugar. *PLoS Genet.* 2005;1(27–35):2005.

60. Kanarek RB. Availability and caloric density of the diet as determinants of meal pattern in cats. *Physiol Behav.* 1975;15:611–618.

61. Hirsch EC, Dubose C, Jacobs HJ. Dietary control of food intake in cats. *Physiol Behav.* 1978;20:287–295.

62. Castonguay TW, Giles TC, Harrison JE, Rogers QR. Variations in sucrose concentration and their effect of food intake in the domestic cat. *Abstr Soc Neurosci.* 1987;13:464.

63. Reisin E, Alpert MA. Definition of the metabolic syndrome: current proposals and controversies. *Am J Med Sci.* 2005;330:269–272.

64. Diabetes UK. Type 2 diabetes & obesity: a heavy burden. London: Diabetes UK; March 2005.

65. Shaw DI, Hall WL, Williams CM. Metabolic syndrome: what is it and what are the implications? *Proc Nutr Soc.* 2005;64: 349–357.

66. Marchesini G, Moscatiello S, Di Domizio S, Forlani G. Obesity-associated liver disease. *J Clin Endocrinol Metab.* 2008;93(11)(suppl 1):S74–S80.

67. Calle EE, Thun MJ. Obesity and cancer. *Oncogene.* 2004;23:6365–6378.

68. German AJ, Ryan VH, German AC, et al. Obesity, its associated disorders and the role of inflammatory adipokines in companion animals. *Vet J.* 2010;185:4–9.

69. Kealy RD, Lawler DF, Ballam JM, et al. Effects of diet restriction on life span and age-related changes in dogs. *J Am Vet Med Assoc.* 2002;220:1315–1320.

70. Salt C, Morris P. Associations between longevity and body condition in domestic dogs. In *Proceedings of the*

WALTHAM International Nutritional Sciences Symposium 2013: from pet food to pet care: bridging the gap, p. 52. http://www.waltham.com/dyn/_assets/_pdfs/winss/FINALWINSSProceedings2013.pdf Accessed January 23, 2015.

71. Feldhahn JR, Rand JS, Martin G. Insulin sensitivity in normal and diabetic cats. *J Feline Med Surg.* 1999;1:107–115.

72. Tvarijonaviciute A, Ceron JJ, Holden SL, et al. Effects of weight loss in obese cats on biochemical analytes relating to inflammation and glucose homeostasis. *Domest Anim Endocrinol.* 2012;42:129–141.

73. Zoran DL, Rand JS. The role of diet in the prevention and management of feline diabetes. *Vet Clin North Am Small Anim Pract.* 2013;43:233–243.

74. Brown DC, Conzemius MG, Shofer FS. Body weight as a predisposing factor for humeral condylar fractures, cranial cruciate rupture and intervertebral disc disease in cocker spaniels. *Vet Comp Orthop Traumatol.* 1996;9(2):38–41.

75. Kealy RD, Olsson SE, Monti KL, et al. Effects of limited food consumption on the incidence of hip dysplasia in growing dogs. *J Am Vet Med Assoc.* 1992;201:857–863.

76. Impellizeri JA, Tetrick MA, Muir P. Effect of weight reduction on clinical signs of lameness in dogs with hip osteoarthritis. *J Am Vet Med Assoc.* 2000;216:1089–1091.

77. Wolk R, Shamsuzzaman ASM, Somers VK. Obesity, sleep apnea, and hypertension. *Hypertension.* 2003;42:1067–1074.

78. Bach JF, Rozanski EA, Bedenice D, et al. Association of expiratory airway dysfunction with marked obesity in healthy adult dogs. *Am J Vet Res.* 2007;68:670–675.

79. Manens J, Bolognin M, Bernaerts F, et al. Effects of obesity on lung function and airway reactivity in healthy dogs. *Vet J.* 2012;193:217–221.

80. Mosing M, German AJ, Holden SL, et al. Oxygenation and ventilation characteristics in obese sedated dogs before and after weight loss: a clinical trial. *Vet J.* 2013;198:367–371.

81. Henegar JR, Bigler SA, Henegar LK, et al. Functional and structural changes in the kidney in the early stages of obesity. *J Am Soc Nephrol.* 2001;12:1211–1217.

82. Trayhurn P, Wood IS. Adipokines: inflammation and the pleiotropic role of white adipose tissue. *Br J Nutr.* 2004;92:347–355.

83. Appleton DJ, Rand JS, Sunvold GD. Plasma leptin concentrations are independently associated with insulin sensitivity in lean and overweight cats. *J Feline Med Surg.* 2002;4:83–93.

84. Raffan E, Holden SL, Cullingham F, et al. Standardized positioning is essential for precise determination of body composition using dual-energy X-ray absorptiometry. *J Nutr.* 2006;136(suppl 7):1976S–1978S.

85. German AJ, Holden SL, Bissot T, et al. Changes in body composition during weight loss in obese client-owned cats: loss of lean tissue mass correlates with overall percentage of weight lost. *J Feline Med Surg.* 2010;10:452–459.

86. German AJ, Holden SL, Moxham GL, et al. A simple reliable tool for owners to assess the body condition of their dog or cat. *J Nutr.* 2006;136(suppl 7):2031S–2033S.

87. German AJ, Holden SL, Bissot T, et al. Use of starting condition score to estimate changes in body weight and composition during weight loss in obese dogs. *Res Vet Sci.* 2009;87:249–254.

88. Marshall WG, Hazewinkel HAW, Mullen D, et al. The effect of weight loss on lameness in obese dogs with osteoarthritis. *Vet Res Commun.* 2010;34:241–253.

89. Flegal KM, Kit BK, Orpana H, Graubard BI. Association of all-cause mortality with overweight and obesity using standard body mass index categories: a systematic review and meta-analysis. *JAMA.* 2013;309:71–82.

90. Parker VJ, Freeman LM. Association between body condition and survival in dogs with acquired chronic kidney disease. *J Vet Intern Med.* 2011;25:1306–1311.

91. Finn E, Freeman LM, Rush JE, et al. The relationship between body weight, body condition, and survival in cats with heart failure. *J Vet Intern Med.* 2010;24:1369–1374.

92. German AJ, Holden SL, Wiseman-Orr ML, et al. Quality of life is reduced in obese dogs but improves after successful weight loss. *Vet J.* 2012;192:428–434.

93. Deagle G, Holden SL, Biourge V, et al. Investigating long-term outcomes of weight management in obese cats. In *Proceedings of the WALTHAM International Nutritional Sciences Symposium 2013: from pet food to pet care: bridging the gap*, p. 49. http://www.waltham.com/dyn/_assets/_pdfs/winss/FINALWINSSProceedings2013.pdf Accessed January 23, 2015.

94. German AJ, Holden SL, Bissot T, et al. Dietary energy restriction and successful weight loss in obese client-owned dogs. *J Vet Intern Med.* 2007;21:1174–1180.

95. Gosselin J, McKelvie J, Sherington J, et al. An evaluation of dirlotapide to reduce body weight of client-owned dogs in two placebo-controlled clinical studies in Europe. *J Vet Pharmacol Ther.* 2007;30(suppl 1):73–80.

96. Weber M, Bissot T, Servet E, et al. A high protein, high fiber diet designed for weight loss improves satiety in dogs. *J Vet Intern Med.* 2007;21:1203–1208.

97. German AJ, Holden SL, Bissot T, et al. A high protein high fibre diet improves weight loss in obese dogs. *Vet J.* 2010;183:294–297.

98. Servet E, Soulard Y, Venet C, Biourge V. Ability of diets to generate "satiety" in cats. *J Vet Intern Med.* 2008;22:1482.

99. Cameron KM, Morris PJ, Hackett RM, Speakman JR. The effects of increasing water content to reduce the energy density of the diet on body mass changes following caloric restriction in domestic cats. *J Anim Physiol Anim Nutr.* 2011;95:399–408.

100. Alexander JE, Colyer A, Morris PJ. The effect of reducing dietary energy density via the addition of water to dry diet, on body weight, energy intake and physical activity in adult neutered cats. In *Proceedings of the WALTHAM International Nutritional Sciences Symposium 2013: from pet food to pet care: bridging the gap*, p. 50. http://www.waltham.com/dyn/_assets/_pdfs/winss/FINALWINSSProceedings2013.pdf Accessed January 23, 2015.

101. Butterwick RF, Markwell PJ. Changes in the body composition of cats during weight reduction by controlled dietary energy restriction. *Vet Rec.* 1996;138:354–357.

102. German AJ, Holden SL, Mason SL, et al. Imprecision when using measuring cups to weigh out extruded dry kibbled food. *J Anim Physiol Anim Nutr.* 2011;95:368–373.

103. National Research Council. Committee on Animal Nutrition, Subcommittee on Dog and Cat Nutrition: Feeding behavior in dogs and cats. In: *Nutrient requirements of dogs and cats*. Washington, DC: National Academies Press; 2006:21–27.

104. German AJ, Holden SL, Mather NJ, et al. Low-maintenance energy requirements of obese dogs after weight loss. *Br J Nutr.* 2011;106(suppl 1):S93–S96.

CHAPTER

14

Acute Pain and Behavior

Sheilah A. Robertson

INTRODUCTION

In many countries, the number of pet cats equals or outnumbers dogs,[1,2] yet appropriate understanding and treatment of feline pain is still lacking. Most pet cats undergo at least one surgical procedure in their lifetime, usually for neutering. Veterinarians consider surgical procedures in dogs and cats to be equally painful, but treat cats less often.[3] It is important to understand why that is. One reason for the higher level of treatment in dogs may be that their pain-related behaviors are more overt. There is a strong desire to do better, and, as part of their professional oath, veterinarians agree to *protect animal welfare, prevent and relieve animal suffering, and continually improve their professional knowledge.* It is true to say that compared with dogs, pain in cats has been neglected,[4–9] but there are encouraging data showing that this is now changing in many parts of the world.[10–12] However, in the interests of feline welfare, the veterinary profession must strive to do more.[12] One of the main reasons cited for undertreatment of pain in cats is difficulty in its recognition and assessment. Other reasons include a lack of feline-specific data on analgesic agents, fear of drug-related side effects, and the lack of products with market authorization. The focus of this chapter is the recognition and quantification of acute pain in cats.

WHAT IS PAIN?

Pain, as defined by the International Association for the Study of Pain (IASP) Task Force on Taxonomy, is "an unpleasant sensory and emotional experience associated with actual or potential tissue damage, or described in terms of such damage."[13] This implies that pain has both sensory and affective components and is a complex, multidimensional experience. The sensory or, put simply, "ouch" component includes the type of pain and its source, location, and intensity. Pain occurs while one is in a conscious state. It is always unpleasant and aversive, and this underlies its description as an emotion. The affective or emotional component can be thought of as "how it feels" or "how it makes you feel"

and is a negative experience associated with actual harm or the potential for harm. There is a consensus that, as in humans, pain has an emotional component in animals but is more challenging to measure.[14] It is important to understand that pain is always subjective and involves "private states"[14] that are not directly accessible by others; in other words, no one can feel another person's pain. The fact that pain can never be measured directly makes accurate quantification of pain difficult, even in humans who are capable of self-reporting pain, as these reports are still a proxy measure. However, in most situations, "pain is what the patient says it is." An added challenge is the unique experience of each individual; even after the same surgical procedure, humans do not experience the same quality and intensity of pain, nor the same pain-related emotions.

PAIN IN NONLINGUAL POPULATIONS

In order to treat pain it is necessary to look for it, recognize it, and quantify or measure it in some way so that the efficacy of interventions can be assessed. Some subpopulations of humans (e.g., neonates and individuals with cognitive impairment) cannot self-report; therefore, the IASP added the following important caveat to its definition of pain: "The inability to communicate verbally does not negate the possibility that an individual is experiencing pain and is in need of appropriate pain-relieving treatment."[13] Animals also fall into this special category.

Animals are often labeled as nonverbal, but in reality they are nonlingual, as they are in essence lacking only human language. Making conclusions about an animal's pain is challenging, but careful observation of behavior, posture, and facial expressions[15] is currently thought to be the most accurate method. Put simply, in most humans, pain is what the patient says it is, but in animals it is what people say it is. The burden is on clients and the veterinary profession, as their proxy, to ensure that what they are "saying" is not lost in translation. If humans get this wrong, it is possible for an animal to be overtreated but much more likely that it will be undertreated, which will negatively affect that individual's welfare.

PAIN ASSESSMENT TOOLS

"If you cannot measure it, you cannot improve it."
Lord Kelvin

There is no gold standard for assessing acute pain in cats at this time. Several different scoring methods that include physiologic and behavioral variables have been created and used in clinical settings, but until recently most tools or instruments did not undergo rigorous testing for validity. All scoring systems that depend on human observers are subjective to some degree and leave room for error, which could be either under-assessing or overassessing an animal's pain. Creating an objective or empirical tool to capture a subjective state such as an animal's pain has in the past been done by well-intentioned people who have taken intuitive leaps.[16] Focusing on something that makes sense to someone familiar with the species can be a good starting point, but it must be treated as a hypothesis and rigorously tested for validity, reliability, and sensitivity.[16-18]

Physiologic Indicators of Pain

Pain can cause changes in several physiologic parameters, such as heart rate, blood pressure, and respiratory rate. Neuroendocrine secretion may be altered in animals in pain. Therefore, as part of the stress response to anesthesia and surgery, catecholamine and cortisol concentrations have been measured in an attempt to identify objective indicators of pain. β-endorphin, an endogenous opioid, can be released from the adenohypophysis to modify pain and provide some degree of analgesia; therefore, this has also been measured as a correlate or proxy marker of pain in many species.

The University of Melbourne Pain Scale for dogs includes measurement of heart rate and respiratory rate. The authors who developed the scale stated that when combined with assessment of behavioral responses, it could be used reliably to evaluate the degree of pain in dogs after surgery.[19] Conzemius and colleagues[20] found no or only poor correlation between heart rate, respiratory rate, or blood pressure and a visual analogue scale (VAS) or numerical rating scale (NRS) when assessing postoperative pain in dogs. Holton and colleagues[21] assessed pain using a NRS and recorded heart rate and respiratory rate in hospitalized dogs. They included dogs undergoing orthopedic or soft tissue surgery, dogs with medical conditions, and healthy dogs and concluded that in a veterinary practice environment, heart rate and respiratory rate are not useful indicators of pain.

In a controlled research environment using laboratory animal sourced cats, systolic blood pressure was shown to be a good predictor of postoperative pain following ovariohysterectomy.[22] However, when used in a clinical setting, the correlation between pain and easily measured physiologic variables such as heart rate, respiratory rate, and blood pressure has, as in dogs, been disappointing in cats. Smith and colleagues, who conducted both studies, concluded that in cats, objective variables, including heart rate, respiratory rate, and systolic blood pressure, were not consistent indicators of pain in an uncontrolled clinical situation.[23] Brondani and colleagues found a weak correlation between pain scores and systolic blood pressure in cats undergoing ovariohysterectomy.[24] During refinement of a multidimensional composite pain scale for assessing acute postoperative pain in cats, heart rate and respiratory rate were rejected after item analysis.[5]

Pain can result in pupil dilation, but this was not found to be useful for assessing pain in dogs.[21] Mydriasis was not used as a criterion for deciding if rescue analgesia was required following ovariohysterectomy in cats, because opioids produce marked mydriasis in this species.[25] Other factors that influence pupil size include ambient lighting and the use of anticholinergic agents. Fear also causes mydriasis in cats[26]; therefore, pupil size should be considered an insensitive indicator of pain in this species.

Physiologic variables can be affected by many factors other than pain. The stress of a journey to a veterinary practice will alter heart rate, blood pressure, and respiratory rate in most cats,[27] and cats often show behaviors indicative of fear and stress when in a clinical setting, which are accompanied by physiologic changes.[26]

Plasma cortisol and β-endorphins are components of the stress response to anesthesia and surgery, and much effort has gone into trying to correlate these hormones with pain in laboratory and clinical settings. In both a controlled laboratory environment and a clinical setting, cortisol increased in response to surgery (ovariohysterectomy). The increases reported correlated with the duration of surgery and were ameliorated when butorphanol, an opioid analgesic, was given.[22,23] Some studies have shown that, compared with placebo treatment groups, plasma or serum cortisol levels were lower in cats undergoing neutering procedures with or without onychectomy if they received analgesics.[28,29] In another study, there was no difference in plasma cortisol between cats that underwent anesthesia alone and those that underwent anesthesia and had a tenectomy or onychectomy, but differences between surgical and nonsurgical groups could be detected by trained observers blinded to the procedure when they used an interactive VAS and tested the cat's response to palpation.[30] Brondani and colleagues suggested that cortisol may be an indicator of pain in cats, provided they have a period of adaptation to the veterinary practice environment before the surgery is performed.[24] Looking at cortisol concentrations may be useful in a research setting, such as when assessing analgesic agents and when cats have had an opportunity to adapt to the environment; however, it should not be used alone as a measure of pain in cats. It is not a practical tool in a clinical setting, because the results of the assay are not immediately available and cats are unlikely to be acclimated to the environment. β-endorphin concentrations did not differentiate between control cats (anesthesia only) and those that also underwent surgery.[30]

Overall, no single physiologic measurement or neuroendocrine marker has been found to be a sensitive clinical correlate of pain in cats.

Mechanical Threshold Testing

Following surgery or acute injury, changes occur locally, resulting in peripheral or primary sensitization. This leads to a reduction in the noxious stimulus required at the wound to elicit a response by the patient. In some cases, changes in the central nervous system also occur due to the afferent barrage of signals coming from the periphery, resulting in a condition termed *central* or *secondary sensitization*. Central sensitization leads to a decrease in the mechanical threshold required to elicit a response in areas remote from the primary injury. One strategy for measuring pain related to primary sensitization is to quantify the sensitivity of the wound by measuring the stimulus required to produce an aversive response in the patient (e.g., turning to look at the site, turning to bite, or vocalizing). Noxious stimuli include thermal, electrical, and mechanical energy, but the latter is most practical in a clinical setting. Application of mechanical pressure is termed *algometry,* and the level of stimulation needed for a given response is usually inversely proportional to the degree of discomfort.[31]

Mechanical nociceptive threshold testing with devices such as algometers, von Frey filaments, and palpometers has proved a useful technique for measuring both primary (wound) and secondary (remote areas) hyperalgesia in animals. Using a finger-mounted pressure device, Slingsby and colleagues were able to demonstrate a reduction in scrotal hyperalgesia following castration when cats were administered meperidine (pethidine).[32] Testing wound sensitivity is considered a valuable tool by other authors.[5,25,30,33,34] Mechanical devices that accurately measure the applied force (e.g., in Newtons) are valuable research tools (Figure 14-1), but physical palpation is an excellent tool in clinical practice (Figure 14-2).

Gait Analysis and Weight Bearing

Pressure platforms and pressure-sensitive walkways can be successfully used in cats to analyze gait,[35-37] and this may provide an objective method of assessing pain after limb procedures.[36] Acute joint pain alters weight bearing in cats, and total force, contact pressure, and contact area can be measured using pressure mats.[38] This objective technique has been successful in differentiating the use of nonsteroidal antiinflammatory drugs from placebo for provision of analgesia in experimental models of joint pain and supported the assessments made by observers who used a subjective lameness and VAS.[38]

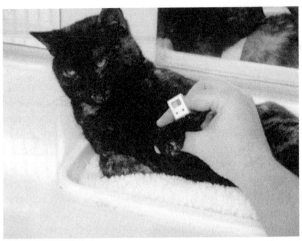

FIGURE 14-1 Algometers or palpometers are useful research tools for measuring the applied force that elicits a response by the patient.

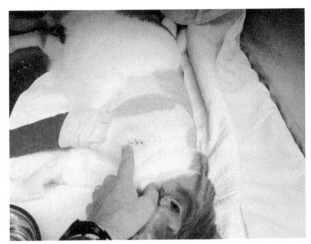

FIGURE 14-2 Palpation is an important clinical technique for assessing sensitivity of wounds.

Activity

It has been hypothesized that both acute and chronic pain may decrease activity in animals, including cats. Accelerometer-based activity monitors worn on a cat's collar have been validated against video analysis of distance moved.[39] These monitors have been used to measure changes in activity related to treatment in cats with degenerative joint disease,[40] but they have not been widely used in acute pain studies.

DEVELOPING PAIN ASSESSMENT TOOLS

Some key points for developing tools to measure subjective states have been proposed[16] that can be applied to quantify acute pain in cats. A scoring system, often termed a tool, scale, or instrument, should have the following attributes:

- *Animal-centric,* in that it is based on a functional and recognizable response by the animal to a specific stimulus, such as surgical castration
- *Anthropocentric,* in that it has a human goal in mind; for example, specific behaviors would be identified to trigger treatment with an analgesic
- *Intuitive,* meaning that observed emotional states are understood using a degree of empathy
- *Empirical,* meaning that the data collected are objective and support predetermined aims; in this case, is pain actually being measured, or something else?

As previously stated, any system that is used must be tested for validity, reliability, repeatability, and sensitivity. Without strictly defined criteria of what to look for and observations made by well-trained and experienced observers, many scoring systems are highly variable, with observers disagreeing about what they see.[41] One scoring system may show an analgesic agent to be effective, whereas another will show the same analgesic to be ineffective. These differences are inevitable if a system is insensitive and results in large interobserver variability.

Pain Scales in Veterinary Medicine

Several scales have been reported in the veterinary literature and advocated for evaluating postoperative pain. However, most have not followed the principles of ethology or the techniques used by researchers who developed the prototype scales used in humans. Some have used anecdotal descriptors of pain behaviors in animals that have not been validated to correlate with injury. Basic unidimensional pain scales include simple descriptive scales (SDSs) or verbal ordinal scales. These usually have three or four descriptors from which to choose, such as "no pain," "mild pain," "moderate pain" and "severe pain," and these categories have been used in feline clinical studies.[42-44] NRSs, or numerical ordinal scales, are similar to SDSs but have numbers assigned for ease of tabulation and analysis. For example, "no pain" could be assigned the number 0 and "very severe pain" the number 5, but various ranges from 0 to 10 have been used. This system implies equal difference or weighting between each category. For example, it is inferred that a score of 8 is twice as painful as a score of 4, which is unlikely to be the case. A further development of this system is a categorized numerical rating or ranking system in which certain categories of behaviors thought to be related to pain are chosen and assigned a value.[30] For example, vocalization could be one category in which "no vocalization" could be assigned a score of 0 and "hissing" a rank of 3; another behavior category could be "activity."

In an attempt to improve on these discontinuous scales, the VAS has been widely used in animals, including cats.[45] This tool consists of a continuous line, anchored at either end with a description of the limits of the scale, such as "no pain" at one end (usually the left) and "severe pain" at the opposite end. The observer places a mark vertically through the horizontal line that he or she thinks correlates to the animal being observed, and this is later translated into a number by measuring the distance of that mark from 0 (no pain). Holton and others[41] compared the use of a simple descriptive, NRS and VAS for assessing pain in dogs following surgery. There was significant observer variability, which was as high as 36%, for all three scales. Although simple to use, these scales are extremely subjective and may not detect small changes in pain. These scales are unidimensional in that they really only assess intensity of pain and do not account for the many other aspects of pain that likely affect an animal, such as pain-related disability, changes in normal behavior, or the dynamic aspects of pain. Purely observational studies without interaction with the animal are likely to lead to erroneous assessments. Inactivity may be a protective mechanism for some types of pain, and pain would not be detected unless there were further assessment and interaction. For example, a cat may remain very still and quiet because it is in pain and may therefore be scored as having minimal pain and thus receive no analgesics. Adding an assessment of dynamic or evoked behavioral responses, such as pain in relation to movement or palpation, is expected to add another valuable dimension to the assessment process and may result in a very different assessment.

One example of this type of scale is an extension of the classic VAS system known as the dynamic and interactive visual analogue scale (DIVAS). With this system, the animal is first observed undisturbed and from a distance. The reason for this is that some animals will not display overt pain behaviors in the presence of a caregiver, but will when they think they are unobserved. This has been documented by the use of video cameras and is likely a protective mechanism against potential predators. The cat is then approached, handled, and encouraged to move around. The surgical incision (or area of trauma), and the surrounding area are then gently palpated, and a final overall assessment of the animal's pain is made. The DIVAS system has been used to assess postoperative pain in cats,[42-44,46,47] and, when performed by one individual unaware of treatments, it detected differences between analgesics and between treated and untreated cats.[46]

It is now accepted that quantitative measurement of behaviors is the most reliable method for assessing pain in animals and that if the methodology used to develop and validate these systems is rigorous, the measurement can be objective with minimal observer bias.[17] The important questions that each of us needs to ask are: What does pain look like in cats? What do cats do when they are in pain? How does this impact their overall well-being? In other words, it is important to look at all facets of pain. Creating these tools and validating them is a time-consuming but worthwhile task.

Principles for the Development of Behavior-Based Composite Pain Scales

Multidimensional composite scales are particularly important when self-reporting is not possible, but they must incorporate components that are proven to be sensitive and specific to pain in the species being studied. Psychometric principles must be used to develop these tools.[18] There is an established process in human medicine for measuring complex constructs such as quality of life, as well as guidelines for choosing items to include in the tool, how to construct a questionnaire, and methods for testing validity, reliability, and sensitivity. The initial components of a scale can be developed by using a detailed behavior ethogram. By using this technique, animals can be observed before and after a surgical procedure, and a control group (no surgery) can also be included. In addition, the frequency of specific behaviors is counted. This was the approach of Waran and colleagues, who used cats undergoing ovariohysterectomy.[48] Another approach is to use scales already described in the literature and ask people who work with the species being studied which words and expressions they think describe behavioral signs of pain. The latter approach was used by Holton and colleagues in dogs[17] and by Brondani and colleagues in cats.[25] Researchers at the University of Glasgow used this approach to develop an acute pain measurement tool for cats.[49] These are only starting points, and the tools must be tested. Knowledge of the normal behavior of the individual being evaluated is important, and deviations from normal behavior may suggest pain. Anxiety, fear, or a combination of these may also be present. Anxiety and fear may be present when an animal is admitted to a veterinary practice, which would also be expected before and after surgery unless the cat rapidly adapts; however, pain behaviors will arise following the procedure. Three approaches to using behavior as a pain assessment tool include asking the following questions (Box 14-1):

- Is the cat's normal behavior maintained before and after a painful event?
- Are normal behaviors lost following a painful event?
- Do new behaviors occur following a painful event?

In dogs, the most vigorously tested behavior-based acute pain scoring system is the Glasgow Composite Measures Pain Scale.[17,18] Similar systems have been and continue to be developed and refined for cats and are discussed in detail below.[5,25,33,49]

BOX 14-1	**Using Behavioral Signs to Assess Pain in Cats**

- Maintenance of normal behaviors
- Loss of normal behaviors
- Development of new behaviors

To date, most pain tools have been developed based on cats undergoing ovariohysterectomy, but different types and sources of pain, such as abdominal versus musculoskeletal or oral pain, may result in different behaviors, which must be considered when developing and using these tools. Work by Brondani and colleagues[5,25,33] to develop a multidimensional composite scale for use in cats following ovariohysterectomy with specific scores for each behavior within a category or domain has greatly improved the ability to measure pain in this species (Table 14-1). Any instrument must be tested for validity, variability, and utility before it can be used with any confidence in a clinical setting. Construct validity can be tested by assuming that analgesics will relieve pain and result in a decreased pain score. Criteria validity can be tested by comparing the new tool with another tool, such as a NRS, and seeing if the scores move in the same direction. Basically, this is done to ensure that the testing is appropriately measuring the intended item, in this case, pain and not something else, such as sedation or residual effects of anesthesia. Variability can be tested by having different observers score the same animal. If the scale is well designed, there will be very little interobserver variability. For clinical use, the tool must have utility, meaning that it should be easy to use, quick to perform, and suitable for different observers, such as veterinarians, nurses, technicians, and other animal care staff, and sometimes owners.

On the basis of current knowledge, it is suggested that the aspects of pain assessment listed in Box 14-2 are important criteria for use in evaluating acute postoperative pain in cats. Each of the items listed in Box 14-2 is described in more detail below. The developers of measurement tools emphasize that it is helpful to record data preoperatively (baseline) for comparison whenever possible. However, there are specific behaviors that occur in cats only following surgery, only when pain relief is inadequate, and likely in cats that have other causes of pain; therefore, even without baseline information, these are still valuable tools for clinical assessment. Examples (videos) and explanations of the behaviors included in the tool developed by Brondani and colleagues[5,33] are available via a dedicated website.[50] The most recently published tool includes many of the same assessment domains but was developed independently and used cats with surgical, traumatic, and medical conditions to test validity.[49]

Other pain scales are available for use in cats, but it must be noted that these have not been vigorously validated. One is the Colorado State University Feline Acute Pain Scale.[51] This scale does incorporate psychological and behavioral assessments, posture, response to palpation, and body tension. Another is the 4A-Vet postoperative pain scale for dogs and cats.[52,53] This is a multidimensional composite scale; however, its validity after translation from French to English has not been confirmed, and it uses the same scale for dogs and cats.

TABLE 14-1   **UNESP-Botucatu Multidimensional Composite Pain Scale for Assessing Postoperative Pain in Cats**[53]

SUBSCALE 1: PAIN EXPRESSION (0 – 12)

Miscellaneous behaviors	Observe and mark the presence of the behaviors listed below	
	A - The cat is laying down and quiet, but moving its tail	A
	B - The cat contracts and extends its pelvic limbs and/or contracts its abdominal muscles (flank)	B
	C - The cats eyes are partially closed (eyes half closed)	C
	D - The cat licks and/or bites the surgical wound	D
	• All above behaviors are absent	0
	• Presence of one of the above behaviors	1
	• Presence of two of the above behaviors	2
	• Presence of three or all of the above behaviors	3
Reaction to palpation of the surgical wound	• The cat does not react when the surgical wound is touched or pressed; or no change from pre-surgical response (if basal evaluation was made)	0
	• The cat does not react when the surgical wound is touched, but does react when it is pressed. It may vocalize and/or try to bite	1
	• The cat reacts when the surgical wound is touched and when pressed. It may vocalize and/or try to bite	2
	• The cat reacts when the observer approaches the surgical wound. It may vocalize and/or try to bite. The cat does not allow palpation of the surgical wound	3
Reaction to palpation of the abdomen/ flank	• The cat does not react when the abdomen/flank is touched or pressed; or no change from pre-surgical response (if basal evaluation was made). The abdomen/flank is not tense	0
	• The cat does not react when the abdomen/flank is touched, but does react when it is pressed. The abdomen/flank is tense	1
	• The cat reacts when the abdomen/flank is touched and when pressed. The abdomen/flank is tense	2
	• The cat reacts when the observer approaches the abdomen/flank. It may vocalize and/or try to bite. The cat does not allow palpation of the abdomen/flank	3
Vocalization	• The cat is quiet, purring when stimulated, or meows interacting with the observer, but does not growl, groan, or hiss	0
	• The cat purrs spontaneously (without being stimulated or handled by the observer)	1
	• The cat growls, howls, or hisses when handled by the observer (when its body position is changed by the observer)	2
	• The cat growls, howls, hisses spontaneously (without being stimulated or handled by the observer)	3

SUBSCALE 2: PSYCHOMOTOR CHANGE (0 – 12)

Posture	• The cat is in a natural posture with relaxed muscles (it moves normally)	0
	• The cat is in a natural posture but is tense (it moves little or is reluctant to move)	1
	• The cat is sitting or in sternal recumbency with its back arched and head down; or the cat is in dorso-lateral recumbency with its pelvic limbs extended or contracted	2
	• The cat frequently alters its body position in an attempt to find a comfortable posture	3
Comfort	• The cat is comfortable, awake or asleep, and interacts when stimulated (it interacts with the observer and/or is interested in its surroundings)	0
	• The cat is quiet and slightly receptive when stimulated (it interacts little with the observer and/or is not very interested in its surroundings)	1
	• The cat is quiet and "dissociated from the environment" (even when stimulated it does not interact with the observer and/or has no interest in its surroundings); the cat may be facing the back of the cage	2
	• The cat is uncomfortable, restless (frequently changes its body position), and slightly receptive when stimulated or "dissociated from the environment"; the cat may be facing the back of the cage	3
Activity	• The cat moves normally (it immediately moves when the cage is opened; outside the cage it moves spontaneously when stimulated or handled)	0
	• The cat moves more than normal (inside the cage it moves continuously from side to side)	1
	• The cat is quieter than normal (it may hesitate to leave the cage and if removed from the cage tends to return, outside the cage it moves a little after stimulation or handling)	2
	• The cat is reluctant to move (it may hesitate to leave the cage and if removed from the cage tends to return, outside the cage it does not move even when stimulated or handled)	3

Continued

TABLE 14-1 UNESP-Botucatu Multidimensional Composite Pain Scale for Assessing Postoperative Pain in Cats—cont'd

Attitude	Observe and mark the presence of the mental states listed below	
	A - Satisfied: The cat is alert and interested in its surroundings (explores its surroundings), friendly and interactive with the observer (plays and/or responds to stimuli) * The cat may initially interact with the observer through games to distract it from the pain. Carefully observe to distinguish between distraction and satisfaction games	A
	B - Uninterested: The cat does not interact with the observer (not interested by toys or plays a little; does not respond to calls or strokes from the observer) * In cats that don't like to play, evaluate interaction with the observer by its response to calls and strokes	B
	C - Indifferent: The cat is not interested in its surroundings (it is not curious; it does not explore its surroundings) * The cat can initially be afraid to explore its surroundings. The observer needs to handle the cat and encourage it to move itself (take it out of the cage and/or change its body position)	C
	D - Anxious: The cat is frightened (it tries to hide or escape) or nervous (demonstrating impatience and growling, howling, or hissing when stroked and/or handled)	D
	E - Aggressive: The cat is aggressive (tries to bite or scratch when stroked or handled) • Presence of the mental state A • Presence of one of the mental states B, C, D, or E • Presence of two of the mental states B, C, D, or E • Presence of three or all of the mental states B, C, D, or E	E 0 1 2 3

SUBSCALE 3: PHYSIOLOGICAL VARIABLES (0 – 6)

Arterial blood pressure	• 0% to 15% above pre-surgery value • 16% to 29% above pre-surgery value • 30% to 45% above pre-surgery value • > 45% above pre-surgery value	0 1 2 3
Appetite	• The cat is eating normally • The cat is eating more than normal • The cat is eating less than normal • The cat is not interested in food	0 1 2 3

TOTAL SCORE (0 – 30)

DIRECTIONS FOR USING THE SCALE

Initially observe the cat's behavior without opening the cage. Observe whether it is resting or active; interested or uninterested in its surroundings; quiet or vocal. Check for the presence of specific behaviors (see "Miscellaneous behaviors" above).

Open the cage and observe whether the cat quickly moves out or hesitates to leave the cage. Approach the cat and evaluate its reaction: friendly, aggressive, frightened, indifferent, or vocal. Touch the cat and interact with it, check whether it is receptive (if it likes to be stroked and/or is interested in playing). If the cat hesitates to leave the cage, encourage it to move through stimuli (call it by name and stroke it) and handling (change its body position and/or take it out of the cage). Observe when outside the cage, if the cat moves spontaneously, in a reserved manner, or is reluctant to move. Offer it palatable food and observe its response.*

Finally, place the cat in lateral or sternal recumbency and measure its arterial blood pressure. Evaluate the cat's reaction when the abdomen/flank is initially touched (slide your fingers over the area) and in the sequence gently pressed (apply direct pressure over the area). Wait for a time, and do the same procedure to assess the cat's reaction to palpation of surgical wound.

* To evaluate appetite during the immediate postoperative period, initially offer a small quantity of palatable food immediately after recovery from anesthesia. At this moment most cats eat normally independent of the presence or absence of pain. Wait a short while, offer food again, and observe the cat's reaction.

Table 14-1 is available for download at http://www.animalpain.com.br/en-us/.

BOX 14-2 Specific Domains to Consider When Assessing Acute Pain in Cats

• Posture and comfort
• Activity and mobility
• Attitude and demeanor
• Response to touch, pressure, and palpation
• Attention to the wound or painful site
• Vocalization
• Facial expression

BEHAVIOR-BASED INDICATORS OF PAIN

Posture and Comfort

Specific postures have been confirmed as indicators of acute pain in many species. A hunched or tense posture is included as a behavioral item in the Glasgow Composite Measures Pain Scale for measuring acute pain in dogs.[17,18] Detailed ethograms have been used to analyze behaviors in cats before and after ovariohysterectomy with the aim of identifying key behavioral indicators of acute pain in cats.[48] In that study, different groups of cats underwent anesthesia without surgery, anesthesia with surgery (ovariohysterectomy) and preoperative analgesics, and anesthesia and surgery with both pre- and postoperative analgesics. The occurrences of specific observations and behaviors such as grooming, head down, curled up in a natural sleeping position, position in the cage, rubbing, hiding, vocalization, and postures such as a tucked or half-tucked position with a tense abdomen were recorded over a 2-hour period before and for 5 hours after anesthesia alone or anesthesia plus surgery. There was a significantly increased frequency of crouched and half-tucked postures in the surgery groups, with a greater frequency in cats that received only preoperative analgesics. In addition, cats that had received only preoperative analgesics turned to look at the incision and physically attended to it (licking) more frequently following surgery. The crouching and half-tucked postures were not seen prior to surgery.[48] Examples of these postures are shown in Figure 14-3, *A* and *B*. The cat in Figure 14-3, *B* is wearing an Elizabethan (E)-collar, which in itself can alter behavior (see below), and the author believes can alter a cat's posture. Therefore, it is important to take this into consideration or to observe the cat with and without the E-collar.

Within the category of posture, the UNESP-Botucatu Multidimensional Composite Pain Scale[54] (see Table 14-1) classifies four postures that are assigned a score of 0, 1, 2, or 3. Cats with natural relaxed postures are scored as 0. Examples of normal postures are shown in Figure 14-4, *A–C*.

Recognizing normal postures and looking for these in a clinical setting is helpful. Figure 14-5, *A* shows an example of a cat in a normal sleeping posture (curled up and relaxed) in its home surroundings. Figure 14-5, *B* shows a cat in a veterinary practice environment adopting a similar position despite severe facial trauma (maxillary and mandibular fractures) and placement of a percutaneous endoscopic gastrostomy tube and intravenous catheters.

A score of 1 is given to cats that may adopt a natural posture but are tense and reluctant to move. Cats that are sitting or in sternal recumbency with their back arched and head down (Figure 14-6, *A* and *B*) or in dorsal or lateral recumbency with the pelvic limbs extended (Figure 14-7, *A* and *B*) or contracted are scored as a 2. Cats that frequently alter their body position and look as if they are trying to find a comfortable posture are assigned a 3, the highest score in this category. Cats that are in other abnormal positions, such as "flat out" (Figure 14-8) or prostrate and tense should be considered in pain, and, although they may not fit exactly into one of the categories, clinical judgment should be used to assign them a score.

Activity

Activity or movement should be assessed. Observe whether the cat moves normally, especially when it gets up or lies down. The "cat stretch" is both a spontaneous and an elicited maneuver. When cats first wake up, they will do a deep stretch (head down, front limbs extended, and hind end held in the air) (Figure 14-9); if they are in pain, this behavior is often absent or restricted. Cats often perform this move when stroked from head to tail by a person (see below). It is usually necessary to open the cage door and allow the cat to leave the cage to fully assess mobility. If there is a step down from the cage to the floor, watch to see if the cat jumps down freely or hesitates or uses a strategy that decreases pain resulting from impact or stretching. It can be helpful to use a toy when assessing activity and demeanor (see below).

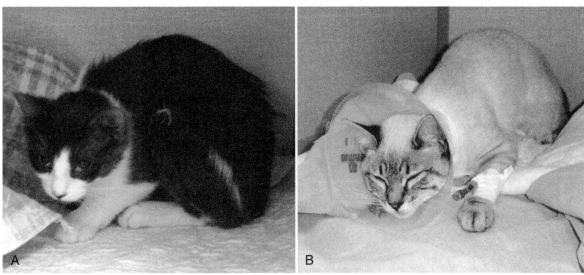

FIGURE 14-3   These cats demonstrate the crouched and half-tucked postures associated with abdominal surgery.[48]

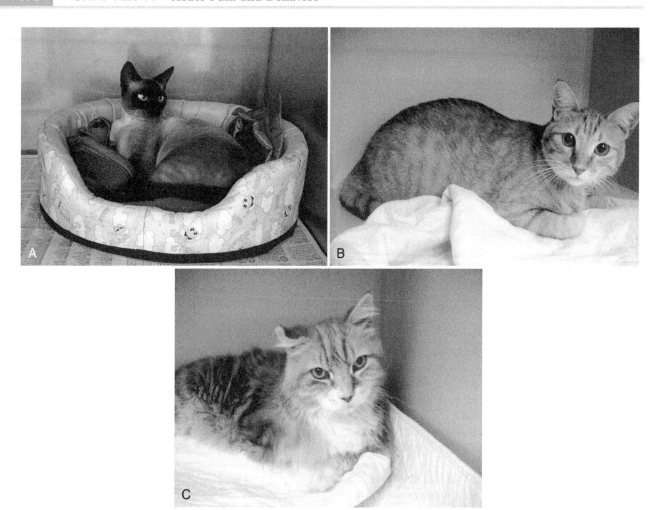

FIGURE 14-4 These cats display normal facial expressions and postures in a veterinary practice environment. (**A,** Courtesy J. T. Brondani)

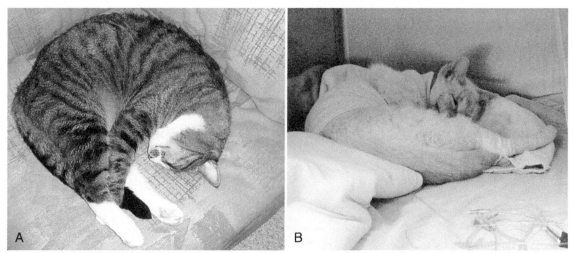

FIGURE 14-5 **A,** This cat is in a normal, curled-up, relaxed posture in its home environment. **B,** This cat is in a similar position, indicating a good level of comfort in a clinical setting following major trauma to its maxilla and mandible.

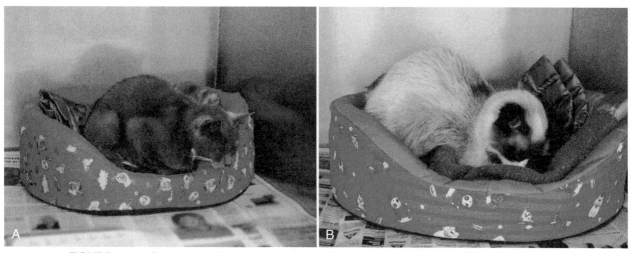

FIGURE 14-6 Cats that are in pain may adopt a sitting or sternal posture with back arched and head down. (Courtesy J. T. Brondani)

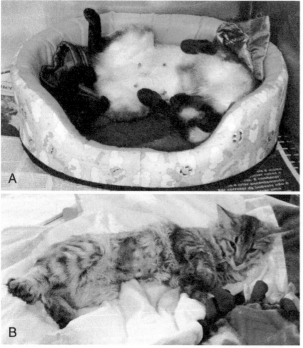

FIGURE 14-7 Cats that adopt a dorsally or laterally recumbent position with the pelvic limbs extended or contracted should be considered in pain. (**A,** Courtesy J. T. Brondani)

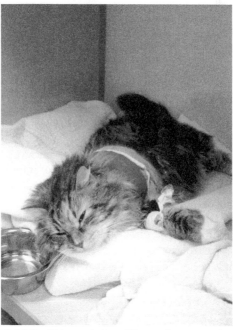

FIGURE 14-8 This cat is in a "flat-out" unnatural position and is tense. In addition, it has a facial expression (half-closed eyes) that suggests a significant level of pain.

Attitude and Demeanor

How an animal interacts with its environment and people may also give important clues as to its degree of pain. Attitude and demeanor encompass psychological elements of pain and are accepted as valid components of pain assessment tools for both dogs and cats.[5,17,18,33] Veterinarians and nurses often use words such as *depressed*, *disinterested*, *indifferent*, *content*, and *happy* in reference to animals and how the animals might feel. The words *satisfied*, *uninterested*, *indifferent*, *anxious*, and *aggressive*

are used in the UNESP-Botucatu Multidimensional Composite Pain Scale[54] (see Table 14-1). Figure 14-10 shows examples of a disinterested cat and one that seems dissociated from its environment and perhaps is trying to hide. The Colorado State University Feline Acute Pain Scale[51] uses the terms *interested*, *less interested*, *curious*, *withdrawn*, and *seeks solitude* in its psychological section.

Unfamiliar surroundings such as a veterinary practice can cause negative emotional states including anxiety and fear as well as adverse effects such as freezing, hiding, and hypervigilance[55] in addition to the physiologic changes described earlier. Hiding is a coping mechanism, and

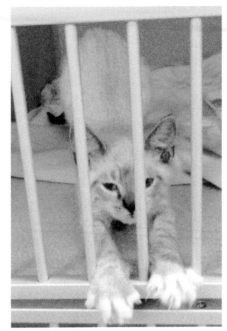

FIGURE 14-9 The classic "cat stretch" is commonly performed by cats upon rising and can be elicited by stroking them from head to tail. These are normal behaviors that may be absent or truncated when a cat is in pain.

providing a hiding place can decrease anxiety and fear by making the cat feel secure. All of these behaviors may also be noted in a cat that is in pain, so they should be evaluated even though they are not specific indicators of pain, and, when taken in context (the cat has had surgery or the cat has some other painful condition), they can be valuable indicators of the cat's overall psychological state. Differentiating between fear, anxiety, stress, and pain can be difficult; this topic is discussed below.

This part of an assessment is especially informative when it is performed before and after a painful procedure so that changes in attitude and demeanor can be documented; this may be loss of normal behaviors or appearance of new behaviors (see Box 14-1). Position in the cage may not be a useful detail to note if considered in isolation or at a single time point. Fearful cats, whether in pain or not, may go to the back of the cage. However, significant findings are a cat that was noted to be at the front of the cage, inquisitive, and engaged in what was going on outside the cage before surgery but is now at the back of the cage (Figure 14-11, *A* and *B*) and a cat whose pain is well managed but is observed at the back of the cage and disinterested in its surroundings after the procedure.

In cats that are not feral, interaction with a caregiver should be assessed. Again, this is more meaningful if the responses before and after a painful event are known. For this reason, it is valuable to do baseline evaluations before surgery. If the cat is being evaluated for pain unrelated to surgery, asking the client about the cat's normal interactions with people can be helpful, and changes from what is normal for that cat can be documented. The Glasgow Composite Measures Pain Scale for acute pain in cats (CMPS-F) includes response to being stroked along the back from head to tail as part of the overall assessment.[49] Positive responses to this maneuver when it is elicited include arching of the back with the tail up and standing on tiptoes, whereas a negative response is no response or aggression. The response to toys can also be included in the evaluation and can be accomplished by observing what the cat does with toys or how it responds to an interactive game with a person. Again, before-after behavior comparisons are valuable.

Response to Touch, Pressure, and Palpation

Following injury, primary sensitization occurs and surgical incisions become hyperalgesic. As previously discussed, testing wound sensitivity is a validated and

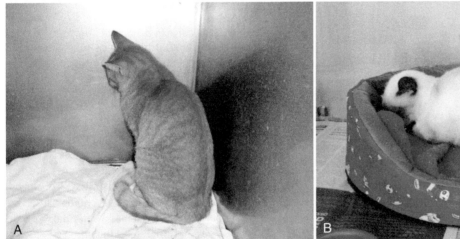

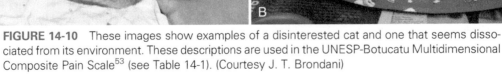

FIGURE 14-10 These images show examples of a disinterested cat and one that seems dissociated from its environment. These descriptions are used in the UNESP-Botucatu Multidimensional Composite Pain Scale[53] (see Table 14-1). (Courtesy J. T. Brondani)

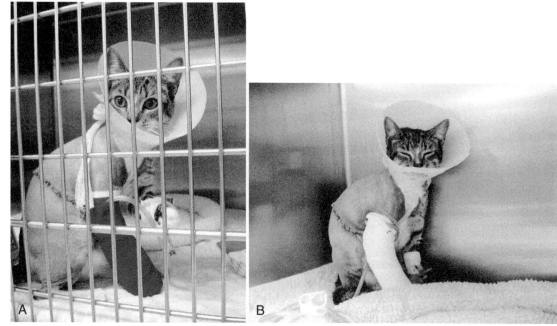

FIGURE 14-11   The cat's position in the cage can be a useful indicator of its emotional state and may be related to pain, but it may be meaningful only if before and after comparisons are made (before and after surgery or before and after analgesic intervention). **A,** This young cat at the front of its cage appears interested in its surroundings, indicating a lack of pain. **B,** The same cat at the back of the cage appears disinterested, is more hunched, and has its eyes half-closed, all indicators that analgesia is not adequate.

objective assessment method.[32] Palpation of the injured area tests evoked pain. With appropriate analgesic use, it should be possible to palpate wounds and the surrounding area. This is an important component of assessment because many animals may be very reluctant to move, owing to their pain, and it could easily be assumed that they are comfortable if no direct interaction takes place. This part of the overall pain assessment should be done after all observational components and after assessing how the cat interacts with the assessor. If the cat has undergone an abdominal procedure (midline incision), the assessor should first touch the flank using two fingers and then the area around the wound (approximately 2 inches [5 cm] from the incision); they should then move close to the wound, noting the cat's response. If there is no response, the procedure should be repeated, but this time the assessor should apply gentle pressure. Palpation of the abdomen, the wound, and the area around the wound will elicit a range of responses, depending on how painful the site is. There may be no response, or the palpation may evoke swishing of the tail, flattening of the ears, crying, hissing, or growling or cause the cat to bite or lash out. When using the UNESP-Botucatu Multidimensional Composite Pain Scale[54] (see Table 14-1), the cat's reactions to palpation of the abdomen and flank and the wound are scored separately, with each scored as 0 (no response), 1, 2, or 3. In this scale, response to palpation represents 20% of the overall possible score. In work by investigators at the University of Glasgow,[49] palpation accounts for 25% of the total score, emphasizing the importance of this aspect of assessment. Although current pain scoring tools for cats have been or are being developed primarily using cats that have undergone ovariohysterectomy, assessment by palpation can be applied to any situation, including wounds in other areas and when other painful conditions are suspected (e.g., acute visceral or limb pain) (Figure 14-12).

There are clearly times when palpation cannot be included in an assessment, such as when working with unsocialized or feral cats. In these situations, the number assigned to this section of the scale should be subtracted from the total possible score and the rest of the assessment performed. When using the UNESP-Botucatu Multidimensional Composite Pain Scale[54] with feral cats, palpation and measurement of blood pressure cannot be performed; therefore, subtract 6 (palpation) plus 3 (blood pressure) from the total possible score (30) and score the cat out of a possible total of 21.

Attention to the Wound or Painful Site

Observing how much attention an animal pays to a painful site is an assessment of spontaneous pain. Descriptions of what a dog does to its wound, such as ignoring, chewing, licking, or rubbing it or looking at it are components of validated pain scales, with each action assigned a score.[17,18] Licking and biting a wound

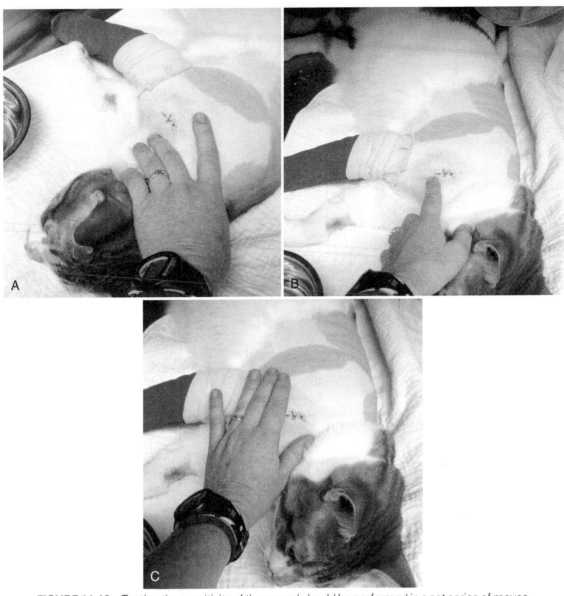

FIGURE 14-12 Testing the sensitivity of the wound should be performed in a set series of moves. **A,** First, touch around the wound. **B,** Second, touch close to the wound. **C,** If no response is elicited, apply pressure to the wound.

are also indicators of pain in cats.[5,33] Cats are fastidious groomers. Therefore it is important to observe cats carefully to differentiate between normal grooming behavior and paying too much attention to a wound by licking it constantly or biting it (Figure 14-13).

Vocalization

Cats have a large and varied vocal repertoire. They may be silent, or they may purr, meow, cry, howl, groan, hiss, or spit. These may be spontaneous or provoked vocalizations. How and why cats purr are controversial topics. Purring occurs when a female cat nurses her kittens and when humans provide social contact, such as petting, stroking, or feeding. Purring is often associated with what are assumed to be pleasurable events and may be a means of communication between adult cats and kittens. However, purring also occurs during more stressful events, such as a physical examination or after an injury. Changes in vocalization such as distress meowing, growling, hissing, and spitting may suggest that the cat is anxious or fearful.[26] Silence, however, does not necessarily mean the cat is not anxious or that it is not in pain.[26] Despite the ambiguity of feline vocalization, it is still widely accepted as a meaningful component of a pain assessment tool. Both spontaneous and evoked vocalizations can be assessed and scored.[5,33,49]

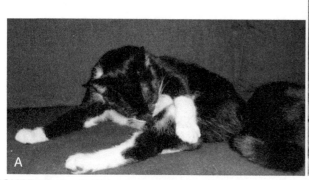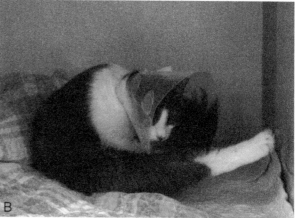

FIGURE 14-13   A, This cat is performing normal grooming of the abdomen. **B,** This cat should be observed carefully for a few minutes to differentiate normal grooming from overattention to the wound.

Facial Expression

As early as 1872, Darwin wrote about the expression of emotions in humans and animals, noting that pain was recognizable through facial expression.[56] Since then, significant effort has been made to validate facial indicators of pain in children and other populations with limited communication ability (e.g., humans with cognitive impairment) by identifying anatomically based facial action units and using a facial action coding system.[57] Facial expression is widely used alone or incorporated into human pediatric clinical and research pain instruments.[58] Pain can be expressed at birth, and it is generally regarded that facial expression of emotions is hardwired and modulated by learning later in life.[59] Infants have a universal primal face of pain, which is a biologically determined ability to display stress and pain.[59] Newborn infants have been videotaped before, during, and after application of a noxious stimulus, such as a heel stick to collect blood. This painful stimulus elicited a facial expression that was characterized by opening of the mouth, drawing in of the eyebrows, and closing of the eyes, with commonality between sexes and different ethnic facial features.[59]

Rodents are widely used in pain research, and there is a need to develop tools that identify spontaneous rather than evoked pain in these species. Mice were videotaped during a classical visceral pain assay, and individual frames of their faces were collected from these tapes and a coding system devised.[60] This work led to the development of the Mouse Grimace Scale. Five facial action units indicative of pain were identified, including an eyelid squeeze, a nose and cheek bulge, and a change in ear and whisker positions.[60] Further work on this scale has confirmed its high accuracy and reliability.

Reliable methods for assessing acute pain in rabbits are lacking, but, as in mice, a Rabbit Grimace Scale has been developed by analyzing still shots of rabbit faces taken from videotapes while the rabbits underwent ear tattooing with or without the use of a topical anesthetic cream.[61] Physiologic (heart rate and blood pressure) and serum corticosterone responses were not different between groups, but facial expressions differentiated the treatment groups reliably. Similar to the results in mice, five facial action units were identified and included orbital tightening, cheek flattening, nose shape, and whisker and ear positions.[61] Closure or semiclosure (slit) of the eyes seems to be a consistent feature of acute pain in infant and adult humans, mice, and rabbits.

Preliminary work on the use of facial expression as an indicator of perception of an acute noxious stimulus has been undertaken in cats in a research setting.[62] Cats were videotaped during thermal and mechanical nociceptive threshold testing. Comparison with baseline images revealed that in response to the thermal stimulus, the palpebral fissure was narrowed; the ears were caudolaterally rotated; and the whiskers were bunched together and flattened against the face. At mechanical threshold, similar changes were observed in the eye and ear, but whisker changes were less apparent.[62] These findings are similar to those in other species. In a clinical setting, changes in facial expression related to acute pain in cats can be noted (Figures 14-14 and 14-15). Several facial expressions, including squinted eyes, were described and included in an initial composite pain score used to evaluate pain in cats undergoing ovariohysterectomy.[25] During subsequent refinements and validation of this composite scale, "partially closed/half closed" or "squinty eyes" is the only facial expression to remain.[5,33] Recent analysis of 78 facial landmarks in pain-free and painful cats has identified six significant factors that differentiate between the two populations and these include ear position and areas around the muzzle and mouth.[63] These features are currently undergoing investigation for validity, reliability and responsiveness in a clinical setting.

Although the behaviors in this section have been described separately, many will be seen concurrently in the same patients. Figures 14-3, *B;* 14-7, *B;* 14-8; and 14-16 show cats with abnormal body postures combined with facial expressions suggestive of pain.

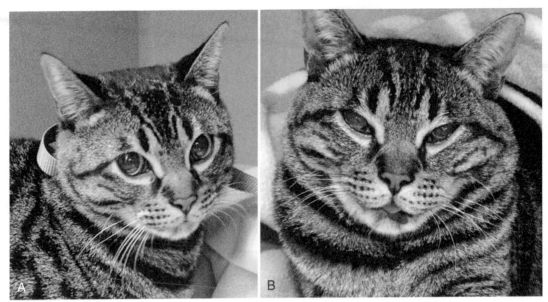

FIGURE 14-14 **A,** The cat's facial expression before surgery. **B,** The cat's squinted, or half-shut, eyes after surgery indicate pain.

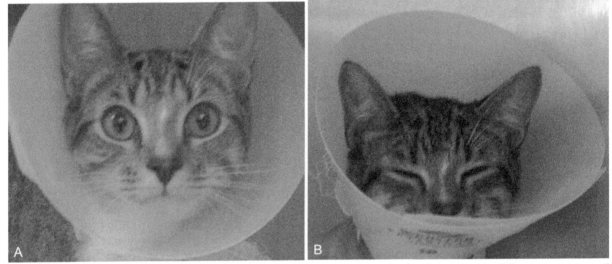

FIGURE 14-15 These images of the same cat show its facial expression when analgesia is adequate **(A)** and when it is not **(B).**

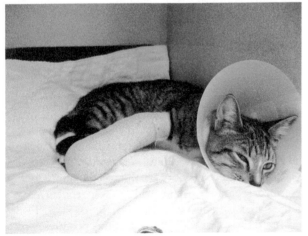

FIGURE 14-16 This cat is showing several indicators of pain. It is in an abnormal posture; it is tense; and its eyes are half-closed.

OTHER FACTORS TO CONSIDER IN AN OVERALL ASSESSMENT

Eating in a clinical environment is a positive sign of well-being. It is often assumed that if a cat is eating, it is unlikely to be in pain, and a cat's willingness to eat is included in some pain assessment scales.[5,33] Appetite or lack of appetite is not a sensitive indicator of pain in cats. Cats in pain will eat, and there are many causes of inappetence or anorexia other than pain. In addition, in the immediate postoperative period and/or due to the nature of the procedure, surgery, or illness, it may not be appropriate to offer the cat food to assess its appetite.

Cats tend to spend a considerable amount of each day sleeping; however, when assessing sleep, the observer must differentiate normal restful sleep from so-called feigned sleep.[64] What feigned sleep looks like has not been well described in the veterinary literature. Cats that are feigning sleep tend to be immobile and apparently asleep for the majority of the time, with little or no time spent awake and exploring their surroundings. In addition, they do not look relaxed while immobile, and, if disturbed, they may show an exaggerated startle response. Feigned sleep is thought to be a passive defense mechanism, and, if not recognized, the negative emotional state of the cat may be underestimated.[65] Cats that are in pain may also feign sleep (SA Robertson, personal observation). This may be because movement is painful and may reflect an overall negative emotional state.

Cats are notorious for disliking bandages and restrictive dressings. Grint and colleagues[34] performed a study to compare pain and wound tenderness in cats undergoing ovariohysterectomy via a flank or midline incision. In an attempt to blind the observers, abdominal bandages were used at the initiation of the study. However, this was soon abandoned because it caused markedly abnormal behaviors, including extreme reluctance to move, abnormal postures, and evasive behaviors.[34] Other behaviors associated with placing bandages include rolling around, and, if a limb is bandaged, even if just to secure an intravenous catheter, the cat may hold its foot in the air and stop placing that foot on the ground, giving the appearance of lameness. This can be temporary or maintained until the bandage or tape is removed. Therefore, the influence of bandages on behavior must also be considered so that the observer is not misled in making the wrong assessment. If possible, the use of bandages should be minimized to avoid stress and provocation of new and abnormal behaviors. If bandages are deemed essential, they should be placed as loosely as possible, and materials that stretch are recommended. If the assessor thinks the bandages are the cause of the observed behaviors, the bandages should be removed if possible and the cat reassessed. As mentioned previously, if a cat has received adequate analgesia, it will ignore the wound and analgesics, not bandages, should be used to prevent a cat from rubbing, licking, or biting a wound. The use of E-collars has also been documented to alter behavior in cats.[66]

Failure to urinate or defecate may cause agitation and restlessness in hospitalized cats. They may have altered elimination patterns due to stress; however, it may be that the litter box that has been provided is inappropriate (too small or difficult to access), or they may have an aversion to the litter provided. Elimination may also be decreased due to lack of exercise while restricted to a cage.[55] In addition, outdoor cats may not rapidly adjust to using a litter box if hospitalized. Therefore, if after a thorough assessment the cat does not appear to be in pain but is displaying abnormal behaviors, rule out other causes such as a full bladder or colon. These examples highlight the importance of good nursing care, not just analgesic intervention for promoting the comfort and well-being of a cat while it is hospitalized.[55]

USING RESPONSE TO TREATMENT AS A DIAGNOSTIC TOOL

Despite the advances in the ability to recognize and assess pain in cats, as well as identification of intervention scores (see below), there are many times when the clinician just is not sure. In these cases, the benefit of the doubt should be given to the patient. One approach to diagnosing pain is to use the response to analgesic intervention as a diagnostic tool. Reevaluate the patient's record, noting what caused the pain, when the cat was last given an analgesic, and whether it was an appropriate choice (drug and dose). It may be that the cat requires another dose of an opioid sooner than expected or that it needs a higher dose or a different analgesic, which could be a different opioid, a different class of analgesic, or a combination of drugs. Following further intervention, the cat should be fully reassessed, and the pain score should be significantly reduced. If it is not, then further investigation is warranted.

IS IT FEAR, STRESS, ANXIETY, PAIN, OR DYSPHORIA?

Pain, fear, stress, and anxiety are all negative emotions; therefore, each must be addressed and minimized in cats under the care of the veterinary practice. The psychological and physiologic effects of these emotions, including but not limited to decreased normal rest and sleeping, hypervigilance, elevated stress hormone levels, hypertension, and tachycardia, impair the recovery process and can confuse clinical assessments. In addition, cats that are labeled as difficult to handle will receive suboptimal nursing.

Distinguishing pain from fear, stress, anxiety, and dysphoria is challenging, but if the cause of the observed behavior changes can be determined, treatment goals can be optimized. Recognition of fear, stress, and anxiety are comprehensively discussed elsewhere in this book. This chapter discusses some of the postures adopted by cats that are fearful that are similar to those adopted by cats in pain. Figure 14-17 shows the facial expressions and body postures associated with fear. Figure 14-18 shows a cat that was fearful before surgery (A) but in pain following surgery (B). The differences in posture and facial expression may be subtle, but, taken in context, they are very helpful for guiding treatment. Figure 14-19 shows an apprehensive or fearful cat prior to a dental procedure for multiple extractions (A, B) and after the procedure (C). The different facial expressions and ear positions should be noted. Figure 14-19, C suggests pain is present; this cat should be further evaluated.

Cats have been described as dysphoric when they resent being handled, are restless or agitated, pace, and vocalize in a plaintive manner.[67] This is distinct from euphoria, which is a positive emotional state and has been defined as a cat that is calm and easy to handle and that shows some or all of the following: purring, kneading

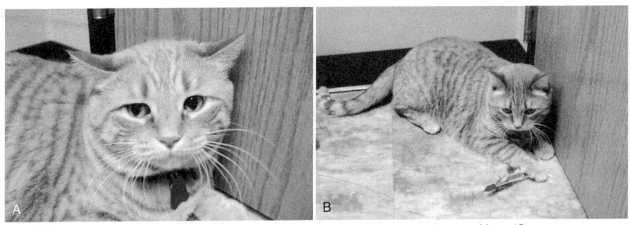

FIGURE 14-17 The facial expression and body posture of this cat are indicative of fear. (Courtesy I. Rodan)

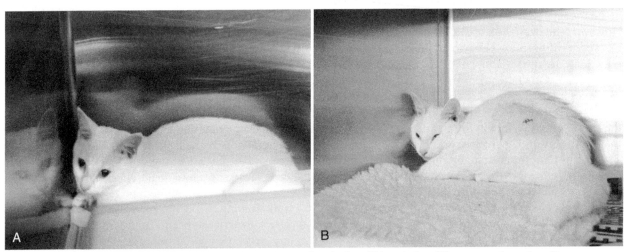

FIGURE 14-18 Photographs of the same cat taken before **(A)** and after **(B)** surgery show the difference in facial expression and body posture of a cat with fear and/or anxiety **(A)** and pain **(B)**.

with its forepaws, rolling, and rubbing its head and body on the cage door.[67] Both dysphoria and euphoria in cats following treatment with opioid drugs have been described. If, after assessment, a cat is deemed comfortable but dysphoric and an opioid has been used for analgesia, then administration of a sedative or tranquillizer is an appropriate intervention. Acetylpromazine, medetomidine, or dexmedetomidine can be used.

UTILITY OF PAIN ASSESSMENT TOOLS

A pain assessment tool is of value to the patient only if the veterinary team uses it. Unless the instrument is designed to be simple to use and quick to complete, the chances of it being used consistently in a busy clinical setting are low. When tools are initially developed, they should be considered prototypes. They may be long and cumbersome, but experience has shown that, with testing and suggestions from end users, they can often be modified and shortened without losing precision. Ideally, the tool should fit on one page or less.[18]

The current UNESP-Botucatu Multidimensional Composite Pain Scale[54] (see Table 14-1) is lengthy and may take too long to complete in some situations. Therefore, efforts should be made to simplify and shorten it. Although not validated, the Colorado State University Feline Acute Pain Scale[51] is popular because it is simple to use and can be completed very rapidly. The newly developed Glasgow CMPS-F fits on one page and will likely become popular in a busy clinical setting.[49]

INTERVENTION

As previously stated, pain assessment tools or instruments should be anthropocentric, meaning that they should have a human goal in mind. The utility of a pain assessment tool is enhanced if a score can be linked to an intervention level that will guide treatment. In dogs, intervention levels have been identified for some composite scales with good agreement among trained and experienced clinicians on when to treat.[18]

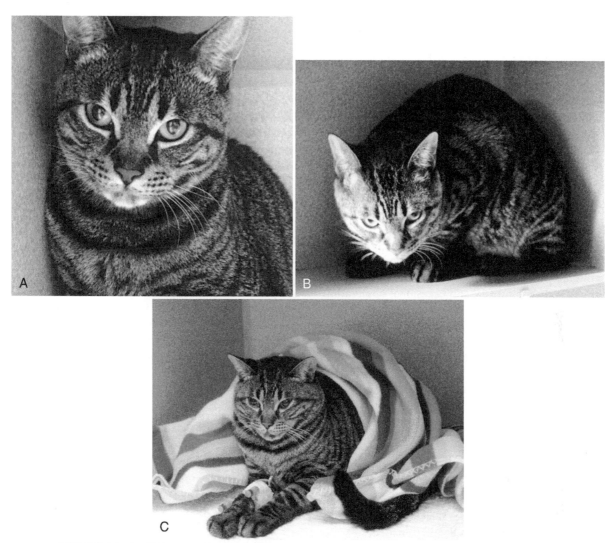

FIGURE 14-19   This cat underwent a dental procedure including tooth extractions. **A** and **B,** Photographs taken before surgery show facial expressions and body postures indicative of early signs of fear or anxiety. **C,** After surgery, the cat's facial expression is more indicative of pain.

Trained observers were used to identify cutoff points for treating cats using unidimensional scales (VAS, NRS, and SDS), and, although there was reasonable agreement,[68] this may not be true for untrained observers. Wide interobserver variability was reported with these scales when used to assess canine pain.[41] Interobserver (different assessors) and intraobserver (single assessor scoring the same videos of cats 2 months apart and in randomized order) reliability and cutoff points for intervention have been reported for the UNESP-Botucatu Multidimensional Composite Pain Scale.[69] Activity, attitude, and miscellaneous behaviors showed moderate inter- and intraobserver reliability, whereas all other scale items showed good to very good reliability. The optimal cutoff point was >7 (out of a possible total of 30). It is hoped that this information will assist in clinical decision making and improving pain management in cats. The suggested

intervention score in the Glasgow CMPS-F is ≥4 (out of 16).[49]

Despite these tools becoming available, it is still important to use clinical judgment or, as Mellor states, "Trust the animal, not the test."[16] This sentiment is echoed by Reid and colleagues, who agree that no animal should be denied analgesic therapy solely on the basis of the results of a pain score; the final decision must be made based on an overall assessment and clinical judgment.[18]

WHEN SHOULD CATS BE ASSESSED, AND WHO SHOULD PERFORM THE ASSESSMENT?

The health status of the animal, the extent of surgery and/or injuries, and the anticipated duration of analgesic drug treatment determine the frequency and intervals of evaluations. In general, evaluations should be made hourly for the first 4 to 6 hours after surgery or injury, provided the animal has recovered from anesthesia, has stable vital signs, and is resting comfortably. Patient response to analgesic therapy and expected duration of analgesic drug treatment will help in determining the frequency of evaluations. For example, if a cat is resting comfortably following the postoperative administration of buprenorphine, it may not need to be reassessed for 2 to 4 hours. Animals should be allowed to sleep following analgesic therapy. Vital signs can often be checked without unduly disturbing a sleeping animal. In general, animals are not awakened to check their pain status; however, this does not mean they should not receive their scheduled analgesics. Continuous, undisturbed observations, coupled with periodic interactive assessments are likely to provide more information than a cursory and occasional observation of the patient through the cage door. In general, the more frequent the observations, the more likely subtle signs of pain or changes in the cat's behavior will be detected. Whichever system is adopted, it must be practical and fit the needs of the veterinary practice.

All veterinarians and animal care staff should be trained to assess pain in cats. The recognition, assessment, and treatment of pain are fundamental components of compassionate veterinary care. Several studies have highlighted the role of veterinary technicians and nurses as patient advocates. In a survey conducted in the United Kingdom, only 8.1% of veterinary practices used a pain scoring system, yet 80.3% of nurses agreed it was a useful clinical tool and 96% of nurses felt their knowledge of pain management could be improved.[70] In Canadian surveys, awareness of pain and its treatment were found to be enhanced in practices that employed a trained veterinary technician.[71,72] Animal care staff are ideally suited to spearhead pain assessment initiatives. They often admit the cat, interact with the cat and client, do the initial preoperative assessment, and oversee the recovery phase of anesthesia. Therefore, they are ideally suited to observing changes in the cat's behavior.

Continued Assessment at Home

Despite advances in pain management, increased understanding of the needs of hospitalized cats, and identification of stressors in this environment, there is no doubt that most clinicians and cat owners agree that the home environment is, in many cases, the best place for cats to complete their recovery. If cats could be asked, they surely would agree. There is little information on behavior changes in cats recovering at home, even following common elective surgery.[66]

Väisänen and colleagues used a questionnaire and a VAS to study owner-assigned assessment of behavior changes and pain in cats recovering at home in the 3 days following ovariohysterectomy or castration.[66] Owners consistently reported changes in their cat's behavior, with a decrease in activity and playfulness, an increase in time spent sleeping, and a change in how the cat moved or its ability to jump being most commonly reported. Owners also commented on changes in facial expression, interrupted stretching, crouched postures, interest in the wound, and aggression toward other cats in the household and felt these were indicators of pain in their cat. These changes were more apparent in females than in males and decreased between day 1 and day 3. An interesting fact reported in this study was the positive correlation between the use of an E-collar (e.g., see Figure 14-3, *B*) and the behavior score, again indicating that aspects other than pain must be taken into account in the overall assessment. This study indicated that owners have an important role to play and can help improve the postoperative care of cats. Owners know their cat best and are likely to pick up even subtle changes in behavior that are overlooked in a clinical setting. Sending clients home with pain assessment tools is recommended. See handout titled **Does My Cat Hurt?**.

SUMMARY

It is the duty of the veterinary profession to prevent and relieve pain in cats, and the ability to do this is greatly enhanced if all veterinary professionals are confident that they can recognize and in some way measure it. Physiologic variables have not proved to be accurate correlates of pain in cats. Unidimensional scales, although simple to use, have limitations and do not assess all the complex sensory and emotional aspects of pain. Multidimensional composite pain scales that are heavily based on both observed and interactive behaviors and include assessment of spontaneous and evoked or dynamic pain are more sensitive and reliable for use in nonlingual species. Current scales for cats show great promise, and others are being developed, modified, and validated. It is hoped these tools will increase the number of cats that receive appropriate analgesic therapy following surgery or injury and enhance the quality of clinical trials. Despite advances in the ability to quantify pain in cats, it will never be an exact science, so using one's clinical judgment is still important. As Mellor states, "Trust the animal, not the test."[16]

ADDITIONAL RESOURCES

American Veterinary Medical Association (AVMA): *U.S. pet ownership & demographics sourcebook,* Schaumburg, IL, 2012, AVMA. https://www.avma.org/kb/resources/statistics/pages/market-research-statistics-us-pet-ownership-demographics-sourcebook.aspx (Accessed January 24, 2015).

4A-Vet postoperative pain scale for dogs and cats. http://www.ncbi.nlm.nih.gov/pmc/articles/PMC3743348/table/tbl3/ (Accessed January 24, 2015).

Colorado State University Veterinary Medical Center: Feline Acute Pain Scale. http://csuanimalcancercenter.org/assets/files/csu_acute_pain_scale_feline.pdf (Accessed January 24, 2015).

International Association for the Study of Pain: IASP taxonomy: pain terms. http://www.iasp-pain.org/Taxonomy (Accessed January 24, 2015).

Pet Food Manufacturer's Association: Pet Population 2014. http://www.pfma.org.uk/pet-population-2014/ (Accessed January 24, 2015).

São Paulo State University: Animal pain. http://www.animalpain.com.br/en-us/ (Accessed January 24, 2015).

ACKNOWLEDGMENTS

The authors are grateful to Juliana Brondani for some of the images used and for commenting on the content of this chapter.

REFERENCES

1. American Veterinary Medical Association (AVMA). U.S. pet ownership & demographics sourcebook, Schaumburg, IL, 2012, AVMA. https://www.avma.org/kb/resources/statistics/pages/market-research-statistics-us-pet-ownership-demographics-sourcebook.aspx Accessed January 24, 2015.
2. Pet Food Manufacturer's Association. Pet Population 2014. http://www.pfma.org.uk/pet-population-2014/ Accessed January 24, 2015.
3. Lascelles B, Capner C, Waterman-Pearson AE. A survey of current British veterinary attitudes to perioperative analgesia for cats and small mammals. *Vet Rec.* 1999;145:601–604.
4. Hansen B, Hardie E. Prescription and use of analgesics in dogs and cats in a veterinary teaching hospital: 258 cases (1983-1989). *J Am Vet Med Assoc.* 1993;202:1485–1494.
5. Brondani JT, Luna SP, Padovani CR. Refinement and initial validation of a multidimensional composite scale for use in assessing acute postoperative pain in cats. *Am J Vet Res.* 2011;72:174–183.
6. Dohoo SE, Dohoo IR. Postoperative use of analgesics in dogs and cats by Canadian veterinarians. *Can Vet J.* 1996;37:546–551.
7. Raekallio M, Heinonen KM, Kuussaari J, et al. Pain alleviation in animals: attitudes and practices of Finnish veterinarians. *Vet J.* 2003;165:131–135.
8. Williams VM, Lascelles BD, Robson MC. Current attitudes to, and use of, peri-operative analgesia in dogs and cats by veterinarians in New Zealand. *N Z Vet J.* 2005;53:193–202.
9. Joubert KE. The use of analgesic drugs by South African veterinarians. *J S Afr Vet Assoc.* 2001;72:57–60.
10. Joubert KE. Anaesthesia and analgesia for dogs and cats in South Africa undergoing sterilisation and with osteoarthritis–an update from 2000. *J S Afr Vet Assoc.* 2006;77:224–228.
11. Hewson CJ, Dohoo IR, Lemke KA. Perioperative use of analgesics in dogs and cats by Canadian veterinarians in 2001. *Can Vet J.* 2006;47:352–359.
12. Farnworth MJ, Adams NJ, Keown AJ, et al. Veterinary provision of analgesia for domestic cats (Felis catus) undergoing gonadectomy: a comparison of samples from New Zealand, Australia and the United Kingdom. *N Z Vet J.* 2014;62:117–122.
13. International Association for the Study of Pain. IASP taxonomy: pain terms. http://www.iasp-pain.org/Taxonomy Accessed January 24, 2015.
14. National Research Council. Committee on Recognition and Alleviation of Pain in Laboratory Animals: Pain in research animals: general principles and considerations. In: *Recognition and alleviation of pain in laboratory animals.* Washington, DC: National Academies Press; 2009:11–29.

15. Flecknell PA. Do mice have a pain face? *Nat Methods.* 2010;7:437–438.
16. Mellor D, Patterson-Kane E, Stafford K. Standardized behavioural testing in non-verbal humans and other animals. In: Mellor DJ, Patterson-Kane E, Stafford KJ, eds. *The sciences of animal welfare.* Chichester, UK: Wiley-Blackwell; 2009:95–109.
17. Holton L, Reid J, Scott EM, et al. Development of a behaviour-based scale to measure acute pain in dogs. *Vet Rec.* 2001;148:525–531.
18. Reid J, Nolan AM, Hughes JML, et al. Development of the short-form Glasgow Composite Measures Pain Scale (CMPS-SF) and derivation of an analgesic intervention score. *Anim Welf.* 2007;16(suppl 1):97–104.
19. Firth AM, Haldane SL. Development of a scale to evaluate postoperative pain in dogs. *J Am Vet Med Assoc.* 1999;214:651–659.
20. Conzemius MG, Hill CM, Sammarco JL, et al. Correlation between subjective and objective measures used to determine severity of postoperative pain in dogs. *J Am Vet Med Assoc.* 1997;210:1619–1622.
21. Holton LL, Scott EM, Nolan AM, et al. Relationship between physiological factors and clinical pain in dogs scored using a numerical rating scale. *J Small Anim Pract.* 1998;39:469–474.
22. Smith JD, Allen SW, Quandt JE, et al. Indicators of postoperative pain in cats and correlation with clinical criteria. *Am J Vet Res.* 1996;57:1674–1678.
23. Smith JD, Allen SW, Quandt JE. Changes in cortisol concentration in response to stress and postoperative pain in client-owned cats and correlation with objective clinical variables. *Am J Vet Res.* 1999;60:432–436.
24. Brondani JT, Luna SP, Marcello GC, et al. Perioperative administration of vedaprofen, tramadol or their combination does not interfere with platelet aggregation, bleeding time and biochemical variables in cats. *J Feline Med Surg.* 2009;11:503–509.
25. Brondani JT, Loureiro Luna SP, Beier SL, et al. Analgesic efficacy of perioperative use of vedaprofen, tramadol or their combination in cats undergoing ovariohysterectomy. *J Feline Med Surg.* 2009;11:420–429.
26. Rodan I, Sundahl E, Carney H, et al. AAFP and ISFM feline-friendly handling guidelines. *J Feline Med Surg.* 2011;13:364–375.
27. Quimby JM, Smith ML, Lunn KF. Evaluation of the effects of hospital visit stress on physiologic parameters in the cat. *J Feline Med Surg.* 2011;13:733–737.
28. Dobbins S, Brown NO, Shofer FS. Comparison of the effects of buprenorphine, oxymorphone hydrochloride, and ketoprofen for postoperative analgesia after onychectomy or

onychectomy and sterilization in cats. *J Am Anim Hosp Assoc.* 2002;38:507–514.

29. Glerum LE, Egger CM, Allen SW, et al. Analgesic effect of the transdermal fentanyl patch during and after feline ovariohysterectomy. *Vet Surg.* 2001;30:351–358.

30. Cambridge AJ, Tobias KM, Newberry RC, et al. Subjective and objective measurements of postoperative pain in cats. *J Am Vet Med Assoc.* 2000;217:685–690.

31. Coleman KD, Schmiedt CW, Kirkby KA, et al. Learning confounds algometric assessment of mechanical thresholds in normal dogs. *Vet Surg.* 2014;43:361–367.

32. Slingsby LS, Jones A, Waterman-Pearson AE. Use of a new finger-mounted device to compare mechanical nociceptive thresholds in cats given pethidine or no medication after castration. *Res Vet Sci.* 2001;70:243–246.

33. Brondani JT, Mama KR, Luna SP, et al. Validation of the English version of the UNESP-Botucatu multidimensional composite pain scale for assessing postoperative pain in cats. *BMC Vet Res.* 2013;9:143.

34. Grint NJ, Murison PJ, Coe RJ, et al. Assessment of the influence of surgical technique on postoperative pain and wound tenderness in cats following ovariohysterectomy. *J Feline Med Surg.* 2006;8:15–21.

35. Lascelles BD, Findley K, Correa M, et al. Kinetic evaluation of normal walking and jumping in cats, using a pressure-sensitive walkway. *Vet Rec.* 2007;160:512–516.

36. Romans CW, Conzemius MG, Horstman CL, et al. Use of pressure platform gait analysis in cats with and without bilateral onychectomy. *Am J Vet Res.* 2004;65:1276–1278.

37. Verdugo MR, Rahal SC, Agostinho FS, et al. Kinetic and temporospatial parameters in male and female cats walking over a pressure sensing walkway. *BMC Vet Res.* 2013;9:129.

38. Carroll GL, Narbe R, Kerwin SC, et al. Dose range finding study for the efficacy of meloxicam administered prior to sodium urate-induced synovitis in cats. *Vet Anaesth Analg.* 2011;38:394–406.

39. Lascelles BD, Hansen BD, Thomson A, et al. Evaluation of a digitally integrated accelerometer-based activity monitor for the measurement of activity in cats. *Vet Anaesth Analg.* 2008;35:173–183.

40. Lascelles BD, DePuy V, Thomson A, et al. Evaluation of a therapeutic diet for feline degenerative joint disease. *J Vet Intern Med.* 2010;24:487–495.

41. Holton LL, Scott EM, Nolan AM, et al. Comparison of three methods used for assessment of pain in dogs. *J Am Vet Med Assoc.* 1998;212:61–66.

42. Steagall PV, Taylor PM, Rodrigues LC, et al. Analgesia for cats after ovariohysterectomy with either buprenorphine or carprofen alone or in combination. *Vet Rec.* 2009;164:359–363.

43. Giordano T, Steagall PV, Ferreira TH, et al. Postoperative analgesic effects of intravenous, intramuscular, subcutaneous or oral transmucosal buprenorphine administered to cats undergoing ovariohysterectomy. *Vet Anaesth Analg.* 2010;37:357–366.

44. Polson S, Taylor PM, Yates D. Analgesia after feline ovariohysterectomy under midazolam-medetomidine-ketamine anaesthesia with buprenorphine or butorphanol, and carprofen or meloxicam: a prospective, randomised clinical trial. *J Feline Med Surg.* 2012;14:553–559.

45. Tobias KM, Harvey RC, Byarlay JM. A comparison of four methods of analgesia in cats following ovariohysterectomy. *Vet Anaesth Analg.* 2006;33:390–398.

46. Lascelles B, Cripps P, Mirchandani S, et al. Carprofen as an analgesic for postoperative pain in cats: dose titration and assessment of efficacy in comparison to pethidine hydrochloride. *J Small Anim Pract.* 1995;36:535–541.

47. Slingsby L, Waterman-Pearson A. Comparison of pethidine, buprenorphine and ketoprofen for postoperative analgesia after ovariohysterectomy in the cat. *Vet Rec.* 1998;143: 185–189.

48. Waran N, Best L, Williams V, et al. A preliminary study of behaviour-based indicators of pain in cats. *Anim Welf.* 2007;16(suppl 1):105–108.

49. Calvo G, Holden E, Reid J, et al. Development of a behaviour-based measurement tool with defined intervention level for assessing acute pain in cats. *J Small Anim Pract.* 2014;55: 622–629.

50. São Paulo State University. Animal pain. http://www.animalpain.com.br/en-us/ Accessed January 24, 2015.

51. Colorado State University Veterinary Medical Center. Feline Acute Pain Scale. http://csuanimalcancercenter.org/assets/files/csu_acute_pain_scale_feline.pdf Accessed January 24, 2015.

52. 4A-Vet postoperative pain scale for dogs and cats. http://www.ncbi.nlm.nih.gov/pmc/articles/PMC3743348/table/tbl3/ Accessed January 24, 2015.

53. Grandemange E, Fournel S, Woehrle F. Efficacy and safety of cimicoxib in the control of perioperative pain in dogs. *J Small Anim Pract.* 2013;54:304–312.

54. São Paulo State University: UNESP-Botucatu Multidimensional Composite Pain Scale. http://www.animalpain.com.br/assets/upload/escala-en-us.pdf Accessed January 25, 2015.

55. Carney HC, Little S, Brownlee-Tomasso D, et al. AAFP and ISFM feline-friendly nursing care guidelines. *J Feline Med Surg.* 2012;14:337–349.

56. Darwin C. The expression of the emotions in man and animals. London: John Murray; 1872.

57. Lucey P, Cohn J, Lucey S, et al. Automatically detecting pain using facial actions. *Int Conf Affect Comput Intell Interact Workshops.* 2009;2009:1–8.

58. Stevens B, McGrath P, Gibbins S, et al. Determining behavioural and physiological responses to pain in infants at risk for neurological impairment. *Pain.* 2007;127:94–102.

59. Schiavenato M, Byers JF, Scovanner P, et al. Neonatal pain facial expression: evaluating the primal face of pain. *Pain.* 2008;138:460–471.

60. Langford DJ, Bailey AL, Chanda ML, et al. Coding of facial expressions of pain in the laboratory mouse. *Nat Methods.* 2010;7:447–449.

61. Keating SC, Thomas AA, Flecknell PA, et al. Evaluation of EMLA cream for preventing pain during tattooing of rabbits: changes in physiological, behavioural and facial expression responses. *PLoS One.* 2012;7:e44437.

62. Herbert GL, Robertson SA, Murrell JC: Changes in the facial expression of cats during nociceptive threshold testing. Presented at the 11th World Congress of Veterinary Anaesthesiology, Cape Town, South Africa, September 23–27, 2012.

63. Holden E, Calvo G, Collins M, et al. Evaluation of facial expression in acute pain in cats. *J Small Anim Pract.* 2014;55:615–621.

64. Griffin B: Getting real: making the ASV standards work for you. Anim Sheltering 38–41, May/June 2011. http://www.animalsheltering.org/resources/magazine/may_jun_2011/getting_real.pdf Accessed January 24, 2015.

65. McCobb EC, Patronek GJ, Marder A, et al. Assessment of stress levels among cats in four animal shelters. *J Am Vet Med Assoc.* 2005;226:548–555.

66. Väisänen MA, Tuomikoski SK, Vainio OM. Behavioral alterations and severity of pain in cats recovering at home following elective ovariohysterectomy or castration. *J Am Vet Med Assoc.* 2007;231:236–242.

67. Robertson SA, Wegner K, Lascelles BD. Antinociceptive and side-effects of hydromorphone after subcutaneous administration in cats. *J Feline Med Surg.* 2009;11:76–81.

68. Brondani JT, Luna SPL, Mama KR, et al. Cut-off point for rescue analgesia of uni-dimensional scales used to assess postoperative pain in cats. In: *Proceedings of the Association of Veterinary Anaesthetists Spring Meeting*; 2013:78.

69. Brondani JT, Luna SP, Minto BW, et al. Reliability and cut-off point related to the analgesic intervention of a multidimensional composite scale to assess postoperative pain in cats. *Arq Bras Med Vet Zootec*. 2013;65:153–162.

70. Coleman DL, Slingsby LS. Attitudes of veterinary nurses to the assessment of pain and the use of pain scales. *Vet Rec*. 2007;160:541–544.

71. Hewson CJ, Dohoo IR, Lemke KA. Factors affecting the use of postincisional analgesics in dogs and cats by Canadian veterinarians in 2001. *Can Vet J*. 2006;47:453–459.

72. Dohoo SE, Dohoo IR. Factors influencing the postoperative use of analgesics in dogs and cats by Canadian veterinarians. *Can Vet J*. 1996;37:552–556.

Chronic Pain and Behavior

Richard Gowan and Isabelle Iff

INTRODUCTION

Advances in veterinary medicine have resulted in an increased life expectancy for feline patients. As cats live longer, the possibility of age-related pathology and diseases increases along with the prevalence of co-morbid conditions.[1] Chronic pain accompanies many of these disease states, with an inherent functional (and emotional) impact on the individual's quality of life. While approaches to the recognition and management of acute pain relief in cats have gained momentum over the past decade, awareness and management of chronic pain has received less attention. There are numerous reasons for this, including poor recognition of the clinical manifestations of chronic pain and a lack of validated methods for assessing it.[2] It is likely that many cats suffer from chronic pain and that practitioners often miss the signs and the opportunity to relieve cats of this debilitating state.

This chapter outlines the current understanding of chronic pain in cats, the difference in pathophysiology of acute and chronic pain, pain recognition, assessment, and quantification in cats, along with current and future management strategies and how such strategies can be integrated in the daily routine. A closer look at several chronically painful conditions in cats is given towards the end of the chapter.

PATHOPHYSIOLOGY OF CHRONIC PAIN

Acute pain is an alarm system of the body and "protects" the body from further harm. Chronic pain has lost the "protective role" and becomes a disease in itself. More detail on terminology can be found below. All the neurophysiologic "pathways" activated in acute pain are involved in chronic pain.

There is no one pain pathway but rather a big pain network. However, to facilitate understanding of the neural structures involved in pain perception and help with choice and combination of treatment, the following will briefly describe the "pain pathway," which **abstracts** how pain is relayed through the body (Figure 15-1).

In the **periphery,** a noxious stimulus causes a depolarization in a nerve fiber. The nerve fibers transmitting pain end in free nerve endings (nociceptors). Nociceptors are small, generally unmyelinated afferent nerve fibers, which are activated by strong mechanical, thermal, or chemical stimuli. Different factors, especially inflammatory mediators, can influence the sensitivity of these nociceptors (peripheral sensitization). The stimulus travels up the afferent nociceptive fibers and enters the dorsal root of the spinal cord. Pain impulses are carried via Aδ (myelinated) and C (unmyelinated) fibers. Aδ fibers produce sharp, pricking pain. C fibers cause a slow burning pain and are found in the viscera as well.

In the **spinal cord** the stimulus is relayed to a secondary neuron, projecting into the higher centers of the brain. The primary (peripheral) neuron synapses on a secondary neuron (wide dynamic range neuron or nociceptive specific neuron) in the spinal cord with the main neurotransmitters at this level being glutamate and substance P. Many factors modulate this signal transmission in the spinal cord, which serves as an important location for the action of analgesic drugs.

Additionally, at this level, the spinal cord can undergo plastic changes resulting in augmentation of the signal. Prolonged or massive stimulation may result in **central sensitization,** augmenting a pain response. This central sensitization can occur within hours, can be measured electrophysiologically as "wind up" and is due to several mechanisms:

1. With prolonged or massive stimulation the NMDA (*n*-methyl-d-aspartate) receptor at the level of the second neuron is stimulated. This receptor produces changes in gene transcription, upregulating receptor sensitivity and receptor numbers, thus increasing the response of the secondary neuron to a giving peripheral input. One could say it increases the "gain" of the system.
2. Recently it has been shown that central sensitization is not purely a neuronal event. Glial cells, which have been considered to have a mainly supportive role in the central nervous system, are activated. This activation has a pivotal role in maintaining chronic pain states.

From the spinal cord, the information is relayed over the thalamus to the brain either directly or indirectly.

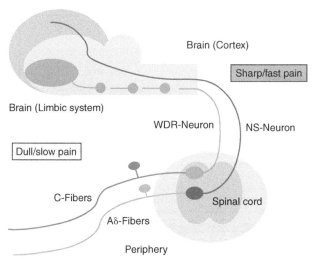

FIGURE 15-1 Graphic representation of the fast and the slow pain pathways.

In the brain stem, branches of the secondary nerve fibers stimulate interneurons and descending projections, which modulate the pain pathway at several levels. Inhibitory interneurons with noradrenaline and serotonin as neurotransmitters trigger modulation of the secondary spinal cord neuron. These systems are called the **descending inhibitory control system.** Spinal interneurons can modulate the secondary neuron in the spinal cord as well.

At the level of the **brain**, the stimulus reaches the sensory cortex describing the sensory discriminative side of pain (where, how much?—commonly mediated through Aδ fibers) and the limbic system related to the motivational-affective aspects (aversive feelings, emotions, suffering—commonly mediated through C fibers) of pain. Both areas in the brain are ultimately responsible for the behavior changes occurring with chronic pain. However, it is mainly the limbic system that is responsible for changes in emotions and emotional well-being.

Chronic Pain and Emotional Well-Being

Any aversive sensory experience may provoke protective reactions, including defensive behavior and learned avoidance. In the context of chronic pain, the perception of pain may result in the modification of behaviors, such as those between the cat and its social and environmental surroundings.[3] Very little is known about the emotional manifestations of pain by animals. While it is difficult to directly evaluate emotional responses in animals, it is reasonable to infer that the pain process and experience in cats may be similar to those in humans, given that both species possess similar neural pathways and neurotransmitters.[3] Emotional well-being has a significant impact on an individual's quality of life and it can be argued that this experience is just as, if not more,

important than the physical and functional outcomes of pain management.

In people it has also been shown that cerebral control can modify the response to pain. Motivation and pain avoidance are contrasting forces shaping an individuals behavior. Motivation (or drive) is defined as being goal oriented: optimizing well-being, minimizing pain and suffering, and maximizing pleasure.[4] For cats, they will be motivated to achieve their survival needs and display their normal species-specific behavior in their environment. However, such needs may be compromised and this may play a critical part in their self-management of chronic pain through adaptive behaviors. For example, cats may choose to forgo enjoyable goals and experiences if these result in unpleasant stimuli such as pain.

As a clinical example, cats enjoy being able to perch and survey their environment; this frequently manifests as jumping up high to sit on a windowsill. However, in cats with degenerative joint disease (DJD) this may cause undue pain in their joints so that they either adapt the manner in which they get up onto the windowsill or choose to cease this pursuit even though it remains a desirable, enjoyable goal (Figure 15-2). Nevertheless, driven by the desire for an overwhelming positive reward (such as a treat or the opportunity to interact with their

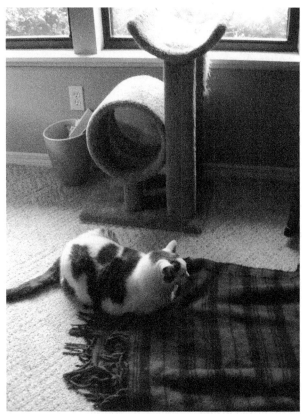

FIGURE 15-2 Although this cat enjoys perching and looking out the window, musculoskeletal disease prevents it from jumping onto the perch. (Courtesy S. Robertson)

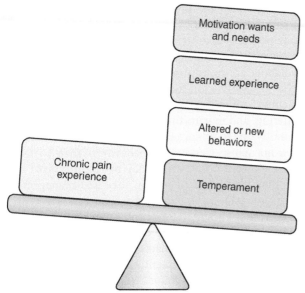

FIGURE 15-3 A cat would likely balance and consider many factors versus the potential for pain experienced. Altered and new adaptive behaviors can minimize or avoid pain. Temperament and learned experiences likely affect what and how these behaviors manifest. Needs and wants act as motivation in the face of pain stimulus, for example, the need to eat versus the want or desire to play are different motivating factors.

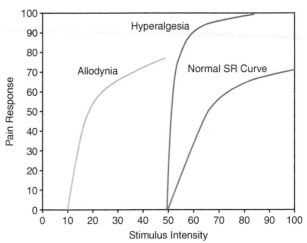

FIGURE 15-4 A representation of central sensitization, hyperalgesia, and allodynia. Normally, increasing nociceptive stimulus elicits an increased magnitude of pain. With central sensitization, the same nociceptive stimulus causes a greater pain response, "hyperalgesia." With allodynia, low or previously nonpainful stimulus elicits a pain response. (Adapted from A. Bergadano, 15th FECAVA Eurocongress/AFVAC/SAVAB/LAK Congress, Lille, France, November 2009)

owner), the cat may still choose to jump up to this same point, despite the presence of pain and debility.

Altered behaviors will therefore be highly variable and depend on the perceived benefit (e.g., food, comfort, security) and enjoyment to the individual as well as the anticipated pain and discomfort. The innate temperament of the cat, learned fear, and other learned behaviors may also influence factors and decisions that cats make in pain avoidance (Figure 15-3).

DEFINITION AND TERMINOLOGY

The International Association for the Study of Pain (IASP) defines pain as "an unpleasant sensory and emotional experience associated with actual or potential tissue damage, or described in terms of such damage. . .the inability to communicate verbally does not negate the possibility that an individual is experiencing pain and is in need of appropriate pain-relieving treatment."[5]

This means that pain is a multidimensional experience with unpleasant sensory, functional, and emotional components.

Terminology

1. **Acute** or **chronic:** chronic pain is arbitrarily defined as pain lasting longer than 1 to 6 months, or pain lasting beyond the expected period of tissue healing and resolution of pathology. However, clinically these

are difficult to differentiate, especially when acute "flare ups" occur during chronic pain states.[6]

2. **Adaptive** or **maladaptive:** to describe the difference between the protective role of pain and the changes which make it an illness, different terms have been used. Pain related to protective reflexes is commonly termed adaptive pain; in the past, the terms protective, nociceptive, or physiologic pain have been used. Maladaptive pain represents abnormal or dysfunctional neurotransmission, serving no physiological protective purpose and has been called pathological pain.[6–8]

3. **Inflammatory, neuropathic,** or **mixed** pain[8]: defined according to the mechanism causing pain. Inflammatory pain refers to pain caused by noxious stimulation of peripheral nerve fibers, and may be somatic or visceral in origin. Neuropathic pain is due to damage or disease affecting the peripheral and/or central nervous systems.[9]

4. **Hyperalgesia** and **allodynia:** hyperalgesia is a heightened pain experience from a known painful stimulus (i.e., pain "amplification"). Allodynia refers to the experience of pain from a nonpainful stimulus (i.e., changes in nerve signaling causes pain to be experienced from a nonpainful stimulus)[9] (Figure 15-4). Both phenomena have been related to central sensitization.

RECOGNITION AND ASSESSMENT OF CHRONIC PAIN

Recognition of Chronic Pain in Cats

It is now widely described and recognized that all animals experience pain and the expression of pain varies with age and species, as well as among individuals. Additionally, certain procedures and conditions commonly assumed to be painful in dogs may be overlooked in cats.[7] Behavioral changes in older cats have been ascribed to old age rather than pain even though it is known that musculoskeletal disorders in cats are common.[7] It is likely that veterinary professionals have been unaware or insensitive to the manifestations of chronic pain in cats. Chronic pain hurts, it impacts physical function, and cats do suffer emotionally: these components all impact an individual's quality of life.

The following thoughts may be important when considering recognition and assessment of chronic pain in cats.

1. Cats cannot communicate the presence and also the quantity of pain and suffering verbally. Verbal communication is the gold standard for assessing pain in people. However, even in people it is recognized, that individuals, who are unable to communicate can suffer from pain.[5] Common examples include small children, sedated individuals in intensive care units and patients suffering from dementia.[10] These patients are commonly assessed by proxy, as is the case with cats.

2. As largely solitary animals, without a pack or colony to protect them, the wildcat ancestors minimized overt displays of vulnerability by adopting behaviors that tend to hide the presence of disease in a survival instinct for self-preservation. In each individual situation, the physiological needs of the cat and the severity of the disease, impairment, or pain will determine the ultimate outcome (Figure 15-5). This theory of self-preservation is used to explain traditional views that cats tend to withdraw and avoid showing overt signs of pain and disease.

3. Chronic pain may also be present in the absence of ongoing clinical disease, persisting beyond the expected course of an acute injury; examples include neuropathic pain after amputation or onychectomy.

4. The difference between "normal" age related changes in behavior and changes related to chronic pain may be very difficult to differentiate. Owners of older animals commonly believe that many behavior changes are a result of aging, rather than a sign of possible pain and disease.

SIGNS OF CHRONIC PAIN IN CATS

As with the presentation of most diseases in cats, the clinical signs of chronic pain may be nonspecific, usually manifesting as changes to normal behaviors, or the development of abnormal behaviors. Pet owners are very familiar with their pet's normal behavior and they may detect changes most easily.[11] However, they may not recognize changes that begin and progress insidiously. Sometimes change is only recognized when pain is minimized or eliminated through appropriate analgesia or when the underlying disease is addressed. The manifestations of pain will also depend on the source and nature of the pain and any accompanying disabilities. Conditions commonly associated with chronic pain are listed in Box 15-1 and are discussed in more detail later in the chapter. Many of the indicators discussed in this chapter have been found in studies looking at DJD, therefore the list may change as further pain states are evaluated.

Altered normal behaviors include changes in:

1. Activity level or performing activities like jumping, playing, using a litter box. Difficulties in using the litter box may lead to inappropriate elimination.[7]
2. Appetite, eating, and drinking behaviors.
3. General mobility, like ease of movement, fluidity of movement, and body posture. This applies mainly to cats with musculoskeletal issues. These manifest as altered lifestyle choices, along with specific alterations to mobility that primarily include alterations in jumping and climbing.[12-14] It is likely that these activities exert most stress on the joints in cats and

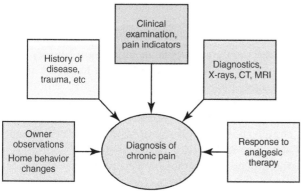

FIGURE 15-5 Multidimensional approach to diagnosing chronic painful conditions in cats.

BOX 15-1	Conditions Often Causing Chronic Pain in Cats

- Chronic musculoskeletal pain (e.g., degenerative joint disease, osteoarthritis)
- Postsurgical (e.g., fibrosarcoma excision, limb amputation)
- Dental and oral pain (e.g., chronic gingivostomatitis)
- Visceral pain (e.g., inflammatory bowel disease, pancreatitis, interstitial cystitis)
- Chronic otitis externa, chronic dermatitis, and pruritic lesions
- Neoplasia-associated pain (e.g., osteosarcoma, lymphoma)
- Neurologic pain (e.g., diabetic neuropathy)

therefore cause most pain. From a behavioral perspective, these changes to normal activities could be viewed as operant conditioning or learned avoidance behaviors. Reduced willingness to jump up or down and reduced height and frequency of jumping minimize any discomfort experienced. In some situations the cat may still be able to exhibit normal behavior, for example, if the desire is for a cat to get on the owner's bed, they may first jump onto a lower bedside table to then gain access to the bed, rather than over-extending themselves by jumping up in one go, but in other situations they will simply forgo the normal behavior. If the clients are not made aware of the significance of these changes, they will probably not understand them as pain-minimizing strategies (Box 15-2).

4. Grooming and coat appearance (e.g., self-scratching, alterations in grooming frequency or intensity).[13]

5. Temperament, mood and demeanor, or sociability with people and animals.[13] Alterations in previously enjoyable interactions and normal behaviors with owners may occur as a result of learned pain avoidance. For example, grooming or stroking the back of a cat suffering chronic painful lumbosacral DJD may elicit a painful or unpleasant stimulus. Even if the cat previously viewed this as desirable, this now painful and aversive stimulus may result in the cat becoming intolerant of the interaction or avoiding it. If cats remove themselves from such painful experiences, this may also reduce the observance and recognition of pain in cats by their owners. Clients may report changes in their cat's mood or an increase in reclusive behavior. It has been found that aggressive behavior patterns may increase in response to pain but may vary between individuals.[15] This is an observation that should also be explored in cats, as veterinarians would be aware that in-clinic aggression in cats is highly variable and may be influenced by innate temperament, learned fear behavior, and

previous painful experiences. A great variety of feline behaviors may occur at the veterinary practice. Physical examinations can be more difficult in cats, with less opportunity to gain reliable physical cues of pain. Behaviors assumed to be pain-associated may in fact be from learned avoidance or an anxiety or fear response. Temperament and behavior further exacerbates the difficulties faced in interpreting physical findings of pain in cats. Multiple studies on DJD in cats have found that only some cats assessed to be in pain were more aggressive, less socially interactive, and less tolerant of physical petting and brushing by owners.[12,16-18] However, temperament assessment was worse in those cats with high radiographic DJD scores and high pain scores in the clinical assessment.[19] It was hypothesized that pain may be the cause of uncooperative or intolerant disposition in the veterinary practice and with the owners at home, and thus be associated with a negative temperament score.[19] Alterations in mood, interactivity, and aggressive tendencies have been shown in some cats suffering from painful DJD, improvements in which are often seen in response to analgesic therapy.[12,13,20] The underlying temperament is associated with an individual's behavioral and emotional response pattern and is regarded as innate rather than learned in people.[21] Pain intensity is no different between personality types, but introverted people have significantly more suffering and illness behavior. Extroverts were more likely to express their suffering, but suffered less from their pain (having better coping mechanisms).[22] This implies the cognitive and emotional process of how pain influences our perceived quality of life is influenced by our innate personality traits.[22] While these human studies are not directly applicable to cats, temperament type (i.e., genetics) further modified by environment and experience, may play a role in an individual cat's perception of pain. Innate temperament may also influence the way in which a cat modifies its behavior in response to pain, impacting its coping mechanisms. Innate temperament traits are accentuated and molded through environmental and life experiences, but no work has been done to investigate how these traits may be affected by stressors such as chronic pain. Pain is an unpleasant sensory and emotional experience and is known to elicit a stress response that will have physical and emotional effects.[23] The influence of the emotional stressors fear and anxiety on various feline behaviors and the effect of potential stressors on the cat's emotional state and its behavior has been studied[24] but as yet there is no comparable work on the way in which chronic pain may affect emotion in cats. Additionally, the interaction between temperament and pain has not been explored in cats. If temperament

---

BOX 15-2   Changes to Behavior and Routine as a Consequence of Chronic Pain in Cats

- More secluded, more time sleeping
- Changed mood, unhappy, withdrawn
- Abnormal interactive patterns, sleep-wake pattern changes
- Aggression towards owners or other animals
- Aggression on manipulation or being touched in places
- Less inclination to play and interact physically
- Reduced appetite or weight loss
- Altered daily activity or routines
- Elimination disorders, missing litter tray

profiles are indeed stable and predictable through life, it would be interesting to assess whether this information could be integrated with the tools for the early detection of pain, and if chronic pain-associated behavior is different in those cats deemed more "extroverted" (i.e., social and friendly personalities) versus those deemed more "introverted" (i.e., less social and unfriendly personalities). The Feline Temperament Score (FTS) is a validated temperament test used to improve compatibility of rehoming cats from adoption shelters to suitable home environments in the United States.[25] Adolescent FTP scores were relatively stable over time and correlated well with behaviors in the new home and towards people. FTP testing may provide accurate insights into and consistent measures of a cat's sociability. Cats with FTP scores suggesting they are less outgoing and less friendly may be inclined to be more aggressive and reclusive in certain tactile interactions with owners or unfamiliar people. The presence of chronic pain may increase the intensity and frequency of undesirable interactions and owners may therefore avoid situations that trigger aggressive responses. In addition, worsening of aggressive behaviors could be an indicator of the development or worsening of underlying chronic pain. On the other hand, cats with FTP scores suggesting they are more sociable and friendly might not display aggressive or reclusive behaviors as readily. These cats might be more easily integrated as part of a family unit and may derive more enjoyment and security from operant conditioned interactions with their owners. These cats may actually seek out the comfort or physical security offered by interactions with people and may perhaps exhibit more easily identifiable behavioral changes associated with pain or disability, due to their stronger desire to maintain pleasurable experiences with their owners.

While some of the aforementioned signs are similar to those of acute pain, common chronic pain signs are less obvious. However, assessing acute pain symptoms may be necessary during "flare ups" of chronically painful conditions. Additional changes may include:

1. Looking at or licking affected areas[11]
2. Facial expression (furrowed brow, squinted eyes, and hanging head)[11]
3. Posture (hunched, tense), abnormal gait, shifting of weight, sitting or lying in abnormal postures[11]
4. Distanced and tense appearance[11]

Chronic Pain in Dogs Versus Cats

As a result of their different evolutionary backgrounds and different levels of interactions with humans, dogs tend to be more overtly expressive when suffering disease or pain. For example, dogs with DJD tend to show many more overt and obvious clinical signs and thus there tends to be a higher recognition of chronically painful conditions in dogs than in cats.[18]

Interactions between dogs and their owners include routines, such as going for regular walks or runs (on and off a leash), playing with a Frisbee, balls, or toys; regular grooming, and so on. With something like musculoskeletal pain, impediments to these routines become apparent to owners, and prompt veterinary evaluation is often sought. In contrast, most cats do not have many interactive exercise routines with their owners and as their primary response to painful stimuli may be simply to withdraw and be less active, any impediment or link to pain may be easily overlooked by owners. Similarly, with a disease such as DJD, cats may choose to avoid situations and activities that result in pain and so learned avoidance can be one reason why lameness is not a common sign of DJD in cats. Additionally, limping is rare in feline DJD because it is commonly a bilateral disease, as opposed to canine DJD.[13]

Diagnosing Chronic Pain in Cats

History and Signalment in Investigating Chronic Painful Conditions

Signalment and accurate history-taking is a vital key to screening and managing patients suffering from chronic painful conditions. Owners are crucial in the recognition and assessment of their pet, as they live with the cat and are more familiar with its normal behavior than a veterinarian who spends 10 to 30 minutes of consultation time with the animal. However, it is important that they are asked the "right" questions in order to recognize pain in their pet and subsequently evaluate its progression and response to treatment (Box 15-3). While owners are often in the best position to perceive

---

BOX 15-3   Behavioral Changes Often Associated With Chronic Painful Musculoskeletal Conditions in Cats

- Reduced height of jumping
- Reluctance to jump up or down
- The use of intermediate points to access usual high places
- Loss of cat-like grace and agility
- Missing landing spots, especially jumping up
- Pulling themselves up onto couches and beds
- Consideration before jumping down from a height
- Heavy landings when jumping down
- Changes to gait, e.g., more stiff and stilted gait
- Lameness is uncommon

changes suggestive of pain, they may not assign significance to their observations until prompted.[12]

It has been suggested that questionnaires filled in by the client can be ideal tools to assist in the recognition and assessment of feline chronic pain, and these have been used by dog owners for pain associated with cancer and DJD.[26,27] Currently, the optimal construction of these tools for cats has not been determined.[11] Any questionnaire should ideally have undergone psychometric testing and validation in the appropriate language. Much of the manifestation of chronic pain in cats is seen in adaptive behavioral, mood, and lifestyle changes and in avoidance mechanisms. The area most researched in cats is chronic pain from DJD, with studies characterizing more specifically the behaviors observed by owners.[16,17] Subsequent studies found that owners were able to assess response to therapies.[12,20] Further work refining client outcomes has subsequently resulted in the publication of the Feline Musculoskeletal Pain Index (FMPI).[14,28,29] This tool is able to discern differences in mobility and quality of life scores between those cats with normal mobility and those affected by DJD.

In people, chronic pain is commonly evaluated by the impact it has on quality of life (QOL). Studies have been conducted on the factors that owners consider to be important for their cat's QOL,[29] and the concept of QOL has been used to assess cats being treated with antiviral agents[30] or suffering from cardiac disease,[31,32] cancer,[33] or diabetes.[34] Recent progress has been made in developing an owner-directed instrument to assess musculoskeletal pain in cats with DJD.[28,35,14] Focusing on function as an outcome may not be the only useful measure of a cat's quality of life because an owner may perceive certain attributes and various household routines as more important than veterinarians necessarily would. Using a combination of objective measures, such as physical/functional outcomes, along with the nonphysical aspects, possibly representing the client's perception of their cat's well-being, may offer the best global assessment of an individual's QOL.

During history-taking, open-ended questions regarding appetite, activity, mobility, mood and temperament, grooming, gait, and changes specific to the home and social environment, including contact with other pets and the owner, can help identify areas of concern. Previous surgical or traumatic events may also prompt further investigation. Behavior changes suggestive of pain such as avoidance or aggressive reactions to physical contact may guide physical and additional examinations (see Box 15-2).

Clients may also be requested to film their pet at home. With the advent of modern mobile phones many people have easy access to a video camera, and filming the cat's gait or abnormal behavior may give clues to the underlying problem. It is also possible to use technology to enable veterinarians to carry out virtual house visits and to see the cat in its home environment in real time without needing to be physically present.

Previous medications, the response, and side effects also form part of this initial assessment.

In the absence of a validated questionnaire, several points/behaviors may be identified after the history-taking, which can then be scored by the owner. These so-called client specific outcome measures (CSOM) are discussed later in this chapter.

Physical and Clinical Investigation

A full physical examination should always be undertaken, but the need for careful assessment of different body systems and the extent of further investigations will be determined in part by suspected underlying disease and/or causes of pain.

Surgical sites should be examined for evidence of ongoing pain and/or sensitization. Palpation of different body parts is an important factor to identify the location of pain. However, the absence of a reaction to palpation *does not* indicate that the animal is not experiencing pain. This may be particularly true for musculoskeletal pain,[19] but generally is valid for all localities of pain. As DJD is common in older cats, an orthopedic examination should be carried out. A thorough examination may elicit apparent pain responses from the musculoskeletal system, but the interpretation and significance of these responses is difficult in cats.[19] Muscle atrophy may indicate limb disuse from pain avoidance behaviors.

Abdominal palpation can assess for visceral pain, but as this pain tends to radiate it may be difficult to locate the exact organ or site involved.[36]

Further Investigations

Further investigations should be performed to identify a physical cause for chronic pain. However, absence of physical disease does not imply that pain is not present. Chronic pain can be persistent without physical changes due to the mechanisms described at the beginning of this chapter. Further tests depend on the suspected nature of chronic pain, and commonly include diagnostic imaging, which may help with the detection of musculoskeletal, dental, aural, intracranial, abdominal, and spinal disease. The pitfalls of pain detection and the significance of radiographic changes in DJD are discussed further in the section on management of DJD pain later in this chapter.

Assessing and Quantifying Chronic Pain in Cats

Assessing and quantifying chronic pain is paramount in the initial evaluation, assessment of treatment success, and in research when evaluating new analgesics. Validated tools and instruments are rare in animals in general, even more so in cats, especially for chronic pain.

Assessing and quantifying chronic pain in cats

Because cats are nonverbal, they require pain scoring by proxy, which is a major confounding factor in feline medicine, as it may introduce owner bias and the owner's perception of the response to treatment. In one study with a hypothesis that physical activity (mobility) would be the most important aspect of quality of life in cats with DJD, it was found that owners instead placed more importance on nonphysical outcomes (60%).[29] Signs such as the cat's perceived comfort and its ability to rest, eat, and groom were particularly significant to owners of older cats, while owners of younger cats considered mobility and ability to play to be more important. Owner perception that reduced physical activity is inevitable during the aging process may help to explain why function and mobility do not seem as important to owners in assessing quality of life, especially in older cats.[29] However, mobility is the functional outcome that many studies of DJD-associated pain have focused on as a means of measuring response to therapy. There is currently no clinically accessible validated objective measure to assess the efficacy of treatment modalities. Tremendous steps have been made towards the establishment of a valid assessment tool for cats suffering with DJD, and the FMPI has come close to being proven as valid for assessing the response to analgesic treatment, but requires reassessment before complete validation.[35,14] While such measures are valuable, they are only one possible tool in the clinical monitoring of pain and currently have not been developed for pain associated with DJD.

Client Specific Outcome Measures (CSOM)

An important pain monitoring tool that can be used in the veterinary practice setting is client specific outcome measures (CSOM). Their clinical use has been reported in dogs and cats.[35,37,38]

CSOM are generated based on the initial history-taking where three to four problematic/abnormal activities or behaviors are identified. These simple client observations can be transcribed in a visual analogue scale of 0 to 10 or simple yes/no answers comparing before and after therapy. A template of a CSOM is listed in Table 15-1. An example of a CSOM used by one of the authors (II) for a cat with chronic back pain, likely from DJD of the lumbar vertebrae, is given in Figure 15-6. These assessments can help monitor and quantify responses to therapies. Either they are completed by the client on a weekly basis ("pain diary") or the client can score the CSOM when at the veterinary practice for follow-up visits. Besides CSOM, daily or weekly video diaries can also be used to assess treatment response.

Activity Monitors and Kinetic Force Measurement Devices

Other options for monitoring pain management currently under further scrutiny are activity monitors and pressure sensitive kinetic force measurement devices.[35,38–41] Activity monitors (accelerometers) can be worn by cats and have been used to detect increases in mobility in individuals with DJD when treated with meloxicam, and in a study assessing a therapeutic diet for osteoarthritis.[38,41] A further study found that the activity monitor was more specific for activity at night, both in detection of reduced mobility and in improvements when meloxicam was administered.[40] While activity assessment is an important aspect of assessing DJD pain, this may not necessarily be of importance in other forms of chronic pain and so far these tools have been useful in a research setting. In veterinary practices, the measures of quality of life that incorporate behavioral and lifestyle modifications that occur in response to chronic pain continue to be extremely important.

For kinetic force measurement devices, peak vertical force (PVF) measures show promise in a research

---

TABLE 15-1 Example of a Client-Specific Outcome Measurement Tool*

Physical Activities to Monitor	Normal	Slightly Below Normal	Worse Than Normal	Markedly Worse Than Previously	Unable to Perform Anymore
1.					
2.					
3.					
Nonphysical Parameters to Monitor	Normal	Slightly Below Normal	Worse Than Normal	Markedly Worse Than Previously	Unable to Perform Anymore
4.					
5.					

*Instructions: Select three specific physical behaviors or activities (e.g., jumping onto the bed or play) and two nonphysical parameters (e.g., grooming or eating) that the client could observe their cat doing routinely and that they consider important to their cat's quality of life. Clients should be urged to consider current behaviors that have changed in comparison to those usual in the cat's adult life, and then record changes if analgesic therapy is instituted.

Pain Diary for "Flexi." Please score each activity with a number between 0 and 10. Zero (0) means there are no problems/activity is normal; 10 means there are extreme problems/activity is abnormal. Please score Flexi once weekly, always on the same day, taking into account the whole past week

Date	4-3	4-8	4-15	4-22	4-29	5-15	5-27	6-10
Buckling left hind leg when urinating	8	6	4	4	2	0	0	0
Buckling left hind leg on stairs	8	6	6	4	2	0	0	0
Falling over when walking	4	4	4	1	1	0	0	0
Lying outside on veranda				0	0	0	0	0
Comments		NSAID		Acupuncture		Acupuncture	Acupuncture, NSAID, EOD	

FIGURE 15-6 Client specific outcome measures (CSOM) for a cat with chronic back pain. The client scored the cat initially on a weekly basis. The activities have been chosen after the initial history-taking/examination. One CSOM was added when the client mentioned on a follow-up appointment that the cat was lying outside again with the other cats, which she has not been doing when in pain. *EOD*, Every other day; *NSAID*, nonsteroidal anti-inflammatory drug.

setting for objective validation of therapeutic efficacy.[40] This is important to evaluate efficacy of pain management using drugs or other modalities for clinical use.

Quantitative Sensory Testing

Quantitative sensory testing (QST) describes the use of psychophysical tests of the skin, mucosa, or muscle tissue to assess pain pathways. They test nociception and changes in nociception semiquantitatively and can help identify the type and intensity of neuropathic pain identified as areas of hyperalgesia or allodynia.[14] While the potential to use QST in clinical veterinary medicine is great, there are no easy-to-use, validated, and simple tests currently available.[42]

Acute Pain Scales

Although acute pain scales may seem useful in a clinical setting, they are not useful to detect chronic pain states.[43] Measures of acute pain may be helpful when diagnosing acute "flare ups" during chronic pain conditions. More information on acute pain scoring can be found in Chapter 14.

Analgesic Trials

Due to anatomical and physiologic similarities, one can assume that pain is present in conditions deemed painful in humans. Where chronic pain is suspected on clinical grounds but cannot be proven, or further investigations to confirm its presence are inappropriate or refused, an appropriate analgesic trial could and in most cases should be instituted. Using a CSOM measurement tool, the response and changes in behavior can be assessed. These assessments and any observed changes will help to determine if pain is present and may help in assessment of analgesic efficacy (see Figure 15-5).

"Assessment" and Education of the Client

Every initial consultation should address the expectations and concerns of the cat owner. Clients may mistakenly believe that older cats are "just slowing down" or 'just getting old' when they see altered behaviors. While this might be true in some situations, altered behaviors should at least prompt the search for potential underlying pain. With DJD, for example, clients commonly hold the mistaken belief that their cats do not experience pain because lameness and obvious changes to gait are uncommon.[12,44] However, if questions are asked about general mobility and jumping activity, the clients can start to recognize the significance of their cat's adaptive behavior. Many clients remain unaware of the important connection between pain and the alterations in behavior in cats, until they are educated about cats' coping and adaptive strategies.

Through the shift in focus from treatment to early disease detection and "wellness" programs, cat owners can be better educated and become more proactive. It remains critical that veterinary professionals teach clients that subtle changes in a cat's routine are significant and that they may reflect physical and/or emotional problems. With greater awareness, clients will know when to seek veterinary attention, allowing for earlier detection and management of disease processes.

Frequent visits at the start of treatment to check for treatment success and possible side effects of medication will help to evaluate a benefit to risk ratio that both the veterinarian and the client agree upon. Many clients may be hesitant to institute therapies due to fear of toxicity or due to disbelief their cat may be suffering pain. Client monitoring of changes to mobility may help convince them of the need for continued therapy. Sometimes it is not until the analgesic therapy is ceased that clients will notice the decline in activity.

If the expected treatment outcomes have not been met, a reassessment of therapy, outcomes, and expectations should be undertaken. Not all improvements may be quantifiable as outward physical and behavioral signs, such as changes to mobility. Often there are non-physical changes in the cat's life that may have improved its quality of life even when expected functional targets are not achieved. Clients may describe their cat as just being happier, resting more comfortably, having a better mood, and showing sociability changes. These criteria are equally, if not more, important to many cat owners, and perhaps to the cats themselves. This is why it is important to individualize both expectations of pain management in each patient and consistently review their progress. Minimizing pain, maximizing functional and emotional well-being, and balancing the risks of pharmaceutical management are the clinical challenges of effectively managing chronic pain in feline patients.

PAIN MANAGEMENT

General Thoughts and Concepts

It is the desire of every veterinarian (and owner) to relieve suffering, maintain or improve quality of life, and where possible, extend duration of the life of animals under their care. Providing appropriate analgesic therapy is a critical part of avoiding suffering and improving quality of life. Professional knowledge of the use of analgesic drugs has expanded enormously in dogs and cats over recent years, and while much still has to be learned, a growing body of data exists about the management of both acute and chronic pain syndromes. In general, knowledge in cats lags behind that in dogs, and this is worsened by the fact there are few compounds registered for long-term use in controlling pain in cats.

Multimodal (combining different treatment modalities) and combination drug therapy will often lead

to better clinical outcomes and a reduction in the likelihood of adverse drug events. Effective pain management in human medicine employs an interdisciplinary approach to the relief of pain and improvement in the quality of life of those living with chronic pain. The typical pain management team includes medical practitioners, surgeons, clinical psychologists, physiotherapists, occupational therapists and nurses. Similarly in the veterinary setting it is important to involve specialists, including those with expertise in analgesia, behavioral medicine, and rehabilitation medicine; veterinary nurses and technicians; and the client in an attempt to achieve a more integrated approach to managing the chronic pain patient, monitoring efficacy of treatment, and providing surveillance for adverse events.

A multimodal approach to managing chronic pain seems intuitive to most. It balances pharmacological and nonpharmacological resources to minimize patients' discomfort, improve their ability to maintain their quality of life in their environment, and potentially alter the progression of the underlying disease mechanisms. For example, with DJD, this may include the use of a nonsteroidal antiinflammatory drug (NSAID), in combination with a therapeutic diet, a weight loss program, and environmental modification to maintain access to an individual's household resources (Figure 15-7).

The duration of treatment will vary in each individual, but will be guided by the history and disease processes, the presenting clinical signs, and the response to therapy. The aim may not always be to eliminate pain, but rather to normalize the pain sensitivity in some situations (i.e., down regulation of central sensitization). This is important in setting realistic therapeutic goals with clients, as controlling chronic pain proves difficult even in people.[45]

Pain is certainly not static, with acute flare-ups (often termed breakthrough pain) occurring throughout the course of the disease. During these periods, add-on dosing of analgesics and/or increasing the dose of the

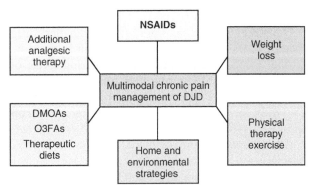

FIGURE 15-7 Multimodal pain management, for example, a clinical approach to managing chronic musculoskeletal pain from degenerative joint disease.

current drug therapy may be appropriate. If episodes of breakthrough pain become more prevalent, therapeutic options should be reassessed with increased doses, further combination drug therapy (CDT), or multimodal avenues being pursued.

There may be some debate as to the best order of application of pharmacological or nonpharmacological methods in a multimodal approach. It is the authors' opinion that using pharmacological strategies first counters two key factors in effectively and quickly managing chronic pain. First, the nonpharmacological (NP) modalities may have a slow onset of action of weeks to months. Secondly, chronic pain may have already led to central sensitization, therefore further delaying adequate analgesics may lead to worsening maladaptive pain processes. Selecting proven base analgesics such as NSAIDs as a first choice may therefore be warranted to effectively manage chronic feline pain. This will provide some immediate relief while instituting long-term nonpharmacological multimodal strategies.

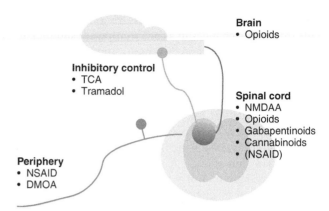

FIGURE 15-8   Graphic demonstrating the level of action on the pain pathway of different drugs used to treat chronic pain in cats. Note that especially at the level of the spinal cord, the drugs may act on different receptors and still be used for combination drug therapy. *DMOA,* Disease modifying agent; *NMDAA,* NMDA receptor antagonist; *NSAID,* nonsteroidal antiinflammatory drug; *TCA,* tricyclic antidepressant.

PHARMACEUTICAL PAIN MANAGEMENT OPTIONS

The lack of scientific data and objective means of assessing chronic pain, as well as a relative paucity of feline-specific data on the use of different analgesic drugs has undoubtedly contributed to poor provision of analgesia for chronic pain in feline patients. Some available knowledge is anecdotal, but even this can still be valuable as the need for long-term pain relief becomes more apparent, and the veterinary profession waits for more solid studies to be undertaken to guide clinical decisions in the future.

An understanding of the pathophysiology of pain and where certain drugs interact with the pain "pathway" may help to explain the possible actions of some of the drugs used (Figure 15-8). This will result in a more targeted application of analgesics in certain clinical settings when managing individual patients with suspected chronic pain.

Veterinarians routinely practice combination drug therapy (CDT) to effectively manage pain in an acute setting, using drugs, which act at differing levels of the pain "pathway." The same logic can be applied when managing patients suffering chronic painful conditions. Currently, the practice of CDT has been largely based on clinical experience.

The rationale for employing CDT is based on the following theoretical principles:
- Potential synergism in a multifaceted approach to analgesia
- Overwhelming clinical evidence of the efficacy of CDT in acute pain management
- Potential for individual reductions in drug dose and associated risks of adverse drug reactions
- Targeted therapy for the different mediators of central and peripheral pain

It is interesting to note that in the control of chronic pain in humans, pain reduction averages about 30% in half of the patients enrolled and despite reduction in pain scores, this does not always correlate to improved function.[45] This suggests that commonly prescribed analgesic modalities in people often fail to adequately control pain and improve function, and points to the increased attention paid to evaluating CDT in controlling chronic pain in people.[46]

While many compounds have good short-term pharmacokinetic data available, which is an excellent starting point, often (though not always) expert opinion and clinical experience is relied on for recommendations for long-term therapy. Adding to these difficulties is the difference in registration, availability, and prescribing habits of therapeutics between different countries and geographic regions (e.g., meloxicam is not registered for long-term use cats in the United States, but is in Europe and Australasia). Due to current limitations, much of what is prescribed on a daily basis to manage chronic feline pain effectively is either off-label or contra-label usage. Additionally, very little is known about drug interactions of medications used to treat chronic pain in cats.

Only a few drugs are available in "cat-friendly" formulations and off-label drugs commonly come in sizes and tastes which cats do not take voluntarily. Special compounding and strategies to make it easy for the client to administer drugs are important. Changing medication to ensure that the client can administer pharmacotherapy to the cat on a daily basis, especially for long-term treatment, may be necessary and may be more important than giving the perfect choice of analgesic. Commonly, animals with chronic pain are older animals suffering from concurrent disease, precluding the use of certain drugs.

Any animal prescribed long-term medication should have regular veterinary check ups, which may include blood and urine analysis to detect changes early. The exact timing of reevaluations depends on the disease and the individual patient.

Dose recommendations for commonly used analgesics in cats are summarized in Tables 15-2 and 15-3.

Nonsteroidal Antiinflammatories

Nonsteroidal antiinflammatory drugs (NSAIDs) are the mainstay of effectively managing certain types of chronic pain in humans, cats, and dogs, especially those associated with tissue inflammation.[47,48] NSAIDs interact variably with cyclooxygenase and lipoxygenase enzymes (COX-1, COX-2 and LOX). Inhibition of these enzymes affects the breakdown of arachidonic acid into the prostanoids responsible for the transmission and mediation of pain and inflammation in the periphery.[49] The homeostatic importance of COX enzymes is widely known and their inhibition causes adverse events when administering NSAIDs in small animals.[47,50] In general, NSAID use in cats is more of a concern due to their relatively decreased rate of glucuronidation, but while this affects the pharmacokinetics of some NSAIDs, others are metabolized via oxidative pathways, which may lead to more predictable pharmacokinetics and/or an increased safety profile.[51] There is an extensive literature review regarding the use of NSAIDs in cats by Lascelles et al, along with descriptions of their pharmacology and pharmacokinetics.[47]

Currently meloxicam is the only NSAID registered for long-term use in cats for the control of chronic musculoskeletal pain in Europe and Australia, and there is also published clinical data on its long-term use in both on- and off-label contexts in cats. It is hoped that in due time studies supporting the efficacy and safety of long-term use of other NSAIDs, such as robenacoxib, will emerge. Additionally, local rules and regulations (as well as availability) may affect the ability of a clinician to use one or more of these drugs. Despite licensing/registration differences, there is a growing body of evidence supporting the long-term safety and clinical efficacy of certain NSAIDs in managing chronic pain associated with musculoskeletal disease.[12,49,52,53] It is worth

---

TABLE 15-2 Nonsteroidal Antiinflammatory Drugs Currently Registered for Cats (varies globally)

Product	Dosage	Days of Registered Use	Licensed Indications
Meloxicam	0.1 mg/kg PO, loading 0.05 mg/kg PO q 24 hrs	Indefinite	Acute postoperative pain and for chronic musculoskeletal pain
Robenacoxib	1-2 mg/kg /kg PO q 24 hrs	Up to 11 days	For surgical and musculoskeletal pain relief
Tolfenamic acid	4 mg/kg PO q 24 hrs	Up to 3 days	Treatment of febrile syndromes
Ketoprofen	1 mg/kg PO q 24 hrs	Up to 5 days	Relief of acute painful disorders
Tepoxalin	No registered dose	n/a	Anecdotal use in cats for acute and chronic pain management

n/a, Not applicable; *PO*, by mouth; *q*, every.

TABLE 15-3 Additional Drugs That Can be Used for the Control of Chronic Painful Conditions in Cats, Especially in Combination Drug Therapy Modalities

Drug	Suggested Dose	Comments
Tramadol	1-4 mg/kg PO q 12-24 hrs	Used to manage moderate to severe pain in people. Used often in conjunction with an NSAID. Some reports in cats
Amantadine	2-5 mg/kg PO q 24 hrs	Potentiates analgesic effects in combination with NSAIDs, gabapentin or opiates, antagonizes central sensitization
Gabapentin	5-20 mg/kg PO q 12-24 hrs	Effective in managing neuropathic pain in people. Pharmacokinetic studies in cats
Pregabalin	1-2 mg/kg PO q 12-24 hrs	Effective in managing neuropathic pain in people, expensive
Metamizole (Dipyrone)	20 mg/kg PO q 8-12 hrs	Licensed in some countries to treat acute pain, anecdotal use in cats for chronic pain
Amitriptyline	0.5-2.0 mg/kg PO q 24 hrs	First line therapy for managing chronic neuropathic pain in people

NSAIDs, Nonsteroidal antiinflammatory drugs; *PO*, by mouth; *q*, every.

pointing out that dosages of some long-term studies may differ from the label dose. The COX-2 preferential (e.g., meloxicam) and COX-2 specific NSAIDs (e.g., robenacoxib) theoretically offer improved safety profiles compared with nonselective NSAIDs. However, no "safe" NSAID exists, as all have the potential for adverse effects if used inappropriately, if given at an excessively high dose, and/or if given for a prolonged period of time. There are numerous considerations to adhere to when prescribing NSAIDs, especially to older cats. Judicious patient selection and client education is of critical importance. Establishing the health profile of an individual and the relative stability of any concurrent diseases prior to instituting therapy is prudent. More extensive consensus guidelines covering the long-term use of NSAIDs in cats have been published and are freely available online (see Additional Resources at the end of the chapter).[49]

A common dilemma facing veterinarians managing older cats is that these patients often suffer chronic painful disorders as well as chronic kidney disease. Chronic kidney disease (CKD) is currently a labeled contraindication for the use of all NSAIDs. This should not totally preclude the use of NSAIDs, but rather a cautious and considered approach in their prescription is warranted. There are two clinical retrospective studies evaluating the long-term use of NSAIDs in cats with concurrent CKD.[52,53] In another study, meloxicam did not have an effect on glomerular filtration rates in euvolemic cats with reduced renal mass equivalent to International Renal Interest Society IRIS stage 2 and 3 CKD.[54] The results of this study were consistent with the hypothesis that glomerular filtration rates of cats with normal or reduced renal function are not dependent on cyclooxygenase function in euvolemic states. This serves to illustrate that with judicious patient screening, regular monitoring, client information and education, hydration maintenance, and appropriate dose selection, NSAIDs may be used in cats with CKD.

It is common practice to reduce the dose for longterm NSAID administration. For meloxicam, doses between 0.01 mg/kg and 0.03 mg/kg PO every 24 hours have been reported.[49,52,53] It is suspected that these lower empiric dose rates were selected to reduce the potential for adverse events, balancing the perceived risk with client observed clinical response. There are no controlled studies assessing the effects of dose length, dose titration, or how reduced dose frequency affects chronic pain control in cats. Studies in dogs with DJD support the prolonged use of NSAIDs in managing chronic pain, as it has been shown that with prolonged and consistent use, there was a continued positive clinical effect.[48] Downward dose titration of NSAIDs has been found to be effective in certain individual dogs and consistent levels of analgesia have been shown to deliver more effective pain control.[48,55] Similarly, a study in people found that continuous administration of NSAIDs resulted in significantly better pain management than intermittent or pulse dosing.[56] Dose titration is therefore a common sense approach to using NSAIDs in cats long term, but while there is good evidence that efficacy of meloxicam in managing DJD is maintained at doses below the official label dose, this may not be true of all cats or other diseases, especially where pain may be more severe.

When used for certain types of pain or in association with other types of medication, NSAIDs may not be appropriate. In humans, NSAIDs are believed to be relatively ineffective at managing neuropathic pain.[46] The employment of multimodal therapy and CDT is of benefit in the clinical management of patients suspected of suffering pain refractory to NSAIDs and neuropathic pain, for example patients with significant spinal DJD. Furthermore, for management of neoplasia or certain other conditions (such as inflammatory bowel disease), glucocorticoids may be an important part of therapy. The use of glucocorticoids is one of the recognized contraindications to using NSAIDs and in such cases alternative approaches to the provision of analgesia should be sought.

The authors regard NSAIDs as the base modality for controlling chronic pain as they have the most evidence of safety and efficacy supporting their rational use. However, they are often best used in a multimodal setting and/or in CDT (Box 15-4).

Tramadol

Tramadol acts at two levels of the pain "pathway". It works as a serotonin and noradrenaline reuptake inhibitor on the level of the descending inhibitory control system and the first metabolite O-desmethyltramadol

---

BOX 15-4   Guidelines for Safe Long-Term Prescription of Nonsteroidal Antiinflammatory Drugs (NSAIDs) in Cats

- Thoroughly assess relative patient suitability for NSAIDs
- Ensure accurate dosing based on lean body weight
- Use reduced doses according to intercurrent disease state
- Give clear client NSAID information home handouts
- Give clear labeled dosing instructions
- Give the drug with or shortly after food
- Cease immediately if any vomiting, diarrhea or inappetence
- Titrate to lowest effective dose or dose interval according to response
- Use concurrently with multimodal therapies

(ODM) acts on μ-opioid receptors. The pharmaco-kinetics of tramadol in cats show production of large amounts of ODM.[57,58] Tramadol has a high bioavail-ability of 93% and a long half-life of 4.5 hours suggesting twice daily administration is appropriate.[59] It has been used in conjunction with an NSAID in cats with DJD, without additional improvement compared with an NSAID alone.[60] However, when used alone in cats with DJD it improved scores on one sensory test as well as increased night-time activity.[61] The suggested dose rate for long-term tramadol use in cats is 1 to 3 mg/kg twice daily. However, increased doses of tramadol as a one time oral administration of 4 mg/kg in thermal thresh-old testing increased both the magnitude and duration of action, and in a simulation a dose of 4 mg/kg every 6 hours was calculated to produce maximum effect.[62] However, euphoria, mydriasis, sedation, salivation, and facial itch have been reported in animals without pain at doses between 1 and 4 mg/kg.[62] Therefore, dose and/or frequency may need to be altered for more severe pain, especially in acute flare-up situations. As with other modes of chronic analgesia, dose titration and/or combination drug therapy is ideal.

Possible side effects include sedation, euphoria/dys-phoria, mydriasis, and gastrointestinal effects such as anorexia, vomiting, and constipation. It is not recom-mended to use tramadol in conjunction with other drugs acting on serotonin reuptake (e.g., amitriptyline). One of the authors often uses tramadol for an NSAID dose-sparing effect. Combinations of low dose tramadol compounded into capsules with varying doses of gaba-pentin have also had anecdotal success, although seda-tion may be seen (e.g., 1 mg/kg tramadol + 3 mg/kg gabapentin once to twice daily).

Tramadol is extremely bitter tasting as a tablet or liq-uid, making compliance in cats a major problem. Com-pounding the medication into capsules is an effective strategy, but strong flavored pastes and liquids may also be useful.[63]

Buprenorphine

Opioids are important in the management of acute pain. Buprenorphine is well absorbed when administered by the oral transmucosal route in cats.[64] The use of opioids for chronic pain is not recommended as first-line treat-ment in people,[65] however it seems to have its place in the management of cancer pain.[66] Buprenorphine does not seem to be suitable for DJD pain in cats. In the authors' opinion, the tendency of opioids to cause depen-dence and tolerance make them less suited for chronic administration to cats, however they may be used as adjuncts during periods of breakthrough pain. Bupre-norphine is under special legislation in most countries and over-the-counter prescription is not possible in all countries.

Gabapentin

Gabapentin is an antiepileptic, but has been used in people to treat chronic pain.[67] One mechanism of action of gabapentin is its binding to voltage gated calcium channels, inhibiting the release of excitatory neurotrans-mitters important at the level of the spinal cord.[68]

The pharmacokinetics of gabapentin has been described in cats. The half-life was roughly 3 hours.[69] Gabapentin failed to show an antinociceptive effect in an experimental thermal threshold model at oral doses ranging from 5 to 30 mg/kg, however this model may not reflect clinical pain states.[62] Gabapentin has been used as an adjunctive to treat acute pain at a dose of 10 mg/kg for 2 weeks.[70] It has also been used in a case series of three cats with clinical signs suggestive of chronic neuropathic pain at 6.5 mg/kg orally, twice daily for several months.[68] Clinical efficacy was judged to be successful with cessation of other analgesic med-ication possible. One of the authors (RG) has used gaba-pentin with apparent good to excellent efficacy in managing long-term musculoskeletal, neuropathic, and neoplasia related pain in cats, mostly in combina-tion with an NSAID.

An effective target dose has been suggested at 10 mg/kg twice to three times daily, with a dose range suggested of 3 to 30 mg/kg, with dose titration based on efficacy and side effects. Sedation may be observed on initiating therapy.

The taste of gabapentin seems not to be overly aver-sive as cats will often take portions of an opened cap-sule mixed into their food. The liquid formulation of gabapentin should not be used because it contains xyli-tol. However, a compounded liquid can be formulated. One of the authors (RG) has good success using a com-pounded liquid solution, starting with a dose of 2 mg/kg twice daily with titrating doses upward over a week or two, until a dose of 10 mg/kg twice daily is achieved. Dose frequency may be reduced over time, followed by eventual reduced dose titration to effect.[9] The drug is eliminated via renal excretion and dose adjustments and caution should be employed in cats with renal impairment. Gabapentin shows interesting promise for controlling pain in cats, with controlled studies assessing its efficacy required.

Pregabalin

Pregabalin is a gabapentinoid with similar actions to gabapentin in modulation of central sensitization, and it is used to manage neuropathic pain in people.[71] Based on a single-dose pharmacokinetic study in six cats, a dose of 1 to 2 mg/kg orally twice daily has been sug-gested to treat seizures in cats.[72] There are no clinical reports assessing the analgesic effects of pregabalin in the veterinary literature. Further clinical trials are war-ranted to assess both the long-term safety and efficacy of pregabalin in cats. The most common side effect observed in people and cats is sedation.[72] Unlike gabapentin, it is not available as a generic medicine, making it much more expensive than gabapentin.

Other anticonvulsants like phenobarbital and diazepam have been used as treatment for feline hyperesthesia syndrome.[73] Diazepam used in humans with rheumatoid arthritis does not improve clinical signs and induces side effects,[74] and no reports of its use in neuropathic pain were found. Reports about analgesic effects of phenobarbital are limited to experimental studies,[75] and no clinical studies have been found. There is a potential that observed effects are due to sedation.

Amantadine

Amantadine is an oral N-methyl-D-aspartate (NMDA) receptor antagonist acting against central sensitization at the level of the spinal cord. It is used to control chronic painful neuropathic syndromes in people.[76] The pharmacokinetics of amantadine have been described in cats and the recommended dose is 3 to 5 mg/kg orally once a day, but no studies exist looking at its long-term use.[77] In one small study, the addition of amantadine reduced the antinociceptive dose of opiates required in some cats.[78] Amantadine is not expected to exert analgesic effects alone and in humans it is used to enhance the analgesic effects of NSAIDs and opiates.[76] In dogs with painful osteoarthritis refractory to NSAID management, the addition of amantadine to meloxicam significantly improved the physical activity scores compared with NSAIDs as a sole therapy.[37]

Amantadine seems to have clinical promise and anecdotally has been used in cats to improve analgesia in combination drug therapy.[79]

Amitriptyline—Tricyclic Antidepressants

Tricyclic antidepressants (TCAs) are serotonin reuptake inhibitors and work on the descending inhibitory system of the pain pathway. They are considered first line therapies to help manage chronic pain in people.[80] The doses used are generally lower than those used to manage depression in people. Drugs such as amitriptyline might show similar benefits in the management of cats with chronic neuropathic pain syndromes and are worthy of further investigation.

There is no research assessing the effects of amitriptyline or other TCAs on chronic feline pain. It is commonly suggested as part of a multimodal management of recurrent bouts of painful feline interstitial cystitis.[81] The current recommended dose of amitriptyline is 0.5 to 2 mg/kg orally once a day. There are anecdotal reports of clinical efficacy in managing chronic painful conditions in cats when combined with an NSAID or in managing pain from inflammatory bowel disease in cats along with corticosteroid administration,[9] as well as a case report where it was used as an adjunct in the multimodal management of a cat with suspected pain after amputation.[82] One of the authors (RG) has experienced good clinical control of chronic pain and sensitivity in several patients with severe otitis externa, where the use of NSAID's was contraindicated or ineffective alone.

Cannabinoids

Cannabinoids are used in people to control chronic pain.[83] Cannabinoids are substances binding to the cannabinoid receptors, which modulate inflammation as well as pain pathways at the level of the spinal cord.[84] Palmitoylethanolamide (PEA) is an endocannabinoid, which is used as a nutritional supplement in conjunction with hesperidin and glucosamine for urological disorders in cats in Italy.[85] Theoretically, PEA may be an interesting choice to manage inflammation and pain in animals.[86] However, thus far it has not been scientifically evaluated in cats. The recommended dose as a supplement is 10 mg/kg (range 7.5 to 15 mg/kg).[85]

Maropitant

Maropitant is a neurokinin (NK)-1 receptor antagonist acting as an antiemetic. However, this receptor is also involved in the pathophysiology of pain as a receptor for substance P in the central nervous system. In humans, NK-1 receptor antagonists have not been useful as an analgesic.[87] It has been shown to improve pain scores in mice after visceral surgery and to reduce minimal alveolar concentration of sevoflurane during ovarian ligament stimulation.[11,88] It may be used as part of CDT to reduce nausea and vomiting related to visceral pain or from side effects of other drugs. It is commonly used by one of the authors (II) to treat chronic visceral pain.

Corticosteroids

Corticosteroids are potent antiinflammatory drugs acting on the arachidonic acid pathway. However, they are also hormones, which have an effect throughout the whole body. While their use may be indicated in severe inflammatory pain, consideration should be given to the fact that loss of muscle mass and side effects may counteract potential benefits. The authors do not recommend the use of corticosteroids as a primary tool in treating pain in cats.

Local Injection Therapy

Epidural and intraarticular application of steroids, activated plasma, or neurotoxins has been described in humans and animals, however no documentation regarding their use in cats has been found.

Nutraceuticals and Disease Modifying Osteoarthritis Agents

Polysulfated Glycosaminoglycans

Polysulfated glycosaminoglycans (PSGAGs) are injectable products characterized as disease modifying osteoarthritis agents (DMOAs). Their exact mechanism of efficacy is unknown. Studies have demonstrated efficacy greater than placebo for managing cases of canine osteoarthritis.[67] Although anecdotal clinical experience suggests they may have some efficacy in cats with DJD, there are no clinical data either supporting nor refuting the efficacy and use of PSGAGs in cats. The authors' preference is to use a proven analgesic therapeutic along with a regular DMOA or oral nutraceutical in managing cases of painful DJD.

Nutraceuticals

Nutraceuticals are food additives or supplements that are purported to have disease modifying potential in osteoarthritis and other conditions. There are at least 30 nutraceuticals with potential DMOA claims.[89] The most popular include glucosamine, chondroitin, omega-3 fatty acids, avocado, soya bean, and green lipped muscle extracts.

A systematic review of veterinary literature concluded that the evidence of efficacy of nutraceuticals in alleviating clinical signs of arthritis was poor, with the exception of a study looking at a diet in dogs (omega-3 fatty acids).[90]

This highlights the lack of available scientific data for cats, but also the poor body of evidence supporting these agents—the placebo effect and owner inferred bias affects many study outcomes in the use of nutraceuticals.[90] The list of neutraceutical agents purported to help with osteoarthritis or other painful conditions constantly grows, but as these products are not subject to the same rigorous efficacy and safety testing as pharmaceuticals, claims over apparent efficacy should be treated with caution and high quality clinical trials are required to assess efficacy. Generally, they are likely to be more effective early in the course of mild disease. In reality, painful osteoarthritis in cats is often diagnosed later in the course of the disease. While the use of nutraceutical supplements is generally regarded as safe, they may actually do harm if used in place of proven analgesic therapy for chronic painful conditions. Veterinarians should aim to provide effective and safe analgesia to improve the quality of life of patients, and current knowledge suggests nutraceuticals alone may not be adequate for osteoarthritis-associated pain (although they might be used in a multimodal approach to managing pain in some patients).

Glucosamine and Chondroitin

These are nutraceutical supplements often recommended in veterinary medicine for the management of osteoarthritis. More recent studies in people have failed to show any clinical efficacy in pain reduction or disease modification for these agents in osteoarthritis.[91]

Omega-3 Fatty Acids

Omega-3 fatty acid dietary supplementation has been shown to have a measurable effect on clinical signs of osteoarthritis in dogs and people.[90,91] More recently a study in cats has demonstrated similar clinical findings. Cats were administered high levels of omega-3 fatty acids versus placebo in a controlled study.[92] A therapeutic diet containing multiple DMOAs including omega-3 fatty acids, glucosamine, chondroitin, and green lipped muscle extract demonstrated clinical efficacy in both CSOM and objective activity counts.[41] Therefore, dietary changes might be a valuable addition in managing pain in cats with DJD.

NONPHARMACEUTICAL MANAGEMENT

Physical and Rehabilitation Therapies

This area of pain management is slowly being accepted as an option in managing feline patients suffering painful musculoskeletal and neurological debilities as it has been in dogs and people.[93] Exercise and rehabilitation programs have been shown to effectively decrease pain and improve function in people.[94] Exercise and home rehabilitation techniques can be incorporated into the treatment plan for cats suffering musculoskeletal pain.[93] Cats can be trained to accept controlled exercise such as treadmill walking to improve limb strength and some will even take to hydrotherapy.[93,95] These are best supervised by a suitably trained animal physiotherapist. Passive range of motion exercises and massage techniques can easily be taught to clients to aid in improved joint mobility and relief of muscle pain often associated with osteoarthritis. These have the added benefit of enhanced interaction between the owner and the cat and have very few if any deleterious effects when performed appropriately. Other options such as laser, heat, or cold therapy may be useful in some patients.[93] Weight loss is one of the cornerstones of therapy to reduce painful musculoskeletal disease in people and dogs, and it is logical that gradual weight reduction in overweight cats would also be of benefit. As with most modalities, there are no controlled studies assessing the efficacy or suitable application of these therapies in cats.

It is likely that a multimodal approach with adequate pharmacologic control of chronic pain will lead to and aid in the ability to exercise and to benefit from

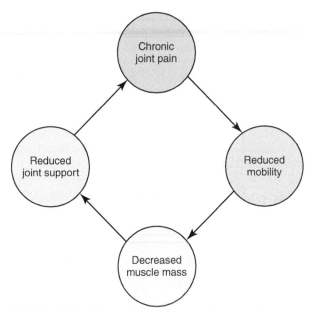

FIGURE 15-9 The cycle of chronic joint pain. Analgesic and physical therapies produce synergism in effectively managing chronic musculoskeletal pain. Adequate pain control can increase the willingness to exercise. Increased exercise can further reduce chronic pain by strengthening muscles and improving joint support.

rehabilitation. This increase in mobility and muscle strength will in turn lead to a reduction in pain experienced (Figure 15-9).

Lifestyle and Environmental Management Strategies

Improvements in the psychological and emotional state of people with chronic pain have modest benefits for the pain they experience.[96] The medical literature describes people suffering from chronic pain being at increased risk of emotional disorders such as anxiety, depression, and anger.[96] Chronic pain is also known as a stressor on the body that can increase cortisol levels which in turn can exacerbate disease states and therefore worsen pain.[97] It is possible in cats too, that chronic pain is an individualized experience, and is influenced by a cat's emotional and psychological state.

Environmental Enrichment

Environmental enrichment and positive experiences may play a key role in a multimodal approach to effective management of chronic pain and well-being.[98] As with rehabilitation, physical activity has not only physical benefits, but also affects the emotional well-being of people[94] and this may be true for cats as well. Regular exercise and play not only provides joint strengthening exercise for cats with DJD, it provides pleasurable experiences and mental stimulation for the cat.

Behavior Therapy

Operant behavioral therapy is a psychological intervention often used to help people effectively reduce chronic pain behaviors.[99] The aim in people is to reduce many maladaptive behaviors such as limping, avoidance, and inactivity and to help reinforce healthy adaptive behaviors such as activity and increased engagement.[99] Similar mechanisms of operant behavioral therapy could be effective in managing quality of life and encouraging healthy coping behaviors in cats. Reinforcing pleasurable experiences and making some environment modifications will help maintain these, along with reducing negative pain experiences. Referral to a veterinary behavioral medicine specialist would be appropriate to implement this part of the treatment approach.

Establishing what is important for the cat in the eyes of the owner is likely to be key to improving specific conditioned routines for the individual. Getting each client to define these not only helps to monitor response to treatment, but also to identify aspects that can be used to enrich their cats lives more specifically. Establishing more routines may help improve a cat's sense of well-being in its environment and reduce vulnerability it may feel due to pain or debility.

Environmental Modification

Chronic musculoskeletal pain may cause enough of an inhibitory negative stimulus that some cats may no longer seek pleasurable or desirable aspects of their environment that they otherwise would under pain free circumstances. Simple home modifications can be made to limit the pain or discomfort involved in accessing preferred or important places in the environment that may otherwise be difficult to access. This may be achieved, for example, by using a ramp, stairs, or extra intermediary levels to allow cats access to desired perching or resting spots. The aim is for cats to maintain use of their environment and resources with less strain and less pain and this approach can form part of behavioral and exercise therapy (Figure 15-10).

The provision of easily accessible soft, warm places to rest may also have a physical benefit in managing musculoskeletal pain.[93] Infrared heat beds, warmth in a sunny spot, and other heat emanating devices could be useful tools in improving environmental as well as physical well-being of cats.

House soiling can be associated with physical disease (e.g., musculoskeletal disease) (Figure 15-11) and pain can limit the cat's ability to access the litter box. It is therefore important to ensure that litter boxes are placed in easily accessible locations (e.g., the cat does not have to negotiate stairs to get to the box) and have at least one low side to enable the cat to enter and exit the box

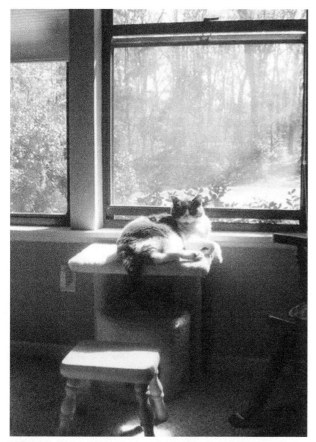

FIGURE 15-10   This cat was unable to reach its favorite spot (seen in Figure 15-2) until a step stool was provided so it could reach its perch. (Courtesy S. Robertson)

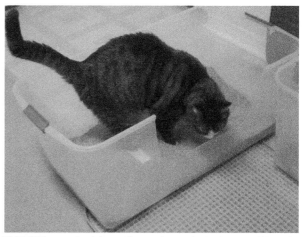

FIGURE 15-12   Manually cutting a hole into a side of a large plastic box to make the entry into the litter box lower and facilitate access. (Courtesy S. Robertson)

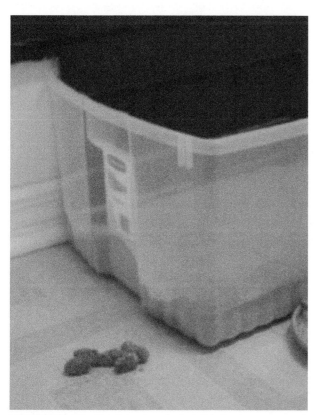

FIGURE 15-11   Painful musculoskeletal disease may result in inability to get into the litter box and house soiling. (Courtesy S. Robertson)

without difficulty (Figure 15-12). Similarly, easy access should be maintained in relation to essential resources such as food and water (Figures 15-13 and 15-14).

Pheromones and Grooming

Poor coat quality is a nonspecific finding in many cats suffering chronic painful or debilitating health conditions. These cats may lose the physical ability or motivation necessary to groom, where this may have previously occupied a large part of their pleasurable home routine. Gentle regular grooming and stroking, particularly around the head, face and neck, can increase the release of certain neurotransmitters that in people have been shown to improve mood and reduce pain.[94,100] Regular grooming is another pleasurable conditioned routine that can maintain the human-cat bond and improve a cat's well-being. Similarly the use of synthetic feline facial pheromone may improve the emotional health of some cats in a stressful (physical or emotional) behavioral setting.[101,102] It may lead to improved grooming, eating, and social interaction (i.e., emotional well-being) and therefore could form part of a multimodal pain management plan.

Acupuncture

Acupuncture has been used as a primary and complementary treatment option for managing pain in people for many years and has more recently gained popularity in veterinary medicine. The hypothesized modes of pain relief from acupuncture can be explained via several neurophysiological modalities.[103] There is evidence to support its use in managing chronic pain in people and in dogs.[104,105] There are no clinical trials that prove or disprove the analgesic effects of acupuncture in cats. As the nature of acupuncture therapy is an individualized treatment, it is difficult to standardize treatment protocols and therein lays an inherent problem in assessing the efficacy of acupuncture. It is both authors' clinical perspective that acupuncture is valuable in multimodal analgesic settings, improving the perceived quality of life

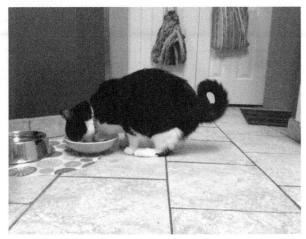

FIGURE 15-13 Note this cat's uncomfortable stance while eating caused by degenerative joint disease. (Courtesy M. Scherk)

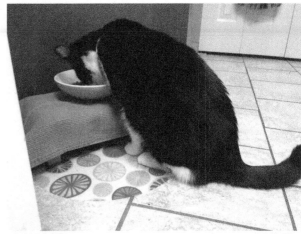

FIGURE 15-14 Raising the food onto a low shelf allows the cat to sit normally and eat comfortably. (Courtesy M. Scherk)

of cats suffering chronic pain (Figure 15-15). Owner observations of improved appetite, better mood, and increased mobility are common.

Surgical Management in Chronic Pain

Obviously, if a primary inciting cause of chronic pain can be surgically corrected or ameliorated, this should be considered as the preferred treatment option; for instance, extraction of teeth affected with painful resorptive lesions. The importance of adequate perioperative pain control for cats in chronic pain cannot be overstated. Adequate preemptive and postoperative analgesia, as well as adequate tools for assessing analgesic adequacy, should reduce the incidence of chronic maladaptive postsurgical pain in our feline patients.

Surgical management of chronic painful musculoskeletal disorders in cats has historically been unrewarding, in particular the arthrodesis of joints chronically affected by DJD.[106] Joint debridement and removal of osteochondral bodies may relieve some associated pain. Joint replacements have become the gold standard in humans to ameliorate chronic pain from DJD, especially when medical options can no longer provide adequate comfort or function. It has also shown promise in dogs undergoing hip replacements.[107] A small case series of three cats receiving hip replacements reported excellent functional long-term clinical outcomes.[108] For cats, commonly femoral head osteotomy is recommended, however it is recognized that for some cats total hip replacement may offer the best choice regarding function.[108] Historically, it has been assumed cats managed well with femoral head ostectomy.[109] Longitudinal studies comparing DJD, long-term pain, and functional outcomes would be required to see whether cats truly managed well with these traditional measures.

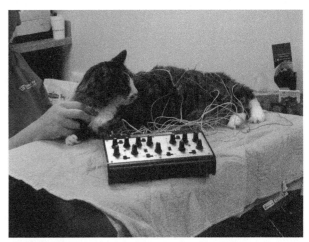

FIGURE 15-15 Acupuncture is a very comfortable and often relaxing procedure for the feline patient and is an excellent component of a pain management protocol. (Courtesy S. Robertson)

Stem Cell Therapy

The use of adipose derived mesenchymal stem cell therapy (AD-MSC) in the management of painful osteoarthritis is a relatively new technique in veterinary medicine. Clinical improvement has been reported in several small reports in dogs receiving AD-MSC therapy for osteoarthritis.[110-112] The mechanisms for these observed improvements are currently unknown, but are likely mediated through analgesic and antiinflammatory effects. It is suspected that cell-based therapy does not result in regeneration of joint tissues. Regenerative medicine is the ultimate goal of therapy for many diseases including DJD, but further studies are essential to gauge the true efficacy and functionality of this form of AD-MSC therapy.

Radiation Therapy

Radiation therapy can be administered as a form of treatment for cancer pain as well as for management of DJD. Palliative radiation therapy has been used to alleviate pain in a variety of tumors, with success rates between 66% and 74%, lasting an average of 3 to 5 months with minimal signs of acute radiation reactions. Palliative protocols utilize 1 to 4 fractions (radiation therapy doses) of radiation. Bone tumors treated by radiation therapy carry the risk of a pathological fracture. In people there is evidence that radiation therapy can be used to treat chronic DJD, however it is currently unclear how many patients benefit from the treatment.[112]

MANAGEMENT OF SPECIFIC CHRONIC PAINFUL DISEASES

The potential medical causes of chronic pain are many and varied. The following summary of some of those conditions highlights the need for a multi-disciplinary approach to cases of chronic pain. In some cases it may be appropriate to involve veterinary specialists such as dentists, gastroenterologists, endocrinologists, oncologists, dermatologists, internists, orthopedic specialists, and surgeons in the management of these patients.

Degenerative Joint Disease and Musculoskeletal Pain

There have been many good studies on aspects of feline DJD over the past two to three decades and this literature deserves particular attention. DJD, also called osteoarthritis, is associated with the progressive destruction of cartilage, subchondral bone, ligaments, and/or joint capsule in affected joints. In chronic cases, it commonly has inflammatory and neuropathic components.

Prospective reports of the prevalence of DJD in cats suggest it is an exceedingly common radiographic finding, with studies reporting the radiographic prevalence of appendicular DJD of 61% to 91% and axial skeletal DJD of 55% to 92%.[12,16–18,20] These estimates are much higher than the previous reported prevalence of 22% to 64% from retrospective studies,[12,16,17] often based on convenience sampling rather than a true cross-sectional study. In all studies, the reported prevalence increased with age. The most commonly affected joints are the hips, elbows, stifles, and tarsus for appendicular DJD. The distal thoracic spine had the highest prevalence of radiographic lesions, but the distal lumbar and lumbo-sacral regions were most severely affected and most often associated with clinical signs (Figure 15-16, *A*, and *B*).

Radiographic features of feline DJD differ from those reported in dogs, with cats having a tendency to form less periarticular new bone and the new bone differing in appearance to DJD in dogs.[18,44,114] Poor correlation

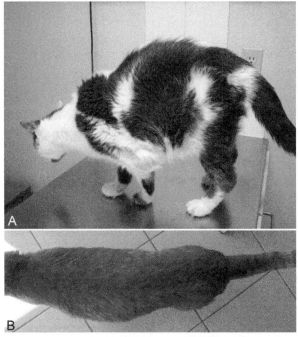

FIGURE 15-16 **A,** An arthritic senior cat exhibiting a typical posture associated with painful chronic musculoskeletal disease. **B,** Note the cat's narrow hind end consistent with degenerative joint disease in the hips. (**A,** Courtesy S. Little **B,** Courtesy I. Rodan)

has been observed comparing macroscopic evaluation of cartilage with radiographs.[114] Meniscal mineralization is also a common radiographic finding of feline stifles, with their significance often debated, however these findings seem to correlate well with medial compartment cartilage DJD.[114,115]

Traditionally, radiographic findings of feline DJD have been thought to correlate poorly to the presence of clinical signs and pain, with only 33% of joints radiographically affected with osteoarthritis being assessed as painful in one report.[12] This discrepancy is also a well-documented finding in human osteoarthritis and has been shown to exist in several other studies of feline DJD.[18,20,44]

Quantification of such discrepancies showed that pain response to palpation was recorded in 0% to 67% of joints with radiographic DJD changes.[19] Despite this, a lack of pain response had a higher prediction of no DJD changes on radiographs. Elicited pain scores correlated best with the severity of DJD changes in the elbows and the distal spinal segment.[18,19] The presence of crepitus, joint thickening, or an effusion further increased the specificity for the presence of DJD on radiographs. A conclusion was that the absence of pain and clinical joint changes is predictive of radiographically normal joints.[19] Therefore a thorough orthopedic and goniometric examination is a good screening tool, but mostly to help rule out radiographically visible DJD changes, but it must be remembered that some painful joints will show no radiographic changes of DJD either.[19]

These studies serve to highlight the difficulty in being able to accurately diagnose painful DJD in the cat. This is why a multidimensional approach is required (see Figure 15-5). The above indices can be used as indicators of disease, but whether these correlate well to the presence of pain for the individual is uncertain.

Because of these uncertainties, assessing response to therapy as a diagnostic measure of painful musculoskeletal disease in cats is an invaluable tool in many situations. Many times, DJD may be suspected based on signalment, history and physical findings, yet radiographs may not be feasible for financial or health concerns. Conversely, radiographic findings should serve more to help confirm suspicions of DJD in feline patients and not as a direct guide for the appropriate treatment. Indicators used to screen DJD in other species may not be appropriate in cats.[16,17] Many of the early publications highlight the discordance of clinical presentation and the prevalence of radiographic change, making the false assumption that DJD is less common in cats than dogs.[16,17] Common behavioral changes, which can be assessed semiquantitatively, have been identified. CSOMs as well as the use of a structured questionnaire (FMPI) should form the basis for the detection and assessment of chronic musculoskeletal pain in cats.[28,29,35,14]

NSAIDs are the most common drugs prescribed to manage chronic painful DJD in all species, including people, dogs, and cats. As discussed previously, NSAIDs can be very safely employed in most feline patients, but critical to this is patient selection and client education. Their use should form the cornerstone of a multimodal approach to managing pain from DJD where appropriate. If pain relief is deemed inadequate or a patient is considered unsuitable for long-term NSAID administration, then medications such as tramadol, gabapentin, or amantadine could be added or used as sole agents along with combination-drug strategies.

In monitoring and assessing response to a certain modality, one must set realistic goals specific to each cat-owner bond and their household routines. CSOM or video diaries should be used to discuss progress and treatment success with the client. At appropriate recheck intervals, these responses should be reassessed relative to the veterinarian's and the client's expectations. It is these quantifiable benefits that can be weighed against the perceived risk (if any) of medications and will guide any dose titration.

If pain management has been adequate over an extended period of time controlling central sensitization, many patients can be well maintained on titrated doses of NSAIDs, or these can be stopped altogether, and the patient maintained with adjunctive therapies.

Dental and Oral Pain

Many oral and dental conditions cause chronic discomfort and pain in feline patients. Periodontal disease, gingivostomatitis, odontoclastic resorptive lesions, dental and oral fractures, and oral tumors are some commonly encountered examples.[116] Inflammatory conditions of the mouth are very common in cats. Up to 95% of cats older than 2 years may be affected. Anorexia is a common presentation of oral pain, as well as dropping food while eating, hissing and running from food, preference of soft food, and negative changes in temperament. Head shaking, sneezing, repetitive jaw motions while eating, drinking or grooming, and excessive tongue movements have also been observed.[117] However it is important to note that these cats may also show none of the aforementioned signs and eat normally. Medicating these patients orally may present an additional challenge because of the sensitive mouth.

Primary management, such as dental extraction with acute pain management, may resolve much oral discomfort. Removing predisposing factors is a commonly used treatment option and will often remove the underlying etiologic condition. Aggressive concurrent pain management is important. However, despite excellent surgical and/or medical management, some patients may continue to experience oral discomfort due to continued presence of disease and/or neuropathic pain, evident in behaviors suggestive of hyperalgesia. Signs may include difficulty with prehension and dropping of food, pawing at the mouth, or avoidance behavior around the mouth and head. This was evident the case report from Lorenz et al (2012), where two cats responded well after the addition of gabapentin for poorly controlled chronic oral pain after facial trauma.[71] As inflammation of oral/dental disease is an important part of the disease process, NSAIDs are an important mainstay of therapy. Meloxicam may offer an advantage, as it is available as a liquid preparation. Oral transmucosal buprenorphine may be used for severe pain or acute flare-ups. One of the authors (RG) has observed good clinical efficacy in palliative analgesic effects of gabapentin in combination with NSAIDs in cats suffering oral tumors.

Diabetic Neuropathy

Diabetic peripheral neuropathy is a painful and debilitating complication of diabetes mellitus in humans.[57] In an extensive study of diabetic cats,[92] it was found that there were changes to both sensory and motor nerves of the pelvic and thoracic nerves, so it would be logical to anticipate that pain is potentially a component for some cats with diabetes. While overt painful diabetic neuropathy has not been reported in cats, there are anecdotal reports of diabetic cats exhibiting clinical signs pointing towards neuropathic pain, such as changes in interactive behavior or avoidance and a dislike of their paws being touched.[15] One case of a cat with excessive licking after an episode of diabetic motor neuropathy has been treated with gabapentin with success.[2]

In people, the most common drugs used for control of painful diabetic neuropathy are TCAs, gabapentin, and pregabalin.

Feline Interstitial Cystitis

This may often go unrecognized as a cause of chronic neurogenic pain from visceral inflammation, similar to humans.[118] Chronic urinary tract disease is a common problem of cats, and by exclusion of a causative agent and/or cystoscopy, feline interstitial cystitis (FIC) is diagnosed. It can resolve with or without treatment and recurs frequently. Abnormality of urothelial integrity, bladder permeability, glycosaminoglycan GAG expression, and adrenal hypofunction during predisposing stress as well as different central nervous system changes have been described in the affected population of cats. The central nervous system changes include C fibers with increased sensitivity to distension and other altered neural properties, and signs of enhanced noradrenergic output. Abnormal adrenocortical function seems to be present in humans and cats with feline interstitial cystitis (FIC), and a genetic basis has also been postulated. Stranguria, dysuria, overgrooming the perineal region or ventral abdomen, howling when urinating, and pain when picked up are common signs in these cats; a similar human condition has been associated with significant pain. Stress reduction and removal of stressors as well as multimodal environmental modification and synthetic feline facial pheromone are useful in managing FIC.[119-121] Tricyclic antidepressants (e.g., amitriptyline) have been used in the long-term management if environmental modifications and conventional analgesics have not been successful.[122] They have not been compared with placebo and they are not useful to control acute flare-ups. Buprenorphine can be used during acute flare-ups while the management with NSAIDs has been discussed as controversial. Gabapentin, opiates, and NSAIDs have also shown some efficacy in managing interstitial cystitis in people.[118]

Glycosaminoglycan treatment orally or pentosan polysulfate injections have been anecdotally reported, but to date no studies have shown effects greater than placebo. Palmitoylethanolamide pretreatment reduces visceral hyperalgesia in a bladder instillation model in rats and this drug may be useful in the future after undergoing more rigorous clinical testing. Referral to a veterinary dental specialist may need to be considered for some cases.

Chronic Visceral and Gastrointestinal Pain

This broad range of potentially chronic painful gastrointestinal tract (GIT) diseases would include chronic inflammatory enteropathies (IBD), hepatopathies, pancreatitis and constipation. Neoplasia of the GIT would also be included but may mediate pain via additional mechanisms (see section on neoplasia and chronic pain). There is evidence that chronic inflammatory GIT diseases can stimulate local mechanoreceptors that can lead to sensitization and neuropathic visceral pain in people and animals.[123,124] Abdominal pain in people that suffer from chronic IBD can have a profound impact on the quality of life for sufferers.[124] Difficulties in assessing this concept in cats are numerous due to the lack of any sensitive means of detecting and localizing visceral pain (e.g., palpation) and any tools in assessing relative efficacy of therapeutics. However, applying general knowledge of cat behavior and chronic pain, it is logical that improvements in demeanor, activity, and appetite in particular may be useful tools. Another problem is the episodic nature of many of these enteropathies where acute flare-ups are common.

Chronic pancreatitis is a painful condition in humans and it is assumed to be painful in cats.[125] Besides symptomatic therapy, analgesic and antiinflammatory agents for low grade intermittent disease should not be underestimated, but treatment remains challenging. Buprenorphine as well as an NSAID with low potential to cause ulcers in a low dose have been recommended anecdotally.[125] Although controversial, in humans a low dose of pancreatic enzyme in food reduces postprandial pain by reducing pancreatic secretion through a negative feedback effect.

Many cats suffering chronic enteropathies or other chronic inflammatory abdominal disease appear to suffer transient abdominal pain or have variable appetites despite apparent adequate medical management. There may indeed be a neuropathic pain component for some of these cats, as there are anecdotal reports that the addition of amitriptyline improved the behavior and/or appetite of many cats suffering chronic IBD.[9] Acupuncture, TCAs, gabapentin, and pregabalin have shown efficacy in the mediation of visceral neuropathic pain in people.[124] Maropitant may have a place in the management of breakthrough visceral pain, be it due to its antiemetic or its analgesic properties, and anecdotally many veterinarians use it off-label successfully for control of visceral pain.

Neoplasia and Chronic Pain

Pain from neoplasia can be a direct result of the tumor, from treatment of the tumor (chemotherapy or radiation therapy), or as a result of disease caused by the tumor. Pain associated with neoplasms occurs through numerous pathways. Tumors are not highly innervated by sensory neurons, however different tumor related mechanisms may be responsible for pain associated with neoplasia.

Pain from tumors can be visceral, somatic, neuropathic, or quite often mixed.[89] Inflammation surrounding the tumor, local changes in pH, and direct distortion of mechanoreceptors may be responsible for some of the pain.[126] Neuropathic pain can be stimulated by direct damage or inflammation of nerves. Chronic pain also develops due to neoplastic and related cells releasing factors such as prostaglandins and cytokines that stimulate nociceptors.[89] Tumors involving internal organs often cause chronic visceral pain by direct actions on compressive or stretch receptors, release of local nociceptor stimulating factors, ischemia, and damage to local nerves.

All neoplasia in cats should be considered as potentially painful, with adequate analgesia being part of management or palliation for every cat. Clinically, in humans the size, localization, or type of tumor does not predict the severity of pain or even the presence of pain. In a mouse model of bone cancer, pain related behaviors are present before any significant bone destruction is evident. As neoplasia is a progressive and dynamic disease, constant clinical reassessments of a cat's pain should be made in conjunction with its owner. Different tools have been used to assess quality of life in cancer patients ranging from simple questions to multifactorial assessments.[33] As the disease progresses the animal has to be reevaluated on a regular basis to adjust pain relief and discuss euthanasia if this is warranted. In addition regular reassessments following start of treatment (either tumor related or pain related) are warranted.

Management of neoplasia with surgery, chemotherapy, or radiation therapy can relieve discomfort by reducing the size of the tumor, but can also stimulate further pain with the release of factors that mediate pain and cause damage to local nerves.[89] Some chemotherapeutic agents can cause neuropathy and pain when used in humans by interfering with cytoskeletal structures. Motor changes and possible myalgia have been reported in one cat with a vinblastine overdose. Radiotherapy can cause side effects related to healthy tissue around the treatment site. Treating pain associated with these side effects is very important, and an acute radiation score has been described in dogs and correlates well with pain scores.[127] It has been found useful for initiating preemptive analgesia during and after radiation therapy.

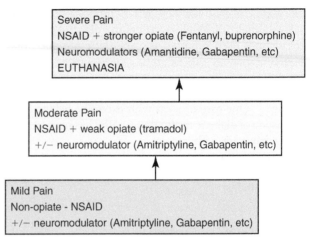

FIGURE 15-17 Stepwise approach to controlling progressive chronic neoplastic pain in cats. (Adapted from the World Health Organization's cancer pain treatment ladder.)

Several types of neoplasia in cats have shown an upregulation in cyclooxygenase-2 (COX-2) expression.[128,129] However, in a clinical setting reduction of growth has been rarely documented, with the exception of transitional cell carcinoma where NSAID (COX-2 inhibitors) have been associated with partial and even complete remission of the tumor.

However, the use of glucocorticoid treatment accompanies many treatment protocols for neoplasia and the use of NSAIDs will be precluded in these cases.

The full range of analgesics could be employed in a combination drug therapy approach to effectively minimize the pain from neoplasia. The World Health Organization (WHO) developed a pain management ladder, providing a step-wise approach to cancer pain of increasing severity (Figure 15-17), which might usefully be adapted for veterinary patients.

Chronic Pain Associated With Surgical Intervention or Trauma

Many of the recent advances in effective and aggressive management of acute pain relief should reduce the incidence of chronic postsurgical pain in cats. This can often be debilitating and historically has been hard to manage. Chronic postsurgical pain can occur after any surgery, but it is usually more common in cases where nerve trauma is involved. Cats suffering postsurgical neuropathic pain may exhibit signs from overgrooming associated or not associated with the surgical site, hyperesthetic-type behaviors, and localized hyperalgesic sensitivity when the affected area is stimulated.[9,68] Examples where this may occur include limb amputations, onychectomy, tumor excision, fracture repair, and chronic skin wound management.[9,82,89]

Post limb amputation neuropathic pain (phantom limb pain) is seldom reported in veterinary literature, with only one report in cats.[82] This may be in part due to the lack of recognition of its potential occurrence and the cat's perceived ability to "cope."[81] Sixty percent of people undergoing surgical or traumatic limb amputation experience neuropathic pain, but most develop signs one year after the procedure. This may be due to peripheral sensitization from regenerating nerve endings or central sensitization.[130] In dogs, reports of phantom limb pain document onset after approximately 40 days.[131]

Onychectomy remains a controversial topic and is banned as a cosmetic procedure (i.e., for human benefit) in many countries. Studies assessing long-term outcomes report mixed findings regarding the prevalence and significance of long-term pain and behavioral influence. Clinical perspectives vary, but there is no doubt some cats suffer from chronic lameness postsurgery.[132] Whether this is due to pain or changed functionality is unknown, but if it is affecting only a proportion, it is more likely to be pain-associated. These cats may also exhibit more aggressive avoidance tendencies or signs suggestive of neuropathic pain; shaking and flicking, overgrooming or chewing their feet, and dislike of their feet or limbs being touched.[9] Thorough preoperative and postoperative pain management may markedly impact the incidence of chronic neuropathic pain. Despite ideal presurgical and postsurgical analgesia, some cats are still afflicted with signs suggestive of chronic neuropathic pain and it is possible that genetics, temperament, and environmental factors may predispose certain individuals to this phenomenon.[132]

Tricyclic antidepressants, gabapentin, and pregabalin along with NSAIDs, amantadine, and opiates are effective in the management of postsurgical and traumatic neuropathic pain in people.

Other Painful Conditions

Dermatological Disease, Slow Healing Wounds, and Burns
Case reports describing the management of painful dermatological diseases, slow healing wounds, and burns can be found in the literature.[2]

Feline Hyperesthesia Syndrome
The term feline hyperesthesia syndrome has been used to describe cats with such symptoms as twitching skin, sensitivity around the tail and spine, biting, licking, and automutilation as well as personality change.[133] There is currently only limited evidence for this condition and it may be a reflection of undiagnosed dermatologic or neurologic disease or behavior problems and is therefore not further discussed.

Miscellaneous Conditions
Other conditions presumed to be chronically painful in cats, but for which no reports were found in the literature, include congestive heart failure, thromboembolism, otitis, constipation, corneal disease, and glaucoma.

INTEGRATION OF CHRONIC PAIN MANAGEMENT IN PRACTICE

Veterinary literature over the past two decades has revealed that cats do indeed frequently suffer from chronic painful conditions, appreciation of which has been sadly lacking in the past. However, a heightened awareness of pain, a focus on quality of life, a good perception of feline behavior, and the tools which are available to clinicians, help to recognize when pain may be an important component of clinical disease. An increasing knowledge of drug therapy in cats also provides more options for pain management than ever before.

Armed with the knowledge of feline behavioral pain language, veterinary staff and, more importantly, cat owners can be better informed about relevant behavioral changes. This has already been done successfully with many diseases, so that clients are more aware that certain signs or behavioral changes might represent serious underlying illness and disease. Clients often present their cats for routine health examinations and disease detection screening, and many veterinary practices have implemented successful age specific health programs for cats, including senior care programs. These screen for early disease and monitor an individual's health trends as they age. As veterinary professionals have refined these health management tools in their practices, their ability to detect disease earlier, when evidence is still subtle, has also improved. This will also hold true for painful diseases such as DJD.

It is through these programs, and through staff proactivity in engaging with clients, that they can be made aware of the subtle changes their cat may display in an attempt to minimize the debilitating effect of chronic pain. Client information sheets are extremely useful, as are pictures and videos of cats in pain, for example, arthritic cats. These can highlight the changes that clients often associate with slowing down and getting older, but may actually be disease- or pain-associated. Many clients do not perceive these as pain-related changes, and it may take time for the clients to begin to observe their cat at home with a different critical viewpoint as a result of the new information (Figure 15-18).

The knowledge that has been gained from studies into DJD and how pain behaviors may manifest in cats can be applied to other conditions known to be

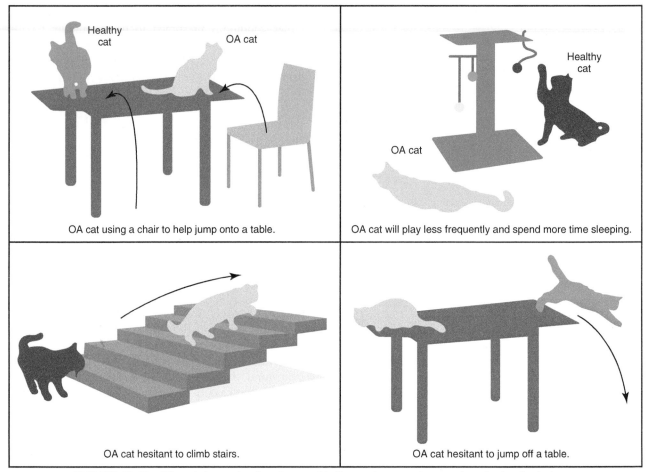

OA cat using a chair to help jump onto a table.

OA cat will play less frequently and spend more time sleeping.

OA cat hesitant to climb stairs.

OA cat hesitant to jump off a table.

FIGURE 15-18 Client information handouts with illustrations can be used to depict the behaviors cat owners should be made aware of. Clients should identify several factors relating to mobility specific to their cat and their home environment to monitor during therapy. *OA*, Osteoarthritis. (Courtesy Boehringer Ingelheim)

associated with chronic pain. Building the knowledge basis of how chronic pain manifests in feline patients, how it affects their quality of life, and what measures can be put in place to manage this pain is essential in the modern veterinary practice.

SUMMARY

Modern veterinary science has helped to extend the longevity of feline patients. Along with this longevity have come the increased chances of age-associated diseases and comorbid diseases. Chronic pain can be part of many of these processes, such as DJD and neuropathic pain associated with chronic disease of the visceral organs. Despite the advances made, it is likely that the prevalence of chronic pain suffered by cats is still being underestimated. Further studies will help to refine the ability to screen for pain and monitor response to therapy. With this growing awareness, future studies will be able to guide the veterinary profession more effectively through this new field of integrated chronic pain management and healthcare.

Analgesic modalities are not equally effective in each individual patient, highlighting the complex nature of chronic pain and why pain control modalities should be routinely reevaluated for clinical efficacy. The lack of adequate pain control in chronic pain has significant effects on physical and emotional well-being and the perceived quality of life.[29]

It is a rewarding clinical challenge to manage the quality of life of feline patients. Ensuring quality of life is central to the role of the veterinarian, but this is still an art form rather than one of robust science. A pain free existence is desirable, with studies indicating most clients would forego some life expectancy for improved quality of life.[31] Many clinical decisions have potential for adverse effects, but balancing quality of life with potential negative outcomes is essential. A lack of exact knowledge of pain and analgesics should not prevent veterinarians from striving for the best outcomes for their patients. Withholding analgesia out of concern for potential adverse effects may inadvertently increase the risk of ongoing pain affecting quality of life. Therefore taking an informed, conscientious risk may be preferable for some patients.

ADDITIONAL RESOURCES

Consensus guidelines on the long-term use of NSAIDs in cats. http://jfm.sagepub.com/content/12/7/521.

Feline Musculoskeletal Pain Index, http://www.cvm.ncsu.edu/docs/cprl/fmpi.html.

REFERENCES

1. Gunn-Moore D. Considering older cats. *J Small Anim Pract.* 2006;47:430–431.
2. Robertson SA, Lascelles BDX. Long-term pain in cats: how much do we know about this important welfare issue? *J Feline Med Surg.* 2010;12:188–199.
3. Liebeskind JC, Paul LA. Psychological and physiological mechanisms of pain. *Annu Rev Psychol.* 1977;28:41–60.
4. Pintrich PR. An achievement goal theory perspective on issues in motivation terminology, theory, and research. *Contemp Educ Psychol.* 2000;25:92–104.
5. International Association for the Study of Pain: Definition of pain. http://www.iasp-pain.org/Education/Content.aspx?ItemNumber=1698#Pain Accessed October 5, 2014.
6. Meintjes RA. An overview of the physiology of pain for the veterinarian. *Vet J.* 2012;193:1–5.
7. AAHA/AAFP Pain Management Guidelines Task Force Members, Hellyer P, Rodan I, et al. AAHA/AAFP pain management guidelines for dogs and cats. *J Feline Med Surg.* 2007;9:466–480.
8. Muir 3rd WW, Woolf CJ. Mechanisms of pain and their therapeutic implications. *J Am Vet Med Assoc.* 2001;219:1346–1356.
9. Mathews KA. Neuropathic pain in dogs and cats: if only they could tell us if they hurt. *Vet Clin North Am Small Anim Pract.* 2008;38:1365–1414.
10. Herr K, Coyne PJ, Key T, et al. Pain assessment in the nonverbal patient: position statement with clinical practice recommendations. *Pain Manag Nurs.* 2006;7:44–52.
11. Mathews K, Kronen PW, Lascelles D, et al. Guidelines for recognition, assessment and treatment of pain. *J Small Anim Pract.* 2014;55:E10–E68.
12. Clarke SP, Bennett D. Feline osteoarthritis: a prospective study of 28 cases. *J Small Anim Pract.* 2006;47:439–445.
13. Bennett D, Morton C. A study of owner observed behavioural and lifestyle changes in cats with musculoskeletal disease before and after analgesic therapy. *J Feline Med Surg.* 2009;11:997–1004.
14. Benito J, Depuy V, Hardie E, et al. Reliability and discriminatory testing of a client-based metrology instrument, feline musculoskeletal pain index (FMPI) for the evaluation of degenerative joint disease-associated pain in cats. *Vet J.* 2013;196:368–373.
15. Camps T, Amat M, Mariotti VM, et al. Pain-related aggression in dogs: 12 clinical cases. *J Vet Behav Clin Appl Res.* 2012;7:99–102.
16. Hardie EM, Roe SC, Martin FR. Radiographic evidence of degenerative joint disease in geriatric cats: 100 cases (1994–1997). *J Am Vet Med Assoc.* 2002;220:628–632.
17. Godfrey DR. Osteoarthritis in cats: a retrospective radiological study. *J Small Anim Pract.* 2006;46:425–429.
18. Lascelles BD, Henry 3rd. JB, Brown J, et al. Cross-sectional study of the prevalence of radiographic degenerative joint disease in domesticated cats. *Vet Surg.* 2010;39:535–544.
19. Lascelles BD, Dong YH, Marcellin-Little DJ, et al. Relationship of orthopedic examination, goniometric measurements, and radiographic signs of degenerative joint disease in cats. *BMC Vet Res.* 2012;8:10.
20. Slingerland LI, Hazewinkel HAW, Meij BP, et al. Cross-sectional study of the prevalence and clinical features of osteoarthritis in 100 cats. *Vet J.* 2011;187:304–309.
21. Rothbart MK, Ahadi SA, Evans DE. Temperament and personality: origins and outcomes. *J Pers Soc Psychol.* 2000;78:122–135.
22. Wade JB, Dougherty LM, Hart RP, et al. A canonical correlation analysis of the influence of neuroticism and extraversion on chronic pain, suffering, and pain behavior. *Pain.* 1992;51:67–73.
23. Mellor DJ, Cook CJ, Stafford K. Quantifying some responses to pain as a stressor. In: Moberg GP, Mench JA, eds. *The biology of animal stress: Basic principles and implications for animal welfare.* Oxon, UK: CABI Publishing; 2000:171–198.
24. Levine ED. Feline fear and anxiety. *Vet Clin North Am Small Anim Pract.* 38:Oxon, UK: CABI Publishing; 2008:1065–1079.
25. Siegford JM, Walshaw SO, Brunner P, Zanella AJ. Validation of a temperament test for domestic cats. *Anthrozoos.* 2003;16:332–351.
26. Brown DC, Boston RC, Coyne JC, Farrar JT. Development and psychometric testing of an instrument designed to measure chronic pain in dogs with osteoarthritis. *Am J Vet Res.* 2007;68:631–637.
27. Hielm-Björkman AK, Rita H, Tulamo RM. Psychometric testing of the Helsinki chronic pain index by completion of a questionnaire in Finnish by owners of dogs with chronic signs of pain caused by osteoarthritis. *Am J Vet Res.* 2009;70:727–734.
28. Zamprogno H, Hansen BD, Bondell HD, et al. Item generation and design testing of a questionnaire to assess degenerative joint disease-associated pain in cats. *Am J Vet Res.* 2010;71:1417–1424.
29. Benito J, Gruen ME, Thomson A. Owner-assessed indices of quality of life in cats and the relationship to the presence of degenerative joint disease. *J Feline Med Surg.* 2012;14:863–870.
30. Hartmann K, Kuffer M. Karnofsky's score modified for cats. *Eur J Med Res.* 1998;3:95–98.
31. Freeman LM, Rush JE, Oyama MA, et al. Development and evaluation of a questionnaire for assessment of health-related quality of life in cats with cardiac disease. *J Am Vet Med Assoc.* 2012;240:1188–1193.
32. Reynolds CA, Oyama MA, Rush JE, et al. Perceptions of quality of life and priorities of owners of cats with heart disease. *J Vet Intern Med.* 2010;24:1421–1426.
33. Tzannes S, Hammond MF, Murphy S, et al. Owners 'perception of their cats' quality of life during COP chemotherapy for lymphoma. *J Feline Med Surg.* 2008;10:73–81.
34. Niessen SJ, Powney S, Guitian J, et al. Evaluation of a quality-of-life tool for cats with diabetes mellitus. *J Vet Intern Med.* 2010;24:1098–1105.
35. Benito J, Hansen B, DePuy V. Feline musculoskeletal pain index: Responsiveness and testing of criterion validity. *J Vet Intern Med.* 2013;27:474–482.

36. Bergadano A. Diagnosis of chronic pain in small animals. *Companion Anim Pract.* 2010;20:61–68.

37. Lascelles BD, Gaynor JS, Smith ES, et al. Amantadine in a multimodal analgesic regimen for alleviation of refractory osteoarthritis pain in dogs. *J Vet Intern Med.* 2008;22:53–59.

38. Lascelles BD, Hansen BD, Roe S, et al. Evaluation of client-specific outcome measures and activity monitoring to measure pain relief in cats with osteoarthritis. *J Vet Intern Med.* 2007;21:410–416.

39. Moreau M, Guillot M, Pelletier JP, et al. Kinetic peak vertical force measurement in cats afflicted by coxarthritis: data management and acquisition protocols. *Res Vet Sci.* 2013;95:219–224.

40. Guillot M, Moreau M, Heit M, et al. Characterization of osteoarthritis in cats and meloxicam efficacy using objective chronic pain evaluation tools. *Vet J.* 2013;196:360–367.

41. Lascelles BD, DePuy V, Thomson A, et al. Evaluation of a therapeutic diet for feline degenerative joint disease. *J Vet Intern Med.* 2010;24:487–495.

42. Brown DC. Quantitative sensory testing: A stimulating look at chronic pain. *Vet J.* 2012;193:315–316.

43. Langford DJ, Bailey AL, Chanda ML, et al. Coding of facial expressions of pain in the laboratory mouse. *Nat Methods.* 2010;7:447–449.

44. Lascelles BDX. Feline degenerative joint disease. *Vet Surg.* 2010;39:2–13.

45. Turk DC. Clinical effectiveness and cost-effectiveness of treatments for patients with chronic pain. *Clin J Pain.* 2002;18:355–365.

46. Mao J, Gold MS, Backonja MM. Combination drug therapy for chronic pain: A call for more clinical studies. *J Pain.* 2011;12:157–166.

47. Lascelles BDX, Court MH, Hardie EM, Robertson SA. Nonsteroidal anti-inflammatory drugs in cats: a review. *Vet Anaesth Analg.* 2007;34:228–250.

48. Innes JF, Clayton J, Lascelles BDX. Review of the safety and efficacy of long-term NSAID use in the treatment of canine osteoarthritis. *Vet Rec.* 2010;166:226–230.

49. Sparkes AH, Heiene R, Lascelles BD, et al. ISFM and AAFP consensus guidelines on the long-term use of NSAIDs in cats. *J Feline Med Surg.* 2010;12:521–538.

50. Khan SA, McLean MK. Toxicology of frequently encountered nonsteroidal anti-inflammatory drugs in dogs and cats. *Vet Clin North Am Small Anim Pract.* 2012;42:289–306.

51. Grudé P, Guittard J, Garcia C, et al. Excretion mass balance evaluation, metabolite profile analysis and metabolite identification in plasma and excreta after oral administration of [14C]-meloxicam to the male cat: preliminary study. *J Vet Pharmacol Ther.* 2010;33:396–407.

52. Gowan RA, Baral RM, Lingard AE, et al. A retrospective analysis of the effects of meloxicam on the longevity of aged cats with and without overt chronic kidney disease. *J Feline Med Surg.* 2012;14:876–881.

53. Gowan RA, Lingard AE, Johnston L, et al. Retrospective case-control study of the effects of long-term dosing with meloxicam on renal function in aged cats with degenerative joint disease. *J Feline Med Surg.* 2011;13:752–761.

54. Surdyk KK, Brown CA, Brown SA. Evaluation of glomerular filtration rate in cats with reduced renal mass and administered meloxicam and acetylsalicylic acid. *Am J Vet Res.* 2013;74:648–651.

55. Wernham BG, Trumpatori B, Hash J, et al. Dose reduction of meloxicam in dogs with osteoarthritis-associated pain and impaired mobility. *J Vet Intern Med.* 2011;25:1298–1305.

56. Strand V, Simon LS, Dougados M, et al. Treatment of osteoarthritis with continuous versus intermittent celecoxib. *J Rheumatol.* 2011;38:2625–2634.

57. Pypendop BH, Ilkiw JE. Pharmacokinetics of tramadol, and its metabolite O-desmethyl-tramadol, in cats. *J Vet Pharmacol Ther.* 2007;31:52–59.

58. Cagnardi P, Villa R, Zonca A, et al. Pharmacokinetics, intraoperative effect and postoperative analgesia of tramadol in cats. *Res Vet Sci.* 2011;90:503–509.

59. KuKanich B. Outpatient oral analgesics in dogs and cats beyond nonsteroidal antiinflammatory drugs. *Vet Clin North Am Small Anim Pract.* 2013;43:1109–1125.

60. Monteiro B. Klinck MP, Moreau M, Guillot M et al. Analgesic efficacy of meloxicam as a transmucosal oral spray formulation, alone or its combination with tramadol, in cats with naturally occurring osteoarthritis. *Anaesthesia and Analgesia.* January 2015;42(1):27.

61. Monteiro B. Klinck MP, Moreau M, et al. Analgesic efficacy of tramadol administered orally for two weeks in cats with naturally occurring osteoarthritis. *Vet Anaesth Analg.* January 2015;42(1):p26.

62. Pypendop BH, Siao KT, Ilkiw JE. Thermal anti-nociceptive effect of orally administered gabapentin in healthy cats. *Am J Vet Res.* 2010;71:1027–1032.

63. Ray J, Jordan D, Pinelli C, Fackler B. Case studies of compounded Tramadol use in cats. *Int J Pharm Compd.* 2011;16:44–49.

64. Robertson SA, Lascelles BD, Taylor PM, Sear JW. PK-PD modeling of buprenorphine in cats: intravenous and oral transmucosal administration. *J Vet Pharmacol Ther.* 2005;28:453–460.

65. Cheung CW, Qiu Q, Choi SW, Moore B. Chronic opioid therapy for chronic non-cancer pain: a review and comparison of treatment guidelines. *Pain Physician.* 2014;17:401–420.

66. Portenoy RK, Ahmed E. Principles of opioid use in cancer pain. *J Clin Oncol.* 2014;32:1662–1670.

67. Attal N, Cruccu G, Baron R, et al. EFNS guidelines on the pharmacological treatment of neuropathic pain: 2010 revision. *Eur J Neurol.* 2010;17:1113–e88.

68. Lorenz ND, Comerford EJ, Iff I. Long-term use of gabapentin for musculoskeletal disease and trauma in three cats. *J Feline Med Surg.* 2013;15:507–512.

69. Siao KT, Pypendop BH, Ilkiw JE. Pharmacokinetics of gabapentin in cats. *Am J Vet Res.* 2010;71:817–821.

70. Vettorato E, Corletto F. Gabapentin as part of multi-modal analgesia in two cats suffering multiple injuries. *Vet Anaesth Analg.* 2011;38:518–520.

71. Tesfaye S, Vileikyte L, Rayman G, et al. Painful diabetic peripheral neuropathy: consensus recommendations on diagnosis, assessment and management. *Diabetes Metab Res Rev.* 2011;27:629–638.

72. Cautela M, Dewey CW, Schwark W, et al. Pharmacokinetics of oral pregabalin in cats after single dose administration. *J Vet Intern Med.* 2010;24:739.

73. Rusbridge C, Heath S, Gunn-Moore DA, et al. Feline orofacial pain syndrome (FOPS): a retrospective study of 113 cases. *J Feline Med Surg.* 2010;12:498–508.

74. Richards BL, Whittle SL, Buchbinder R. Muscle relaxants for pain management in rheumatoid arthritis. *Cochrane Database Syst Rev.* 2012;1, CD008922.

75. Tremont-Lukats IW, Megeff C, Backonja MM. Anticonvulsants for neuropathic pain syndromes: mechanisms of action and place in therapy. *Drugs.* 2000;60:1029–1052.

76. Hewitt DJ. The use of NMDA-receptor antagonists in the treatment of chronic pain. *Clin J Pain.* 2000;16:S73–S79.

77. Siao KT, Pypendop BH, Stanley SD, Ilkiw JE. Pharmacokinetics of amantadine in cats. *J Vet Pharmacol Ther.* 2011;34:599–604.

78. Siao KT, Pypendop BH, Escobar A, et al. Effect of amantadine on oxymorphone-induced thermal antinociception in cats. *J Vet Pharmacol Ther.* 2011;35:169–174.
79. Robertson SA. Managing pain in feline patients. *Vet Clin North Am Small Anim Pract.* 2008;38:1267–1290.
80. Dharmshaktu P, Tayal V, Kalra BS. Efficacy of antidepressants as analgesics: a review. *J Clin Pharmacol.* 2013;52:6–17.
81. Chew DJ, Buffington CA, Kendall MS, et al. Amitriptyline treatment for severe recurrent idiopathic cystitis in cats. *J Am Vet Med Assoc.* 1998;213:1282–1286.
82. O'Hagan BJ. Neuropathic pain in a cat post-amputation. *Aust Vet J.* 2007;84:83–86.
83. Davis MP. Cannabinoids in pain management: CB1, CB2 and non-classic receptor ligands. *Expert Opin Investig Drugs.* 2014;23:1123–1140.
84. Hesselink JM, Hekker TA. Therapeutic utility of palmitoylethanolamide in the treatment of neuropathic pain associated with various pathological conditions: a case series. *J Pain Res.* 2012;5:437–442.
85. Urys product information. http://www.innovet.it/en/?pid=2&prd_az=sr&prd_v=9 Accessed October 8, 2014.
86. Re G, Barbero R, Miolo A, Di Marzo V. Palmitoylethanolamide, endocannabinoids and related cannabimimetic compounds in protection against tissue inflammation and pain: potential use in companion animals. *Vet J.* 2007;173:21–30.
87. Hill R. NK1 (substance P) receptor antagonists – why are they not analgesic in humans? *Trends Pharmacol Sci.* 2000;21:244–246.
88. Niyom S, Boscan P, Twedt DC, et al. Effect of maropitant, a neurokinin-1 receptor antagonist, on the minimum alveolar concentration of sevoflurane during stimulation of the ovarian ligament in cats. *Vet Anaesth Analg.* 2013;40:425–431.
89. Fox SM. Chronic pain in small animal medicine. London, UK: Manson Publishing; 2010, pp. 164–173.
90. Vandeweerd JM, Coisnon C, Clegg P, et al. Systematic review of efficacy of nutraceuticals to alleviate clinical signs of osteoarthritis. *J Vet Intern Med.* 2012;26:448–456.
91. Wandel S, Jüni P, Tendal B, et al. Effects of glucosamine, chondroitin, or placebo in patients with osteoarthritis of hip or knee: network meta-analysis. *BMJ.* 2010;341:c4675–c4675.
92. Corbee RJ, Barnier MMC, van de Lest CHA, Hazewinkel HAW. The effect of dietary long-chain omega-3 fatty acid supplementation on owner's perception of behaviour and locomotion in cats with naturally occurring osteoarthritis. *J Anim Physiol Anim Nutr.* 2012;97:846–853.
93. Sharp B. BSAVA Manual of Canine and Feline Rehabilitation, Supportive Care and Palliative Care. In: Lindley S, Watson P, eds. British Small Animal Veterinary Association; 2010:90–113, Physiotherapy and physical rehabilitation. London, United Kingdom.
94. van Tulder M, Malmivaara A, Hayden J, Koes B. Statistical significance versus clinical importance. *Spine.* 2007;32:1785–1790.
95. Lindley S, Smith H. BSAVA Manual of Canine and Feline Rehabilitation, Supportive Care and Palliative Care. In: Lindley S, Watson P, eds. British Small Animal Veterinary Association; 2010:114–122 Hydrotherapy. London, United Kingdom.
96. Gatchel RJ, Peng YB, Peters ML, et al. The biopsychosocial approach to chronic pain: scientific advances and future directions. *Psychol Bull.* 2007;133:581–624.
97. Robinson RC, Garofalo JP, Gatchel RJ. Decreases in cortisol variability between treated and untreated jaw pain patients. *J Appl Biobehav Res.* 2006;11:179–188.
98. Ellis SLH. Environmental enrichment: practical strategies for improving feline welfare. *J Feline Med Surg.* 2009;11:901–912.
99. Osborne TL, Raichle KA, Jensen MP. Psychologic interventions for chronic pain. *Phys Med Rehabil Clin N Am.* 2006;17:415–433.
100. Lindley S. BSAVA Manual of Canine and Feline Rehabilitation, Supportive Care and Palliative Care. In: Lindley S, Watson P, eds. British Small Animal Veterinary Association; 2010:85–89, An introduction to physical therapies London, UK.
101. Gunn-Moore D. A pilot study using synthetic feline facial pheromone for the management of feline idiopathic cystitis. *J Feline Med Surg.* 2004;6:133–138.
102. Griffith CA, Steigerwald ES, Buffington CAT. Effects of a synthetic facial pheromone on behavior of cats. *J Am Vet Med Assoc.* 2000;217:1154–1156.
103. Karavis M. The neurophysiology of acupuncture: a viewpoint. *Acupuncture Med.* 1997;15:33–42.
104. Gaynor JS. Acupuncture for management of pain. *Vet Clin North Am Small Anim Pract.* 2000;30:875–884.
105. Habacher G, Pittler MH, Ernst E. Effectiveness of acupuncture in veterinary medicine: systematic review. *J Vet Intern Med.* 2006;20:480–488.
106. Staiger BA, Beale BS. Use of arthroscopy for debridement of the elbow joint in cats. *J Am Vet Med Assoc.* 2005;226:401–403.
107. Marcellin-Little DJ, DeYoung BA, Doyens DH, DeYoung DJ. Canine uncemented porous-coated anatomic total hip arthroplasty: results of a long-term prospective evaluation of 50 consecutive cases. *Vet Surg.* 1999;28:10–20.
108. Liska WD, Doyle N, Marcellin-Little DJ, Osborne JA. Total hip replacement in three cats: surgical technique, short-term outcome and comparison to femoral head ostectomy. *Vet Comp Orthop Traumatol.* 2009;22:505–510.
109. Grierson J. Hips, elbows and stifles: common joint diseases in the cat. *J Feline Med Surg.* 2012;14:23–30.
110. Black LL, Gaynor J, Gahring D, et al. Effect of adipose-derived mesenchymal stem and regenerative cells on lameness in dogs with chronic osteoarthritis of the coxofemoral joints: a randomized, double-blinded, multicenter, controlled trial. *Vet Ther.* 2007;8:272–284.
111. Black LL, Gaynor J, Adams C, et al. Effect of intra-articular injection of autologous adipose-derived mesenchymal stem and regenerative cells on clinical signs of chronic osteoarthritis of the elbow joint in dogs. *Vet Ther.* 2008;9:192–200.
112. Vilar JM, Batista M, Morales M, et al. Assessment of the effect of intraarticular injection of autologous adipose-derived mesenchymal stem cells in osteoarthritic dogs using a double blinded force platform analysis. *BMC Vet Res.* 2014;10:143.
113. Keller S, Müller K, Kortmann RD, et al. Efficacy of low-dose radiotherapy in painful gonarthritis: experiences from a retrospective East German bicenter study. *Radiat Oncol.* 2013;8:29.
114. Freire M, Robertson I, Bondell HD, et al. Radiographic evaluation of feline appendicular degenerative joint disease vs. macroscopic appearance of articular cartilage. *Vet Radiol Ultrasound.* 2011;52:239–247.
115. Freire M, Brown J, Robertson ID, et al. Meniscal mineralization in domestic cats. *Vet Surg.* 2010;39:545–552.
116. Niemiec BA. Oral pathology. *Top Companion Anim Med.* 2008;23:59–71.
117. Reiter AM, Mendoza KA. Feline odontoclastic resorptive lesions: an unsolved enigma in veterinary dentistry. *Vet Clin North Am Small Anim Pract.* 2002;32:791–837.
118. Buffington CAT. Visceral pain in humans: lessons from animals. *Curr Pain Headache Rep.* 2001;5:44–51.

119. Phatak S, Foster HE. The management of interstitial cystitis: an update. *Nat Clin Pract Urol.* 2006;3:45–53.

120. Buffington C, Westropp J, Chew D, Bolus R. Clinical evaluation of multimodal environmental modification (MEMO) in the management of cats with idiopathic cystitis. *J Feline Med Surg.* 2006;8:261–268.

121. Westropp JL, Kass PH, Buffington CAT. Evaluation of the effects of stress in cats with idiopathic cystitis. *Am J Vet Res.* 2006;67:731–736.

122. Kraijer M, Fink-Gremmels J, Nickel RF. The short-term clinical efficacy of amitriptyline in the management of idiopathic feline lower urinary tract disease: a controlled clinical study. *J Feline Med Surg.* 2003;5:191–196.

123. Jergens AE, Moore FM, Haynes JS. Idiopathic inflammatory bowel disease in dogs and cats: 84 cases (1987–1990). *J Am Vet Med Assoc.* 1992;201:1603–1608.

124. Srinath AI, Walter C, Newara MC, Szigethy EM. Pain management in patients with inflammatory bowel disease: insights for the clinician. *Therap Adv Gastroenterol.* 2012;5:339–357.

125. Xenoulis PG, Suchodolski JS, Steiner JM. Chronic pancreatitis in dogs and cats. *Compendium.* 2008;30:166–181.

126. Mantyh PW, Clohisy DR, Koltzenburg M, Hunt SP. Molecular mechanisms of cancer pain. *Nat Rev Cancer.* 2002;2:201–209.

127. Carsten RE, Hellyer PW, Bachand AM, LaRue SM. Correlations between acute radiation scores and pain scores in canine radiation patients with cancer of the forelimb. *Vet Anaesth Analg.* 2008;35:355–362.

128. Bommer NX, Hayes AM, Scase TJ, Gunn-Moore DA. Clinical features, survival times and COX-1 and COX-2 expression in cats with transitional cell carcinoma of the urinary bladder treated with meloxicam. *J Feline Med Surg.* 2012;14:527–533.

129. Borrego JF, Cartagena JC, Engel J. Treatment of feline mammary tumours using chemotherapy, surgery and a COX-2 inhibitor drug (meloxicam): a retrospective study of 23 cases (2002–2007). *Vet Comp Oncol.* 2009;7:213–221.

130. Nikolajsen L, Jensen TS. Phantom limb pain. *Curr Rev Pain.* 2000;4:166–170.

131. Grant IA, Iff I. Possible phantom limb pain in 2 dogs after amputation for osteosarcoma. Italy: Abstract at ESVONC Turin; 2010, p. 61.

132. Patronek GJ. Assessment of claims of short- and long-term complications associated with onychectomy in cats. *J Am Vet Med Assoc.* 2001;219:932–937.

133. de Lorimier LP. Feline hyperesthesia syndrome. *Compendium.* 2009;31:E4.

Feline Orofacial Pain Syndrome

Clare Rusbridge and Sarah Heath

INTRODUCTION

Feline orofacial pain syndrome (FOPS) is characterized by behavioral signs of severe oral discomfort. This condition is seen in a variety of feline populations, although Burmese cats predominate, suggesting a genetic basis for this neuropathic pain disorder. Dental pain, for example permanent teeth eruption and periodontal disease, can trigger the condition. Environmental factors can exacerbate the condition and individuals with poor social coping strategies in multicat households appear to be more vulnerable. Affected cats are presented most commonly with pawing and mutilation of the mouth especially the tongue. In many patients discomfort is elicited by movements of the mouth such as eating, drinking, or grooming. The apparent pain is typically unilateral and can be episodic with variable pain-free intervals. The syndrome is often recurrent, and with time may become unremitting, with up to 10% of the cases being euthanized as a consequence of the condition.

PATHOPHYSIOLOGY

Neuropathic Pain

FOPS is considered a neuropathic pain disorder, that is, pain caused by a lesion or disease of the somatosensory nervous system.[1] Pain can be divided into three categories: physiological, inflammatory, and neuropathic. Physiological pain, such as the pain in response to a needle prick, serves to protect an animal from injury. Inflammatory pain is a consequence of tissue damage, for example tooth ache. However, if the nociceptive system becomes sensitized then the pain may change to neuropathic which serves the animal no purpose and is a disease in itself. A defining characteristic of neuropathic pain is abnormal somatosensory processing in the peripheral or central nervous system. The pathophysiology is complex and incompletely understood. However, there are three pivotal phenomena intrinsic to development.[2]

1. **Central sensitization.** The process of "wind-up" by which sensory information about pain is amplified on its way to the brain with a consequent elevated perception of pain. The spinal cord and medullary dorsal horn (pars caudalis) has a pivotal role in pain perception and "wind-up." The dorsal horn receives sensory information from the periphery, including light touch, proprioception, vibration, temperature, and pain. This information is sent from receptors of the skin, bones, joints, mucosa, and teeth through sensory neurons whose cell bodies lie in the dorsal root ganglion. All primary afferents in the dorsal horn use glutamate as their main excitatory neurotransmitter. Many of the unmyelinated C fiber nociceptors contain and secrete neuropeptides such as substance P and calcitonin gene related peptide. The target for substance P is the tachykinin NK1 receptors. These and the glutamate NMDA receptors are pivotal to generate wind-up and amplification of the nociceptive message that arrives from peripheral nociceptors.[3] Consequently pharmacological agents which antagonize glutamate and the release of neuropeptides in the dorsal horn may be effective for management of the pain.
2. **Central disinhibition,** that is, an imbalance between the excitatory and inhibitory side of the nervous system so that there is reduced inhibition to the spinal cord dorsal horn. The descending inhibitory control of the dorsal horn is GABAergic, serotonergic–noradrenergic, and opioidergic[4] and consequently pharmacological agents with this action may be effective analgesics.
3. **Phenotypic change** of mechanoreceptive Aβ-fibers (light touching) in the deeper laminas of the dorsal horn which become activated and produce substance P so that input from them is perceived as pain (tactile allodynia). In the situation of FOPS the unique neuroanatomy of the teeth may predispose this physiological change.

Neuroanatomy of Orofacial Pain: The Trigeminal Nociceptive System

Trigeminal Nerve

Nociception of the face and oral cavity is mediated by the trigeminal nerve. Two of the three main divisions,

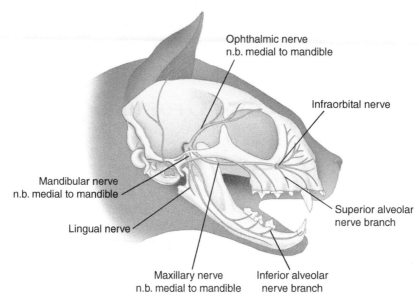

FIGURE 16-1   Lateral aspect of the feline skull illustrating the trigeminal nerve.

the maxillary and the mandibular, serve the oral cavity (Figure 16-1). The maxillary branch innervates teeth and mucosa of the maxilla, the upper lip, superior eyelid, lateral nose, maxillary sinus, and nasopharynx. The mandibular division innervates the teeth and mucosa of the mandible, temporomandibular joint, rostral tongue, the skin covering the mandible, and is also motor to the masticatory muscles.[5,6]

Teeth

The unusual neuroanatomy of the teeth may explain why dental disease is such an important trigger for FOPS (see Figure 16-1). The upper jaw is supplied by the rostral, middle, and caudal superior alveolar nerves, all branches of the infraorbital nerve which in turn is a branch of the maxillary nerve. The lower jaw is supplied by the inferior alveolar nerve which is a branch of the mandibular nerve.[7] Pulpal, periodontal, and buccal gingival margin fibers from an individual tooth generally travel together.[7] The majority of nociceptive information is transmitted by small unmyelinated polymodal C fibers and larger mechanothermal A-δ fibers.[8]

However, in the tooth there are also large numbers of fast conducting large A-β fibers which penetrate the dentine from the pulp cavity.[8] These are responsive to changes in the flow of the plasma-like fluid in the dentinal tubules which is affected by environmental stimuli such as hot, cold, osmotic, mechanical, and drying.[9] They are responsible for the sensation of sharp pain whereas the slower C fibers are associated with a dull ache.[10] This high density of large fibers is quite different from skin nociception and presumably is a necessary adaption as the teeth provide sensory feedback vital for coordinating jaw and neck movement for a variety of behaviors, including biting, mastication, and grooming[11,12] and also contribute information as to whether a bolus of food is suitable for swallowing.[8] However, it is possible that this high density of large fibers may predispose to a chronic pain state. One of the hallmarks of neuropathic pain is upregulation of mechanoreceptors and the development of allodynia—in other words, pain from a stimulus which is not normally painful such as movement, touch, or temperature change (Table 16-1). Another important difference between trigeminal versus

TABLE 16-1	Pain Terms as Defined by the International Association for the Study of Pain Task Force on Taxonomy[1]	
Pain	**Characteristics**
Nociceptive pain	Pain that arises from actual or threatened damage to nonneural tissue and is due to the activation of nociceptors
Nociceptor	A high-threshold sensory receptor of the peripheral somatosensory nervous system that is capable of transducing and encoding noxious stimuli
Neuropathic pain	Pain caused by a lesion or disease of the somatosensory nervous system
Neuralgia	Pain in distribution of nerve or nerves
Allodynia	Pain due to a stimulus that does not normally provoke pain

spinal nociception is the response of the trigeminal system to injury of its target tissue. Following pulpal inflammation, sensory neurons undergo sprouting, meaning that their receptive fields become larger.[13,14] There are also significant changes in expression of ion channels receptors[15] and neuropeptides.[13,16] Central sensitization can be triggered from the inflammation of a single tooth.[17] These changes explain why toothache is so debilitating and painful.[6,18,19]

Tongue

Nociception of the rostral two-thirds of the tongue is mediated through the lingual nerve branch of the mandibular nerve (trigeminal) whereas nociception in the caudal third of the tongue is mediated by the lingual branch of the glossopharyngeal nerve.[5] There is convergence of nociceptive inputs in the nucleus of the solitary tract in the medulla.[20] The clinical signs of FOPS are more suggestive of trigeminal pain as mutilation seems to be to the rostral tongue; however, this may simply be due to ease of access, and a glossopharyngeal pain syndrome cannot be ruled out. In humans glossopharyngeal neuralgia causes intermittent, lancinating pain, involving the posterior tongue and pharynx, with radiation to deep ear structures.[21]

Trigeminal Ganglion

The trigeminal ganglion (Figure 16-2) is located in the trigeminal canal on the rostromedial aspect of the petrosal part of the temporal bone, and contains the majority of the cell bodies of trigeminal afferents, although there are also some located in the mesencephalic trigeminal nucleus.[22]

Central Trigeminal Pathways

Understanding the link between psychological stress and physical pain requires a basic understanding of the central processing of nociceptive information. Nociceptive fibers from tooth pulp and oral cavity ascend to the spinal trigeminal nucleus and the principal sensory trigeminal nucleus in the pons[23–25] (Figure 16-3). From there fibers project into the thalamus[25,26] and from there ascend

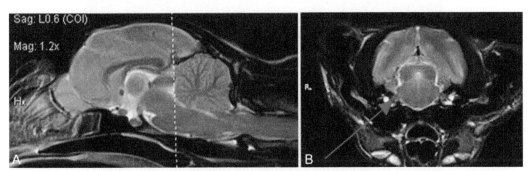

FIGURE 16-2   T2-weighted midsagittal and transverse magnetic resonance images from a Burmese cat. **A,** A dotted line indicates the "cut" of the transverse images which is at the level of the pons and the trigeminal nerve root. **B,** An arrow indicates the trigeminal ganglion. (Imaging courtesy Eli Jovanovik, Fitzpatrick Referrals)

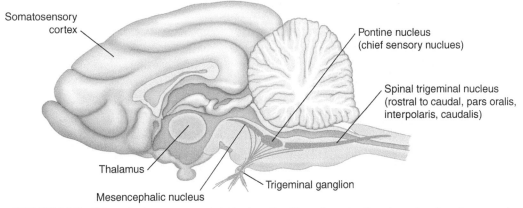

FIGURE 16-3   Trigeminal sensory nuclei. Nociceptive fibers from tooth pulp and oral cavity ascend to the dorsomedial region of all three subnuclei of the spinal trigeminal nucleus (in particular pars oralis but also pars interpolaris and pars caudalis) and the principal sensory trigeminal nucleus in the pons. From there fibers project to the contralateral medial geniculate complex, caudal thalamus, and ventrocaudal medial thalamus. Projections from the thalamus ascend to the primary and secondary somatosensory cortex.

to the primary and secondary somatosensory cortex. These projections to the somatosensory cortex are likely implicated in the sensory-discriminative aspects of pain. There are also projections to the ipsilateral dysgranular insular cortex, ipsilateral external lateral parabrachial nucleus, dorsal thalamus, and dorsal basolateral amygdala which may have a role in the affective–motivational aspects of pain (Figure 16-4).[26]

Pain Matrix

The pain matrix is a theoretical concept often used to understand the neural mechanisms of pain in health and disease.[27] Anatomically the pain matrix is an extensive cortical network including the somatosensory, insular, cingulate, frontal, and parietal areas (see Figure 16-4). Functionally it describes three domains of pain processing in the central nervous system: 1) the sensory discriminative dimension dealing with the localization and severity of

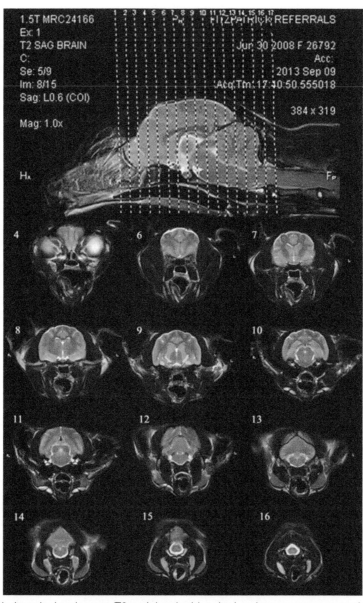

FIGURE 16-4 The central trigeminal pathways. T2-weighted midsagittal and transverse magnetic resonance images from a Burmese cat. Dotted lines and numbers indicate the "slice" of the transverse images. Slice 4, frontal lobe (pain matrix). Slice 6, parietal lobe with somatosensory cortex (purple) (pain matrix). Slice 7, somatosensory cortex (purple) and cingulate gyrus (pink) (pain matrix). Slice 8, cingulate gyrus (pink) and dorsal thalamus (dark blue) (pain matrix). Slice 9, cingulate gyrus (pink) and amygdala (lilac) (pain matrix); caudal (blue) and ventrocaudal (light blue) thalamus (projection pathways). Slice 10, insular area (pink) (pain matrix); mesencephalic nucleus and tract of the trigeminal nerve (orange) Slice 11, trigeminal nerve (yellow) and mesencephalic nucleus of the trigeminal nerve (orange). Slice 12, trigeminal nerve (yellow) and pontine sensory nucleus (dark red). Slices 13–16, spinal trigeminal nucleus (red).

pain; 2) an affective–motivational dimension dealing with the emotional response to pain; and 3) a cognitive dimension.[28] Pain is not just an unpleasant sensory and emotional experience but something that demands a behavioral response to the danger to the body tissue. Due to the dependence on survival, pain demands the brain's attention affecting other cortical processing and other body systems including the immune system, the hypothalamus-pituitary-adrenal axes, the sympathetic nervous system, and the reproductive system.[29] When pain becomes chronic, the efficacy of the pain matrix is improved, meaning that less input, both nociceptive and non-nociceptive, is required to produce pain.[29]

Genetic Susceptibility

A genome-wide association study on Burmese cats affected with FOPS suggested three loci associated with the disease. Two of the loci contain promising candidate genes that are expressed in the central nervous system and have been implicated in migraine and neuropathic pain syndromes in humans and rodents.[30] Further sequencing is in process. The possible connection to migraine is interesting as it is thought that migraine headache is a manifestation of activation of the trigeminovascular system in genetically susceptible individuals.[31] In addition, migraine headache, like FOPS, is affected by environmental factors including stress.[31,32]

CLINICAL SIGNS AND COURSE

FOPS is characterized by oral discomfort and behavioral signs of pain, including face and tongue mutilation (Figure 16-5). Affected cats are most commonly presented with exaggerated licking and chewing movements, with pawing at the mouth (Figure 16-6). More severe cases have mutilation of tongue, lips, and buccal mucosa. Signs are often episodic, typically unilateral and triggered in many cases by mouth movements such as chewing, drinking, or grooming. FOPS may occur in bouts over a period of weeks or months, with subsequent spontaneous remission that may last months or years. Over time, however, the attacks can become more frequent and pain apparently more sustained. Retrospective analysis of cases reveals a peak incidence in immature Burmese cats (6 months or younger), with 75% of the affected cats having recurrent or on-going problems. Failure to adequately control the pain can result in the euthanasia of some cases.[33]

TRIGGERS OF FOPS

Oral Pain

Eruption of Permanent Teeth
The incidence of post traumatic trigeminal neuralgia is surprisingly low given the anatomical considerations above, the prevalence of feline periodontal disease, and the number of dental procedures performed on cats, often with suboptimal analgesia. It has been suggested that this is because the trigeminal system is programmed for a pain event and loss of innervated structures during postnatal development, that is, the eruption and loss of the deciduous teeth.[34] Normal primary tooth shedding and permanent tooth eruption are accompanied by degenerative changes, then remodeling in brain stem trigeminal nuclei.[35,36] Some of the nerves which supply the pulp of a deciduous tooth are retained to supply its permanent successor.[37] This neuronal plasticity is particularly interesting since it is this biological event which is associated with the first FOPS event in many Burmese cats with a suspected inherited predisposition.[33] Affected cats are typically presented at 5 to 7 months of age when the canines and/or molars are erupting, with acute behavioral signs of oral discomfort and attempted or actual tongue and buccal mucosal mutilation. Signs resolve spontaneously when "teething" is complete; however, many of these cats will have a recurrence of signs as adults.[33]

Periodontal Disease
Periodontal disease, especially odontoclastic resorptive lesions, are important triggers of FOPS in adult cats (Figure 16-7). Odontoclastic resorptive lesions (also-known as neck lesions, cervical line lesions, cervical lesions) are extremely common in the feline population and are characterized by root resorption and dentin exposure and are mediated by large multinucleated odontoclast cells. The tooth erosion may not be immediately apparent as the lesion is often covered by a circular area of inflamed and highly vascular gingiva. The teeth most commonly affected are the upper fourth premolar, lower molar, and lower third premolar, but all teeth except the incisors are predisposed.[38,39] The authors hypothesize that the associated suppurative inflammation and unique neuroanatomy of the teeth, in particular the large numbers of fast conducting large A-β fibers penetrating the (exposed) dentine, predisposes development of a neuropathic pain state in genetically susceptible cats. Experimentally, exposure of dentin for 1 to 2 weeks in the dog induces an inflammatory reaction in the pulp,[40] and electrophysiological studies have demonstrated sensitization of the intradental A-fibers in particular in the nerve fibers innervating cervical dentin.[41,42] These changes included increased sensitivity to hydrodynamic stimulation, and spontaneous firing of action potentials.[41,42]

Mouth Ulceration
There have been occasional cases of FOPS associated with mouth ulceration, for example from feline

respiratory virus infection (feline calicivirus and feline herpesvirus).[33]

Neuropathic Pain, Cognition, and Stress

Pain affects cognition and vice versa. In rodent models, chronic pain impairs learning and memory, interrupts attention, and affects decision making. Humans with orofacial pain are more susceptible to psychopathological disorders[43] and anxiety.[44] This impairment occurs on a molecular level due to neuroinflammation affecting the cortical "emotion–pain circuitry" of the amygdala, cingulate, insula, and prefrontal cortex.[43,45,46] Conversely, cognitive processes and emotional state can modulate pain through the descending pathways[47] and chronic exposure to stressful stimuli, for example social stress, induces immune responses in various areas of the brain and spinal cord, and the resulting neuroinflammation triggers sensory hypersensitivity.[46,48]

Stress* has consistently been shown to be a factor that contributes to the maintenance and amplification of the severity of pain, and recent studies have suggested that this is mediated through the noradrenergic locus coeruleus nucleus which coordinates many components of the stress response, as well as nociceptive transmission.[49] Consequently animals in pain may be more predisposed to stress-related behavioral disorders, and chronic stress may trigger or worsen behavioral signs of pain. Therefore a holistic approach must be taken when investigating and treating a pain disorder. This applies to FOPS and also to other painful diseases. For example, chronic pelvic/visceral pain disorders such as interstitial cystitis and inflammatory bowel disease are recognized, in humans, to comprise neuropathic and emotional components.[28,50] A retrospective study found that for one in five FOPS cases, environmental factors influenced the disease expression and individuals with poor social coping strategies in multicat households appear to be more vulnerable.[33]

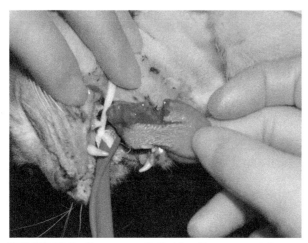

FIGURE 16-5 Tongue mutilation in a Burmese cat. In case of severe mutilation surgical repair may be required and the cat may also require parental nutrition until the tongue lesions have healed. The etiology in this case was thought to be a combination of social conflict with a sibling and placement (together) in a cattery. (Courtesy Jamie Finney MVB, MRCVS, Abbeycroft Veterinary Centre)

COMPARISON WITH HUMAN OROFACIAL PAIN SYNDROMES

According to the International Headache Society Classification,[51] **trigeminal neuralgia** is characterized by brief, electric-shock-like pains, is abrupt in onset and termination, and is limited to the distribution of one or more divisions of the trigeminal nerve. Pain is typically unilateral and occurs spontaneously but is also often triggered by mouth movements and/or touch to certain areas of the mouth or face, especially the

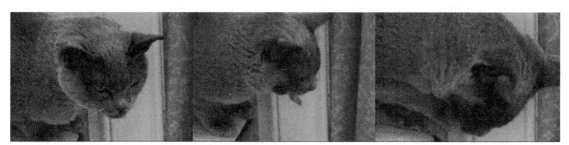

FIGURE 16-6 Video stills from a Burmese cat with feline orofacial pain syndrome (FOPS) demonstrating apparent tongue discomfort and pawing at the mouth. In this case the etiology was undetermined. The FOPS behavior was triggered by tongue movements associated with grooming. Video footage, courtesy Mrs. Nicolle, is available at http://www.veterinary-neurologist.co.uk/FOPS/

---

*Stress is defined as collective physiological and emotional response to any stimulus that disturbs an individual's homeostasis.[28]

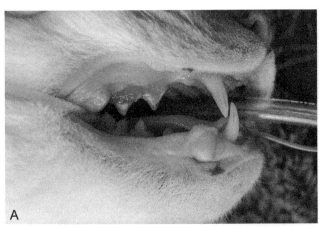
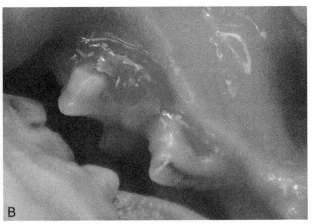

FIGURE 16-7   Feline odontoclastic resorptive lesions (FORL) in a domestic shorthair cat. **A,** Note the area of inflamed and hyperplastic gingiva on the upper third premolar. **B,** Inspection under this tissue revealed erosion of the surface of the tooth. Good quality dental radiographs are paramount when investigating the etiology of feline orofacial pain syndrome (FOPS). (Courtesy Dr. Anne Fawcett, Sydney Animal Hospitals Inner West)

nasolabial fold and/or chin. Like FOPS, trigeminal neuralgia has an exacerbating and remitting course with patients exhibiting shorter periods of remission as they age. Periods of complete remission are highly unusual for neuropathic pain syndromes and this feature distinguishes trigeminal neuralgia from other pain disorders. Inherited susceptibility is a contributory factor in some cases, with a familial occurrence reported in 4.1% of patients with unilateral trigeminal neuralgia and 17% of patients with bilateral trigeminal neuralgia.[52] Classical trigeminal neuralgia is most often caused by microvascular compression at the trigeminal root entry to the brainstem. Symptomatic trigeminal neuralgia is caused by a structural lesion other than vascular compression, for example demyelination associated with multiple sclerosis. **Persistent idiopathic facial pain** (atypical facial pain) is a persistent facial pain that does not have the characteristics of cranial neuralgias and cannot be attributed to a different disorder. Diagnostic tests such as neurological examination, radiographs, magnetic resonance imaging (MRI), and computed tomography (CT) are unremarkable. Unlike trigeminal neuralgia, the pain is described as deep, poorly localized, and is long lasting, often persisting throughout the day and occurring daily. Generally it is limited to one particular area on one side of the face. Like FOPS, the pain may be initiated by surgery or injury to the face, teeth, or gums, but subsequently persists without any demonstrable local cause. A subcategory of persistent idiopathic pain is **atypical odontalgia,** which is characterized by continuous pain in the teeth or in a tooth socket after extraction in the absence of any identifiable dental cause. **Glossopharyngeal neuralgia** is characterized by paroxysmal pain in the area of the ear, base of the tongue, tonsillar fossa, or beneath the angle of the jaw. Like trigeminal neuralgia, pain is provoked by trigger factors such as swallowing, talking, or coughing and it can have a remitting and relapsing course. **Burning mouth syndrome** is described as an intraoral burning sensation for which no medical or dental cause can be found. It is characterized by daily pain with the discomfort persisting for most of the day. If the pain is confined to the tongue then it is termed *glossodynia*. Patients may also describe subjective dryness of the mouth, paraesthesia, and altered taste.

DIAGNOSIS

There is no definite diagnostic test for FOPS, and the diagnosis is made on the basis of appropriate signalment, elimination of other explanations, and identification of contributory causes (Box 16-1).

BOX 16-1   Criteria Supporting a Diagnosis of Feline Orofacial Pain Syndrome (FOPS)

1. Signs suggesting unilateral oral pain
2. No deficit of facial sensation
3. Pain evoked by triggers such as mouth movement (eating, drinking, grooming)
4. Exaggerated response—it is not normal to mutilate and this behavior in itself would suggest a disorder of sensory processing
5. Failure to respond to routine analgesia (nonsteroidal antiinflammatory drugs and opioids) and dental treatment
6. Appropriate signalment—Burmese cat or cross

History-Taking

When investigating a FOPS case it is paramount to spend some time establishing the cat's environment and social interactions, especially with other cats. This behavioral history-taking needs to be extensive and to include information about the cat, its social environment, both feline and human, and its physical environment. In some cases the general practitioner may feel able to do this but in others the possibility of referral to a veterinary behaviorist or other suitably qualified animal behaviorist may need to be considered. History-taking must also include exploring the previous medical history and this is obviously within the remit of the general practitioner.

Information about the cat's physical environment is relevant in cases of both single and multicat households. Cats have a fundamental need to be in control and to be able to access vital resources freely and immediately. It is important to determine locations of water, food, resting sites, and latrines and to observe the layout of the property in terms of the ability of the cat(s) to traverse their territory without running the gauntlet of other cats. Where the cats have access to outdoors it will be important to have information about the siting of cat flaps or the way in which the cat gains access to the outdoor world if a flap is not available. Points of entry and exit need to be freely accessible, and in multicat households and neighborhoods, restriction of movement through the territory can be a significant source of stress.

Since social stress is a very important factor in many cases of FOPS it is essential to investigate feline relationships within multicat households and also to ask questions about interactions between neighborhood cats. Asking clients to closely observe their cats over a 7-day period in order to detect affiliative behavioral interactions such as allogrooming and allorubbing will help to establish how many social groups of cats are residing within the household. It has been shown that owners are often unaware of tension between household cats when that tension is passive in nature, and it is vital that veterinary practices do not rely solely on the clients' perception of their cats' relationships when determining the possibility of social tension being a factor in cases of FOPS (see Chapter 26).

Information about visual access points, from which the resident cat(s) can observe the outdoor environment and neighborhood cats can potentially visually intrude into the house, is extremely important since social stress can result from visual as well as actual invasion of the core territory. Questions should be asked to determine whether neighborhood cats are able to lurk within gardens, on top of sheds, fences, or walls, and restrict the resident cat's free access to its outdoor environment (see Chapter 26).

House visits are ideal to enable the veterinarian to fully understand the layout of the home and neighborhood and thereby identify potential sources of stress, but for many practices this is not an option. Modern technology has opened up the possibility of virtual house visits through applications such as Facetime and Skype and these should be considered as a way of maximizing the ability to adequately investigate the role of stress in FOPS cases, but also in any medical cases where compromising of normal feline behavior within the domestic environment plays a role (see Chapter 12).

Clinical Examination

Orofacial pain can occur because of a disease of many tissues, such as the meninges, cornea, tooth pulp, oral/nasal mucosa, and temporomandibular joint.

It is important to differentiate FOPS from trigeminal neuropathy. Most trigeminal neuropathies will result in a sensory deficit to the skin and eye, and so it is essential to check facial and corneal sensation (Figure 16-8). Motor trigeminal deficits will result in atrophy of the masticatory muscle and decreased jaw tone. As the trigeminal nerve is in close proximity to other neural structures, it is unusual to see a trigeminal lesion in isolation, and there may also be facial muscle paralysis and dry eye (facial nerve); Horner's syndrome (sympathetic supply to the eye); head tilt and other vestibular signs (vestibular nerve), depressed mental status, and paresis (brainstem) (Figure 16-9). In contrast, in FOPS the neurological findings are normal. The mouth should be inspected carefully because of the association of FOPS with odontoclastic resorptive and other oral lesions and also to determine if there are alternative explanations for the discomfort. Odontoclastic resorption lesions are characterized by a zone of inflamed gingiva over the lesion. The area of inflammation is generally

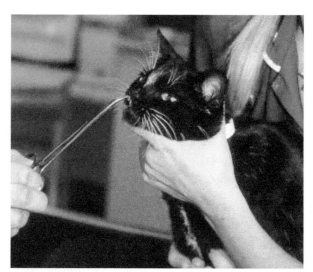

FIGURE 16-8 Assessing facial sensation in a cat. Using artery forceps the skin is tickled or lightly squeezed in several sites including the nostrils, the lips, and the ears. Intact facial sensation is indicated by facial muscle movement, that is, ear twitch or lip retraction and a behavioral response

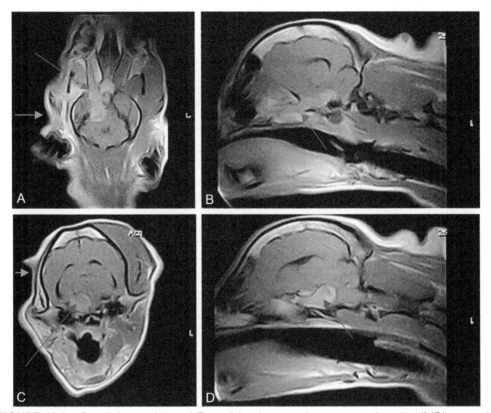

FIGURE 16-9 Gadolinium enhanced T1-weighted magnetic resonance imaging (MRI) scans in multiple planes (**A,** dorsal at level of skull base; **B,** parasagittal at level of infraorbital canal; **C,** transverse at level of pons; **D,** midsagittal,) from an 11-year-old West Highland White terrier that was initially presented with a right-sided corneal ulcer and subsequently developed a right-sided head tilt. Neurological examination also revealed a right-sided Horner's syndrome with reduced tear production (dry eye). There was right sided facial nerve paralysis and absent facial sensation also on the right. There was also extensive atrophy of the right masticatory muscles, depressed mental status, and a right-sided hemiparesis. The MRI scan demonstrates the extensive masticatory muscle atrophy *(green arrow)* and suggests a trigeminal nerve root tumor. The thickened and gadolinium contrast enhanced maxillary branch of the trigeminal nerve can be appreciated extending through the infraorbital canal *(red arrow)*. At the level of the trigeminal nerve root there a large mass compressing the pons *(blue arrow)*.

circular and is highly vascular and edematous. Introduction of a probe can reveal a depression in the sulcus area and is typically associated with pronounced gingival bleeding (see Figure 16-7).[39]

Laboratory Testing

There are no specific hematological or serum biochemistry abnormalities in the case of FOPS. However, it is important to obtain at least a minimal database to rule out contributory systemic disease and identify if there is any contraindications to medical management. In addition, determining the cat's retroviral status is recommended.

Diagnostic Imaging

Dental radiographs are a pivotal part of a diagnostic workup for a FOPS case. Radiographs are best performed with a dental x-ray machine and ideally full mouth intraoral radiographs should be obtained, although an

idea of status can be ascertained initially by the right and left mandibular premolar and molar views.[53] A full mouth series would include a parallel technique for lateral views of the caudal mandibular dentition; a bisecting angle technique for all maxillary and the rostral mandibular teeth; lateral views of the canines, premolars and molars; mesio-distal or rostro-caudal views of the incisors and canines; and oblique views of the maxillary fourth premolars. The changes associated with odontoclastic resorptive lesions are usually obvious (Figure 16-10) and characterized by lysis of tooth tissue, typically in the sulcus at the cemento-enamel junction; however, early cases may be difficult to spot and the radiograph should be examined carefully against a strong light with a magnifying glass or by enlargement of digital radiographs.[39] MRI (see Figures 16-2, 16-4, and 16-9) is useful to rule out other causes of trigeminal disease and is unremarkable in the instance of FOPS.

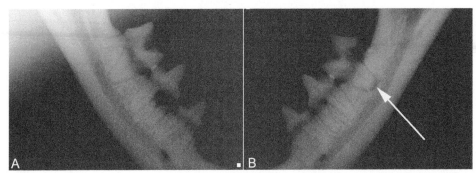

FIGURE 16-10 Lateral radiographs of the mandibular premolars from a 6.8-year-old neutered female Burmese cat that was presented with a third of five episodes of feline orofacial pain syndrome (FOPS). In this instance she was found to have a generalized grade 2 gingivitis (bleeding on probing) with a number of 'missing' teeth. Dental radiographs confirmed odontoclastic resorptive lesions on a premolar and molar tooth. In addition there is marked gingival recession and horizontal bone loss, and a periapical abscess of the rostral root of the left molar (arrow). Treatment included surgical extractions of all cheek teeth distal to the canines in addition to oral medication with phenobarbital for 2 weeks after the procedure. Other FOPS episodes this cat suffered were at 5 months old (erupting permanent canine teeth); 5.5 years old (oral ulceration); 7.5 years old (attendance at a cat show) and 8 years (stay in a cattery). (Courtesy Lisa Milella BVSc, DipEVDC, MRCVS)

MANAGEMENT

Figure 16-11 illustrates the diagnostic and management approach to FOPS. Until discomfort can be controlled, mutilation may need to be prevented by using an Elizabethan collar and/or paw bandaging or plastic nail caps such as "Soft Claws" or "Soft Paws". If this approach is taken it must be remembered that using barrier methods of this sort can be a source of stress and therefore the stress reduction part of the management approach will be all the more important.

Stress Reduction

Any systemic or environmental influences should be addressed. Clients need to be informed about the interplay between pain and stress and understand the need to implement behavioral as well as physical treatment for these cases. Optimizing the home environment from a feline perspective will involve understanding the fundamental principles of feline behavior, such as the need to be in control and to have free and immediate access to resources at all times. Using house plans similar to those used in the investigation of primary behavioral disorders such as house soiling (see Chapter 24) will help the veterinarian to identify problems associated with the distribution of the cat's five essential feline resources—food, water, resting places, latrines, and points of entry and exit into the territory. The plans can also be helpful in discussions with the client as to how the distribution can be optimized. In households where more than one social group is identified, the importance of establishing distinctly separate resource stations must be explained (see Chapter 26) and in multicat neighborhoods it may be necessary to prevent visual intrusion through the use of blinds or temporary frosting on the windows and to prevent physical intrusion through the use of microchip operated cat flaps. The resident cat will need a safe and secure core territory and the ability to access hideouts and places of elevation in order to control stress. Use of commercially available feline facial pheromone F3 within the home environment can be useful as a means of increasing the sensation of safety, but will only be beneficial when used alongside environmental modifications (see Chapter 18). The use of pharmacological approaches to stress management may also need to be considered, and these are discussed in the section on pharmacological treatment of FOPS.

Periodontal Disease

In many cats, dealing with the dental disease together with supplying appropriate analgesia results in resolution of the signs, but it is important to apply the most appropriate management regime as inappropriate treatment may perpetuate or even trigger FOPS. There have been many cases of FOPS that have developed following routine dental treatment and extractions. In particular atomization of tooth roots (burring away the roots) should only be performed with a high speed hand piece and by an experienced operator. Damage to vital structures including the sensory nerve can occur if the alveolar bone is compromised. One of the characteristics of neuropathic pain is persistent pain in the absence of or after the initial inciting cause is removed, and some cases of FOPS do not resolve after the predisposing causes are addressed. Referral to a veterinary dental

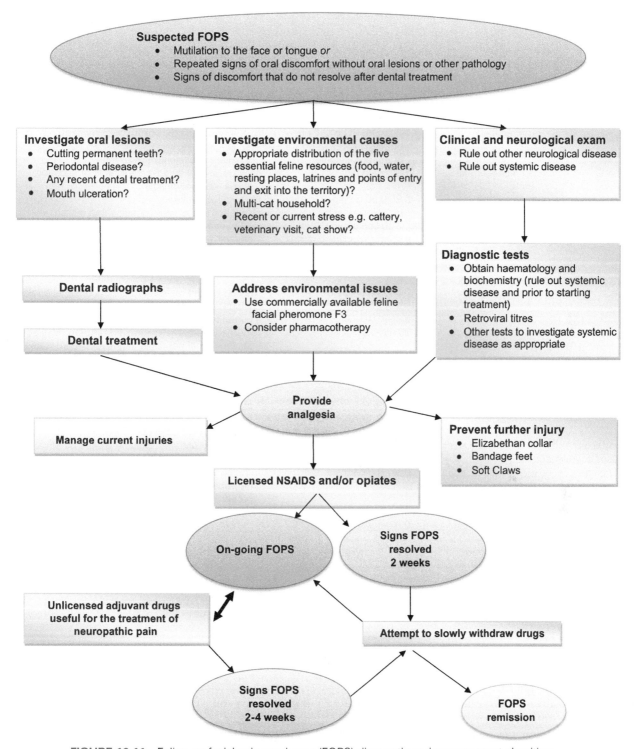

FIGURE 16-11   Feline orofacial pain syndrome (FOPS) diagnostic and management algorithm.

specialist is recommended if the expertise and equipment are not available to extract teeth correctly or to treat FOPS.

Pharmacological Treatment of FOPS

First line analgesia for FOPS should be with licensed nonsteroidal antiinflammatory drugs (NSAIDs) and opioids. However, because neuropathic pain involves disordered somatosensory nervous system processing, this therapy is insufficient in many cases. Drugs used for treating neuropathic pain target the mechanisms of "wind-up," that is, decreasing excitation or increasing inhibition (Table 16-2). Unfortunately, many agents available for treating neuropathic pain in humans have not been established for use in the cat

TABLE 16-2 **Adjuvant Analgesics for Treatment of Neuropathic Pain in the Cat**

Target	Drug	Dose	Notes
DECREASING EXCITATION			
Glutamate	Gabapentin	3-10 mg/kg q 12-24 hrs	Oral suspension is sweetened with xylitol and therefore not recommended. Smallest capsule size is 100 mg; however it is possible to obtain compounded preparations.
	Pregabalin	1-5 mg/kg PO q12-24 hr titrating up based on effect and sedation	In humans binds to receptor with more affinity and for longer. Smallest capsule size is 25 mg.
	Phenobarbital	1-3 mg/kg bid	May be limited by adverse effects of sedation, ataxia, and polyphagia.
NMDA Receptor	Ketamine	0.25-0.50 mg/kg IV loading dose followed by 2-20 µg/kg/min CRI	Hospitalized patients. Often combined with lidocaine and morphine.
Sodium channel	Lidocaine	0.25 mg/kg loading dose followed by 0.6-1.5 mg/kg/hr (10-25 µg/kg/min) CRI	Hospitalized patients. Often combined with ketamine and morphine.
	Amitriptyline	0.5-2.0 mg/kg sid	May be limited by adverse effects of sedation and weight gain. Psychotropic properties may be useful for FOPS associated with anxiety.
	Carbamazepine	25 mg bid	In humans carbamazepine is first line (and licensed) for trigeminal neuralgia, however oxcarbazepine associated with less adverse effects.
DECREASING INHIBITION			
GABA receptor[54]	Phenobarbital	1-3 mg/kg bid	May be limited by adverse effects of sedation, ataxia, and weight gain.
	Diazepam	0.1-0.5 mg/kg sid-bid	May be limited by adverse effects of sedation, ataxia, and weight gain.
Noradrenalin (locus coeruleus)	Dexmedetomidine	40 µg/kg IV or IM	Hospitalized patients. May be limited by adverse effects of sedation.[55]
Serotonin	Fluoxetine	0.5-1.0 mg/kg sid	In humans SSRI are less useful for treating neuropathic pain, however psychotropic properties may be useful for FOPS associated with anxiety.
Opioid	Buprenorphine	0.02 mg/kg transbuccal tid-qid	May be limited by anorexia.[56]
	Butorphanol	0.2-1.0 mg/kg qid	Limited bioavailability and duration.[57,58]

Note that none of these drugs have been assessed for dosage or efficacy in FOPS, therefore empirical doses and efficacy reflect dose recommendations for other painful conditions and the experience of the authors. None of the drugs are licensed for treating neuropathic pain in the cat. All cats receiving long-term adjuvant analgesics should have periodic blood sampling to assess serum biochemistry with hematology.

bid, Twice a day; *CRI,* constant rate infusion; *FOPS,* feline orofacial pain syndrome; *IM,* intramuscular; *IV,* intravenous; *PO,* by mouth; *qid,* four times a day; *sid,* once a day; *SSRI,* selective serotonin reuptake inhibitors; *tid,* three times a day.

either because the pharmacokinetics are unknown or that they have already been established as unsuitable. Based on the limited information and studies performed to date then the most logical oral adjuvant analgesic for oral therapy is phenobarbital or gabapentin.[33] For acute management of hospitalized cases, other drugs such as parental phenobarbital and/or constant rate infusion of lidocaine, ketamine, morphine, and/or dexmedetomidine may be useful. When the physical signs of FOPS have been brought under control it is important to continue to assess the potential for stressors within the cat's environment and the level of anxiety that the cat is experiencing. It is always advisable to address the social and environmental stressors on an ongoing basis, but there may be some cases where medication to reduce anxiety is necessary while optimization of the environment is achieved. In such cases treatment with selective serotonin reuptake inhibitors (SSRIs) may be considered (see Chapter 19).

ACKNOWLEDGMENTS

The authors are grateful to Penny Knowler for assistance in figure preparation, to Drs. Christine Hawke and Anne Fawcett for their helpful comments on dental management, and to Dr. Richard Malik for reading and commenting on the manuscript.

REFERENCES

1. Merskey H, Bogduk N. *Pain terms, a current list with definitions and notes on usage, classification of chronic pain.* 2nd ed. Seattle: IASP Press; 1994.
2. Woolf CJ, Mannion RJ. Neuropathic pain: aetiology, symptoms, mechanisms, and management. *Lancet.* 1999;353 (9168):1959–1964.
3. Herrero JF, Laird JM, Lopez-Garcia JA. Wind-up of spinal cord neurones and pain sensation: much ado about something? *Prog Neurobiol.* 2000;61(2):169–203.
4. Todd AJ, ed. *Neuronal circuits and receptors involved in spinal cord pain processing.* Seattle: ISAP Press; 2009.
5. Evans HE, De Lahunta A. Cranial nerves. In: *Miller's anatomy of the dog.* 4th ed. St Louis: Elsevier Saunders; 2013:708–730.
6. Fried K, Bongenhielm U, Boissonade FM, Robinson PP. Nerve injury-induced pain in the trigeminal system. *Neuroscientist.* 2001;7(2):155–165.
7. Robinson PP. The course, relations and distribution of the inferior alveolar nerve and its branches in the cat. *Anat Rec.* 1979;195(2):265–271.
8. Takemura M, Sugiyo S, Moritani M, et al. Mechanisms of orofacial pain control in the central nervous system. *Arch Histol Cytol.* 2006;69(2):79–100.
9. Andrew D, Matthews B. Displacement of the contents of dentinal tubules and sensory transduction in intradental nerves of the cat. *J Physiol.* 2000;529(Pt 3):791–802.
10. Narhi M, Jyvasjarvi E, Virtanen A, et al. Role of intradental A- and C-type nerve fibres in dental pain mechanisms. *Proc Finn Dent Soc.* 1992;88(Suppl 1):507–516.
11. Dessem D, Luo P. Jaw-muscle spindle afferent feedback to the cervical spinal cord in the rat. *Exp Brain Res.* 1999;128 (4):451–459.
12. Narhi M, Hirvonen T, Jyvasjarvi E, Huopaniemi T. Reflex responses in the digastric and tongue muscles to stimulation of intradental nerves in the cat. *Proc Finn Dent Soc.* 1989;85 (4–5):383–387.
13. Byers MR, Narhi MV. Dental injury models: experimental tools for understanding neuroinflammatory interactions and polymodal nociceptor functions. *Crit Rev Oral Biol Med.* 1999;10(1):4–39.
14. Byers MR, Wheeler EF, Bothwell M. Altered expression of NGF and P75 NGF-receptor by fibroblasts of injured teeth precedes sensory nerve sprouting. *Growth Factors.* 1992;6(1):41–52.
15. Li YQ, Li H, Wei J, et al. Expression changes of K+ -Cl- co-transporter 2 and Na+ -K+ -Cl- co-transporter1 in mouse trigeminal subnucleus caudalis following pulpal inflammation. *Brain Res Bull.* 2010;81(6):561–564.
16. Bowles WR, Withrow JC, Lepinski AM, Hargreaves KM. Tissue levels of immunoreactive substance P are increased in patients with irreversible pulpitis. *J Endod.* 2003;29 (4):265–267.
17. Hargreaves KM. Orofacial pain. *Pain.* 2011;152(suppl 3): S25–S32.
18. Cave NJ, Bridges JP, Thomas DG. Systemic effects of periodontal disease in cats. *Vet Q.* 2012;32(3–4):131–144.
19. Cohen LA, Harris SL, Bonito AJ, et al. Coping with toothache pain: a qualitative study of low-income persons and minorities. *J Public Health Dent.* 2007;67(1):28–35.
20. Katz DB, Nicolelis MA, Simon SA. Nutrient tasting and signaling mechanisms in the gut. IV. There is more to taste than meets the tongue. *Am J Physiol Gastrointest Liver Physiol.* 2000;278(1):G6–G9.
21. Moretti R, Torre P, Antonello RM, et al. Gabapentin treatment of glossopharyngeal neuralgia: a follow-up of four years of a single case. *Eur J Pain.* 2002;6(5):403–407.
22. Lazarov NE. Comparative analysis of the chemical neuroanatomy of the mammalian trigeminal ganglion and mesencephalic trigeminal nucleus. *Prog Neurobiol.* 2002;66 (1):19–59.
23. Shigenaga Y, Okamoto T, Nishimori T, et al. Oral and facial representation in the trigeminal principal and rostral spinal nuclei of the cat. *J Comp Neurol.* 1986;244(1):1–18.
24. Marfurt CF. The central projections of trigeminal primary afferent neurons in the cat as determined by the tranganglionic transport of horseradish peroxidase. *J Comp Neurol.* 1981;203(4):785–798.
25. Azerad J, Woda A, Albe-Fessard D. Physiological properties of neurons in different parts of the cat trigeminal sensory complex. *Brain Res.* 1982;246(1):7–21.
26. Barnett EM, Evans GD, Sun N, et al. Anterograde tracing of trigeminal afferent pathways from the murine tooth pulp to cortex using herpes simplex virus type 1. *J Neurosci.* 1995;15 (4):2972–2984.
27. Iannetti GD, Mouraux A. From the neuromatrix to the pain matrix (and back). *Exp Brain Res.* 2010;205(1):1–12.
28. Clauw DJ, Ablin JN. The relationship between "stress" and pain: Lessons learned from fibromyalgia and related conditions. In: Castro-Lopes J, ed. *Current Topics in Pain: 12th World Congress on Pain.* Seattle: ISAP Press; 2009:245–270.
29. Moseley GL. A pain neuromatrix approach to patients with chronic pain. *Man Ther.* 2003;8(3):130–140.
30. Gandolfi B, Rusbridge C, Malik R, Lyons LA, eds. You're getting on my nerves! Feline orofacial pain syndrome. In: *7th International Conference on Advances in Canine and Feline Genomics and Inherited Diseases 2013*; September 23–27, 2013, Boston.
31. Noseda R, Burstein R. Migraine pathophysiology: Anatomy of the trigeminovascular pathway and associated neurological symptoms, cortical spreading depression, sensitization, and modulation of pain. *Pain.* 2013;154(suppl 1):S44–S53.
32. Mollaoglu M. Trigger factors in migraine patients. *J Health Psychol.* 2013;18(7):984–994.
33. Rusbridge C, Heath S, Gunn-Moore DA, et al. Feline orofacial pain syndrome (FOPS): a retrospective study of 113 cases. *J Feline Med Surg.* 2010;12(6):498–508.
34. Bennett GJ. Neuropathic pain in the orofacial region: clinical and research challenges. *J Orofac Pain.* 2004;18(4):281–286.
35. Westrum LE, Johnson LR, Canfield RC. Ultrastructure of transganglionic degeneration in brain stem trigeminal nuclei during normal primary tooth exfoliation and permanent tooth eruption in the cat. *J Comp Neurol.* 1984;230 (2):198–206.
36. Westrum LE, Canfield RC. Normal loss of milk teeth causes degeneration in brain stem. *Exp Neurol.* 1979;65(1):169–177.
37. Brenan A. Innervation of the dental pulp during tooth succession in the cat. *Brain Res.* 1986;382(2):250–256.
38. Ingham KE, Gorrel C, Blackburn J, Farnsworth W. Prevalence of odontoclastic resorptive lesions in a population of clinically healthy cats. *J Small Anim Pract.* 2001;42 (9):439–443.
39. Johnston N. Acquired feline oral cavity disease Part 2: Feline odontoclastic resorptive lesions. *In Pract.* 2000;22:188–197.
40. Hirvonen T, Ngassapa D, Narhi M. Relation of dentin sensitivity to histological changes in dog teeth with exposed and stimulated dentin. *Proc Finn Dent Soc.* 1992;88(suppl 1):133–141.
41. Narhi M, Yamamoto H, Ngassapa D, Hirvonen T. The neurophysiological basis and the role of inflammatory reactions in dentine hypersensitivity. *Arch Oral Biol.* 1994;39 (Suppl:23S–30S).

42. Narhi M, Kontturi-Narhi V, Hirvonen T, Ngassapa D. Neurophysiological mechanisms of dentin hypersensitivity. *Proc Finn Dent Soc.* 1992;88(suppl 1):15–22.

43. Low LA. The impact of pain upon cognition: what have rodent studies told us? *Pain.* 2013;154(12):2603–2605.

44. McNeil DW, Au AR, Zvolensky MJ, et al. Fear of pain in orofacial pain patients. *Pain.* 2001;89(2–3):245–252.

45. Buffington AL, Hanlon CA, McKeown MJ. Acute and persistent pain modulation of attention-related anterior cingulate fMRI activations. *Pain.* 2005;113 (1–2):172–184.

46. Rivat C, Becker C, Blugeot A, et al. Chronic stress induces transient spinal neuroinflammation, triggering sensory hypersensitivity and long-lasting anxiety-induced hyperalgesia. *Pain.* 2010;150(2):358–368.

47. Weissman-Fogel I, Moayedi M, Tenenbaum HC, et al. Abnormal cortical activity in patients with temporomandibular disorder evoked by cognitive and emotional tasks. *Pain.* 2011;152(2):384–396.

48. Feuerstein M, Sult S, Houle M. Environmental stressors and chronic low back pain: life events, family and work environment. *Pain.* 1985;22(3):295–307.

49. Bravo L, Alba-Delgado C, Torres-Sanchez S, et al. Social stress exacerbates the aversion to painful experiences in rats exposed to chronic pain: The role of the locus coeruleus. *Pain.* 2013;154(10):2014–2023.

50. Labat JJ, Riant T, Delavierre D, et al. Approche globale des douleurs pelviperineales chroniques: du concept de douleur d'organe a celui de dysfonctionnement des systemes de regulation de la douleur viscerale. [Global approach to chronic pelvic and perineal pain: from the concept of organ pain to that of dysfunction of visceral pain regulation systems]. *Prog Urol.* 2010;20(12):1027–1034.

51. Headache Classification Committee of the International Headache Society (IHS). The International Classification of Headache Disorders, 3rd edition (beta version). *Cephalalgia.* 2013;33(9):629–808.

52. Pollack IF, Jannetta PJ, Bissonette DJ. Bilateral trigeminal neuralgia: a 14-year experience with microvascular decompression. *J Neurosurg.* 1988;68(4):559–565.

53. Heaton M, Wilkinson J, Gorrel C, Butterwick R. A rapid screening technique for feline odontoclastic resorptive lesions. *J Small Anim Pract.* 2004;45(12):598–601.

54. Stoyanova II. Gamma-aminobutiric acid immunostaining in trigeminal, nodose and spinal ganglia of the cat. *Acta Histochem.* 2004;106(4):309–314.

55. Porters N, Bosmans T, Debille M, et al. Sedative and antinociceptive effects of dexmedetomidine and buprenorphine after oral transmucosal or intramuscular administration in cats. *Vet Anaesth Analg.* 2014;41(1):90–96.

56. Robertson SA, Lascelles BD, Taylor PM, Sear JW. PK-PD modeling of buprenorphine in cats: intravenous and oral transmucosal administration. *J Vet Pharmacol Ther.* 2005;28(5):453–460.

57. Carroll GL, Howe LB, Slater MR, et al. Evaluation of analgesia provided by postoperative administration of butorphanol to cats undergoing onychectomy. *J Am Vet Med Assoc.* 1998;213 (2):246–250.

58. Wells SM, Glerum LE, Papich MG. Pharmacokinetics of butorphanol in cats after intramuscular and buccal transmucosal administration. *Am J Vet Res.* 2008;69 (12):1548–1554.

PART 6

Management and Treatment of Undesirable Behaviors

Understanding Emotions

Christos Karagiannis and Sarah Heath

INTRODUCTION

All mammals, including human and nonhuman animals like cats, monitor their circumstances, evaluate them, and act through defined subcortical brain circuits with different neurobiological bases, the primal emotional systems.[1] These brain circuits, as a first step, represent the individual's filters which filter the stimuli from the external world to create an internal representation of any circumstance, and as a second step, activate the trigger for the resulting behavioral response. Consequently, the activation of these brain circuits is responsible for the majority of the behavioral actions. However, as a behavioral action can be the same for different emotional systems, the role of the veterinarian working in a behavioral context is to diagnose the underlying etiology of the behavior in order to modify it and not just to focus on the modification of the unwanted or problematic behavior *per se*. From a clinical perspective, when conversing with any client about their pet cat, it is common to hear descriptions of the animal's behavior which incorporate a recognition of emotional state. Comments such as "he really likes that" or "she is scared of him" indicate that clients consider their pet to have emotional responses which are not dissimilar from their own (Figure 17-1). However, animal's emotions involve scientifically identifiable physiological and behavioral components and are not only an anthropomorphic description by the animal's owners.

The study of animal behavior has progressed significantly in recent years, and within a scientific context researchers also discuss animal emotions in terms of multifactorial states with physiological and behavioral components. Because conscious expression of emotion in people is usually achieved through speech, there has been a tendency in the past to dismiss other species as being less emotionally complex than ourselves. However, there are other potential methods to investigate emotional states and recent interest in studying cognitive components of emotions in animals has helped to increase our understanding of both production and companion animals at an emotional level.[2] Working in a veterinary context, an appreciation of the emotional

responses of patients is crucial if their behavior is to be understood and their welfare safeguarded.

Understanding the Emotional Responses of Feline Patients

The need to understand emotional states pervades every part of feline practice, influencing everything from how to approach and handle feline patients in consultations and during hospitalization, to making diagnoses and selecting treatment regimes for both medical and behavioral cases. When clinicians are faced with a pet cat with a behavioral problem, it is important to understand that simply modifying the unwanted behavior without addressing the underlying emotional motivation is like treating a medical symptom without investigating the underlying disease state. Neither are good practice and both present potential threats to the welfare of the patient concerned. As veterinary practitioners, it is necessary to approach behavioral cases through an internal medicine paradigm and to use exactly the same clinical skills to reach an accurate diagnosis. In addition, it is increasingly recognized that emotional state and physical health are inextricably interlinked and therefore an emotional diagnosis may also be an important part of the clinical approach to a range of feline medical conditions. An understanding of the emotional responses of feline patients is therefore the cornerstone of good feline practice.

EMOTIONS

One of the main objections to the discussion of emotions in the context of companion animals has been related to the fact that human understanding of emotions is based on the study of the phenomenological experience of humans through the analysis of what people verbally report. The question is therefore raised: how is it possible to discuss the emotions of nonhuman animals if they are not able to describe them verbally?

The first part of the answer to that question is that emotions are not the same as "emotional feelings" as understood in human terms. Emotions are motivational–emotional systems which mediate instinctual

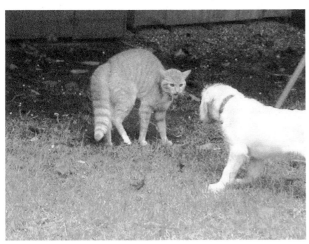

FIGURE 17-1   Owners will readily label certain behaviors in their pet cats according to the emotion they feel is involved—for example in this situation the owner would say that this cat is "scared of the puppy."

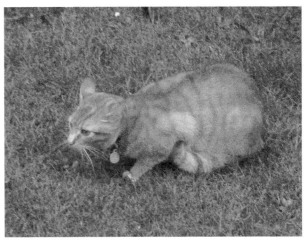

FIGURE 17-2   Defensive behavior is shown by the retraction of the ears and piloerection. If the perceived threat advances, more intense signals such as arching of the back, hissing, and unsheathing of the claws may follow.

emotional arousal.[3] The second part of the answer comes from behavioral and affective neuroscientific studies, which study those instinctual emotional arousals that are displayed naturally as well as in response to deep brain stimulation.[4]

Nowadays, despite important progress in human brain imaging and some early steps towards mapping emotions in humans, the use of similar techniques such as positron emission tomography (PET) and functional magnetic resonance imaging (fMRI) is still in its infancy in animal studies.[5]

One of the first neuroanatomical and behavioral discriminations in the motivational–emotional systems of cats was made by Siegel et al,[6] who studied phenomenally similar aggressive behaviors and described different motivations and different distinct neural circuits. Cats' brain areas were stimulated with electrical stimuli and systemic and intracerebral injections and the displayed behaviors were monitored. Stimulation of the medial hypothalamus was associated with defensive behavior (piloerection, retraction of the ears, arching of the back, marked pupillary dilatation, vocalization–hissing, and unsheathing of the claws), whereas stimulation of the perifornical lateral hypothalamus was associated with quiet-biting predatory attack behavior (stalking, quiet-biting), which was a very similar reaction to natural behavior (Figures 17-2 and 17-3).[6]

From an affective neuroscientific perspective,[3] adapted and developed from Pankseep,[1] the motivational–emotional systems can be classified into different systems.

The Desire System

The arousal of this system induces cats to be intensely interested in exploring their world and increases the potential of seeking and consummatory activity. It

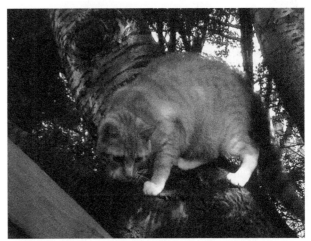

FIGURE 17-3   Predatory attack is preceded by alert stalking behavior.

eventually allows cats to eagerly anticipate and find all kinds of resources they need for survival, such as water, food, warmth, and coolness.[4] Predation is a manifestation of the arousal of the desire system focusing on finding food resources and it is not a different motivational–emotional system (Figure 17-4). Consequently, solitary object play and not social play is triggered by the desire system, as it promotes appetitive learning and learning to predate, and thereby increases cats' excitability when they are about to get what they desire, for example a cat playing with a string (Figure 17-5).[7]

The desire system can be incorrectly conceptualized as simply the "reward" or "pleasure" system, but in reality it appears to be a general purpose neuronal system that coaxes cats to move to places where they have more potential for finding and consuming the resources needed for survival.[4] Furthermore, the desire system promotes learning by assimilating predictive reward relationships

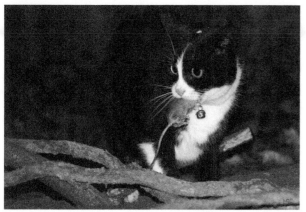

FIGURE 17-4 Predation is a manifestation of the arousal of the desire system. (Courtesy A. Dossche)

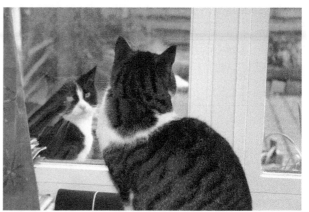

FIGURE 17-6 The sight of other cats in the garden can trigger the frustration system. (Courtesy A. Dossche)

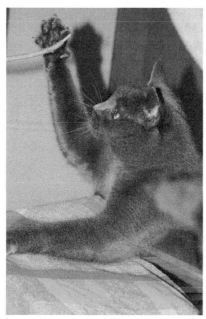

FIGURE 17-5 The desire system in action. (Courtesy A. Dossche)

in the world.[8] For that reason, if this motivational–emotional system is damaged, animals become terminally unmotivated and can die "in the midst of plenty."[4]

The critically important neurochemicals in the activation of this system are dopamine, glutamate, opioids, and neurotensin.[9]

The Frustration System

The frustration system attempts to curtail an animal's freedom of action[4] and integrates the personal significance of a failure to meet expectations, obtain resources, or retain control.[3] This system intensifies and accelerates behavioral responses and is associated with aggressive behaviors when cats do not have control over a situation, are irritated, or restrained. It also helps cats to defend themselves by arousing fear in their opponents.[4] For example, when a cat is fussed for a prolonged period of time it may be irritated (frustrated) and may

need to adapt active strategies to avoid the irritation, like hissing, scratching, or biting the person who pets it. At other times, if the cat cannot directly solve the problem, it may attempt to resolve it by directing its behavioral response toward something other than the cause of the problem. In these cases the frustration is focused on the thwarting of the behavior rather than the cause of it, and is often referred to as *redirected behavior*. For example, when two cats live indoors and one of them sees a strange cat in the garden through the window it may enter a frustrated state (Figure 17-6). If the indoor cat had access to the garden it could run outside and chase, threaten, or swipe out at the strange cat if it did not retreat, but because it is forced to remain inside and the window blocks access to the outside, the cat can becomes frustrated. If at that moment the second cat of the household comes near, the first cat may attack it.[3]

Behavioral differences between the frustration system and the fear–anxiety system were found in a study of Scottish wildcats, which will be discussed later in this chapter.[10]

The key neuromodulators associated with activation of the frustration system are dopamine, glutamate, substance P, and acetylcholine, whereas the main neuromodulator for the inhibition of this system is neuropeptide Y.[9]

The Fear–Anxiety System

The fear–anxiety system relates to the preservation of comfort provided by predictable access to essential resources and the management of threats to personal or resource security[3] (Figure 17-7). When this system is stimulated intensely, the circuit leads cats to flee or avoid the situation, but with weaker stimuli, cats may exhibit a freezing or inhibited behavioral response.[4] If cats are not able to choose either avoidance or inhibition strategies, a more active response, a repulsion response, may be adopted. For example, many cats that are not familiar with young children may be afraid of them and may feel the urge to avoid them in order to be secure. If the children run towards the cat and try initiating play, the cat may need to protect itself and indicate through active

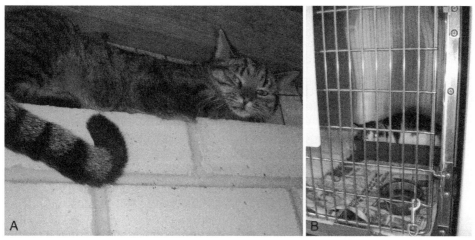

FIGURE 17-7   These two cats are showing behavior consistent with the fear–anxiety system. **A,** The cat is elevating and hiding within its rescue center enclosur. **B,** The cat is hiding within the litter box in a veterinary hospitalization cage. Both cats are using a combination of avoidance and then inhibition to manage a perceived threat to their personal security.

repulsion responses, such as hissing or scratching, that the cat needs more space in order to feel secure. In a clinical context it is important to remember that this system can be triggered if cats visit an environment where they have been frightened in the past, such as the veterinary practice. In this context the cat is anticipating a potential negative event and may start to show behavioral responses prior to exposure to the actual stimulus, for example becoming agitated on entering the parking lot of the veterinary practice or being aggressive to the owners when they are just placing the cat carrier next to the cat at home. This fear–anxiety system intrinsically helps animals to avoid dangers and it is more adaptive to feel anticipatory fear (anxiety) than to be attacked and harmed.[4]

Recently there has been interest in the role of facial expressions in differentiating between underlying emotional motivations for behavioral responses. A preliminary behavioral study of Scottish wildcats by Finka et al[10] examined the spontaneous facial responses of cats related to the fear–anxiety system and the frustration system. In one situation a person approached the cat, creating a stimulus associated with the fear–anxiety system, and in a second situation the cat was briefly denied access to food at feeding time, a situation associated with the frustration system. In the first situation, the fear–anxiety system, the position of the cats' ears was more downwards, whereas during the second situation, the frustration system, the cats rotated both ears and showed more right ear rotator bias.[10] More research is needed to fully understand subtle postural and facial signals, which may help to differentiate between emotional motivations. However, it is recognized that visual signaling is an important part of the communication system of the cat and it is important to remember to monitor these signals when interacting with cats in the veterinary context and when diagnosing motivations for behaviors that clients find problematic.

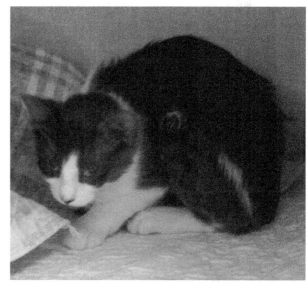

FIGURE 17-8   The pain system is related to the maintenance of body integrity and functioning, and is both a distinct sensation and a motivation. (Courtesy S. Robertson)

The important neurochemicals in the activation of the fear–anxiety system are glutamate, diazepam-binding inhibitor, corticotrophin releasing hormone, cholecystokinin, and alpha-melanocyte stimulating hormone.[9]

The Pain System

The pain system is related to the maintenance of body integrity and functioning, and is both a distinct sensation and a motivation (Figure 17-8).[11] The activation of this system is a response to the environmental stimuli which are related to actual or potential tissue damage.[3] One clinical situation in which it is important to differentiate between the fear–anxiety system and the pain system is when cats develop anxiety associated with the anticipation of a painful condition, such as an injection during vaccinations. This behavior is activated by the fear–anxiety system rather than the pain system since fear/anxiety of pain is not the same as pain *per se* and those conditions are represented by two different motivational–emotional systems.

The main neuromodulators for the pain system are glutamate, neurokinins A and B, and substance P, whereas the main neuromodulators for the inhibition of this system are GABA and opioids.[11]

The Panic–Grief System

The two previously discussed motivational–emotional systems are related to how individual cats protect themselves and their resources, but this next system is related more to the protection of the species rather than the individual. It relates to the safeguarding of the survival of kittens and therefore to the protection of the genetic survival of the species. Before they are able to protect themselves, kittens start to exhibit powerful emotional arousals indicating desperate needs for nurturing care (Figure 17-9). This is most clearly reflected in the intense meowing—"crying"—of lost kittens or those left alone in unfamiliar places. The primary function of separation meowing is to alert queens to seek, retrieve, and vigorously attend to her kittens' needs.[4] This panic–grief system is related to protection provided by others and is reflected in a need for social contact.[3] This system in kittens is a functional system to protect them and while it is less commonly activated in adult cats, who are solitary survivors and show a high level of self-sufficiency, this system can be activated in some adult cats when they are socially isolated or when they are away from an attachment figure. In those cases, the cat's isolation can be problematic for both the cat and the owner, especially in cases where cats become distressed and start showing behavioral signs of separation distress such as defecation outside of the litter tray.[12]

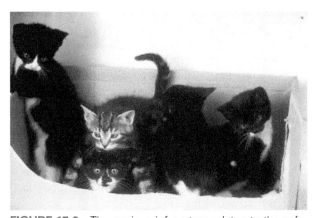

FIGURE 17-9 The panic–grief system relates to the safeguarding of the survival of kittens.

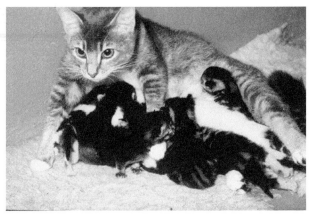

FIGURE 17-10 The care system is involved in the bonding between a queen and her kittens.

The significant neurochemicals in the activation of the panic–grief system are corticotropin-releasing hormone and glutamate, whereas those in the inhibition of this system are opioids, oxytocin, and prolactin.[9]

The Care System

In order for queens to be motivated to invest enormous amounts of time and energy in their offspring there needs to be a strong bond between her and her kittens (Figure 17-10). The motivational–emotional system referred to as the care system is dedicated to maintaining the bonds to the individual kittens through recognizable parental care or nurturance toward others.[3] This system is triggered shortly before the young are born through well-described hormonal changes (increasing estrogen, prolactin, and oxytocin and declining progesterone). The behavioral effects of this system are that the queen takes care of her kittens after their birth and for a long period of time until they are capable of looking after themselves. The mother's hormonal alterations facilitate maternal moods and intense social attraction and bonding with the offspring.[4]

Oxytocin, prolactin, dopamine, and opioids are the key neuromodulators associated with the activation of the care system.[9]

The Lust System

Prior to activation of the care system there is the need for motivation of dimorphic sexual urges which are mediated by specific brain circuits.[4] This brain circuit, which is named the lust system, organizes the specific reproductive needs, ranging from the attraction or the selection of a partner through courtship, to any potential bond, to mating with a sexual partner.[3] Within a domestic setting where the majority of cats are neutered and usually at a prepubertal stage of development the relevance of the lust system and the care system are minimized but they do need to be considered within a breeding environment (Figure 17-11).

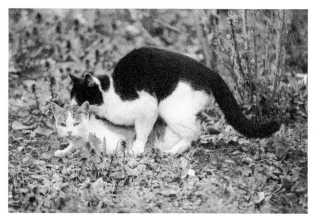

FIGURE 17-11   The lust system is involved in attraction and selection of sexual partners. (Copyright © iStock.com)

The important neurochemicals in the activation of the lust system in both genders are steroids, vasopressin, oxytocin, luteinizing releasing hormone, and cholecystokinin.[9]

The Social Play System

Cats are often considered to be aloof and solitary animals, but they are social mammals and they do need to develop various social skills, including among others being able to be part of a social group. A specific brain circuit that can give some information to individuals about their own social competence and potential in relation to others is the social play system.[3] This system is more likely to be activated in kittens who play with each other or with their parents than it is in adult cats once they are past social maturity (Figure 17-12). Young individuals have intense urges for physical play[4] in order to build up their social skills safely without agonistic encounters.[3] Social play (rough-and-tumble play) must be discriminated from object play (exploration) as the brain circuits are different and distinct, and the play styles serve different needs. Social play is activated by the social play system and, as discussed earlier, object play is activated by the desire system.

The main neuromodulators for the social play system are glutamate, opioids, and acetylcholine, whereas the main neuromodulators for the inhibition of this system are the opioids.[9]

CONCLUSION

As described in the previous paragraphs, there are eight different motivational–emotional systems that serve specific biological needs, that is investigation for resources (desire system), access to the resources and the defense of them (frustration system), avoidance of threat and harm (fear system), social attachment (panic–grief system), sexual partnering (lust system), parental behavior (care system), avoidance of tissue damage (pain system) and the

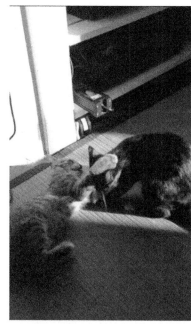

FIGURE 17-12   The social play system is activated in kittens when they play with one another.

opportunity for motor and cognitive clarification of future social behaviors (play system).[2] However, a behavior can be triggered by more than one emotion as emotional responses are not mutually exclusive and more than one may occur at any given time within an individual.[13] For example a cat that reacts adversely to clinical examination by the veterinarian, may be due to a combination of frustration (due to the physical manipulations) and pain. On the other hand, not all behaviors are activated by symbolic emotional elements. For example, remarkable predictable nonharmful events can often trigger a relatively unemotional response, which through repetition can become habitual.[3] Table 17-1 contains a brief description of the role of each motivational–emotional system, examples of related behavioral problems, and a summary of the main neuromodulators associated with each system.

The clinical implications within the context of feline veterinary practice are far reaching. Understanding and identifying the underlying motivational–emotional systems which are responsible for feline behavior, be that problematic behavior presented by the client, unwanted behavioral responses within the veterinary practice, or behavioral complications of medical conditions, is essential. It will enable clinicians to learn to handle feline patients appropriately and to offer appropriate treatment, both medical and behavioral, which can lead to lasting results. Simply managing or suppressing unwanted behavioral responses runs the risk of masking important emotional changes and creating the potential for more serious behavioral and medical consequences in the future. Understanding emotions is therefore essential if the welfare of feline patients is to be respected and safeguarded.

TABLE 17-1 The Role of Each Motivational–Emotional System with Examples of Related Behavioral Problems and the Main Associated Neuromodulators of Each System

Motivational-Emotional System	Role of System	Examples of Possible Related Behavioral Problems	Neuromodulators*
Desire system	Investigation for resources	Meowing during the night (attention seeking)	Dopamine, glutamate, opioids, neurotensin
Frustration system	Access to the resources and the defense of them	Aggressive behavior while being petted	Dopamine, glutamate, substance P, acetylcholine Inhibition: neuropeptide Y
Fear–anxiety system	Avoidance of threat and harm	Toileting out of the litter box due to previous negative experiences (social or painful)	Glutamate, diazepam-binding inhibitor, corticotrophin releasing hormone, cholecystokinin, alpha melanocyte stimulating hormone
Pain system	Avoidance of tissue damage	Rapid change of cat's behavior, typical with increased aggressive behavior or hypoactivity	Glutamate, neurokinins A and B, substance P Inhibition: GABA, opioids
Panic–grief system	Social attachment	Separation related problems	Corticotrophin-releasing hormone, glutamate Inhibition: opioids, oxytocin, prolactin
Care system	Parental behavior	Poor parenting (e.g., queen rejecting her litter)	Oxytocin, prolactin, dopamine, opioids
Lust system	Sexual partnering	Urine marking (when intact animals involved)	Steroids, vasopressin, oxytocin, luteinizing releasing hormone, cholecystokinin
Play system	Opportunity to practice motor and cognitive skills and learn appropriate social behaviors	Inappropriate interactions with other cats	Glutamate, opioids, acetylcholine Inhibition: opioids

Adapted from Mills et al, 2013.[3]

REFERENCES

1. Panksepp J. *Affective neuroscience: the foundations of human and animal emotions.* New York: Oxford University Press; 1998.
2. Paul ES, Harding EJ, Mendl M. Measuring emotional processes in animals: the utility of a cognitive approach. *Neurosci Biobehav Rev.* 2005;29:469–491.
3. Mills D, Braem Dube M, Zulch H. Principles of pheromonatherapy. In: *Stress and Pheromonatherapy in Small Animal Clinical Behavior.* Chichester, UK: Wiley-Blackwell; 2013:37–68.
4. Panksepp J, Wright JS, Döbrössy MD, Schlaepfer TE, Coenen VA. Affective neuroscience strategies for understanding and treating depression from preclinical models to three novel therapeutics. *Clin Psychol Sci.* 2014;2:472–494.
5. Berns GS, Brooks AM, Spivak M. Functional MRI in awake unrestrained dogs. *PLoS One.* 2012;7:e38027.
6. Siegel A, Roeling TA, Gregg TR, Kruk MR. Neuropharmacology of brain-stimulation-evoked aggression. *Neurosci Biobehav Rev.* 1999;23:359–389.
7. Panksepp J, Moskal J. Dopamine and SEEKING: subcortical "reward" systems and appetitive urges. In: Elliot A, ed. *Handbook of Approach and Avoidance Motivation.* New York: Taylor & Francis; 2008:67–87.
8. Wright JS, Panksepp J. An evolutionary framework to understand foraging, wanting, and desire: the neuropsychology of the SEEKING system. *Neuropsychoanalysis.* 2012;14:5–39.
9. Panksepp J. Emotional endophenotypes in evolutionary psychiatry. *Prog Neuropsychopharmacol Biol Psychiatry.* 2006;30:774–784.
10. Finka L, Ellis SLH, Wilkinson A, Mills D. The development of an emotional ethogram for Felis silvestris focused on FEAR and RAGE. *J Vet Behav.* 2014;9:e5.
11. Craig AD. A new view of pain as a homeostatic emotion. *Trends Neurosci.* 2003;26:303–307.
12. Stella JL, Lord LK, Buffington T. Sickness behaviors in response to unusual environmental events in healthy cats and cats with FIC. *J Am Vet Med Assoc.* 2011;1:67–73.
13. Mills D, Karagiannis C, Zulch H. Stress—its effects on health and behavior: a guide for practitioners. *Vet Clin N Am Small Anim Pract.* 2014;44:525–541.

Use of Pheromones in Feline Practice

Theresa L. DePorter

INTRODUCTION TO PHEROMONATHERAPY

People read newspapers to become aware of important events in the world; similarly, cats read the semiochemical messages left in the environment by other cats. Just as words on a page are messages intended to be read some time after they were written, cats apply pheromones to surfaces to communicate a message to be received by another cat at a later time. Pheromonatherapy allows the clinician to encode a favorable message into the cat's environment and thus influence the bias of the cat's emotional response.

UNDERSTANDING PHEROMONES

A semiochemical is a chemical substance that conveys a message from one organism to another, so as to influence the behavior of the recipient.[1] The term semiochemical is derived from the Greek word "semion," meaning "a sign."[2] Allelomones are semiochemicals produced by one species but affecting members of another species. Pheromones are semiochemicals that exert an influence on individuals of the same species.[3] Pheromone signaling substances are contained in bodily fluids such as urine, sweat, specialized exocrine glands, and mucous secretions of genitals (Figure 18-1). Our understanding of the physiological, behavioral, and molecular aspects of pheromones is based on research in many species from insects to mammals. The chemical diversity of pheromones ranges from small volatile molecules to sulfated steroids to large families of proteins. These compounds are classified as pheromones based on their binding to specific receptors and subsequent influence on behavior rather than on similarity of molecular structure. In mammals, pheromones are detected by the vomeronasal (or Jacobson's) organ, located at the rostral end of the hard palate within the nasal cavity. Here molecules bind to specific receptors, which mediate effects within the limbic system. (For more detail, see Chemosensory Systems and the Detection of Pheromones.)

Types of Pheromones

Pheromones are classified as having either releaser or primer effects. Releaser pheromones trigger a specific behavior. For example, sexual pheromones are releasers. Sows in estrus respond to 3α-androstenol and 5α-androstenone, two steroid pheromones found in the saliva of boars, by exhibiting immobility, a rigid, motionless pose that reflects the degree of the sow's reproductive readiness. This is an example of a releasing effect, triggering a specific behavior. Primer pheromones are more common and are the more clinically relevant pheromones to be considered here. Primer pheromones induce modification of the emotional state and are beneficial as an adjunct to other forms of behavior therapy and environmental modification. Primer pheromones, such as facial, interdigital, and appeasing pheromones, induce delayed effects that are modulated through the activation of the neuroendocrine limbic system, including the amygdala, the fear and emotional control center of the brain. Receptors for pheromones are generally present only in the species producing the pheromone; therefore the effect is specific to each species. Appeasing pheromones, produced by the mammalian mother in the first few days after giving birth, are perceived by neonates and play a role in their attraction and attachment to their mother. Currently, appeasing pheromones are best represented by the commercially available canine product Adaptil, which induces a feeling of well-being and a greater sense of safety and comfort. A feline appeasing pheromone marketed as Feliway MultiCat is also now available in the United States.

Like natural pheromones, synthetic pheromone analogues bind to vomeronasal receptors and mediate their effects in the limbic system. Therefore synthetic analogues may be applied in the environment to convey specific messages intended for the patient. Cats may react to their environment based on input from multiple sensory and learned inputs, and semiochemical perception is just one of those. The comforting effect of pheromones cannot completely overcome intense conflicting messages of extreme fear or distress from other senses and perceptions.

Pheromone producing regions in the cat

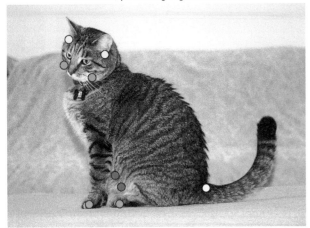

O Periaural regions
◑ Cheeks
◔ Foot pads
● Intermammary sulcus
○ Tail base

FIGURE 18-1 Pheromone signaling substances are released from a number of specialized exocrine glands around the body.

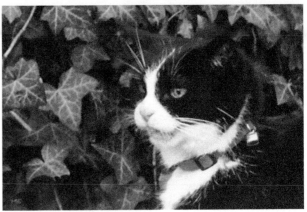

FIGURE 18-2 This cat is displaying the "gape expression" or "flehmen response." (Courtesy A. Dossche)

CHEMOSENSORY SYSTEMS AND THE DETECTION OF PHEROMONES

Pheromones are received by the vomeronasal organ (VNO), a paired tubular structure located just above the hard palate near the internasal septum. The VNO connects to the nasal cavity and, in some species such as the dog and cat, also to the mouth by an incisive duct. In ruminants and horses, the "flehmen response" is accomplished by closing the nostrils, curling the lip away and inhaling deeply to draw air into the passageway of the VNO. Cats display a response called the "gape" to gather pheromones into the passageways. The gape expression follows olfactory investigation and is characterized by a tongue lick to the nose, followed by the cat's gazing in a thoughtful, preoccupied fashion while the upper lips are raised slightly and fluffed with the mouth slightly open (Figure 18-2).[4] Generally air flow in the respiratory passages does not come in contact with the specialized epithelium; instead the molecules are drawn into the lumen in response to a pumplike action of the surrounding vascular tissue. Specialized receptor neurons line the lumen of the VNO; and information is relayed via afferent neurons to the olfactory bulb, amygdala, and ventromedial hypothalamus. In addition to the familiar pathways of the VNO, specialized semiochemical chemosensory receptors in the olfactory system trigger the cascade of molecular and electrical events which appear to have an intrinsic effect on emotional processing and ultimately influence the social familiarity, motivational impulses, and emotional bias behavior of the recipient animal.

PREVENTATIVE AND THERAPEUTIC APPLICATIONS OF PHEROMONES

Cats communicate with other cats by leaving semiochemical messages called pheromones in the environment, which other cats "read" in much the same way as people obtain information by reading a newspaper or book. What if it were possible to speak "cat"? What if it were possible to write a message in cat language, send it to the cats, and influence their behavior? Pheromonatherapy is the art of leaving an encoded feline-friendly message in the environment by introducing a synthetic analogue of natural pheromones. These communications should convey peace and comfort; these semiochemicals should enhance the cats' emotional well-being, not just change their behavior.

Despite generations of cats living alongside humans, feline domestication is incomplete. Yet cats are becoming ever more popular as pets around the world. Cats are naturally suspicious of novelty; and as human environments change dramatically the need for cats to have a sense of safety and security may be higher than ever.[5] Cats' adaptability and plasticity may be exceeded by the variability and complexity of modern domestic life, which may result in problematic feline behaviors.

Cats are now the number one pet in many parts of the world; in North America, there are 81.7 million owned cats compared with 72 million owned dogs. Nearly one half of cat-owning households (49%) already own two or more cats, and 35.4 million U.S. households own at least one cat.[6] Cats are increasing not only in the number of pets in total, but also in density per home, with an average of 2.1 cats per household. The trends in some parts of the world to restrict cats to an indoor lifestyle further challenges their ability to adapt not only to people, but also to complex inter-cat relationships. Cats are naturally socially independent and lack the inherent skills needed to reconcile with one another once hostilities have tainted feline friendships.

Certainly some cats are less reactive, more tolerant, and have better reconciliation skills and these cats may get along with housemate cats readily. But in general, cats don't mediate and resolve poor relationships on their own, by nature. Hope for peaceful reconciliation lies not in using punishment for cats that are aggressive, but in understanding natural interactions, facilitating reconciliation, modulating semiochemical environmental communications, reducing fear, and improving the cat's emotional well-being. Cats naturally may communicate fear and distress signals and leave these messages in the environment, and these distress messages may cause or perpetuate feline hostilities. Prevention of cat-to-cat hostilities is much more efficient than treatment (for more detail about inter-cat conflict see Chapter 26).

PHEROMONE DISPENSING OPTIONS

Cats apply natural pheromones by bunting, rubbing, rolling, or scratching on household surfaces, people, or other animals. In order to mimic these natural actions, synthetic analogues of natural pheromones are available commercially in spray, diffuser, and towelette forms and may be utilized to achieve the desired effects. A spray formulation allows for the targeting of specific or strategic locations. Timing may also be adjusted to provide the optimal effect when it is necessary and most beneficial. Care should be taken to apply the product well away from the cat. Some cats find the alcohol carrier substance used in the spray to be aversive; in these cases, the pheromone message will be best received once the substance has evaporated. Also, it is important that the cat does not feel threatened or intimidated during the application of the spray. Some cats are frightened by the spritzing sound and may leave the area, but that is not the intended or desired effect. A convenient pheromone impregnated towelette is also available in some countries and is suitable for many applications such as wiping on the inside of a carrier before transport. The intent is to apply the pheromone to the environment before introducing the cat so the cat may detect the semiochemical information upon initial investigation and develop a perception of safety in that environment. The spray and wipe formulations are convenient and have the advantage of being portable, but they must be reapplied often in the environment for a continuous effect. Therefore in circumstances where a sense of well-being is desired in a specific location, the electronic diffuser may be the best choice.

The diffuser contains a facial pheromone formulation that affects only cats—it has no effect on humans or other animals. The product takes action when a cat sniffs and inhales it. Most people cannot detect or smell the product, but some sensitive individuals may notice a slight odor, which often dissipates within the first 24 hours. Ceva's diffuser is made from nonflammable plastic for use specifically with Feliway refill vials. The diffuser is plugged into an electrical outlet (complying with local standards specific for regional applications in Europe, Japan, Australia, and other countries, with 110 to 240 V), and in some countries a power indicator light confirms that the diffuser is working. Once the carrier oil reaches a volatile temperature the pheromone is diffused into the cat's living environment, with a coverage area of 50 to 70 m^2 (500 to 700 sq. ft). The diffuser should be plugged in continuously and not be unplugged or moved repeatedly. Each vial is designed to last 28 days (U.S.) or 30 days (U.K.), but due to variations in home environments (e.g., humidity, air flow, and temperature) some may diffuse more rapidly or slowly. In some countries a 60 day refill is also available. In some devices the wick retains some liquid even when the diffuser bottle appears dry and in others the wick may dry out before all of the liquid has been used up and it is important for owners to be advised to replace refill vials (28 day or 56 day refills available in the United States) in accordance with manufacturer recommendations. The Feliway Diffuser is tested and approved by Underwriters Laboratories (UL) but only when used with Feliway refill vials. Finding an optimal location for the diffuser is accomplished by selecting an area that includes the cat's favored resting places. It is also important to ensure that there is plenty of space around the diffuser device and in particular to avoid placing the device beneath any cold surfaces such as shelves or tables since these can cause the evaporating oil to condense quickly and prevent the pheromone from being distributed into the environment. Feline thoroughfares such as hallways, eating locations and litter boxes may not be optimal locations for semiochemical messages. Strategic dosing of pheromones involves placement where the messages may be investigated and deciphered in a relaxed state. The diffusers may be used throughout shelters, boarding facilities, and veterinary practices to provide a continuous comforting message for incoming feline visitors.

PREVENTATIVE AND TREATMENT APPLICATIONS USING FACIAL PHEROMONES

Pheromones may be useful preventatively or as a treatment for specific behavior problems. Five feline facial pheromones, designated F1 to F5, have been identified in cats. The F3 fraction is the pheromone deposited by the cat when facial-marking and chin-rubbing on either objects or people. This creates a familiar, comforting scent of "self" in the environment.[7,8] The synthetic analogue of the F3 fraction is marketed under the trade name Feliway. The F4 fraction of the feline facial pheromone complex is believed to be utilized for allo-marking and recognition in feline social greetings. The synthetic analogue of the F4 fraction is marketed in some countries under the trade name Felifriend.

Preventative and Treatment Applications of the F3 Fraction of Feline Facial Pheromone Complex

Applications for pheromones remain the most studied modality for behavioral interventions and there are numerous studies on efficacy of Feliway for reduction of urine marking (Box 18-1).[9–21] Preventative applications should be applied while the cat is still in a lowered state of arousal, before learning negative associations and before stress coping strategies have been initiated. Behaviors such as urine marking, aggression, or scratching may be refractory or extremely difficult to eliminate from the animal's routine once initiated. It is more difficult to assess the beneficial effect of preventative measures: like a good vaccination program, the evidence of success lies in lack of manifestations of problems or disorders.

The occurrence of urine marking is related to social territorial communication and manifestation of stress. Feliway spray applied onto previously marked areas has been shown to reduce urine marking in 74% to 91% of households and to eliminate urine marking in 33% to 52% of households.[18–22] In a recent meta-analysis, there was significant reduction or improvement in urine marking by at least 90% using fluoxetine, clomipramine, or Feliway.[9] Even cats with a long history of urine marking may be improved with application of Feliway in the locations in which urine marking has occurred. Difficult cases may require a combination of environmental modifications, behavioral therapies, medications and pheromones to sufficiently reduce the incidence of urine marking (see Chapter 24).[23]

Veterinary practices, catteries, boarding facilities and shelters for cats may utilize pheromones to enhance the health and welfare of feline visitors. In a placebo-controlled trial, using cats hospitalized for evaluation of lower urinary tract disease, synthetic F3 pheromone was shown to promote grooming behaviors and increased interest in food.[24] Further, the 24-hour food consumption was significantly higher for cats that were offered a cage containing a Feliway-treated carrier for hiding, as compared with those given only Feliway.[24] Another placebo-controlled trial evaluated the effects of F3 analogue alone, or in combination with acepromazine as a premedication before catheterization. F3 analogue was found to have additional calming effects on cats when combined with acepromazine, and to a lesser degree cats that were not given acepromazine. A synthetic analogue feline facial pheromone (FFP) may make cats calmer but does not reduce struggling for intravenous catheterization.[24a] The cats in the Feliway and acepromazine treatment group also appeared more relaxed in the cage based on head postures and position within the cage.[25] While at a veterinary practice, cats may be inundated with odors such as disinfectants, rubbing alcohol, blood, or even air fresheners which cause the cat to be fearful or distressed. The odors and messages from unfamiliar and distressed felines are likely to convey messages of panic and fear to other cats. Cats can be quite distressed by these messages, much as people at an airport would be distressed to read about a plane crash or terrorist-related event—the threats may not be present but the real or perceived fear is conveyed by communications and results in real emotional distress. Feline patients may benefit from the steady messages from diffusers placed throughout the veterinary practice. Pheromones should be applied to towels, bedding, or other materials a cat will encounter by spraying about 15 minutes in advance of handling or confinement.

The application of the Feliway spray to the cat carrier in advance of travel has also been shown to reduce anxiety related physical signs (e.g., vomiting, urination, defecation) and behavioral signs which are associated with car travel.[26] In some countries, a new convenient wipe formulation is available which may also be used to apply Feliway to the inside of a carrier or a veterinary hospitalization cage. Feliway has also been demonstrated to facilitate introduction into new environments by improving appetite and reducing urine spraying and roaming.[27] As stress can have a profound effect on both behavioral and physical health including cardiac, dermatologic, gastrointestinal, and urinary, Feliway may be a useful adjunctive therapy in reducing the underlying stress that contributes to conditions such as feline idiopathic cystitis.[28]

Mini Case Example: Controlling Urine Marking

A cat was treated for urine marking on furniture by provision of a urine-marking box, daily fluoxetine, and use of Feliway diffusers applied in a urine-marked location. Meals and toys were provided in the urine-marked

---

BOX 18-1   Applications for Feliway

- Adjusting to a new home (e.g., new kitten, new cat, or multi-cat household)
- New experiences (e.g., first car ride, first grooming, or first exposure to noises)
- Stressful events (e.g., fireworks, storms, holidays, parties)
- Changes in cat's environment (e.g., remodeling, renovations, redecorating)
- Veterinary visits, shelters, or boarding
- Carrier transportation and travel
- Urine marking
- Territorial scratching
- Loss of appetite due to stress
- Change in normal behavior due to stress

location. When all environmental factors were stable, the cat did not urine-mark the furniture. However, when the cat experienced stress due to cats outside the house, he sprayed multiple times per day in the urine-marking box; and if the Feliway diffusers were accidentally allowed to empty, he sprayed the furniture as well. The client hoped medication could be discontinued even though the stress threshold for urine marking was low. Additional Feliway diffusers were added throughout the home. The diffusers were plugged in at different times of the month so the presence of Feliway in the home was maintained even if the owner forgot to replace one promptly. Motion activated devices were used in the yard as deterrents to cats outside the house. The cat was successfully weaned off medication.

Preventative and Treatment Applications of the F4 Fraction of Feline Facial Pheromone Complex

The synthetic analogue of the F4 fraction of the feline facial pheromone complex, marketed under the trade name Felifriend, is believed to be utilized for facilitating feline social greetings. In countries where it is available, Felifriend is marketed as a spray designed to be applied directly to human palms and wrists and distributed thoroughly by rubbing the hands together. Felifriend may be utilized by caretakers in shelters or veterinary practices or anyone who will be handling an unfamiliar cat. Felifriend does contain an alcohol carrier which cats may find offensive, so care must be taken to allow evaporation of the alcohol prior to approaching the cat. Holding the treated hands about 20 cm in front of the cat for one minute will enable the cat to recognize the handler as a familiar person and perceive subsequent interactions to be less threatening. It is important that the subsequent interactions do not betray the trust instilled by the semiochemical communication. In compliance with AAFP/ISFM Feline-Friendly Handling Guidelines,[29] the cat should be made to feel safe, at ease, and comfortable in all handling interactions. Felifriend is best applied before initial interactions and certainly before any negative interactions or stresses have begun. For this reason it is probably best limited to use for cats that are naïve in their interactions rather than those that have already built up a body of negative experiences when being handled by humans.

It has been suggested that it may be useful to apply Felifriend to the flanks of dogs or other cats to facilitate social interaction when introducing the cat to unfamiliar pets (Box 18-2). It is recommended that Felifriend be applied to a cloth and the cloth applied to the flanks of the unfamiliar pet rather than using the spray directly onto the animal which runs the risk of startling the cat. Again, application before arousal or escalation of distress is important and many behaviorists would not recommend using this product in cases of established inter-cat tension. One veterinary situation

---

> **BOX 18-2   Applications for Felifriend**
>
> - Introductions or reintroductions to people and animals, including other cats
> - New experiences involving handling (e.g., first grooming or first exposure to the veterinarian)
> - Medical procedures (e.g., physical examination, vaccinations, venipuncture, acupuncture)
> - Maintenance or grooming (e.g., bathing, nail trims, or medicating)
> - Shelter or boarding situations with novel caretakers

where Felifriend may be helpful is when one cat from a multi-cat household has had to be separated for health reasons and is being reintroduced. This would only be appropriate if the relationships within the household had been positive prior to the period of enforced separation.

Mini Case Example: Calming a Fearful Cat

Bella, a 2-year-old F/S tortoiseshell domestic shorthair, presented for her annual health examination and routine vaccination. The client was late for the appointment because Bella had been difficult to catch, and both client and cat were quite upset. Bella was crouched in the back of the carrier, hissing and swatting, while the client questioned the technician about the necessity of vaccinations. The technician applied Felifriend to her hands, then covered the carrier with a towel misted with Feliway and played comforting bioacoustic music, "Through a Cat's Ear" in the examination room. As she discussed the importance of the annual examination and vaccination, she held her hands just inside the door to the carrier for 1 minute. After that time, Bella could be gently lifted from her carrier. She crouched but did not hiss. A Feliway towelette was placed inside Bella's carrier. The remainder of Bella's appointment experience was positive and pleasant by implementation of low-stress cat-handling techniques.

Preventative and Treatment Applications Using Appeasing Pheromones

Appeasing pheromones are released by the mother while nursing her offspring and serve to enhance bond formation while comforting and reassuring the neonates. Synthetic analogues of appeasing pheromones have been widely utilized in canines to reduce anxiety and promote feelings of comfort and well-being. Adaptil (formerly D. A.P.) is a synthetic analogue of the canine-appeasing pheromone and has similar effects on older puppies and adult dogs. It has been effectively used to help puppies adapt to new homes; reduce fear and anxiety in puppy classes, the veterinary practice, shelters, and during car travel; improve long-term socialization; and, in conjunction with behavior therapy, treat separation anxiety and noise phobias.[30–37]

Cat-appeasing pheromones are produced in the mammary sulcus of the queen. Product analogues, derived from the pheromones of especially nurturing queens, hold promise for facilitation of cat-to-cat and cat-to-human interactions. A new diffuser product called "Feliway MultiCat" is an appeasing pheromone and actually does not share any of the pheromones found in the similarly named feline facial pheromone product Feliway (Box 18-3). Ultimately it may be determined that Feliway MultiCat offers broad benefits for cats as Adaptil does for dogs but at the time of publication, only a few studies and anecdotal reports are available and the product is only available in the United States.

One case report series suggests the cat-appeasing pheromone product (now Feliway MultiCat) may be useful for fearful cats. The treated cats remained longer in social situations, displayed prolonged and intensified human attention interactions, and were more open to meeting people and fled less urgently.[38] Cat-appeasing pheromones may also be a promising new treatment to reduce social tension among cats with a history of aggressive interactions.[39,40] One family reported anecdotally of their cats' responses to a test formulation of a cat-appeasing pheromone (IRSEA, France). During the period of the pheromone diffuser treatments, their cats experienced less social tension, characterized by an increase in the time the cats spent in relatively close proximity, more tolerance of agonistic displays, quicker recovery following encounters, and overall reduced tension.[40,41] Further, owners observed that the cats were more affectionate and interactive with human family members. The cats displayed more bunting and rubbing; they solicited attention more often, especially at bedtime; and they slept with family members more frequently and for longer periods.

A placebo-controlled study including 45 households presenting for aggression between familiar housemate cats showed that a cat-appeasing pheromone, Feliway

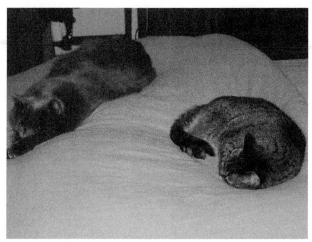

FIGURE 18-3 Cats that display aggression toward familiar housemates will often avoid interactions, due to fear of injury or hostility, by alternating their use of favored spaces and access to preferred resources. These cats had avoided each other; but as the social tension reduced, the owner was able to get a picture of them sleeping in relative proximity. Notice these cats are not relaxed and while social tension has improved it has not resolved at this point and there is still more work to be done.

MultiCat, (Ceva Sante Animale, Libourne, France) reduced aggression, even within the first 7 days of treatment. Aggression between familiar cats is a common problem (Figure 18-3) and may persist for months or years, forcing cat owners either to rehome a cat or permit the cats to live in a chronic state of distress due to social conflict.[42]

Mini Case Example: Resolving Intercat Aggression

Max, a 7-year-old MN DSH, and Sassy, a 7-year-old FS DSH, presented for aggression between housemate cats which had continued for 5.5 years since their first introduction. When Sassy was adopted 7 years previously, Max immediately began chasing, swatting, and cornering Sassy. Sassy would flee, back up to a wall with flattened ears and hiss and wait for people to help her get away from Max. Other times she would hide and avoid interactions with Max. Visitors were also a target of Max's aggression, and most people were afraid of Max. The family was given instructions to avoid punishment and startle techniques for Max's undesirable behaviors. Strategies to redirect his behavior were described. After two months using Feliway MultiCat, a cat appeasing pheromone diffuser product, the owners reported his aggression was reduced, they observed an "incredible change in Max without changing his personality. He just seems to be a happier cat." The family has observed brief "nose-touching" between the cats which was never observed previously.

BOX 18-3 Applications for Feliway MultiCat Diffuser

- Introductions or reintroductions to people and animals, especially other cats
- Resolution or prevention of social conflict between familiar housemate cats in multi-cat households
- Prevention of social conflict between housemate cats following medical procedures (e.g., dentistry) or grooming.
- Benefits for the single cat may include reduced anxiety and enhanced social relationships with other species but have not been fully explored at the time of this printing.

PREVENTATIVE AND TREATMENT APPLICATIONS USING SYNTHETIC FELINE INTERDIGITAL SEMIOCHEMICAL

A synthetic feline interdigital semiochemical (FIS) may be useful for the induction of scratching behavior in cats. Though scratching is a normal part of the feline repertoire, undesirable scratching behavior is the second most common behavior problem reported by cat owners.[43] Motivation for scratching has long been explained as a means of sharpening claws and maintaining the system that allows claw extension and withdrawal, but this does not reveal the entire motivation for this behavior. Scratching provides important visual and olfactory communication of both immediate and long-term social messages.[44,45] Scratching can be used for territorial marking by depositing chemical signals released by the plantar pad glands and by leaving "signs" on the scratched surface (Figure 18-4). In a crossover clinical trial of 19 laboratory-housed cats, a synthetic analogue of the feline interdigital semiochemical (FIS), was shown to modify the scratching behaviors of cats considering the latency, duration, and frequency of scratching after treatment compared with placebo.

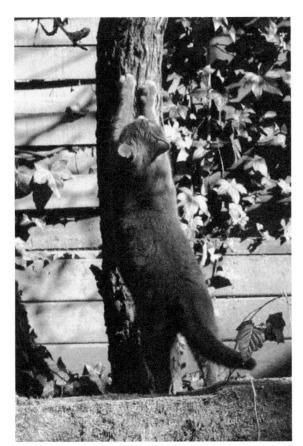

FIGURE 18-4   Scratching can be used for territorial marking by depositing chemical signals and leaving "signs" on the scratched surface. (Courtesy A. Dossche)

Feliscratch may provide a unique mechanism to encourage scratching in locations that owners consider desirable, while Feliway may be applied to locations the owners consider undesirable for scratching. This pheromone management strategy would provide the cat with guidance and encouragement for scratching on a surface the owner prefers. Currently Feliscratch is not widely available or distributed (BIOSEM Labs, Paris, France).

COMMERICAL PHEROMONATHERAPY

The advent of commercial pheromones provides opportunities to attempt to influence behavior solely by exposing the animal to the product. However in natural circumstances, relatively minuscule amounts of pheromones are released and the resulting influence on behavior occurs within a multisensory context. The naturally released pheromone is associated with the sights, sounds, and presence of the sender to deliver a complex multidimensional message. For example, boar pheromones are produced in the saliva while the boar also sniffs, noses, attempts to mount, and sings a "courting song" comprised of a series of soft guttural grunts. The result is a multisensory message to solicit the sow's reproductive attention. A lactating female cat produces her own blend of appeasing pheromones from the intermammary sulcus, conveying a sense of security and motherly reassurance to her offspring, a message further enhanced by her licking, suckling, and auditory signals. Collectively these messages communicate maternal commitment and safety to the kittens.

Commercial pheromones are synthetic analogues of molecular blends derived from natural samples. Samples are collected from several individuals, ideally animals that display superior semiocommunication-related behaviors when interacting socially. These samples must be carefully and accurately obtained, then analyzed by gas chromatography and mass spectroscopy. Based on analysis of the chromatogram, the product is artificially synthesized. Biological screening plus clinical trials are necessary for confirmation of efficacy of the end product. The product concentration will necessarily be much higher than naturally occurring pheromones. Some emerging products include claims that the product is a "natural" formulation rather than a synthetic analogue. However, one must wonder how many cats must be housed in order to obtain this natural formulation. A clear understanding of the complexities of harvesting natural pheromones illuminates the absurdity of such claims. Ceva Santé Animale (Libourne, France) continues to be the world leader in behavior products and research assessing suitable applications. A review has been written which provides summaries of the latest developments in the field of pheromonatherapy and serves as a practical reference guide.[46]

Understanding the derivation and the natural applications of pheromones helps elucidate the appropriate applications and possible misapplications. If a cat is terrified and simultaneously detects a semiochemical message conveying comfort and tranquility, one can imagine this may be confusing or disconcerting to the feline psyche. Pheromone products are therefore best applied to influence a behavioral response; they are not intended to completely control a specific action sequence or response. A complete understanding of the pet's motivation to perform the undesirable behaviors is essential to the consideration of intervention strategies. For example, a client requests help to alleviate her cat's scratching on her couch. It is important to understand the cat's motivation for scratching. A cat that feels safe and comfortable in the environment may scratch less overall. But if the cat is startled or squirted with water for scratching, then the cat's anxiety or comfort level in the environment will not be improved but indeed worsened. The cat should be provided acceptable places to scratch and gently redirected to another activity instead of scratching.

Commonly Asked Questions About Synthetic Pheromones

- **Can feline pheromones affect people or dogs?**
  Each pheromone exerts a species-specific effect. The behavior of other animals in the home may change, but would be indirectly mediated by the change in the cat's behavior as influenced by the pheromones.
- **Do synthetic pheromones cause any side effects?**
  There are no known detrimental effects of synthetic analogue pheromones. Feliway, Feliway MultiCat and Felifriend are designed especially for cats, are nonsedative, have no effect on people or any other animals, and can be used in conjunction with supplements or medications. Some collar products contain scents which may be bothersome to cats (e.g., florals) and thus may be annoying. Collars that have a powdery residue have been reported to cause skin irritation in some cats.
- **Do synthetic pheromone diffusers produce an odor?**
  Most people do not notice any detectable odor or scent. New diffusers may smell slightly for the first 24 hours. Generally this may be related to dust in the air or dust which has settled on the diffuser during a period of nonuse. If the environment is very dusty, then the odor may persist. If the device is used continuously for long periods of time, it should be replaced every 6 months or every 6 refills.
- **How long do synthetic pheromones need to be used to control a behavior?**
  Many cats may benefit from long-term applications of pheromones. Necessity will vary from case to case

based on individual personality, coping strategies, and the presence of daily or occasional stressors. Pheromones may be used continuously or intermittently without any detrimental effects or development of tolerance.

THE FUTURE OF PHEROMONATHERAPY

The extent to which scent communication and deposition of pheromones is important to cats is well understood but probably underestimated. Pheromonatherapy provides the opportunity to "speak to the cat" regarding safety, well-being, and social communication. These messages should be used responsibly to provide for the cats' mental, emotional, and physical welfare without simultaneously misleading or deceiving the cat. Applications for pheromones remain the most studied modality for behavioral interventions. Since the concept of utilizing a facial pheromone was first introduced at a symposium in 1996, the veterinary community response has ranged from skepticism to first-line panacea for all undesirable feline behaviors.[47] The clinician should identify the problem behaviors, evaluate the ethological motivations, formulate a diagnosis, and execute a complete behavior modification program, recommend environmental modifications that are key in feline understanding, and review key symptoms that the client can monitor in order to assess progress over time. Behavioral studies may include client observations and interpretations of behavioral signs of fear or distress (e.g., vocalizations, inappetance, or avoidance) and somatic signs (e.g., fleeing, urination, salivation, or scratching). Assessment of response for clinical cases necessitates reliance on client perceptions of improvement and the impact of learning or introduction of new stressors. Evidence and clinical trials for the effectiveness and application of feline pheromones are numerous and the dedicated reader should contact Ceva for a reference guide that includes detailed abstracts and proceedings for these studies.

The future of pheromonatherapy includes new synthetic analogue formulations with considerations for a diverse range of applications and contexts to improve the welfare of the cat by speaking the cat's language and sharing messages of trust and comfort.

ADDITIONAL RESOURCES

Horwitz D, Mills D. *BSAVA Manual of Canine and Feline Behavioural Medicine.* BSAVA; 2009.

Landsberg GM, Hunthausen WL, Ackerman LJ. *Behavior Problems of the Dog and Cat.* Edinburgh: Saunders/Elsevier; 2013.

Mills D, Braem Dube M, Zulch H. *Stress and Pheromonatherapy in Small Animal Clinical Behaviour.* Chichester: Wiley Blackwell; 2013.

American Association of Feline Practitioners has recommended guidelines for Feline-Friendly Handling.

The Cat Friendly Practice (CFP) program contains the tools for practices to integrate a feline perspective and embrace the standards needed to elevate care for cats. http://catfriendlypractice.catvets.com/

The CATalyst Council program provides resources and tips for owners taking their cat to the veterinarian. http://www.catalystcouncil.org/resources/video.

International Cat Care—a charity dedicated to improving the lives of all cats. http://www.icatcare.org/search/gss/pheromone.

REFERENCES

1. Mills DS, Braem Dube M, Zulch H. *Stress and Pheromonatherapy in Small Animal Clinical Behaviour.* Chichester: Wiley-Blackwell; 2013.
2. Wyatt TD. *Pheromones and Animal Behaviour – Communication by Taste and Smell.* Cambridge: Cambridge University Press; 2003.
3. Tirindelli R, Dibattista M, Pifferi S, Menini A. From pheromones to behavior. *Physiol Rev.* 2009;89:921–956.
4. Houpt KA. *Domestic Animal Behavior for Veterinarians and Animal Scientists.* Ames, IA: Wiley-Blackwell; 2011.
5. Hargrave C. Pheromonatherapy and animal behaviour: providing a place of greater safety. *Companion Animal.* 2014;19:60–64.
6. American Veterinary Medical Association. *U.S. Pet Ownership and Demographic Sourcebook.* Schaumburg IL: AVMA; 2012.
7. Pageat P, Gaultier E. Current research in canine and feline pheromones. *Vet Clin North Am Small Anim Pract.* 2003;33:187–211.
8. Rodan I, Sundahl E, Carney H, et al. AAFP and ISFM feline-friendly handling guidelines. *J Feline Med Surg.* 2011;13:364–375.
9. Mills DS, Redgate SE, Landsberg GM. A meta-analysis of studies of treatments for feline urine spraying. *PLoS One.* 2011;6:e18448.
10. Pageat P. Functions and uses of the facial pheromones in the treatment of urine marking in the cat. In: *Proceedings of the XX1st Congress of the World Small Animal Veterinary Association*; 1996, Jerusalem.
11. Pageat P. Experimental evaluation of the efficacy of a synthetic analogue of cat's facial pheromones (Feliway*) in inhibiting urine marking of sexual origin in adult tom-cats. *J Vet Pharmacol Ther.* 1997;20(suppl 1):169.
12. White JC, Mills D. Efficacy of synthetic feline facial pheromone (F3) analogue (Feliway) for the treatment of chronic non-sexual urine spraying by the domestic cat. In: *Proceedings of the first International Conference on Veterinary Behavioural Medicine*; 1997, Birmingham.
13. Frank D, Erb HN, Houpt KA. Urine spraying in cats: presence of concurrent disease and effects of pheromone treatment. *Appl Anim Behav Sci.* 1999;61:263–272.
14. Hunthausen W. Evaluating a feline facial pheromone analogue to control urine spraying. *Vet Med.* 2000;95:151–156.
15. Ogata N, Takeuchi Y. Clinical trial a feline pheromone analogue for feline urine marking. *J Vet Med Sci.* 2001;63:157–161.
16. Mills DS, White JC. Long-term follow up of the effect of a pheromone therapy on feline spraying behaviour. *Vet Record.* 2000;147:746–747.
17. Mills DS, Mills CB. Evaluation of a novel method for delivering a synthetic analogue of feline facial pheromone to control urine spraying by cats. *Vet Record.* 2001;149:197–199.
18. Frank D, Erb HN, Houpt KA. Urine spraying in cats: presence of concurrent disease and effects of pheromone treatment. *Appl Anim Behav Sci.* 1999;61:263–272.
19. Ogata N, Takeuchi Y. Clinical trial of a feline pheromone analogue for feline urine marking. *J Vet Med Sci.* 2001;63:157–161.
20. Hunthausen W. Evaluating a feline facial pheromone analogue to control urine spraying. *Vet Med.* 2000;95:151–156.
21. White JC, Mills DS. Efficacy of synthetic feline facial pheromone (F3) analogue (Feliway) for the treatment of chronic non-sexual urine spraying by the domestic cat. In: Mills DS, Heath SE, Harrington LJ, eds. *Proceedings of the First International Conference on Veterinary Behavioural Medicine, Birmingham, UK, April 1–2.* Potters Bar: Universities Federation for Animal Welfare; 1997.
22. Mills DS, Redgate SE, Landsberg GM. A meta-analysis of studies of treatments for feline urine spraying. *PLoS One.* 2011;6:e18448.
23. Landsberg GM, Hunthausen WL, Ackerman LJ. Behavior problems of the dog and cat. Edinburgh: Saunders/Elsevier; 2013.
24. Griffith CA, Steigerwald ES, Buffington T. Effects of synthetic facial pheromone on behavior of cats. *J Am Vet Med Assoc.* 2000;217:1154–1156.
24a. Rand JS, Kinnaird E, Baglioni A, et al. Acute stress hyperglycemia in cats is associated with struggling and increased concentrations of lactate and norepinephrine. *J Vet Intern Med.* 2002;16:123–132.
25. Kronen PW, Ludders JW, Hollis NE, et al. A synthetic fraction of feline facial pheromones calms but does not reduce struggling in cats before venous catheterization. *Vet Anaesth Analg.* 2006;33:258–265.
26. Gaultier E, Pageat P, Tessier Y. Effect of a feline appeasing pheromone analogue on manifestations of stress in cats during transport. In: *Proceedings of the 32nd Congress of the International Society of Applied Ethology* Clermont-Ferrand: ISAE; 1998.
27. Pageat P, Tessier Y. Usefulness of the F3 synthetic pheromone Feliway in preventing behaviour problems in cats during holidays. In: *Proceedings of the 1st International Conference on Veterinary Behavioural Medicine*; 1997, Birmingham.
28. Gunn-Moore DA, Cameron ME. A pilot study using synthetic feline facial pheromone for the management of feline idiopathic cystitis. *J Feline Med Surg.* 2004;6:133–138.
29. Rodan I, Sundahl E, Carney H, et al., AAFP and ISFM feline-friendly handling guidelines. *J Feline Med Surg.* 2011;13:364–375.
30. Mills DS, Ramos D, Estelles MG, Hargrave C. A triple blind placebo-controlled investigation into the assessment of the effect of Dog Appeasing Pheromone (DAP) on anxiety related behaviour of problem dogs in the veterinary clinic. *Appl Anim Behav Sci.* 2006;98:114–126.

31. Tod E, Brander D, Wran N. Efficacy of a dog appeasing pheromone in reducing stress and fear related behaviour in shelter dogs. *Appl Anim Behav Sci.* 2005;93:295–308.

32. Levine ED, Ramos D, Mills DS. A prospective study of two self help CD based desensitization and counter-conditioning programmes with the use of Dog Appeasing Pheromone for the treatment of firework fears in dogs *(Canis familiaris)*. *Appl Anim Behav Sci.* 2007;105:311–329.

33. Taylor K, Mills DS. A placebo controlled study to investigate the effect of Dog Appeasing Pheromone and other environmental and management factors on the reports of disturbance and house soiling during the night in recently adopted puppies *(Canis familiaris)*. *Appl Anim Behav Sci.* 2007;105:358–368.

34. Siracusa C, Manteca X, Cuenca R, et al., Effect of a synthetic appeasing pheromone on behavioral, neuroendocrine, immune, and acute-phase perioperative stress responses in dogs. *J Am Vet Med Assoc.* 2010;237:673–681.

35. Gaultier E, Bonnafous L, Bougrat L, et al., Comparison of the efficacy of a synthetic dog-appeasing pheromone with clomipramine for the treatment of separation-related disorders in dogs. *Vet Rec.* 2005;156:533–538.

36. Estelles MG, Mills DS. Signs of travel-related problems in dogs and their response to treatment with dog-appeasing pheromone. *Vet Rec.* 2006;159:140–148.

37. Gaultier E, Bonnafous L, Vienet-Lague, et al., Efficacy of dog appeasing pheromone in reducing behaviours associated with fear of unfamiliar people and new surroundings in newly adopted puppies. *Vet Rec.* 2009;164:708–714.

38. DePorter TL. Exploration of possible clinical applications for cat appeasing pheromone: multiple case review. In: *9th International Veterinary Behaviour Meeting*; 2013, Lisbon.

39. Cozzi A, Monneret P, Lafont-Lecuelle C, et al., The maternal Cat Appeasing Pheromone: exploratory study for the effects on aggressive and affiliative interactions in cats. In: *Proceedings of the 7th International Veterinary Behaviour Meeting*; 2009, Edinburgh, Scotland.

40. DePorter TL. Case report: role of cat appeasing pheromone in the resolution of conflict between familiar felines. In: *Interdisciplinary Forum for Applied Animal Behavior.* 2013. San Diego. http://ifaab.org/2013/abstracts2013.htm

41. DePorter TL. Case report: Role of reconciliation in the resolution of conflict between familiar felines. In: *18th Annual Meeting of the ESVCE European Society of Veterinary Clinical Ethology*; 2011, Avignon, France.

42. DePorter TL, Lopez A, Ollivier E. *Evaluation of the efficacy of a new pheromone product versus placebo in the management of feline aggression in multi-cat households.* Denver, CO, USA: In Proceedings AVSAB/ACVB annual congress; 2014.

43. Heidemberger E. Housing conditions and behavioral problems of indoor cats as assessed by their owners. *Appl Anim Behav Sci.* 1997;52:345–364.

44. Casey R. Management problem in cats. In: Horwitz DF, Mills DS, eds. *BSAVA Manual of Canine and Feline Behavioural Medicine.* 2nd ed. Gloucester BSAVA; 2009:98–110.

45. Bradshaw J, Casey RA, Brown SL. *The Behaviour of the Domestic Cat.* Oxfordshire, UK: CABI; 2012.

46. Bowen J, Gunn-Moore D, Heath S, Mills D. *Comprehensive References.* Ceva; 2011 [Available by request from Ceva Sante Animale as an e-publication or book].

47. Frank D, Beauchamp G, Palestrini C. Systematic review of the use of pheromones for treatment of undesirable behavior in cats and dogs. *J Am Vet Med Assoc.* 2010;236:1308–1316.

Tools of the Trade: Psychopharmacology and Nutrition

Theresa DePorter, Gary M. Landsberg, and Debra Horwitz

INTRODUCTION

Psychotropic agents may aid in improving or resolving problem behaviors, abnormal behaviors, or behaviors that are manifestations of natural feline behavior when these are occurring as a result of emotional disturbance in the individual and when behavioral and environmental modification alone is insufficient. Psychotropic agents should always be used as part of a multimodal program of behavior therapy that considers the natural behavioral repertoire of cats, ethological and motivational considerations, inter- and intraspecies social relationships, and the environmental factors that influence the cats' behavior. Medications exert their major effect by reducing anxiety, fear, arousal, or vigilance; inhibiting aggression; and reducing impulsivity (Figure 19-1). This enables the cat to participate in social interactions or enhances behavior modification. In concert with medication, we must respect the cat's natural social behavior and offer it opportunities to engage in behaviors that are desirable for both the cat and the client. Environmental modifications should focus on fostering a sense of safety, predictability, emotional stability, and physical comfort. Alternatives such as rehoming may need to be considered if social and environmental factors cannot be appropriately addressed in the present home. Behavior modification methods that rely on force, coercion, or punishment increase a cat's fear and anxiety and are not recommended. These might be expedient solutions but can have short- and long-term detrimental effects on the cat's overall welfare as well as increase some undesirable behaviors (e.g., aggression, soiling) or reduce the cat's desire to engage in activities with humans. It is counterproductive and counterintuitive to use medications that alleviate anxiety in conjunction with positive punishment that reduces behaviors by increasing fear. In addition, because the use of medication is intended to improve the cat's welfare, administration strategies must be implemented that do not compromise it. Force-pilling and chase-capture medication strategies must be avoided. The use of psychotropic medications should

always be considered as a way to enhance a cat's overall well-being and welfare while considering the best interests of the individual cat.

This chapter provides an overview of beneficial and commonly used pharmaceutical and nutraceutical tools of the trade. Every effort has been made to focus on the evidence (of which a great deal is lacking in cats) to help guide the general practitioner to make decisions regarding effective application of these tools together with the diagnosis and treatment programs explained in other chapters. Mini case examples are provided to help the clinician make the transition from theory to comfort in real-life applications. The most useful classes of psychotropic medications are reviewed: selective serotonin reuptake inhibitors (SSRIs), tricyclic antidepressants (TCAs), benzodiazepines (BDZs), and azapirones. Other available medications, including monoamine oxidase inhibitors (MAOIs), hormones, antihistamines, anticonvulsants, tranquilizers, antidepressants, neuropeptides, and mood stabilizers, may also be useful to modulate changes in behavior. Suggestions for further study in the area of psychopharmacology are listed in the Additional Resources section at the end of this chapter.

Throughout the chapter, the goal is to provide guidance on stress-free alleviation of anxiety to support an environment of kindness and respect for the cat while facilitating optimal behavior. Natural supplements and dietary options that might be used alone or in conjunction with drugs are also reviewed. The chapter is intended to provide a current reference source for clinicians who want to consider incorporating psychotropic tools into the practice of feline behavioral medicine, rather than to be a detailed account of pharmacology.

SELECTING MEDICATION

Administering Medication

The goal is to administer the appropriate medication without force or stress at an appropriate dose and with the correct dosing interval. Medicating any cat, especially a cat with a behavior problem, poses a number of hurdles, including the practicality of actually

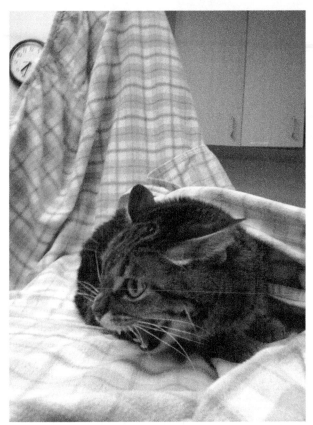

FIGURE 19-1 Selection of medication is based on intended effect and not solely based on diagnosis or manifestation of symptoms. For example, aggressive displays which are normal in one context may represent emotional instability in another context.

administering the prescribed drug to the patient. An open dialogue with cat owners regarding their ability and experience in administering medication is an absolute necessity. The ease with which clients can administer medication to their cat will help to determine what may and may not be achieved.

Drug Selection Considerations

Accurate diagnosis, indications, availability, strength, size, formulation, cost, taste, dosing frequency, and bioavailability are all factors that influence the selection of a medication, the practicality of administration, and whether a therapeutic response can be achieved. If a drug is indicated for the diagnosed disorder, factors to consider include evidence of efficacy, potential benefits and possible risks, and, from a practical standpoint, whether the medication can be safely, effectively, and gently administered. Medicating the patient is further complicated when vigilance, fearfulness, or aggression are a part of the diagnosis and presenting complaint. Therefore, to effectively use medication as an adjunctive component of a treatment program, clinicians must consider strategies for administration and provide client counseling as an integral part of the behavior plan.

Choosing the Right Medication

When choosing the optimal psychotropic agent for feline patients, consider each of the following:

- What is the diagnosis?
- Have social and environmental factors that are contributing to the behavioral condition been adequately addressed?
- Which drug, diet, or supplement might be beneficial for the present condition?
- Is there evidence to support this indication?
- What is known about pharmacokinetics, side effects, and contraindications of the medication in cats?
- What is the appropriate dosage and dosage range for the selected medication, and how frequently should it be administered?
- What are the potential risks with respect to the cat's age, sex, health, and concurrent medications?
- How does the client feel about giving mood-altering medications to the cat?
- Is medication likely to be beneficial in alleviating the behavior problem?
- What is the likelihood of a successful resolution of the behavior problem if medications are not used or the use of medication is delayed?

Administration

- What formulations are available (tablet or liquid)?
- How will the cat take the medication?
- What are the cat's prior experiences with medication and willingness to accept it?

Response and Therapeutic Effect

- Has the desired response to medication been established?
- Have the parameters of the desired response (e.g., occurrence, frequency, intensity) been established?
- What are the characteristics (target behaviors) of a beneficial response?
- When should a response be expected?
- How long might the medication be required, and how should it be withdrawn?

Benefits versus Risks

- What are the risks for the owner, the owner–cat bond, and the cat (i.e., rehoming, euthanasia) if no response is obtained?
- What are the welfare implications for the cat if the behavior problem continues or worsens?
- What are the possible health risks of using medication in this particular patient?
- What are the adverse effects of chronic stress if the environment is compromising feline behavior and cannot be modified effectively?
- Have alternatives to medication been adequately discussed?

Confounding Factors in Assessing Successful Drug Selection and Administration

Although it is tempting to try a therapeutic trial to determine if the target behavior improves, improvement or resolution of a behavior problem in response to a behavioral medication may or may not confirm the diagnosis. Even among pets, the placebo effect may be quite extraordinary and convincing. In some cases, a primary medical condition (e.g., feline idiopathic cystitis or other lower urinary tract disease) can be significantly improved if stress can be reduced through medication. Additionally, psychotropic therapeutics can have multiple effects that might ameliorate signs of anxiety, seizures, and neuropathic pain that could be contributing to the behavior problem. Clomipramine or an SSRI may prove beneficial for the reduction of signs and manifestations of a house soiling problem by altering the frequency of elimination or reducing the cat's anxiety, reactivity, or sensitivity while enhancing the cat's ability to cope. However, if there was an underlying medical condition, the improvement in litter box use could obscure the fact that the pet still has unresolved health issues.

Therefore, it is essential to fully assess medical factors prior to medicating and to address both physical and emotional health concurrently. However, obvious signs of fear or anxiety justify consideration of the immediate use of anxiolytic medications to address the welfare of the cat pending the results of medical diagnostics. Ultimately, successful resolution of a behavior problem following administration of a psychoactive drug may support, but does not definitively confirm, a behavioral diagnosis.

NEUROTRANSMITTERS AS MODULATORS OF BEHAVIOR

Psychotropic agents influence behavior through actions on neurotransmitters and receptors in the central nervous system (CNS). Companion animal behavioral therapeutics focus primarily on serotonin (5-hydroxytryptamine or 5-HT), norepinephrine (noradrenaline), dopamine, acetylcholine, γ-aminobutyric acid (GABA), substance P receptor (neurokinin or NK_1), and excitatory amino acids such as glutamate. Neurotransmission is a complex process that basically results from a dynamic interaction between the neurotransmitter, the presynaptic and postsynaptic receptors, the reuptake pump, and the degradation enzymes.[1] Psychotropic drugs act at varying sites: presynaptically, postsynaptically, and within the synapse itself. Medication can work via a number of modes of action, including enhancing the production and release of the neurotransmitter, blocking the effects of the neurotransmitter at the postsynaptic receptor, exerting an effect on receptors on the presynaptic neuron and/or the postsynaptic neuron, or

blocking the reuptake of the neurotransmitter into the presynaptic neuron. Drugs may also act by inhibiting the breakdown of neurotransmitters within the presynaptic neuron or within the synapse itself.

Complex dynamic relationships exist between the different neurotransmitters. The precise mechanism of action of many drugs and natural therapeutics has not been fully elucidated. In addition, the effects on neurotransmitters and receptors in one species may not necessarily reflect the effects in another species. Therefore, in feline behavioral medicine, because few therapeutic clinical trials have been published, recommendations for use and dosages are often based on anecdotal clinical experience, extrapolation from other species, and rare cases of published pharmacokinetic data. In addition, it is difficult to predict how an individual animal may respond to a selected medication. For human psychiatric patients, medications are often administered on a trial basis while monitoring for beneficial and adverse effects and the same is true in feline patients. Once a medication is selected and administered, its efficacy must be assessed by watching for a decline in clinical signs and an improvement in the cat's emotional health. The goal in administering medication is to improve the cat's well-being and welfare and to change the undesirable behavior while retaining normal social and interactive behaviors. More detailed information about neurotransmitters and their mechanisms of action may be found in the reference texts listed in the Additional Resources section at the end of this chapter.

EVIDENCE FOR USE OF MOOD-ALTERING DRUGS IN CATS

Evidence-based decision making examines the validity of the information, the design of clinical trials, and the application of statistics so that the clinician can select a therapeutic option that best suits the pet, the client, and the problem. However, specific and detailed evidence or algorithms for administration of psychotropic medication in behavioral disorders is lacking in companion animal species, especially cats. Most available information on drug therapy for behavior problems in companion animals comes from case studies and anecdotal clinical experiences of veterinary behaviorists (often on small numbers of cases) and from inferred comparisons between human psychiatric conditions and behavior problems of pets. Although practitioners may be obliged to follow a prescription cascade in some jurisdictions (with licensed drugs for the target species and the approved application used first), there are few licensed products available for cats. Therefore, the best choice based on the evidence available may be a drug that is licensed for another feline application, a drug licensed for cats in another country, or a drug licensed for another species that is in a format that is practical for feline administration. The practitioner must also consider the information in this chapter in light of ongoing and future developments in the field of veterinary behavior and psychopharmacology.

Formulations and Off-Label Applications

In most countries, there are no drugs and very few supplements or dietary options labeled and approved for feline behavior problems. Psychotropic drugs that are not approved for use in cats must be dispensed with full disclosure regarding its off-label use and potential adverse effects and with informed consent provided by the client (Figure 19-2). See the handout titled **Informed Consent for Psychotropic Drug Use for a Cat**. It is recommended that veterinarians have an attorney review any informed consent documents to ensure that they address regulations or restrictions in accordance with local jurisdictions. In the UK, the Veterinary Defence Society provides consent forms for practitioners to use. An informed consent does not absolve the clinician of responsibility, but it does serve to inform the client of the facts and documents the information that has been shared. The medications discussed below are available in formulations for humans or dogs. However, tablet sizes, solutions, flavors, or strengths that are optimal for human or canine patients may not be practical for feline patients. Many of the medications used for cats are conveniently available and affordably priced at human pharmacies, especially when available in generic formulations. Clients may be familiar with these medications from personal experience, which introduces advantages and disadvantages in perception, familiarity, and comfort with drug use; therefore, it may be beneficial to know the client's experiences. In addition, some medications pose risks for human use and abuse, so client familiarity with a drug should be a cause for concern.

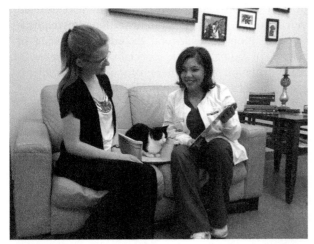

FIGURE 19-2 The veterinary team is responsible for fully discussing of the benefits and side effects of psychotropic medications.

Veterinarians should not ask direct, personal questions regarding human drug use, but instead should actively listen for comments and concerns that reflect the client's personal experiences and may influence the client's decisions regarding the cat's care.

Compounding of Psychotropic Medications

It has become increasingly common for medications to be reformulated into palatable formulations. Compounding might be considered when dose, compliance, or availability is an issue, but it may not be available in all countries. Solubility, stability, absorption, and potency are potential concerns, especially if the medication must be altered or reformulated for administration. Specifically, drugs that are packaged in blister packs, moisture-proof barriers, or light-proof packaging may not be stable if removed from their packaging, nor might they be amenable to compounding into liquid formulations. In addition, drugs that are in delayed-release or enteric-coated form are designed for the human digestive tract; thus, these formulations may not be appropriate for feline use. The same lack of evidence that presents problems for drug selection is exacerbated by compounding. Clinicians must therefore consider all factors, including local and national laws, when determining the formulation prescribed for their patients.

Transdermal Administration

Transdermal delivery of medications has been used for humans (e.g., nitroglycerin) for decades, and newer transdermal options for compounding pet medications are being developed and promoted in some countries. Transdermal medications may seem to be an easy, tolerable, and convenient way to administer psychotropic medications to cats; yet, unfortunately, administration in this manner is not generally recommended, owing to a number of concerns. The permeation enhancers used as transporters increase the fluidity of the stratum corneum, resulting in exfoliation, erythema, and some irritation. Chronic application may increase localized irritation, and there are limited locations, compared with humans, for application (the ear pinna or between the shoulder blades). Dose extrapolation from oral to transdermal formulations is complicated. If skin penetration is poor, minimal amounts of the drug may be absorbed; if a drug is not subjected to the first-pass hepatic metabolism, this may result in quite high or toxic amounts of a drug in the systemic circulation. Practitioners should not allow their comfort with other transdermal formulations, such as methimazole, that have some data for efficacy and absorption to lead them to assume that psychotropic medications share the same efficacy. Studies showing effective dosing, bioavailability, and efficacy are lacking. In one study, the bioavailability of fluoxetine (15% in pluronic lecithin organogel

(PLO) = 150 mg/mL) was approximately 10% when compared with oral dosing.[2] In another study, systemic absorption of amitriptyline and buspirone was found to be negligible (compared with oral dosing).[3] It is not clear if higher doses would achieve therapeutic plasma concentrations; yet, these higher dosages might be quite irritating to cats.

Transdermal applications may also be of concern due to social interactions in cats living in group situations that may groom each other or bunt against family members, thereby transferring the medication from the intended patient to another individual, either feline or human. Inadvertent medicating of children or other household pets with a mood-altering medication may pose serious ethical and medical considerations.

Thus, a cat's failure to respond to a trial of a transdermal psychotropic medication does not define how the cat would respond to an oral formulation. If a client is convinced a "tried" medication did not work, valuable opportunities to intervene are lost. As newer permeation enhancers are offered, the clinician will have to consider if there is sufficient evidence to demonstrate that problems have been sufficiently overcome and that reliable bioavailability assessments have been done. Use of transdermals for psychotropic medications should be used only with great caution and reserved for cases in which other administration options have been exhausted.

CLIENT CONCERNS AND COMPLIANCE

The greatest obstacles in the use of psychotropic medication in cats are clients' resistance to medicating their pet, concerns about side effects, and pet challenges associated with administration of medication. Clients' hesitation to have their cat medicated may be related to negative perceptions, including the assumption that their cat's problem cannot be changed by drugs, belief that administering psychotropic medication will adversely change their cat's personality, belief that psychotropic drugs in general are best avoided, or concerns that, if the medication resolves the problem, their cat may become dependent on the drug for a long time or for life.

To effectively alleviate a feline behavior problem and potentially wean the cat off medication, a multimodal approach is needed, beginning with an accurate diagnosis and integrated with appropriate behavioral and environmental management strategies (as discussed throughout this book). The observable outcomes should also reflect a state of improved emotional well-being for the cat, a cat that is less fearful, more social, and "happier" with people and other pets. The goals of prescribing psychotropic medication are to elevate mood and promote learning rather than to sedate or immobilize. Although some cats may require long-term or even lifelong medication, clients should be assured that decisions are always made on a case-by-case basis and

will be determined by careful observation and response to gradual dose withdrawal. Clients' confidence to begin giving their cat a medication is enhanced when the reasons for its use can be justified and long-term goals are clearly defined. Alternatives to medication should also be openly and fully discussed with the client, especially in cases where social and environmental factors are unable to be addressed satisfactorily from a natural feline behavior perspective. This chapter aims to provide information to help assuage client concerns with evidence and reason in situations where drug therapy is appropriate.

Side Effects: Problems and Perceptions

Many cats experience side effects during the induction period of medication administration. These side effects may be problematic or, in some cases, may actually appear beneficial. For example, a cat's problem behaviors may diminish if the medication evokes a lethargic response. Because these effects are often transient, the client should be advised of these possible effects and understand that they may not last. Furthermore, the occurrence of side effects may provide the clinician with evidence of effective administration, absorption, and metabolism of the medication. It is important to question clients carefully for evidence that the drug is being effectively absorbed and metabolized. For example, many cats given oral fluoxetine or clomipramine experience transient sedation or suppressed appetite, especially during the first week; therefore, the absence of these effects may suggest insufficient absorption and/or poor compliance. If the cat experiences profound undesirable side effects, a dose reduction may be appropriate. Another concern would be raised if the cat seems aloof, withdrawn, or more fearful of the owner, which may be a result of capture and restraint techniques rather than drug-related side effects. Clients should be encouraged to wait for undesirable side effects to pass and not to celebrate the apparent "quick fix" of suppressed behavior. It is advisable to exercise caution when evaluating the effectiveness of medications and switching to an alternative. Unless the medication is dosed at proper therapeutic levels, actually ingested or absorbed, and properly metabolized for a minimum of 4 to 6 weeks, the effectiveness of many psychotropic medications may not be fully appreciated. Premature dose adjustments or switching medications gives the client the false perception that everything has been tried when in fact a full drug trial has yet to be properly completed.

Mini Case Example

A 6-year-old neutered male orange tabby was presented for urine marking. The client reported that the cat enjoyed looking out the window and worried that medication would change her cat's outgoing personality. A detailed description of the cat's behavior revealed a cat that was vigilant and emotionally aroused. Much of the cat's day was occupied by staring out of each window and rushing from window to window, vocalizing in response to the sights and sounds of outdoor cats. It was explained that the cat's vigilant, stress-related window-watching was a symptom of the same emotional response that was contributing to the cat's urine marking, and a program of environmental management was instituted to reduce the cat's ability to look out and to be observed by other cats outside the property. When the environmental modification did not sufficiently reduce the level of vigilance, the option of adjunctive medication to address underlying anxiety was discussed, and the client accepted a trial of medication. The desired outcome measures were reduced vigilance while looking out of windows and reduced urine marking.

Achieving Compliance with Medication Regimens

The efficacy of treatment with psychotropic medication can be achieved (or evaluated) only if the client can successfully and regularly administer the medication. Therefore, at the time of dispensing, it is important to ask the clients about their comfort level in terms of administering medication to their pet and follow up a few days later to inquire whether the client can effectively administer the medication.

The availability of a skilled veterinary technician and/or nurse is invaluable in achieving client compliance in administering medication. These individuals also can provide resources and follow up with the client to ensure success, address concerns, and provide feline behavioral support as required. Some clients may become adept at administering medications directly if properly trained and instructed. Placing the food inside human food or pilling treats (Greenies Pill Pockets; The Nutro Company, Franklin, Tennessee, USA.) may allow some cats to be easily medicated. Crushing the tablet or opening the capsule and placing it inside a tasty human food such as yogurt, cheese, a fish pate, poultry, or anchovy paste may also be successful. Though cats do not taste sweet foods as people do, some cats may accept pills buried in whipped cream. Provided the medication is not in a coated or time release form that should not be crushed, this may be preferable to compounding because the medication can remain in its original form until use. Kittens may actually be trained to accept the handling and manipulation of "pilling" by administering food kibble instead of pills. (Figure 19-3) For more information on administering medications to cats, see handouts titled **How to Pill Your Cat with Kindness: A Cat-Friendly Approach to Medicating** and **Cat-Friendly Medication Administration Techniques**.

Mini Case Example

A cat was treated with 4 mg of fluoxetine (one-half of an 8-mg Reconcile tablet; Elanco Animal Health, Greenfield,

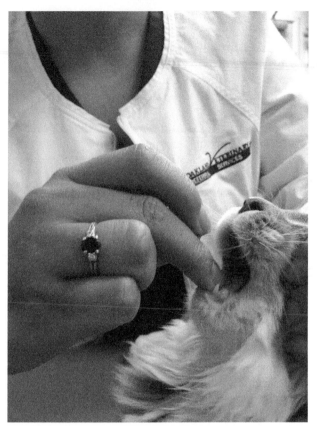

FIGURE 19-3 This cat is being given a piece of dry cat food kibble in the same manner a pill may be administered. By teaching cats this handling procedure before the cat requires medication they can become more amenable to medication throughout their lives.

Ind.) once daily, but the client reported after 5 weeks that her cat was suddenly aloof and distant, so she wanted to stop giving the medication. The cat did not sit with her while she worked on her computer at night as had been his usual routine. Further inquiry revealed that at first the cat would eat the medication when combined with food. Then, after a couple of weeks, the cat did not eat all of the medication, so the client decided to manually pill it, which she reported it "didn't mind." When the cat would walk across the client's computer, the client would be reminded to give the cat a pill. Within a couple of weeks, the cat was no longer walking across her computer. Therefore, the aloofness "side effect" was indeed due to the administration process and associated learning, not with detrimental effects of the medication.

DRUG INTERACTIONS AND SEROTONIN SYNDROME

An excessive increase in serotonin can lead to a rare but serious iatrogenic poisoning event described as *serotonin syndrome* or *serotonin toxidrome*.[4] The exact mechanism is not understood and may occur in response to an initial dose of serotonin-enhancing medication following a dose increase, addition of adjunctive medications, or spontaneously following long-term maintenance therapy. Symptoms of serotonin syndrome include tachycardia, tachypnea, agitation, anorexia, hyperpyrexia, irritability, hypertension, diarrhea, seizures, and, potentially, death. Though this condition is rarely reported, as behavioral medication use increases and polypharmacy becomes more common, the condition is likely to become more prevalent. A combination of medications, supplements, or diets that enhance serotonin levels may pose increased risk for serotonin syndrome. Some specific medications that might cause a reaction if combined with psychotropic medications include combining SSRIs or TCAs with each other or with buspirone, tramadol, or metoclopramide. Also be cautious with certain herbal remedies and supplements (e.g., St John's wort or tryptophan). Some of the symptoms of serotonin syndrome may appear similar to the clinical signs being treated; therefore, the clinician must carefully evaluate reported events to determine if agitation is due to unresolved anxiety issues or is indeed a manifestation of an adverse effect.

PRACTICAL MANAGEMENT TOOLS

The art of psychopharmacology for cats goes beyond selecting the medication. Uneasiness with practical considerations, such as how to assess a behavioral outcome and long-term management, may prevent clinicians from using psychoactive agents. Before beginning medications, it is important to consider whether drugs might be needed for short-term or situational use or for long-term administration, when and how long-term drugs might be weaned, and whether a single or multimodal approach might be used. A multimodal approach may obscure which intervention is most successful, but this should not prevent the clinician from combining multiple variables at one time. For example, a diabetic patient may be managed by changes in insulin, diet, exercise, and water intake simultaneously without worry about which intervention helped. Indeed, all aspects of a behavior treatment plan may be essential to achieve a desired outcome, and any single intervention alone may be insufficient.

Situational Interventions

Situational interventions are to be considered for circumstances where the need is immediate but the occurrence of the situation is infrequent. Consider when the cat displays the problem behavior and the periodicity of the problem when evaluating the best medication for intervention. Some cats are anxious during car travel, for veterinary visits, or fearful of strangers, which may be sufficiently infrequent occurrences for which a benzodiazepine might be used in advance of the event. However, if visitors come to the house frequently, the cat might require a maintenance intervention such as mild

anxiety-reducing dietary or supplemental approaches (e.g., Royal Canin Veterinary Diet CALM, Aimargues, France; Composure, VetriSCIENCE Laboratories, Essex Junction, Vt.; or Anxitane, Virbac, Fort Worth, Tex.) or medications that may have a mild to moderate anxiolytic effect (e.g., buspirone).

Short-Term or Long-Term Maintenance and Drug Withdrawal

Medication may be indicated to alleviate recently developed behavior problems. Prompt initiation of an appropriate medication (e.g., benzodiazepines, pheromones) at the right dosage may provide a quick response. Chronic and ongoing problems may require long-term medications such as buspirone, TCAs, or SSRIs. Long-term resolution of behavior problems with mood-altering medications combined with environmental modifications and behavior modification strategies may result in improvement that cannot be ascribed to only one aspect of the program. Further, the right combination allows the cat to learn, develop habits, and formulate associations. In general, the problem should be well resolved and stable for a sufficient period of weeks or months before dose reduction is considered. The quality and acceptability of the new behavior and the impact of other aspects of the program are also factors that should be considered before reducing medication. Stability of behavior also provides opportunities for clients to be successful with other aspects of the behavior modification program. For example, clients may be able to teach their cat to come when called or to perform tricks that can be used for counterconditioning and operantly teaching desirable outcomes. The cat may be able to learn such a task while medicated, but it may be too fearful or suspicious without the support of medication. Task-related goals give clients a clear idea of what they must accomplish before their cat will be taken off medication. This often means weeks or months of maintenance treatment. The clinician should consider the seriousness of the problem, the difficulty with which success was attained, the level of improvement, and the contribution of other aspects of the program to determine if the risk outweighs the rewards for continuing medication. Some cats may benefit from long-term or lifelong medication. If medication alleviates stress, improves the cat's welfare, and enhances its quality of life, or if it is behaviorally abnormal when not on medication, the cat should be monitored with regular medical and behavioral assessments.

Mini Case Example

Paroxetine was prescribed for a domestic shorthair cat for redirected aggression to the client in response to cats outside the home. Three weeks after medication was initiated, the cat became aroused and explosively reactive due to a feral cat's screaming outside the window in the middle of the night. The client called the next day to say the medication wasn't working. What do you do? Continue the medication! This incident doesn't necessarily represent a medication failure. The time to the peak effect of paroxetine may be 4 to 6 weeks, and this event is extreme, beyond the scope of an expectation of responding to medication alone and before the medication has achieved maximal effect.

Mini Case Example

A domestic longhair cat was given 4 mg of fluoxetine daily for urine marking. The clients forget to give the medication on some days, but as long as the cat gets medication at least 6 days per week, there is no urine marking. If the dose is reduced to five doses per week, the cat urine marks. Therefore, calculate the effective dose as 24 mg per week (4 mg × 6 = 24 mg/week) and redistribute the dose to one 8-mg tablet given 3 days per week. This is the same dose, but it is given in a manner that the clients may be better able to manage consistently.

When a Medication Does Not Work: What Next?

If the first medication selected doesn't resolve the target behavior after a suitable period of time and at an adequate dose for that medication to be effective, then the clinician should consider alternatives, including modification of the behavior program; further environmental modifications, reassessing the accuracy of the diagnosis and even the possibility of rehoming; before instituting polypharmacy.

Referral to a board-certified veterinary behaviorist should be considered for refractory cases, particularly if the clinician is not comfortable with polypharmacy strategies. It is also essential that medication be given at a sufficient dose, that the duration be adequate to be effective, and that ongoing outcomes are accurately assessed before alternatives are tried. Multiple, successive subtherapeutic duration trials are not likely to yield a desirable outcome and will diminish the client's trust that a beneficial medication exists. If the cat does not experience side effects, increasing the dose may achieve the desired results. If the cat experiences significant, transient side effects, a dose increase may result in reoccurrence of side effects.

Switching Medications

Ideally, gradual discontinuation of one drug before starting a new drug is optimal; however, depending on the severity of the problem and the tolerance of the clients, more rapid initiation of drug trials may be required. Switching from one SSRI to another SSRI may be done with only a few days without medication, or it may be done cautiously with 1 day in between, whereas there should be a 2-week period between medications when changing from an MAOI to an SSRI or a TCA to avoid potentially toxic effects. A transition from a TCA to an SSRI or vice versa should optimally include a washout period, but it can often be safely accomplished in less time (e.g., a 3-day washout between doses). Transition from one TCA to another may also be accomplished with minimal risk of dangerous side effects. Depending on dose, individual response to medication, length of treatment, and half-life and clearance of the drug being discontinued, a cat may be transitioned from one drug to another with careful monitoring during the transition without major cause for concern. Whenever an optimal washout cannot be achieved, beginning the new medication at the lowest end of the dose range is advisable. Clients should be advised of potential side effects and that the full therapeutic effects of the change may not be achieved for several weeks.

Combination Therapy

Combination therapy should be considered by clinicians experienced in complex behavior cases; however, one of the biggest challenges faced will be in the assessment of the results. Combination of drugs may be beneficial if there might be fewer side effects with both medications than would be experienced with a higher dose of one medication. Combinations may be useful to achieve success in difficult, refractory cases. Once resolution is achieved, each medication dosage should be reduced one at a time to determine which results in regression.

General practitioners should be aware of which drug combinations are possible and should consider referral of complicated or refractory patients to a board-certified veterinary behaviorist.

SSRI or TCA + diet (monitor for serotonin syndrome if diet contains tryptophan)

SSRI or TCA + benzodiazepine[5]

SSRI or TCA + buspirone (monitor for serotonin syndrome)

SSRI, TCA, or benzodiazepine + nutraceutical (monitor for serotonin syndrome if nutraceutical has known effects on serotonin)—no reported concerns with pheromones, Anxitane, or α-casozepine

SSRI, TCA, or benzodiazepine + gabapentin

Medical management should be used in combination with pheromone therapy and environmental management (See Chapter 18, *Mini Case Example: Controlling Urine Marking*).

Gradual Dose Reduction

Often clients and clinicians wonder if the cat needs ongoing medication. Achievement of resolution may have required many weeks or months of treatment and may be the result of complex or multimodal interventions. By attempting a dose reduction trial and monitoring for the return of target behaviors, the cat may be weaned completely off medication or kept on the lowest effective dose determined. Dose reduction of psychotropic medications may reveal how effective the medication was at alleviating the problem by requiring the client to monitor for recurrence of signs. By removing each intervention stepwise, you may wean the cat off the medication, reduce the medication to the lowest effective dose determined, or, in some cases, validate the necessity of the medication. Dose reduction may be further complicated by the per-dose strength of the medication. TCAs and SSRIs have a delayed onset to effect, so although any recurrence associated with dose reduction may be noticed immediately more commonly, the effect may be noticed over the course of several weeks. Dose reduction is ideally managed by a 25% reduction at 4- to 6-week intervals. For medications with a more prolonged duration of effect, a more gradual dose reduction schedule is recommended. For a cat that has been stabilized on medication for a few months, the dose might be reduced gradually for a few weeks, whereas the dose for cats that have been on medication for 1 year or more may be reduced over the course of many months. A long weaning program helps to identify the lowest effective dose. With medications with a longer half-life (i.e., SSRIs), this may best be done by calculating the total dose per week, multiplying by 75%, and then dividing by the available pill size to determine a practical dose reduction scheme over two or three 6-week cycles.

A 5-kg cat is stabilized on paroxetine, one-half of a 10-mg tablet once daily (total dose = 35 mg/week, target dose reduction = 35 mg × 0.75 = 26 mg). The goal is to accomplish a total weekly dose of 26 mg. This would be approximately 5 mg/day given 5 days per week (total weekly dose = 25 mg). Maintain this regimen for 6 weeks. Observe for regression. Repeat.

Monitoring

Feline patients may benefit from psychopharmacological interventions, but care should be taken to consider the target behaviors, the expected onset to efficacy of the medication, and administration methods that are effective and do not cause stress. It is also important to consider safety, evidence of efficacy, mode of administration, dosing intervals, contraindications, and practicality when choosing a drug and to use pharmacological or nutraceutical interventions in combination with environmental management and behavior modification. Because many cats do not adapt well to change, neophobia may actually be the target symptom for medication. Most behavior programs require time, persistence, and patience to be successful. The client should be counseled that once satisfactory improvement is achieved, a gradual dose reduction program can be implemented to find the lowest effective dose or to wean the cat off the medication

entirely. However, some cats may require their medication long-term. Where the environment is compromising feline behavior and cannot be modified, it is useful for clients to realize that changes in behavior may be difficult to achieve. Although neither is an optimal solution, it may result in either the cat being on medication long-term or the possibility of exploring and perhaps implementing alternative housing arrangements. Regular healthcare should incorporate behavioral assessments. Regular age- and health-appropriate laboratory monitoring (complete blood count, serum chemistry, urinalysis) should be required or recommended for patients on long-term medication for any reason, including psychopharmacologic drugs. Adopting these strategies will ensure that the decision to use medication and the decision to continue to use medication can be incorporated into a complete behavior modification strategy that supports the cat's long-term welfare and emotional well-being. The frequency with which cats on long-term medication are monitored must comply with any regional or national professional and legal requirements.

OVERVIEW OF COMMONLY USED PSYCHOACTIVE TOOLS

Psychoactive tools for treating cats include drugs, supplements, and diets. The major drug classes that have relevance for veterinary behavior include longer-acting drugs such as SSRIs or TCAs, alone or combined with situational medications, and those that have a shorter onset of action, including benzodiazepine and azapirones or neuroleptics.

In general, when prescribing medications, beginning at the low end of a dose range and increasing the dose as needed, based on the medication and the problem, is a prudent approach. Similarly, dose adjustments may be made or drugs withdrawn in response to adverse effects. The individual cat's response cannot be predetermined based on a dose chart, and increasing the dose does not always achieve a better response. More is not always better. The clinician must seek the optimal dose by observing the intended effect for each patient. It is also important to note that there are likely to be breed and individual differences, medical conditions, and concurrent use of other drugs that will require dose adjustments or discontinuation in some individuals. Therefore, pet owners should be advised of the expected therapeutic effects and side effects and instructed to report immediately any unexpected change in their cat's health or behavior. New data continue to emerge about psychotropic drug doses and their effects. All clinicians should therefore empirically evaluate all doses to determine whether they are reasonable before using them in their patients. It is the clinician's responsibility to know the local regulations regarding off-label dispensing and to have appropriate consent or release forms signed. A sample release form can be found in the handout titled **Informed Consent for Psychotropic Drug Use for a Cat**.

Selection of a medication is based on a variety of factors, including analysis of evidence, experience, and availability. In this section, the symbols that appear next to drug names are intended to guide the clinician in selecting commonly used medications versus less frequently used options (see detailed descriptions below). Note that these recommendations and applications are based on the authors' collective experience, frequency of use, and comfort with both their safety and effectiveness for behavior-related applications.

* An asterisk next to a drug name indicates common use and general agreement among the authors based on clinical experience and published evidence for its selection.
** A double asterisk indicates occasional use, regional variations in use, or a secondary selection medication. This coding may indicate there is less strength of evidence for use of the drug, but anecdotal experience and author agreement suggest probable applications for difficult or refractory cases.
† A dagger indicates cautious use by general practitioners and even by the authors. Caution may be advised due to rare or infrequent actual clinical experiences, minimal published reports of use, the existence of better alternatives, or a higher potential for adverse effects. These medications should be considered only when primary and secondary choices have been ineffective.

PSYCHOACTIVE DRUGS

Antidepressants

Antidepressants include both the SSRIs and the TCAs, the most commonly prescribed mood-altering medications. The category is designated "antidepressants" based on the early applications of a few drugs in human medicine. Now there are many classes of antidepressants and many new drugs with complicated mechanisms of action. The term *antidepressant* is confusing for veterinary clients, so a simplified comparative discussion may be useful. Although pets are not generally treated for "depression" according to the human diagnostic terminology, they cope with adversity differently. A person with neuropsychological disorders may resolve that life is too overwhelming and elect to withdraw from social interactions. Pets do not have such an option and may be forced to cope with situations they find overwhelming, which is manifested in fear and anxiety. Unlike other medications, such as the benzodiazepines, antidepressants are unlikely to inhibit learning or memory. Although antidepressants are readily absorbed from the

gastrointestinal tract and achieve peak levels within hours, the reuptake inhibition induces downregulation of synthesis of postsynaptic receptors. Therefore, 4 to 8 weeks of therapy is recommended to fully assess these drugs' effects. Some behavioral effects may be seen more quickly, but these rapid-onset effects may be related to sedation. For example, medications such as amitriptyline have a profound side effect profile and may seem to work quite quickly, but this may be due to the sedation effect and not to downregulation of the serotonin receptors. Concurrent use with MAOIs (e.g., selegiline) should be avoided. Antidepressants should be used cautiously in pets with a known history of seizures. Combining antidepressants can result in serotonin syndrome and is not recommended. Serotonin syndrome is a rare toxidrome of serotonergic drugs that is described under the Drug Interactions and Serotonin Syndrome section earlier in this chapter.

Selective Serotonin Reuptake Inhibitors (SSRIs)

Mode of action: SSRIs are selective in their blockade of the reuptake of 5-HT1A into the presynaptic neurons.

Examples: Fluoxetine,* paroxetine,* sertraline,** fluvoxamine,** citalopram,† escitalopram†

Commonly prescribed for: Anxiety, aggression, impulsivity, compulsive/repetitive behavior, urine marking

Effects: Allow a minimum of 4 weeks to assess effect. Long half-lives mean dose changes may not be fully reflected for several weeks. Lethargy and anorexia are the most common side effects and these effects are most pronounced in the first two weeks.

Contraindications/precautions/warnings: Do not use with MAOIs. Avoid or use with caution with other serotonin enhancing medications or supplements.

Practical considerations: SSRIs frequently are considered first-line treatment option for generalized anxiety, urine marking, and lack of impulse control.

How They Work

SSRIs are selective in their blockade of the reuptake of 5-HT1A into the presynaptic neurons. They require a once-daily dosing schedule, which is convenient for clients and feline patients. Because SSRIs primarily affect serotonin receptors without substantially affecting the reuptake of norepinephrine or dopamine, they may cause fewer side effects than TCAs. Fluoxetine is the most widely used and best recognized SSRI. Other SSRIs, such as paroxetine, sertraline, citalopram, and escitalopram, might be considered by comparing their similarities or distinctions from fluoxetine. In cats, the oral absorption of fluoxetine is 100% with a half-life of 34 to 47 hours, and the half-life of the immediate metabolite, norfluoxetine, is 51 to 55 hours.[6] There is evidence for a wide margin of safety in cats (lethal dose >50 mg/kg [22.7 mg/lb] of body weight).[7,8] Cats with anxiety-based behaviors may respond to many medications, but the first option for ongoing or chronic use is often fluoxetine. If there is a partial or incomplete response or a failure to respond to fluoxetine, another SSRI may still prove to be effective. Individual cats' responses may vary, and only a therapeutic trial will allow you to assess a drug's effectiveness. Dosing trials may also reveal a beneficial effect at a higher or lower dose. Although increasing the dose is a logical option if there is an insufficient response and the maximum recommended dose has not yet been reached, some patients may be more responsive to lower doses. However, there is minimal benefit derived from subtherapeutic dosing, and gradually increasing a dose over many weeks or months may create a downregulation at the cellular level that negates the effects of incremental dose adjustments. A partial beneficial response without occurrence of side effects would suggest that a higher dose should be tried, whereas the occurrence of profound side effects and minimal benefits should prompt the clinician to reduce the dose or try another drug in the same or a different category. Other SSRIs merit special consideration. Paroxetine is a novel phenylpiperidine compound that acts as an SSRI. Paroxetine is a more selective and potent SSRI than fluoxetine, sertraline, or fluvoxamine, and, based on studies in humans, its pharmacokinetics are well suited to clinical use.[9] In Europe, fluvoxamine may be prescribed commonly, whereas in North America this medication is less frequently prescribed. Metabolism of paroxetine is unique in that no active metabolites are produced, which may be beneficial for elderly patients or animals with liver or kidney disease. In humans, paroxetine may be more beneficial for alleviation of social tension or social phobias. Citalopram is considered mildly and uniquely histaminic in humans, and escitalopram is used in elderly people because of its low side effect profile; however, use of these drugs in felines has not yet been explored.

Side Effects

Lethargy and anorexia are the most common side effects. Adverse events reported for SSRIs include reduced appetite, weight loss, lethargy, gastrointestinal disturbances, restlessness, sleep disturbances, and alterations in cardiac conduction. These side effects may be more tolerable or may be ameliorated by reduced doses or every-other-day dosing. SSRIs may be preferred over TCAs where cardiac disease, urine retention, increased intraocular pressure, sedation, or anticholinergic effects might be a concern. Paroxetine has mild anticholinergic effects, including constipation in cats. Because SSRIs inhibit cytochrome P450 enzymes, they can lead to increased toxicity when combined with drugs that are metabolized by these enzymes. The therapeutic effect is generally realized 4 to 6 weeks after initiation, although effects might be noted much earlier. Once a

successful resolution of the behavior problem has been achieved, consider modifying the dose interval while maintaining the same total weekly dose. This same strategy may be used during weaning or dose reduction to determine the lowest effective dose. Because of the long half-life of SSRIs, some cats may be maintained on once or twice per week dosing once the target behavior has stabilized. Because the clearance half-lives of fluoxetine and norfluoxetine are prolonged, gradual weaning is not required, but it may be behaviorally advantageous to gradually reduce the dose if the drug is used for longer than 8 to 12 weeks.

Research on Indications for Use

In one study, fluoxetine was shown to be highly efficacious in the treatment of feline urine marking at a dose of 1 mg/kg.[7] In this placebo-controlled study of 17 cats, the cats treated with fluoxetine had a significant decrease in spraying by Week 2, and spraying continued to decrease through Weeks 7 and 8. Two of the cats that did not improve to a level of 70% or greater were given an increased dose of 1.5 mg/kg for Weeks 7 and 8. Recurrence after drug withdrawal was variable, with cats marking the most at baseline most likely to relapse. Many behaviorists may prescribe fluoxetine at 0.5 mg/kg.

Fluoxetine, paroxetine, or sertraline may be effective for urine marking, anxiety, or repetitive conditions. It is very important to take care to distinguish house soiling due to elimination or to medical problems from urine marking, because the former problem may or may not be related to anxiety. Theoretically, some cats may cope better with a behavior modification program or may experience less apprehension about a state of poor litter box hygiene when supported by medication. However, medication should not be used to mask poor environmental conditions, and it is essential that appropriate behavioral and environmental modification as well as basic feline care (such as litter box hygiene) be instituted in conjunction with medication. In one study, researchers compared the efficacy of clomipramine at 0.5 mg/kg per day and fluoxetine at 1 mg/kg per day in cats treated for 16 weeks. The efficacy of the drugs was similar, with treatment of longer than 8 weeks leading to increased efficacy. Return of marking occurred after abrupt drug withdrawal of fluoxetine in most cats, but marking could be controlled if medication was reinstituted.[10]

Tricyclic Antidepressants (TCAs)

Mode of action: Blockade of serotonin and noradrenaline reuptake with varying degrees of anticholinergic, antihistaminic, and α-adrenergic effects

Examples: Amitriptyline,† clomipramine (Clomicalm; Novartis Animal Health, Larchwood, Iowa),* doxepin,** nortriptyline†

Commonly prescribed for: Anxiety, aggression, impulsivity, compulsive/repetitive behaviors, urine marking

Effects: 4 to 6 weeks to assess effect

Contraindications/precautions/warnings: Other than clomipramine, TCAs are not considered a first-line treatment option because their side effect profile is slightly greater than that of SSRIs.

Practical considerations: No specific feline preparation of clomipramine is available, but the 5-mg tablets can be split for use in cats.

How They Work

TCAs block the reuptake of serotonin and noradrenaline. Clomipramine is the most selective inhibitor of serotonin reuptake among the TCAs. It also inhibits noradrenaline reuptake and has mild anticholinergic and antihistaminic effects. TCAs are unlikely to inhibit learning or memory. Although the use of doxepin, imipramine, and amitriptyline has been suggested in the veterinary literature, evidence of their efficacy is lacking. Antidepressants are readily absorbed from the gastrointestinal tract and achieve peak levels within hours; however, the reuptake inhibition initially induces downregulation of postsynaptic receptors. Therefore, 4 to 6 weeks of therapy may be needed to fully assess the effects of these drugs, although some cats improve much more quickly. Concurrent use with MAOIs, such as selegiline, should be avoided. TCAs should be used cautiously in pets with a known history of seizures.[11]

Side Effects

TCAs have varying degrees of anticholinergic, antihistaminic, and α-adrenergic activity, which probably accounts for side effects such as lethargy, dry mouth, or gastrointestinal signs. TCAs are contraindicated in cats with cardiac disease or glaucoma or for cats in which urine retention is a concern.[11] In a study of seven healthy cats selected to evaluate the effect of clomipramine (10 mg/cat once daily for 28 days) on cardiac rhythm, no cardiac abnormalities were detected on electrocardiograms. Similar results have been seen in dogs treated with amitriptyline and clomipramine.[3,12] In the same study, the researchers did detect statistically significant decreases in serum thyroid concentrations (T4, T3, and free T4) between pre- and post-clomipramine administration.[12] Clomipramine should be used cautiously in cats with thyroid disease, as the reduction in serum thyroid concentrations may obscure hyperthyroidism.

Research on Indications for Use

Like the SSRIs, TCAs are used in veterinary practice to reduce anxiety, panic, and impulsivity. In human medicine, TCAs were available before SSRIs but caused undesirable side effects. The search for agents that would inhibit the uptake of 5-HT from the synaptic cleft with fewer undesirable receptor effects resulted in the discovery and development of the SSRI fluoxetine hydrochloride (Prozac; Eli Lilly, Indianapolis, Ind.). Prozac was first introduced in the U.S. market in January 1988 and soon became the world's most widely prescribed antidepressant.[13] In many ways, this trend followed in veterinary medicine as well because many clinicians have found the SSRIs to be more effective, more economical, and more convenient while causing fewer side effects than TCAs. Further, the flexible once daily dosing indicated for SSRIs is more acceptable for both clients and cats. Although older literature, case reports, and texts focus on TCAs, this may indicate drug availability, clinician familiarity, and the higher cost of newly developed alternatives at the time of publication rather than the researchers' actual preferences or the drugs' clinical advantages.[10,14-19] Approved canine products (Clomicalm) divided into cat-sized doses make the costs reasonable and administration more practical. Clomicalm is licensed for canine separation anxiety in combination with a behavior modification program[14] and, in some countries, for canine compulsive and anxiety disorders. In cats, clomipramine may be an effective means of reducing or controlling urine marking, and it is licensed for this use in Australia.[20] On the basis of their use in humans reported in the literature, which may not entirely be extrapolated to cats, amitriptyline and doxepin have substantial antihistaminic properties due to their ability to block H_1 and H_2 receptors. Amitriptyline equally affects H_1 and H_2 receptors, whereas doxepin is much more selective for H_1 receptors. Doxepin has an affinity for H_1 receptors *in vitro* that is 56 times that of hydroxyzine and 775 times that of diphenhydramine.[21,22] Doxepin may be profoundly sedating in cats, and arriving at a dose low enough to avoid sedation while providing sufficient anxiolytic effect is challenging. Its unique antihistaminic properties make doxepin worthy of consideration for cats with allergic or dermatologic disorders. Amitriptyline has also been used as a treatment for urine marking in cats, but reports of its success are anecdotal and no studies of its use in cats have been published. The bitter taste of amitriptyline tablets may cause excessive drooling and frothing at the mouth, resulting in resistance to medication administration in many cats (Figure 19-4). If amitriptyline is selected for use, it is particularly important not to break amitriptyline tablets into pieces. Prolonged administration of bitter tablets such as amitriptyline is not recommended, as the cat's resistance only makes clients engage in stressful cat-catching and forced-pilling, which adds to the traumatic experience. Many cats experience profound sedation with amitriptyline, which might induce social apathy and in turn might indeed reduce a cat's inclination to urine mark, but this is not the intended effect of

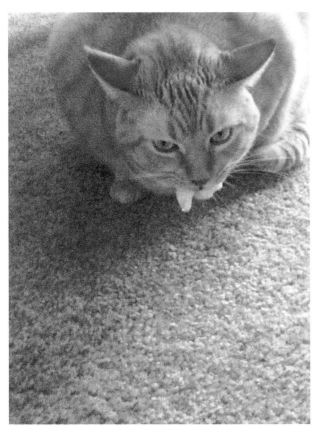

FIGURE 19-4 Cats naturally avoid bitter or unusual tasting foods. Some medications, especially those that are bitter tasting, may cause cats to foam and froth, which can be distressing.

mood-altering medications. Anecdotally, many behaviorists report that they only rarely prescribe amitriptyline. Despite the historical significance of amitriptyline, use of this medication by behaviorists has waned and has largely been replaced by other, more tolerable, more effective, more economical alternatives.

Azapirones

Mode of action: Serotonin 1-A receptor agonists
Examples: Buspirone*
Commonly prescribed for: Anxiety disorders and fear; social tension, timidity, or withdrawal. Effect on social affiliative behavior toward same or other species may be profound.
Effects: 2 to 4 weeks to assess effect
Contraindications/precautions/warnings: Caution with hepatic or renal disorders
Practical considerations: Well tolerated, minimal sedative effect, must be dosed twice daily

How They Work

Buspirone is a serotonin (5-HT1A) receptor agonist and a dopamine receptor (D_2) agonist.[24] It is nonsedating and does not stimulate appetite or inhibit memory. It

may take 1 week or more to achieve effect. Any anxiolytic may cause aggression due to disinhibition.

Side Effects

Gastrointestinal effects are possible, but generally side effects are minimal and mild when they occur. Anecdotally, buspirone is reported to induce friendliness toward people or toward other cats, including a decrease in avoidance and an increase in proximity and seeking human contact with bunting or rubbing. However, when given to a fearful cat, it may lead to disinhibition, resulting in aggression. Therefore, buspirone may be most suited to building the confidence of a fearful victim cat when there are issues with intercat social relationships. Decreased fear would be a desirable effect for cats that have poor cat–human or cat–cat relationships, especially in conjunction with counterconditioning. Improvement in the human animal bond may reduce the risk of relinquishment or euthanasia. Care should be used when combining buspirone with erythromycin or itraconazole, both of which may increase plasma levels of buspirone.

Research on Indications for Use

Buspirone may be useful for mild fear and anxiety and for urine marking in cats. Hart and colleagues examined the effectiveness of buspirone for urine marking and for inappropriate urination in cases where anxiety was a contributing factor, at 2.5 mg/cat twice daily for 2 weeks. If that dose was not sufficient to reduce the cat's urination to the owner's satisfaction, then the dose was increased to 5 mg/cat twice daily. The degree of suppression of urine spraying (100%, 75%, 50%, 25%, or none) was assessed by owner consultation by telephone interview.[10] Buspirone was shown to be effective (>75% reduction) in 55% of the cats treated for urine spraying. When the drug was discontinued after 2 months of treatment, half of the cats resumed urine spraying, and these cats were treated with buspirone for 6 to 18 months. The relapse rate on withdrawal was 53% after 8 weeks of treatment.[23] Buspirone may be useful in combination with SSRIs and TCAs for its potentiating effect with the benefit of minimal side effects; however, caution should be used, especially at higher dosing levels, for signs of serotonin syndrome.[1] Buspirone is not commonly used in Europe; it is more commonly prescribed in North America. Twice-daily dosing and cost are potential downsides, as buspirone may be expensive. Price and availability may be extremely variable between regions and even between pharmacies.

Benzodiazepines

Mode of action: Facilitate the action of the inhibitory neurotransmitter GABA, thus increasing neural inhibition by their agonistic effect on GABA receptors
Examples: Alprazolam,* oxazepam,* lorazepam,* clonazepam,* clorazepate,** diazepam**

Commonly prescribed for: Urine marking, situational anxiety or events (travel, grooming, and veterinary visits), and, less frequently, for ongoing use, such as treatment of a fearful cat with intercat aggression or controlling arousal (and perhaps muscle spasm and seizure focus) in cats with hyperesthesia

Effects: Anxiolytic, sedative, skeletal muscle relaxant, and anticonvulsant effects with an immediate onset of action

Contraindications/precautions/warnings: May disinhibit aggression and/or enhance appetite. Use with caution in cats, as diazepam has been reported to cause rare cases of fatal hepatic necrosis. If a cat becomes listless or anorexic after beginning diazepam, reassess, particularly for liver disease

Caution in cats with hepatic dysfunction: Overdose may cause profound CNS depression

Practical considerations: Useful primarily for the short term or for situational events. Useful for situational combination with other, long-term maintenance drugs. Some cases may have indications for ongoing therapy (expert application).

How They Work

Benzodiazepines potentiate GABA, an inhibitory neurotransmitter. The exact mechanism of action is unknown, but postulated mechanisms include antagonism of serotonin, increased release of and/or facilitation of GABA activity, and diminished release or turnover of acetylcholine in the CNS.[25] Benzodiazepines reduce anxiety, cause muscle relaxation, decrease locomotor activity, and may cause hyperphagia (which may be useful for counterconditioning with food). They may cause paradoxical excitability and can have an amnesic effect on learning and memory. Benzodiazepines reach peak effect shortly after each dose and are therefore useful on an as-needed basis for specific situations or in combination with other drugs.[5] Paradoxical excitability must be distinguished from the anxiolytic effect. Though diazepam is often the most recognized of the benzodiazepines, behaviorists frequently prefer other drugs in this class for applications to reduce stress and anxiety for cats. Some immediate relief with the first dose of benzodiazepines is common. The therapeutic window is often hours in duration but may vary between individuals and between drugs in this class. Clients should observe for the time of onset and the duration of effects and/or benefits for their pet. The elimination half-life of diazepam for cats is 5.5 hours, and for its active intermediate metabolite, nordiazepam, it is 21.3 hours.[25] The elimination half-life of diazepam in humans is 20 to 50 hours for diazepam, and for nordiazepam it is up to 200 hours. This may explain interspecies differences in applications and effectiveness.

Side Effects

Diazepam has been linked with rare cases of hepatotoxicity and death caused by idiopathic hepatotoxicosis within the first week of drug exposure in cats.[26] It is biotransformed into active metabolites that also must be metabolized. Cats do not use glucuronic acid pathways as efficiently as do other species, and this may allow the accumulation of reactive intermediate metabolites in some cats when they are treated with diazepam. As a precaution, baseline blood chemistry tests, especially to measure alanine aminotransferase (ALT) and aspartate aminotransferase (AST), are recommended before starting treatment with benzodiazepines, and values should be rechecked 3 to 5 days later. Medication should be discontinued if there are signs of anorexia or if elevation of ALT and/or AST is detected. Because clonazepam, oxazepam, and lorazepam have no active intermediate metabolites, they may be safer for cats in general and especially for cats with compromised hepatic function. Although there is a great deal of individual variability, clonazepam and oxazepam may also have a longer duration of effect, and may require less frequent dosing, when benzodiazepines are used on an ongoing basis. Benzodiazepines can cause dependency with extended use, resulting in a rebound in the treated behavior when these drugs are discontinued. Gradual withdrawal of medication is suggested to attempt to override this effect.

Research on Indications for Use

Benzodiazepines may be advantageous or preferable whenever a rapid control of anxiety is required. Diazepam has been shown to be effective for feline urine marking. It has been reported to be effective at reducing spraying by 75% or greater in 55% to 74% of cats.[27] Relapse rates of 76% to 91% have been reported after drug withdrawal.[25,27] Twice-daily doses are required with benzodiazepines. They do not appear to be as effective as SSRIs or TCAs, but they are certainly preferable to progestins.[28] Long-term twice-daily use of benzodiazepines may be an option if SSRIs or TCAs are contraindicated or are insufficiently effective, but such use should be approached with caution; in general, benzodiazepines should be viewed as a short-term medication option. They offer an advantage of quicker mode of action and may be considered as a temporary adjunct or alternative for "desperate" cases where a delay in therapeutic effect is intolerable to the clients. Ultimately, the cats may be transitioned to another medication.

Monoamine Oxidase B Inhibitors (MAOBIs)

Mode of action: Irreversible inhibitor of monoamine oxidase with a greater affinity for MAO-B

Examples: Selegiline (Anipryl, Zoetis, Florham Park, N.J.; Selgian, CEVA, Lenexa, Kan.)**

Commonly prescribed for: Cognitive dysfunction or cognitive decline. Also a consideration for emotional disorders (i.e., chronic states of stress or fear)

Effects: 3 weeks is minimum assessment period; it can take up to 6 weeks to demonstrate an effect

Contraindications/precautions/warnings: Should not be used in combination with certain other medications, particularly TCAs, SSRIs, tramadol, metronidazole, prednisone, or trimethoprim sulfa

Practical considerations: Best given in the morning because of their stimulant properties. If a cat with cognitive dysfunction responds favorably to selegiline, this medication should be continued lifelong

How They Work

MAOBIs enhance catecholamine transmission and are licensed for use in dogs in North America for cognitive dysfunction and in Europe for emotional disorders. MAOBIs have been reported to increase the lifespans of healthy mice, rats, and dogs.[29]

Side Effects

Adverse effects may include restlessness, agitation, vomiting, diarrhea, and diminished hearing. Contraindications include known sensitivity and combination with other medications, particularly TCAs (amitriptyline, clomipramine, doxepin), SSRIs (fluoxetine, paroxetine), tramadol, metronidazole, prednisone, and trimethoprim sulfa.[30] Humans who take selegiline are cautioned to avoid cheese because of risks for potentiation of the hypertensive effects of tyramine due to mixed MAOIs or to the metabolite effects, but at clinically relevant doses this is probably not necessary for dogs and cats. However, it may be prudent to avoid giving cheese to a cat taking an MAOBI because an individual's reaction may be based on species or individual variations in ratios of MAO-A and MAO-B receptors and the activity and half-life of intermediate metabolites.[30] Do not give a cat TCAs for at least 2 weeks following discontinuation of selegiline. A 2-week washout period may be sufficient for SSRIs, but some suggest a longer wash out period, even 5 weeks, following discontinuation of drugs belonging to this class.[30] Although selegiline may improve cognitive function and quality of life for aged felines, the potential impact of other medications should be considered carefully.

Research on Indications for Use

There is anecdotal evidence of improvement of signs of cognitive dysfunction in cats with selegiline, and researchers in one small study found no toxicity in cats at doses up to 10 mg/kg.[31] To date, there have been no published studies on the efficacy of selegiline in cats, although there have been reports of its efficacy for cognitive dysfunction and for emotional disorders with signs such as urine marking, depressed appetite, or altered sleep–wake cycles.[32,33]

Other Drugs with Crossover Psychotropic Effects

Gabapentin

Mode of action: Structurally related to GABA, but no known direct actions on GABA or its receptors

Examples: Gabapentin (Neurontin; Pfizer, New York)*

Commonly prescribed for: Hypersensitivity, neuropathic pain, or adjunctive use for anxiety and aggression

Effects: Notable response may occur within days or weeks

Contraindications/precautions/warnings: Well tolerated. Mild adverse effects. Limited information available.

Practical considerations: Similar to pregabalin (Lyrica; Pfizer), which is generally cost-prohibitive at the time of writing

How It Works

Gabapentin is a structural analog of GABA, but it does not alter GABA binding, reuptake, or degradation. It does bind to the $\alpha_2\delta_1$ subunit of presynaptic voltage-gated calcium channels and inhibits calcium influx by way of these channels. Gabapentin inhibits release of excitatory neurotransmitters (substance P, glutamate, norepinephrine) from primary afferent nerve fibers. It may be indicated, particularly as an adjunct to other medications, for refractory seizures, chronic pain, and neuropathic pain. In addition to its anticonvulsant effect, gabapentin may be useful in behavioral therapy for generalized anxiety disorders, impulsivity, mood disorders, phobias, panic disorder, and impulse control disorders, and as adjunctive therapy for compulsive disorders. Gabapentin may be useful as a medication to be given before an examination or veterinary procedure for cats known to react explosively during restraint. Gabapentin has been used as monotherapy or together with SSRIs for impulse control disorders, noise phobias, and self-trauma, in part because of its effect on neuropathic pain. Gabapentin may be dosed up to three times per day for seizure control, whereas for pain control or neuropathic sensations it may be effective when given less frequently, most often twice daily. Peak plasma levels are reported to be about 1.5 to 3 hours with an elimination half-life of about 3 hours.[34] Sedation is the most common side effect, and this may be transient. If effective for reducing pain or reactivity and agitation that may be secondary to pain, this drug may be continued long-term while other pain relievers are reduced or discontinued.

Side Effects

Common adverse events include mild sedation or ataxia. Human oral solution (300 mg/mL xylitol) may create adverse effects related to xylitol, including hypoglycemia, hepatotoxicity, and a false-positive urinary protein dipstick test result, and should be avoided.

Research on Indications for Use

Generally, there is limited information on and variability in suggestions with respect to dosing for gabapentin in cats, but this medication is considered safe and may offer promise as we learn more about its effects in cats.

Maropitant

Mode of action: Neurokinin (NK_1) receptor antagonist, antiemetic

Examples: Maropitant (Cerenia; Zoetis)

Commonly prescribed for: Acute vomiting and the prevention of vomiting

Effects: Reduce nausea and vomiting

Contraindications/precautions/warnings: Maropitant is well tolerated in cats, but limited information is available.

Practical considerations: Best to give a small meal 1 hour before administration of tablets. Avoid prolonged fasting of the cat before dosing. The dissolution of tablets may be delayed by wrapping or embedding the tablets in food or treats. The foil packaging prevents moisture.

How It Works

Maropitant suppresses both peripheral and centrally mediated emesis as an antagonist of the neurokinin-1 (NK_1) receptor, which acts in the CNS by inhibiting substance P, the key neurotransmitter involved in vomiting. In cats, its bioavailability is about 50% following oral administration and 100% following subcutaneous administration. Its terminal elimination half-life is approximately 15 hours.[35]

Side Effects

Maropitant is well tolerated in cats, but limited information is available. Some cats may vomit the pill or hypersalivate after administration. Diarrhea and anorexia have been reported. In one study of 30 cats that received various doses (0.5 to 5 mg/kg subcutaneously for 15 days), maropitant was well tolerated. Localized reactions at injection sites were noted in some cats.[35]

Research on Indications for Use

The primary use and label recommendation for maropitant is the prevention of acute vomiting and the prevention of vomiting due to motion sickness. In fact, some cats that are anxious during car rides may have concurrent motion sickness. Therefore, for a cat that experiences hypersalivation, drooling, or vomiting, this drug is a logical adjunct to treatment for travel-related anxiety. The NK_1 antagonist maropitant citrate (Cerenia) offers a better alternative to acepromazine for this nausea related to travel, without remarkable sedative effects.[35] Orally administered off-label combinations with benzodiazepines might be effective prior to veterinary visits, grooming, or other potentially fear-evoking

events.[36] The mode of action of an NK_1 antagonist suggests that it may alleviate pain- or hypersensitivity-related distress, but further study is needed. In cats, NK_1 substance P receptors in the midbrain periaqueductal gray matter potentiate defensive rage and suppress predatory aggression.[37] Cerenia Injectable Solution is now approved in the United States and the United Kingdom for treatment of vomiting in cats ages 16 weeks and older,[38] but use of tablets or for other indications is still considered off-label use. Maropitant acts in the CNS by inhibiting substance P, the key neurotransmitter involved in vomiting. Substance P is a neuropeptide that is found in the spinal cord and CNS. It is a modulator of nociception involved in signaling the intensity of noxious stimuli. Along with NK_1, substance P is likely involved in the body's response to stress, anxiety, invasion of territory, and noxious or aversive stimuli. NK_1 is present in the hypothalamus, pituitary, and amygdala, which play a role in affective behavior and response to stress. The possible effects of maropitant on feline distress and anxiety have not yet been explored.

Neuroleptics

Mode of action: Neuroleptics are drugs that block dopamine receptors in the brain, causing a nonspecific depression of the CNS, decreased motor function at the basal ganglia, and elevation in prolactin levels with concurrent reduced awareness of external stimuli.

Examples: Acepromazine†

Commonly prescribed for: Tranquilization

Effects: Rapid onset of sedation or immobilization, poor anxiolytic effect

Contraindications/precautions/warnings: Not recommended as a sole agent for anxiety or behavioral applications. Monitor for noise sensitivity and rare cases of increased aggression (most likely a paradoxical effect).

Practical considerations: A lack of antianxiolytic effect and a profound immobilization effect make this a poor choice for alleviation of anxiety and improvement of cat welfare.

How They Work

Neuroleptics are drugs that block dopamine receptors in the brain, causing a nonspecific depression of the CNS and decreased motor function at the basal ganglia, and elevation in prolactin levels with concurrent reduced awareness of external stimuli.[39]

Side Effects

Neuroleptics have been widely used in veterinary medicine as tranquilizers and also to control motion sickness. In addition, they are anticholinergic and should not be used in patients with seizures, liver disease, or heart problems. Other side effects include hypotension (due to α-adrenergic blockade), decreased seizure threshold, bradycardia, ataxia, and extrapyramidal signs such as muscle tremors, muscle spasms, muscle discomfort, and motor restlessness. Traditional application for phenothiazines such as acepromazine do not provide reduction of fear, even if given in sufficient doses to reduce locomotor activity.

Research on Indications for Use

Neuroleptics are not recommended or researched for anxiety-related behavioral applications as a single agent. Phenothiazines are widely used for sedation but are not considered sufficient first-line drugs for behavioral applications, especially not when given alone, because they do not reduce anxiety.[40]

N-Methyl-D-Aspartate Antagonist

Mode of action: N-methyl-D-aspartate (NMDA) antagonist
Examples: Amantadine†
Commonly prescribed for: Pain or allodynia, self-mutilation
Effects: Notable within 1 to 2 weeks
Contraindications/precautions/warnings: Avoid for renal impairment
Practical considerations: Constant or pulsed therapy may be beneficial

How It Works

Amantadine is an NMDA antagonist that may be useful as an adjunctive agent for the management of feline chronic pain, but this drug is not in common use in cats, and there is minimal clinical experience to report. Within the CNS, chronic pain can be maintained or exacerbated when glutamate or aspartate binds to NMDA receptors. Allodynia is a sensation of pain resulting from a normally non-noxious stimulus that may be described in people but must be inferred or speculated in veterinary patients. This hypersensitivity to a benign stimulus may have a profound effect on behavior or social interactions.

Side Effects

Amantadine is primarily excreted unchanged in the urine; therefore, for patients with renal impairment, the dose should be reduced. Side effects, including gastrointestinal effects (i.e., diarrhea or flatulence) or agitations, have been reported when the drug is initiated. Experience in cats is limited. An adverse effect profile has yet to be fully elucidated, but the safety margin appears to be narrow.[39] The toxic dose reported for cats is 30 mg/kg.[39]

Research on Indications for Use

Amantadine alone may not provide good analgesia, but it may be useful in combination with other analgesics (e.g., opiates, nonsteroidal anti-inflammatory drugs) to alleviate chronic pain.[39] It may be used to manage chronic pain or spinal pain, which may be a contributing factor in feline anxiety, human-directed aggression associated with handling, tail mutilation, or hyperesthesia or intercat aggression between familiar housemate cats. Amantadine may be useful for long-term daily therapy, and it may be effective when pulsed for 2-week periods.[41]

Miscellaneous

There are many medications that may be useful for modifying feline behavior which are less frequently used because there is little information other than anecdotal personal communications. These medications include clonidine, trazodone, propranolol, cabergoline, pindolol, cyproheptadine, and mirtazapine. In the future, these medications may gain favor or conversely may be determined to be contraindicated in cats; therefore, these drugs are mentioned but not described in detail in this chapter.

Other drugs with behavioral or psychotropic effects deserve mention. Progestins may alleviate certain behaviors, but at a high risk for serious detrimental side effects, so their use is considered to be outdated and inappropriate. Synthetic progestins, including medroxyprogesterone and megestrol acetate, have been used in cats for problems ranging from aggression to feline urine marking.[42–44] Natural progestins are primarily produced endogenously by the corpus luteum. Progestins have an effect on the secretion of pituitary gonadotropins and also have an antiinsulin effect. Serious medical consequences may result with single or prolonged use of progestins, including adrenocortical depression, mammary hypertrophy, mammary neoplasms, endometrial hyperplasia, diabetes mellitus, hypothyroidism, bone marrow suppression, and pyometra. Other adverse reactions include increased appetite with increases in body weight and/or thirst, depression, lethargy, personality changes, and temporary inhibition of spermatogenesis. The risk of serious deleterious effects must be balanced with all other available treatment options. In the past, progestins have been used misused and overused as a single-agent treatment without understanding or implementation of behavior modification for many animals with undesirable behaviors. Their use should not be considered other than as a last resort when other therapies have failed and after explanation of them to the client and disclosure of safer alternatives.

Cyproheptadine is useful to enhance appetite and may be effective for the control of urine marking, especially in male cats.[42] However, in one comparison study, clomipramine was found to be more effective than cyproheptadine in the control of urine marking.[16,42] Mirtazapine is an excellent choice for appetite stimulation but has not been explored as a behavioral drug in cats, despite its classification as a noradrenaline and specific serotonin agent and its applications for depression and anxiety in people. Beta blockers such as propranolol have been used to reduce the physiological signs of anxiety (heart rate, respiratory rate, gastrointestinal upset) in combination with drugs that diminish behavioral signs. In humans and dogs, pindolol has been used infrequently to accelerate the SSRI response, particularly with paroxetine. At present, there is no information to support the use of pindolol in cats.

COMPLEMENTARY AND ALTERNATIVE MEDICINE (CAM)

The National Center for Complementary and Integrative Health (NCCIH) defines *complementary and alternative medicine*, or CAM, as a group of diverse medical and healthcare practices and products that are not generally considered part of conventional medicine. CAM includes herbal medicines, vitamins, minerals, and other natural products; mind and body medicine, including relaxation exercises and acupuncture; manipulation therapy, including chiropractic and therapeutic massage; and energy healing, including healing touch and homeopathy.

Safety and Efficacy

Ideally, all therapeutic modalities should be subject to the same stringent criteria for safety and efficacy. To receive licensing, drugs must be proven to be safe and efficacious. In addition, toxicity, contraindications, drug interactions, and side effects must be documented. CAM therapies, however, can be marketed as long as they are safe and make no claims with respect to health or disease. Yet, many people put a great deal of trust in these products because of anecdotal claims of efficacy and the fact they are marketed as "all natural." Of course, safety or potential adverse effects are not an issue when the active ingredients are immeasurable, such as in homeopathy or Bach flower remedies. However, efficacy, safety, toxicity, side effects, and contraindications are indeed a concern for natural products with measurable levels of ingredients (botanical/herbal, animal products, nutraceutical, vitamins, minerals).

Another issue for consideration with natural products is dose. For many of the natural therapeutics used in animals, dosages are extrapolated from the human dose (which is based on a 70-kg man). However, as absorption and metabolism vary greatly between species, there can be no assurance that a measured portion of a human dose will be safe or effective in cats. More recently, some of the natural products have been demonstrated to have varying degrees of efficacy in either clinical or laboratory trials or both. Therefore, some natural products could eventually become "conventional" if their efficacy and safety can be validated.

Pros and Cons

- **Client appeal**
  Pro: Natural products provide a level of appeal for clients resistant to pharmacologic and conventional options.
  Con: Clients may choose to use natural therapeutics over evidence-based drug regimens based solely on anecdotal support of efficacy.
- **Palatability and ease of administration**
  Pros: Some natural products, such as L-theanine, are highly palatable to cats. In addition, flavored supplements and therapeutic diets can make administration and compliance more practical.
  Cons: If the pet will not voluntarily consume the supplement or diet, administration may not be practical. In addition, a change in diet may not be clinically appropriate for some cats.
- **Safety**
  Pros: Most natural options have wide safety margins and minimal side effects. In fact, homeopathic remedies are diluted to a level at which the active ingredients are immeasurable. Their high safety margins suggest that these natural products may even be combined with other medications, but evidence for this is lacking.
  Cons: Just because a product is labeled as natural does not mean it is safe. This is particularly true for human products used in pets. For example, depending on dose, α-lipoic acid and garlic may be toxic to cats. In addition, some natural products can contain toxins.[45, 46] If clients do not advise their veterinarian that they are administering these products to their cats, there is the potential for adverse events, such as with the use of ginseng or tryptophan together with products that might enhance serotonin transmission.
- **Availability and cost**
  Pros: Many natural products are available over the counter (OTC); therefore, they are readily available. Some products are relatively inexpensive. Clients may elect to continue using a natural product based on their own interpretation of a beneficial response.
  Cons: Because not all natural products are equal, a higher price might need to be paid to ensure quality (e.g., probiotics, chondroitin sulfate). Some natural products are more expensive than a medication.
- **Efficacy**
  Pros: There are a few natural products that have some demonstrated evidence of efficacy for cats. A benefit may occur promptly with some of these products, whereas a much slower onset of action may be associated with others, such as L-theanine or the CALM diet, which may be effective only after 1 month or longer.

Cons: The efficacy of most natural products has not been demonstrated by scientific method. In addition, there is no standardization and less regulation of OTC products compared with pharmaceuticals. There may be high variability in quality, bioavailability, and concentration between products and manufacturers.

- **Rationale for selecting a nutraceutical instead of a medication**

    Pros: Some cats will take a nutraceutical immediately, and clients may be more accepting of this treatment modality. Clients may also need to feel they have exhausted all other options before administering mood-altering drugs to their cats. If the cat's anxiety or reactivity is reduced, the cat may be more accepting of medication options. Dietary options provide cat-friendly ways to administer anxiolytics to cats.

    Cons: Generally, natural products may be less potent than prescribed pharmaceuticals, so case selection is important. If a nutraceutical with insufficient potency is selected, the cat's behaviors may worsen during the time period when the natural option is administered. The cat's problems may worsen and/or the client's confidence in your recommendations may diminish.

Examples of CAM Approaches

α-Casozepine
How It Works
α-Casozepine (α-S1 tryptic casein) is a tryptic hydrolysate of α-S1 casein, a protein in cow's milk. Its activity may be similar to the anxiolytic effects of benzodiazepines. It is purported to have an affinity for GABA$_A$ receptors in the brain.[47]

Uses
α-Casozepine is used to treat fear, anxiety, stress, and related behavior problems in cats.

Side Effects
α-Casozepine has no known or reported side effects or contraindications.

Indications and Research
In a placebo-controlled study in cats, α-casozepine significantly improved cats' fear of strangers, contact with familiars, general fear, fear aggression, and autonomic signs.[47] The daily dose is a minimum of 15 mg/kg, and an effect is generally expected within 15 to 30 days.

Tryptophan
Mode of Action
Tryptophan is an essential amino acid and the biochemical precursor of serotonin, and it is obtained only through the diet. Tryptophan also functions as a biochemical precursor for niacin and melatonin.

How It Works
Tryptophan is converted to serotonin and therefore addition of tryptophan to the diet, along with the necessary coenzymes for conversion, might increase serotonin level or enhance its transmission to stabilize mood and reduce anxiety and impulsivity. However, for dogs, it has been suggested that in order for tryptophan supplementation to be effective, other large amino acids should be reduced, either in the diet or by addition of high levels of carbohydrate, such as pasta or rice, to create a relative reduction in circulating levels to decrease competition for the carrier that transports protein into the brain.[48]

Uses
Tryptophan may be used as adjunct to treat feline anxiety and stress-related behavior problems. There is minimal evidence to support use as a single agent.

Side Effects
There is some concern that supplementation with tryptophan (or 5-HT) might increase the risk of serotonin syndrome (discussed below) if used concurrently with other products that increase serotonin or enhance its transmission. Therefore, concurrent use with SSRIs, buspirone, tramadol, or other products that might increase serotonin level should be avoided. If it is considered absolutely necessary, then active monitoring for gastrointestinal or neurologic signs that might be consistent with serotonin syndrome would be prudent.

Indications and Research
In one placebo-controlled study on the effectiveness of dietary supplementation with L-tryptophan for stress-related behaviors in cats living in multicat homes, researchers demonstrated statistically significant reductions of observed stress-related behaviors, such as vocalization, agonistic behaviors, house soiling, destructive household scratching, and agonistic interactions.[49] In addition, although caution should be exercised (see "Side Effects" heading above), the use of tryptophan in combination with an SSRI might increase the serotonin pool in pets that are not sufficiently responding to the effects of the SSRI alone. In humans, in a review of the empirical research into the role of tryptophan in depression, focused on dietary methods to influence tryptophan levels, researchers suggested that empirical evidence for improving mood through dietary manipulation of tryptophan is lacking and that it is difficult to change plasma tryptophan levels through diet alone.[50]

Stress Management Veterinary Diets
Currently, the only dietary stress management product available is the Royal Canin Veterinary Diet CALM.

How They Work

The CALM formula provides a nutritionally complete and palatable diet that includes three unique calming nutrients to help reduce pet anxiety and provide stress relief. The first, α-casozepine, is an amino acid chain derived from milk. Additionally, CALM contains L-tryptophan and nicotinamide (vitamin B_3), which are known stress relievers.

Uses

Stress management diets are used for fear, anxiety, stress, and related behavior problems.

Side Effects and Contraindications

There are no specific side effects, unless the diet itself is contraindicated because of other medical priorities (see "Tryptophan" section above).

Indications and Research

The potential for reducing stress, stress-related behaviors, and anxiety with a diet might greatly improve ease of administration and compliance. The period to effect for the diet has not been determined, but presumably a minimum of 3 weeks would be required to ascertain if the diet is beneficial. Evidence for potential efficacy is discussed under the individual ingredients (α-casozepine and L-tryptophan). There are currently no published data for cats that the combination of ingredients in the diet has benefits over the individual ingredients themselves. There is no specific published evidence related to the use of CALM in cats but one paper has been published regarding its use in relation to anxiety related behaviors in dogs.

L-Theanine

How It Works

L-Theanine is a product that is naturally found in green tea, which is a structural analog of glutamate, an excitatory neurotransmitter. Thus, it may block the effects of glutamate and increase GABA, an inhibitory neurotransmitter.

Uses

L-Theanine is used to treat fear, anxiety, stress, and related behavior problems in cats.

Side Effects

Side effects have not been reported.

Indications and Research

One particular advantage of using L-theanine (Anxitane) is that it is highly palatable for most cats. In a pilot trial in cats, emotional disorders, including signs of unacceptable elimination, fear aggression, fear of humans, and physical manifestations of anxiety, showed improvement after 30 days.[51] The cat dose is one-half of a 50-mg tablet twice daily.

Mini Case Example

In one case where two feral cats in a household were barely approachable and rarely left the security of a remote bedroom and rarely came out from under the bed, it was not possible to administer medication to the cats. As an alternative approach, L-theanine tablets were placed under the owner's bed daily for 2 weeks. The optimal dose was determined to be one small tablet per day. Eventually, some of the pills were gone each day, though it was not certain which cats ate the Anxitane or if one cat ate it all. The drug's safety profile suggests this would be safe up to five times this dose. The safety and palatability allowed the Anxitane to be administered in a less regulated, unsupervised manner. In response to the Anxitane, together with a comprehensive behavior program to address the cats' environmental and social needs, the target behaviors decreased promptly.

Fatty Acids

Mode of Action

Polyunsaturated fatty acids—especially the most well recognized, docosahexaenoic acid (DHA)—play an important role in maintaining neuronal integrity and enhancing energy use by neurons. They are incorporated into many tissues for structural and signal function and are essential for early brain and retinal development. They may also improve early learning.[52] It has been reported that cats lack the liver capacity to synthesize longer-chain omega-3 and omega-6 fatty acids.[53]

Use

Polyunsaturated fatty acids are used to facilitate healthy brain and retinal development and learning in kittens, to improve cognitive abilities in senior cats, and help to manage issues of fear and anxiety.

Side Effects

High doses of polyunsaturated fatty acids should be avoided because of the potential for gastrointestinal effects, altered immune function, altered platelet function, and weight gain. Whereas a safe upper limit for dogs is suggested to be 370 mg/kg of body weight of combined eicosapentaenoic acid (EPA) and DHA, a safe upper limit for cats has not yet been established.[54]

Indications and Research

Providing polyunsaturated fatty acid supplements for the nursing queen and her kittens may be of particular importance for healthy brain development. Fish oil supplementation may also be beneficial to improve cognitive function in aging cats.[55,56]

Melatonin

How It Works

Melatonin is synthesized from serotonin in the pineal gland. It plays a role in the regulation of circadian rhythms and the sleep–wake cycle, with high levels secreted into the circulation during the night and low levels during the day. Melatonin may increase serum prolactin and growth hormone, and in the long term it may reduce luteinizing hormone. It is also a free radical scavenger.

Uses

In countries where it is available, melatonin is used for sleep cycle disorders and may be used for anxiety.

Side Effects

There have been no reported side effects of using melatonin.

Indications and Research

Although controlled studies of melatonin are lacking, it has been reported to be useful in the treatment of anxiety, fear, and sleep cycle disorders in dogs and cats. In cats, the dose may range from 1.5 to 3 mg per cat (although doses up to 12 mg have been reported).[39] Melatonin is not available in all countries.

Pheromones

Pheromones provide a safe, natural, effective option for use alone or in combination therapy. They exert an influence on the amygdala by way of the vomeronasal organ.[57] There is extensive literature on the use and efficacy of pheromones for feline behavior therapy. These therapies are covered in Chapter 18. Pheromones modulate behavior by mechanisms that are different from those of the medications and supplements discussed herein. They provide the general practitioner with options for very safe augmentation strategies.

Catnip

How It Works

Catnip exerts its influence on the CNS through the olfactory bulb, but not the vomeronasal organ.[58] The active ingredient in catnip (Nepeta cataria) is the essential oil nepetalactone, which is a terpene composed of two isoprene units with a total of 10 carbons. Catnip or catmint produces an apparent euphoric or hallucinogenic reaction in about 50% to 75% of cats, and responsiveness is reported to be an autosomal dominant trait beginning at about 8 weeks of age. Affected cats may exhibit a range of behaviors, including sniffing, licking, and chewing the plant, head shaking, chin and cheek rubbing, head rolling, and body rubbing. This reaction lasts for 5 to 15 minutes and then may be initiated again for another hour or more. Catnip is available as a leaf,

but liquid and aerosol forms are also available. Volatile oils appear to exert a cholinergic effect, which may account for some of their psychoactive properties.

Uses

Catnip is used for enrichment, reinforcement-based training, response substitution, and counterconditioning.

Side Effects

Supplementation is not entirely without risk, as catnip intoxication has been reported.[59] In addition, if the behavioral response is undesirable for the cat or the client, its use should not be continued.

Indications and Research

When cats that are responders sniff even a small amount of catnip, they may begin to headshake, lick, chew, or rub up against the catnip, and then start to twitch, salivate, and roll on the ground, for up to 15 minutes. The response resembles elements of oral/appetitive, playful, predatory, and sexual behaviors.[58] In cats that have a positive response, catnip might be used as positive reinforcement for training, response substitution (engaging the cat in an alternative acceptable behavior), enrichment, and counterconditioning. For example, catnip may be applied in common areas of the home where cats may come together. Catnip naturally redirects the cats to a pleasant, playful emotional state and may be useful for facilitation of social interactions.

Homeopathy and Bach Flower Remedies

How They Work

Homeopathy is based on the principle that a substance (plant, animal, mineral) that causes symptoms in a healthy individual will cure that disease ("like cures like") by administration of a remedy that is diluted beyond measurable amounts. Although the amount is undetectable after dilution, the remedy is said to contain vibrational energy essences that match the patterns in the ailing patient. Homeopathy has no scientifically plausible mechanism of action, and researchers in two randomized placebo-controlled trials of homeopathic remedies for canine noise phobias found no evidence of efficacy.[45,60,61] Bach flower remedies are a form of vibrational energy made from springwater infused with wildflowers preserved in 27% brandy or glycerin. Bach remedies are homeopathic dilutions. Unlike homeopathy, however, the energizing stops when the remedy is finished; therefore, further dilution does not potentiate the remedy's effects.

Uses

Homeopathy and Bach flower remedies have many purported uses for anxiety, stress, and behavior problems. These agents can be obtained in manufactured and combination remedies (e.g., the Rescue Remedy;

Directly from Nature, Thousand Oaks, Calif.) or can be individually designed to treat the cat's specific clinical presentation.

Side Effects

Other than potential effects of the preservative if brandy is used, the products are safe because the ingredients are not measurable and increasing doses are considered to have decreasing potency. Owner's may disregard label directions and give large amounts of these remedies which may cause cats to experience sedation effects of the alcohol.

Indications and Research

Homeopathy, though it has no scientifically plausible mechanism of action, is growing in popularity. Evidence is lacking for behavioral indications, and it is possible cats may be deprived of appropriate, evidence-based treatment while clients are tempted to explore homeopathy.[45,60,61]

Miscellaneous

Other herbs and nutraceuticals that may have behavioral effects include valerian, St John's wort, and kava, but evidence is lacking for their indications, doses, and safety. Cognitive supplements, including *S*-adenosylmethionine are discussed in Chapter 25 on senior behavior and cognitive dysfunction. Senior cats that are presented with behavior problems may benefit from cognitive function-enhancing supplementation, even when primary cognitive dysfunction is not diagnosed.

ADDITIONAL RESOURCES

Crowell-Davis SL, Murray T. *Veterinary Psychopharmacology.* Ames, IA: Wiley-Blackwell; 2005.

Crowell-Davis SL, Landsberg GM. Pharmacology and pheromone therapy. In: Horwitz DF, Mills D, eds. *BSAVA Manual of Canine and Feline Behavioural Medicine.* 2nd ed. Gloucester, UK: British Small Animal Veterinary Association (BSAVA); 2009.

Landsberg G, Hunthausen W, Ackerman L. *Behavior Problems of the Dog and Cat.* 3rd ed. Oxford: Saunders; 2013.

National Center for Complementary and Integrative Health (NCCIH) homepage. https://nccih.nih.gov/ Accessed February 1, 2015.

Overall KL. *Manual of Clinical Behavioral Medicine for Dogs and Cats.* St Louis: Elsevier; 2013.

Papich MG. *Saunders Handbook of Veterinary Drugs.* 3rd ed. St Louis: Elsevier; 2011.

Plumb D. Plumb's Veterinary Drug Handbook. 7th ed. Ames, Iowa: Wiley-Blackwell; 2011.

Stahl SM. *Stahl's Essential Psychopharmacology.* 3rd ed. Cambridge, UK: Cambridge University Press; 2007.

Stahl SM. The Prescriber's Guide. 3rd ed. Cambridge, UK: Cambridge University Press; 2009.

REFERENCES

1. Stahl SM. *Stahl's Essential Psychopharmacology.* 3rd ed. Cambridge, UK: Cambridge University Press; 2007.
2. Ciribassi J, Luescher A, Pasioske KS, et al. Comparative bioavailability of transdermal versus oral fluoxetine in healthy cats. *Am J Vet Res.* 2003;64:994–998.
3. Mealey KL, Peck KE, Bennett BS, et al. Systemic absorption of amitriptyline and buspirone after oral and transdermal administration to health cats. *J Vet Intern Med.* 2004;18:43–46.
4. Gillman PK. Triptans, serotonin agonists, and serotonin syndrome@ (serotonin toxicity): a review. *Headache.* 2010;50:264–272.
5. Crowell-Davis SL, Seibert LM, Sung W, et al. Use of clomipramine, alprazolam and behavior modification for the treatment of storm phobias in dogs. *J Am Vet Med Assoc.* 2003;222:744–748.
6. Papich MG. *Saunders Handbook of Veterinary Drugs: Small and Large Animal.* 3rd ed. Philadelphia: Elsevier/Saunders; 2011.
7. Pryor PA, Hart BL, Bain MJ, Cliff KD. Causes of urine marking in cats and effects of environmental management on frequency of marking. *J Am Vet Med Assoc.* 2001;219:1709–1713.
8. Stark P, Fuller RW, Wong T. The pharmacologic profile of fluoxetine. *J Clin Psychiatry.* 1985;46:7–13.
9. Boyer WF, Feighner JP. An overview of paroxetine. *J Clin Psychiatry.* 1992;53(suppl):3–6.
10. Hart BL, Cliff KD, Tynes VV, Bergman L. Control of urine marking by use of long-term treatment with fluoxetine or clomipramine in cats. *J Am Vet Med Assoc.* 2005;226:378–382.
11. Crowell-Davis S, Murray T. Tricyclic antidepressants. In: *Veterinary Psychopharmacology.* Ames, IA: Blackwell; 2006:179–206.
12. Martin KM. Effect of clomipramine on the electrocardiogram and serum thyroid concentrations of healthy cats. *J Vet Behav.* 2010;5:123–129.
13. Wong DT, Perry KW, Bymaster FP. Case history: the discovery of fluoxetine hydrochloride (Prozac). *Nat Rev Drug Discov.* 2005;4:764–774.
14. King JN, Simpson BS, Overall KL, et al. Treatment of separation anxiety in dogs with clomipramine: results from a prospective, randomized, double-blind, placebo-controlled, parallel-group multicenter clinical trial. *Appl Anim Behav Sci.* 2000;67:255–275.
15. Tynes VV, Hart BL, Pryor PA, et al. Evaluation of the role of lower urinary tract disease in cats with urine marking behavior. *J Am Vet Med Assoc.* 2003;223:457–461.
16. Kroll T, Houpt KA. A comparison of cyproheptadine and clomipramine for the treatment of spraying cats. In: Overall KL, Mills DS, Heath SE, Horwitz D, eds. *Proceedings of the 3rd International Congress on Veterinary*

Behavioural Medicine. Potters Bar, UK: Universities Federation for Animal Welfare; 2001:184–185.

17. Dehasse J. Feline urine spraying. *J Appl Anim Behav Sci*. 1997;52:365–371.

18. Landsberg G, Wilson AL. Effects of clomipramine on cats presented for urine marking. *J Am Anim Hosp Assoc*. 2005;41:3–11.

19. King JN, Steffan J, Heath SE, et al. Determination of the dosage of clomipramine for the treatment of urine spraying in cats. *J Am Vet Med Assoc*. 2004;225:881–887.

20. Seksel K, Lindeman MJ. Use of clomipramine in the treatment of anxiety-related and obsessive-compulsive disorders in cats. *Aust Vet J*. 1998;76:317–321.

21. Bernstein JE. Effect of doxepin hydrochloride on acute and chronic urticaria. *J Invest Dermatol*. 1982;78:353–354.

22. Kaplan HI, Sadock J, eds. *Pocket Handbook of Psychiatric Drug Treatment*. 2nd ed. Baltimore: Williams and Wilkins; 1996.

23. Hart BL, Eckstein RA, Powell KL, Dodman NH. Effectiveness of buspirone on urine spraying and inappropriate urination in cats. *J Am Vet Med Assoc*. 1993;203:254–258.

24. Crowell-Davis SL, Murray T. Azapirones. In: *Veterinary Psychopharmacology*. Ames, IA: Blackwell; 2006:111–118.

25. Crowell-Davis SL, Murray T. Benzodiazepines. In: *Veterinary Psychopharmacology*. Ames, IA: Blackwell; 2006:34–71.

26. Center SA, Elston TH, Rowland PH, et al. Fulminant hepatic failure associated with oral administration of diazepam in 11 cats. *J Am Vet Med Assoc*. 1996;209: 618–625.

27. Marder AR. Psychotropic drugs and behavioral therapy. *Vet Clin North Am Small Anim Pract*. 1991;21:329–342.

28. Cooper L, Hart BL. Comparison of diazepam with progestin for effectiveness in suppression of urine spraying behavior in cats. *J Am Vet Med Assoc*. 1992;200:797–801.

29. Knoll J. (−)Deprenyl (selegiline) a catecholaminergic activity enhancer (CAE) substance acting in the brain. *Pharmacol Toxicol*. 1998;82:57–66.

30. Crowell-Davis SL, Murray T. Monoamine oxidase inhibitors. In: *Veterinary Psychopharmacology*. Ames, IA: Blackwell; 2006:134–147.

31. Ruehl WW, Griffin D, Bouchard G, Kitchen D. Effects of L-deprenyl in cats in a one month dose escalation study [abstract 206]. *Vet Pathol*. 1996;33:621.

32. Landsberg G. Therapeutic options for cognitive decline in senior pets. *J Am Anim Hosp Assoc*. 2006;42:407–413.

33. Dehasse J. Retrospective study on the use of selegiline (Selgian) in cats. New Orleans. Presented at the American Veterinary Society of Animal Behavior annual meeting, New Orleans, LA, 1999.

34. Siao KT, Pypendop BH, Ilkiw JE. Pharmacokinetics of gabapentin in cats. *Am J Vet Res*. 2010;71:817–821.

35. Hickman MA, Cox SR, Mahabir S, et al. Safety, pharmacokinetics and use of the novel NK-1 receptor antagonist maropitant (Cerenia) for the prevention of emesis and motion sickness in cats. *J Vet Pharmacol Ther*. 2008;31:220–229.

36. Hart BL. Behavioral indications for phenothiazine and benzodiazepine tranquilizers in dogs. *J Am Vet Med Assoc*. 1985;186:1175–1180.

37. Gregg TR, Siegel A. Differential effects of NK1 receptors in the midbrain periaqueductal gray upon defensive rage and predatory attack in the cat. *Brain Res*. 2003;994:55–66.

38. Zoetis: Cerenia online brochure. https://www.zoetisus.com/products/pages/cerenia/pdf/Cerenia_Combo_PI_May2012.pdf Accessed February 2, 2015.

39. Plumb D. *Plumb's Veterinary Drug Handbook*. 7th ed. Ames, Iowa: Wiley-Blackwell; 2011.

40. Overall KL. Pharmacological approaches to changing behavior and neurochemistry. In: *Manual of Clinical Behavioral Medicine for Dogs and Cats*. St Louis: Elsevier; 2013:474–475.

41. Stein B. *VASG Dog & Cat Anesthesia & Pain Management Support*. http://www.vasg.org/ Accessed February 2, 2015.

42. Schwartz S. Use of cyproheptadine to control urine spraying in a castrated male domestic cat. *J Am Vet Med Assoc*. 1999;215:501–502.

43. Voith VL, Marder AR. Canine behavioral disorders. In: Morgan RV, ed. *Handbook of Small Animal Practice*. New York: Churchill Livingstone; 1988:1033–1043.

44. Hart BL. Objectionable urine spraying and urine marking in cats: evaluation of progestin treatment in gonadectomized males and females. *J Am Vet Med Assoc*. 1980;177:529–533.

45. Overall K, Dunham A. Homeopathy and the curse of the scientific method. *Vet J*. 2009;180:141–148.

46. Landsberg G, Hunthausen W, Ackerman L. Complementary and alternative therapy for behavior problems. In: *Behavior Problems of the Dog and Cat*. 3rd ed. Oxford, UK: Saunders; 2013:139–149.

47. Beata C, Beaumont-Graff E, Coll V, et al. Effect of alpha-casozepine (Zylkene) on anxiety in cats. *J Vet Behav Clin Appl Res*. 2007;2:40–46.

48. DeNapoli JS, Dodman NH, Shuster L, et al. Effect of dietary protein content and tryptophan supplementation on dominance aggression, territorial aggression, and hyperactivity in dogs. *J Am Vet Med Assoc*. 2000;217:504–508.

49. Pereira GG, Fragoso S, Pires E. Effect of dietary intake of L-tryptophan supplementation on multihoused cats presenting stress related behaviours. In: *BSAVA Congress 2010 Scientific Proceedings: Veterinary Programme* Gloucester, UK: British Small Animal Veterinary Association (BSAVA); 2010.

50. Soh NL, Walter G. Tryptophan and depression: can diet alone be the answer? *Acta Neuropsychiatr*. 2011;23:3–11.

51. Dramard V, Kern L, Hofmans J, et al. Clinical efficacy of L-theanine tablets to reduce anxiety-related emotional disorders in cats: a pilot open-label clinical trial [abstract 7]. *J Vet Behav*. 2007;2:85–86.

52. Heinemann KM, Bauer JE. Docosahexaenoic acid and neurologic development in animals. *J Am Vet Med Assoc*. 2006;228:700–705.

53. Filburn CR, Griffin D. Effects of supplementation with a docosahexaenoic acid-enriched salmon oil on total plasma and plasma phospholipid fatty acid composition in the cat. *Int J Appl Res Vet Med*. 2005;3:116–123.

54. Lenox CE, Bauer JE. Potential adverse effects of omega-3 fatty acids in dogs and cats. *J Vet Intern Med*. 2013;27:217–226.

55. Pan Y, Araujo JA, Burrows J, et al. Cognitive enhancement in middle-aged and old cats with dietary supplementation with a nutrient blend containing fish oil, B vitamins, antioxidants and arginine. *Br J Nutr*. 2013;110:40–49.

56. Cupp CJ, Jean-Philippe C, Kerr WW, et al. Effect of nutritional interventions on longevity of senior cats. *Int J Appl Res Vet Med*. 2007;5:133–149.

57. Tirindelli R, Dibattista M, Pifferi S, Menini A. From pheromones to behavior. *Physiol Rev*. 2009;89:921–956.

58. Hart BL, Leedy MG. Analysis of the catnip reaction; mediation by olfactory system, not vomeronasal organ. *Behav Neural Biol*. 1985;44:38–46.

59. Hornfeldt CS. *Nepeta cataria* (catnip) 'poisoning' in cats. *Vet Pract Staff*. 1994;6(1):7.

60. Cracknell NR, Mills DS. A double-blind placebo-controlled study into the efficacy of a homeopathic remedy for fear of firework noises in the dog (*Canis familiaris*). *Vet J*. 2008;177:80–88.

61. Cracknell NR, Mills DS. An evaluation of owner expectation on apparent treatment effect in a blinded comparison of 2 homeopathic remedies for firework noise sensitivity in dogs. *J Vet Behav*. 2011;6:21–30.

PART 7

Approaching Problem Behavior within the Veterinary Practice

Providing Feline-Friendly Consultations

Eliza Sundahl, Ilona Rodan, and Sarah Heath

INTRODUCTION

The adoption of "feline friendly" protocols and procedures can have a profound effect on the overall experience of the veterinary visit for everyone involved. Many clients will avoid coming to the practice with their pets because of a previous negative experience and this is detrimental to the cat's welfare. For many cat owners their perception that their pet "hates" to go to the veterinarian significantly influences their own emotional response to the experience and they report that they get stressed just thinking about a visit.[1] The frequency of visits to veterinary practices is significantly lower for feline than canine patients.[2] By developing a better understanding of the cat and its emotional responses, veterinary practices can create an environment that encourages clients to return regularly and to be more receptive to pursuing the veterinary care that the cat needs.

Injuries sustained during cat handling have been shown to be the leading cause of reported employee insurance claims in a veterinary practice.[3] Preventing negative feline emotion is the key to reducing unwanted behavioral responses in the veterinary practice, including aggression, and thereby decreasing the risk of injury and stress for clients, patients, and practice staff.

THE PRACTICE CULTURE

Veterinary professionals have a great opportunity to reshape client perceptions and improve the cat's experience, but in order to do so it is necessary to ensure that the practice understands the visit from a feline perspective. In order to establish a feline-friendly practice culture it is necessary to address some important questions:

- Can team members recognize fear in feline patients?
- Have they been taught specific feline-friendly handling techniques?
- Do certain team members make comments or use body language that exacerbates the negative veterinary experience for fearful cats?
- Are they willing to accept the change to understanding the visit from the cat's perspective?

Team members deserve education that not only improves the experience of the cat, but also keeps them safer and makes their job more enjoyable.

It is important for team members to resist the urge to respond to a cat's behavior in a negative manner. Staff training should focus on viewing the world from a feline perspective and recognizing and preventing the subtle signs of fear in cats. It is not helpful for staff members to use words such as *mean* or *evil* when describing feline patients, as this will tend to foster a negative perception and is likely to lead to situations where personnel lose their patience and become angry with cats that are actually displaying behaviors caused by fear, anxiety, or pain. A staff member should be able to replace annoyance or anger about an animal's behavior with strategies that are based on understanding the emotional state of the patient. When veterinary professionals reduce the cat's perception of threat, the result is a much improved and safer experience for all concerned.

Many veterinary practices have a team member who is called upon to help with cats—a "cat advocate." These individuals are great resources and should be encouraged to facilitate the necessary changes in the practice to improve feline consultations. Unfortunately, in many practices, there are also members of staff, even veterinarians, who are uncomfortable with cats and find working with them particularly challenging.[4] Such individuals may resist efforts to change a practice culture especially if they are unconvinced of the role that fear is playing in the difficult behaviors of their patients. It is therefore important to take time to educate everyone within the practice about normal feline behavior and communication and to give them sound scientific reasoning for the changes that are being suggested. The aim is to educate the whole team, from receptionist to practice owner, so that they better understand the feline patients and learn to handle them respectfully. A whole-team approach is vital if there is to be successful implementation of feline-friendly procedures.

Fear and Anxiety

Fear is an emotional response to an immediate stressor, whereas *anxiety* is defined as the emotional anticipation of an adverse event that may or may not be real.[5] A feline handler needs to be aware of both of these states to improve the cat's experience at the present moment, as well as to prevent potential anxiety during future visits.

There are numerous reasons why the cat may be fearful when it is brought to the veterinary practice. Fear can begin at home if the carrier is brought out only for veterinary visits and can be worsened by the way in which the cat is placed into it, often by shoving and force. In an effort to get a cat into a carrier, a favored person, acting out of character from the feline perspective, often chases and corners the cat. The cat is then taken on a fear-inducing car ride that ends at the veterinary practice, where everything is unfamiliar and often threatening. (For more information on how to habituate the cat to the carrier and change this experience, see Chapters 5 and 9.)

If strategies to reduce the impact of these events are not put in place, fear can not only escalate during the current visit but may also contribute to anxiety during future visits. For example, when a cat is not given an opportunity to utilize its natural coping strategies of hiding and retaining a sense of control during a veterinary visit, its state of emotional arousal will remain high and its fear will be perpetuated. Anxiety then develops during future visits as a result of the significant memories of the previous frightening experience. A similar negative association can develop if the cat experienced pain during a previous visit. For example, a cat that underwent a pain-inducing examination or a procedure without sufficient analgesia will have memories of the painful experience and become anxious during future visits as a result. The anticipatory nature of the anxious state will result in the cat being ready to defend itself, and it may enter the practice already displaying apparently aggressive behaviors such as screaming, lunging, or attacking.

To prevent feline fear and anxiety, it is essential to understand the cat's natural behavior and to recognize how these emotional states are both triggered and manifested. The most successful feline interactions within the context of a veterinary practice involve using the cat's own coping behaviors to the best advantage.[6,7]

What Does Fear Look Like?

In the face of a perceived threat, cats will respond to their emotional state by displaying behavioral responses which are associated with the so called "fight or flight" response. These responses have been classified into four general categories sometimes referred to as *freeze, fiddle/fidget, flee,* or *fight*.[8] The more current terminology of inhibition, appeasement, avoidance, and repulsion, better describes the spectrum of behaviors that a cat may display. These behavioral responses are manifested in a variety of ways that will vary from cat to cat. Furthermore, cats may show more than one response and may alter their reaction as a threatening situation develops. In adulthood, cats have very limited appeasement strategies and will usually select the more passive responses of avoidance (fleeing) and inhibition (freezing), if available. When these responses are not successful or the cat is prevented from using them, it will resort to the more active repulsion responses (fight). For more information see Chapters 12 and 17.

The behavior of the inhibited or "freezing" cat often leads to a misinterpretation that it is a compliant cat. Learning to recognize features such as the hunkered down posture and head position, dilated pupils, and retracted ears, can distinguish an inhibited cat from one showing comfort with the environment (Figure 20-1). When in an aroused emotional state, cats may display displacement behaviors such as repositioning, pacing, or licking. These behaviors may occur in conjunction with any of the behavioral responses. For example, a cat may show avoidance, run away from a threat, and then sit and groom itself, or a cat may show repulsion, hiss and spit, and then begin to lick (Figure 20-2). The presence of behavioral responses such as inhibition, avoidance, and repulsion are indicative of the cat's negative emotional state and should not be

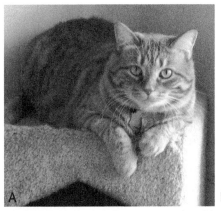
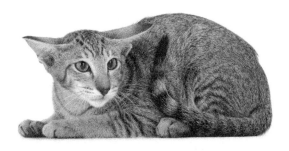

A B

FIGURE 20-1 It is important to be able to distinguish between the posture of a contented cat **(A)** and one that is demonstrating an inhibited behavioral response to negative emotion such as fear **(B)**.

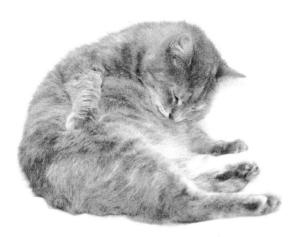

FIGURE 20-2 When cats are in an aroused emotional state they can display displacement behaviors such as grooming. (Copyright © iStock.com)

ignored (Figure 20-3). When displacement behaviors are being demonstrated it is important to act to protect the cat from the perceived threat and to ensure that its environment, both physical and social, is meeting its behavioral needs.

The apparently aggressive cat is usually a fearful cat that has been denied the opportunity to use other, more appropriate coping strategies and has therefore progressed into a more heightened state of emotional arousal. When potential defense strategies of avoidance (flight) and inhibition (freeze) prove unsuccessful for achieving safety, the cat will be forced to use the defense strategy of repulsion (fight) instead.[8] The challenge is to identify behaviors that indicate fear earlier on so that steps can be taken to encourage the cat to use the more acceptable defense strategies of avoidance and inhibition and thereby avoid the consequences of defensive aggressive behavioral responses. Understanding the cat's normal behavior and how it responds to fear helps form the foundation on which to build strategies that will result in less fear and hence less fear-associated aggression. Veterinary practices often miss opportunities to defuse escalating negative emotions. For example, hiding is a basic feline coping strategy when a cat feels threatened.[9] The simple act of allowing a cat to feel hidden can often allow it to cope with its surroundings sufficiently to prevent further arousal.[9] Loss of control is another fundamental stressor in the feline world, and

How Do Cats Demonstrate a Negative Emotional State?

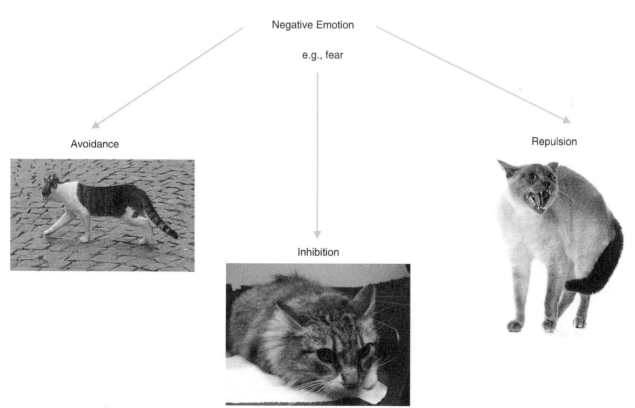

Negative Emotion

e.g., fear

Avoidance

Inhibition

Repulsion

FIGURE 20-3 Cats are solitary survivors and self-protection is paramount. When experiencing negative emotion, such as fear, they will opt for the more passive behavioral responses of avoidance and inhibition if these are available. When this is not possible they will select repulsion. Understanding the body and facial posturing associated with these behavioral responses will increase understanding of cats and help prevent additional patient fear and human injury.

the use of forceful restraint can therefore have the paradoxical effect of making cats harder to handle. Many veterinary professionals have been taught to forcibly restrain cats in order to control them. However, normal feline behavior predicts that cats will become more fearful and suspicious about their surroundings as their sense of control is decreased.[10] Forceful handling is therefore a trigger for negative emotional arousal and fosters the adoption of defensive behavioral strategies. Use of preventive measures to maintain a low level of emotional arousal in feline patients and to favor positive emotional states is the key to successful veterinary visits.

It is important to understand that defense strategies have developed as a survival mechanism in the face of a perceived threat. Therefore, when these defensive behaviors are present, it must be assumed that the cat feels threatened. Such a threat is likely to be wholly unintentional on the part of the veterinary staff. However, it is the perception of the cat that is important, and early and accurate recognition of its emotional state and early intervention to maximize its ability to use its natural coping strategies are the key to a veterinary visit that is successful for everyone involved.[8] Early signs of fear may be difficult to recognize because the signs may be subtle; therefore it is essential to provide an education program for all members of staff.

In the veterinary environment there are various techniques which can be used when cats are demonstrating signs of negative emotion, such as fear or anxiety. One aim is to induce a more positive emotional response, for example, by offering toys or treats, or asking the clients to interact with their cat. The other is to encourage the cat to use natural behavioral responses to deal with the negative emotion, such as allowing hiding places to be used. Either of these approaches can help to ameliorate stress and de-escalate the situation before the cat resorts to the more problematic defense strategy of repulsion.

In view of the solitary survivor status of the cat, it is logical that they will make every effort to protect themselves in a potentially threatening situation. Avoidance is therefore a natural and obvious feline response to a fearful situation, but the veterinary context is one in which escape is often not possible because the examination or procedure needs to go ahead. With the escape response thwarted, the cat may select an inhibition response and make every effort to hide. These cats will be more compliant if allowed to do so. Alternatively the cat may switch from avoidance to a repulsion response. At the beginning of an interaction the cat is still motivated to avoid overt confrontation and its body language can change from subtle posturing to more overt bluffing. Cats may use piloerection to increase their perceived body size and hiss and vocalize threats designed to avoid a physical confrontation. This behavioral display should signal to the veterinary staff that it is time to de-escalate the situation by offering options for the cat to stay hidden, such as covering with a towel. If the cat's warnings are not heeded and the veterinary staff insist on continuing with the procedure this will be perceived as an escalation of threat and the cat will have no choice other than to engage in physical confrontation.

It is important to remember that animals may respond in different ways when they are forced to deal with negative emotions such as fear and anxiety. Each cat will have a different threshold or emotional capacity which influences its ability to cope and remain in a more positive and relaxed state.

HANDLING PRINCIPLES BASED ON UNDERSTANDING OF THE CAT

Handling plans are necessary to prevent or decrease a cat's negative arousal state. Plans that are based on the inherent coping mechanisms of the cat are the most beneficial. Providing a predictable environment in terms of both physical space and routine is very important to help prevent fear.[10] Allowing cats to have a sense of "being invisible" can help minimize their anxiety, especially when they are presented with unfamiliar surroundings (Figure 20-4). The cat can have a safe place to

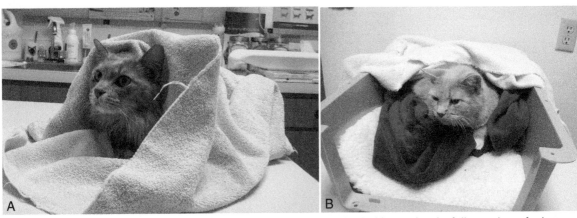

FIGURE 20-4 Providing towels can give a perception of being hidden and make feline patients feel more secure.

hide that still allows observation and examination while helping them maintain covert behavior.

Veterinary staff need to recognize that, as each cat has a different tolerance level and will react in its own way, handling efforts must integrate what is known about normal feline behavior as it applies to the individual cat. Table 20-1 provides the most important points to bear in mind to understand the cat and to apply to prevent cats' fear and improve feline visits. More detailed discussion of normal cat behavior can be found in the other chapters in this book (see Chapters 3 and 4).

Initial Contact

The information given to a cat owner prior to their visit to the practice is the first step in creating a less stressful visit. Implementing feline-friendly handling strategies begins with the initial client contact. When a new client contacts the practice to make an appointment, staff should be trained to ask about the client's previous experiences. If the client indicates that past visits have been unpleasant for them or their pet, take the time to help them understand what to do in the future to help alleviate fear and anxiety. Provide written resources,

either online or in brochure form, on how to make the carrier familiar in the home, thus reducing the cat's fear (for more information, see Chapter 9).

Team members working at the front desk should be trained to identify fearful patients through their initial questions and to flag these appointments so that the rest of the staff are prepared from the start of the consultation to take steps to prevent escalation of fear. It is important to document in the cat's health record that it is fearful during veterinary visits, and information about the most successful handling techniques for that individual patient should also be recorded. Preparations should be made to de-escalate anxiety and fear before the need arises.

Appropriate choice of carrier is an important factor in reducing potential stress associated with the veterinary visit. It is important to advise clients whose cats have had issues in the past that an inexpensive alternative carrier, such as a plastic one that can be taken apart in the middle, can facilitate appropriate handling and make a significant difference to their pet's stress levels (Figure 20-5).

Most cats brought into a veterinary practice are more comfortable remaining inside their carriers. Even those

TABLE 20-1 Understanding Feline Behavior Provides Tools to Prevent Fear	
Normal Feline Behavior and Communication	**Tools to Prevent Fear by Understanding the Cat**
The feline social system: Cats are less likely to interact with unfamiliar cats or other animals and will tend to avoid them	Provide an environment where cats do not have to see unfamiliar cats or other animals: • Cover the carrier with a towel or blanket • Get the cat into the examination room as soon as possible • Keep the cat in the examination room for the exam and sample collection • Arrange wards with back-to-back or side-to-side cages so that cats cannot see unfamiliar animals
Cats in the same social group rub and groom each other, preferably on the head and neck	Massage or pet under the chin, in the cheek area, and between the ears
Cats prefer the familiar	• Habituate the cat to the carrier at home • Habituate the cat to car rides or other travel • Habituate the cat to mock home exams and home maintenance procedures • Bring to the veterinary visit familiar bedding, toys, and so forth that the cat likes • Provide "fun" vet visits
Cats need to have a sense of control	• Allow the cat to choose to come out of the carrier whenever possible • Examine the cat where the cat wants to be and in its preferred position • Provide places to hide and places up high in boarding and hospital wards • Restrict the number of handlers and always use minimal restraint
Cats learn best through positive reinforcement and rewards	Reward or positively reinforce desired behavior Do not punish; rather, ignore or redirect undesired behavior
Cats use olfactory communication and are sensitive to smells in their environment. Pheromones are used for communication	Avoid strong smells Do not use alcohol for sample collection Install feline synthetic pheromone analog diffusers in the veterinary practice and use the spray where appropriate
Vision: Cats are alerted to rapid movements Staring at the cat is a threat	Move slowly to obtain quicker results Work with the patient from behind or from the side Do not look directly at a frightened cat; do "winky" eyes
Hearing: Cats' hearing is superior to ours	Speak in soft voices Keep cats away from loud noises (e.g., centrifuges, washers, dryers)
Touch: Cats are sensitive to touch	Restrict tactile interactions to the head and neck Do not hold feet tightly

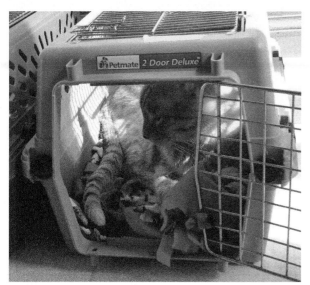

FIGURE 20-5 This carrier can be taken apart and the lid can be lifted off. This allows the cat to remain in the carrier and removes the need for any confrontation or struggling associated with bringing the cat out onto the examination table or wherever the cat wants to be.

that dislike it when they are at home find the ability to hide within the carrier comforting and are attracted by the scent reminders of home. This makes it a secure place to be and offers a preferred alternative to sitting on the examination table, where the cat feels totally exposed to the challenging environment of the consulting room.

Forcing a cat out of its carrier in order to carry out an examination or treatment precipitates fearful responses, including escalation to fear-induced "aggression". Zippered, canvas, soft-sided carriers often require a cat to be forcibly removed, as performing the examination while the cat is within them is very difficult. As stated above, hard-sided carriers that can be partially disassembled are preferable so that the cat can be examined and treated within the safety of the bottom half of its own carrier. Be sure that clients understand that the key aspect of this type of carrier is that the top half can come off, not just that there is an opening in the top. Clients should check the latches and screws of this type of carrier every time they use it to be sure that they are functioning well. It is not unusual for cat carriers to remain unused for long periods of time and it is important that the client has checked the carrier before the cat goes inside. Latches need to snap securely, and screws and bolts need to be free-moving so that they can be taken apart easily. The noise of people struggling to open the carrier can be threatening to the cat inside.

Clients should be advised to place familiar blankets or towels from home in the carrier to increase familiarity and give a sense of security. Asking clients to bring an extra towel with the cat's scent for use during handling in the veterinary practice can further reduce fear. The application of a synthetic feline facial pheromone analog such as Feliway, either in spray or wipe form can add to a

sense of security. Due to the fact that the pheromone is suspended in alcohol the spray should be applied approximately 10 to 15 minutes prior to the cat going into the carrier to avoid any aversive effects of the scent of the evaporating alcohol.[11] See Table 9-1 in Chapter 9 for a list of recommended videos that will help clients to prepare for a visit to the veterinarian, including information on choosing an appropriate carrier.

Preparing the Veterinary Practice

Unfamiliar scents, sounds, sights, or tactile contact can cause significant feline fear. In order to increase the sensation of familiarity in the practice, synthetic facial pheromone diffusers should be used in every room where cats may go. The pheromone has a species-specific effect and will therefore be of no benefit in dog-, avian-, or small mammal–only rooms, but it is important to consider ways of managing stress for these species as well in their respective areas of the practice. It can be beneficial to spray feline synthetic pheromones on fabric items, such as the towels that may be used in handling, remembering to do so a minimum of 10 to 15 minutes before intended use because of the alcohol carrier. If a veterinary practice is being built from scratch, it is advisable to use building materials such as solid doors and sound dampening materials to minimize noise. However, in most situations, there is little or no opportunity to redesign or modify the building itself, and noise in the veterinary practice can be minimized by taking other simple steps, including using soft voices, avoiding dropping screws and bolts onto the top of the carrier when taking it apart, and reducing the risk of sudden or loud noises due to items used in the examination room, such as equipment that is placed on counters or bangs against the carrier. Providing background sound has been recommended as a means of improving a positive emotional state and "white noise" or calming music such as "Through a Cat's Ear," may be useful. More information on this topic can be found in Chapter 22. It is beneficial to eliminate the sight of other animals by providing separate waiting and caging areas, but where this is not possible, the use of towels and screens to minimize visual contact will be beneficial. A designated cat waiting area can allow a range of opportunities to reduce stress, for example by providing seating designed to prevent cats from seeing each other (see Chapter 9 for more details). It is helpful to use an efficient appointment system so that a cat does not have to stay in a waiting area and can ideally be taken directly into an examination room. Feline stress can be further reduced by considering the texture of the consulting table surface and using materials that offer a tactile appeal, such as fleece, towels, and small blankets. These materials can also allow burrowing or other comforting behaviors. Laminate consulting table surfaces are preferable to stainless steel, but if stainless steel is the only option, it can be covered with a soft towel or fleece with a nonslip material underneath (see Chapter 21 for more details). Such a surface will offer a more acceptable tactile experience for the cat, and it will also minimize other potential sources of alarm and stress associated with a stainless steel table, such as reflections, a cold surface, slipping, and noise.

Effective hygiene control not only reduces risk of cross-infection but also helps to limit unwanted communication between feline patients, which can serve to increase arousal and anxiety. For this reason, it is important to clean areas where the cat has rubbed to eliminate secretions from scent glands as well as the surface where the cat has been standing and depositing scent information from its pads. Hand washing not only cleans but also can help to eliminate feline social odors and prevent the veterinary staff from inadvertently passing messages from cat to cat. It can also be helpful to use lint rollers liberally between patients to remove cat hair deposited on the clothing of the veterinary staff that might also carry these significant feline odors.

The design and layout of the examination room will be a contributing factor when deciding how to devise an appropriate approach for performing the exam (see Chapter 10). Although offering hiding places is an important tenet of low-stress handling, the hiding places need to facilitate the exam and not work against the objective of keeping the cat as calm as possible. The ideal feline examination room will have minimal furniture and will have built-in seating and work surfaces with sides that go completely to the floor.

It is important to structure the consulting room so that there are no potentially inaccessible hideouts that the cat could conceal itself in. In a traditional examination room, there may be a table or seating with legs, both of which can create potential hiding places which cats will gravitate towards when they come out of the travelling carrier. When there are several pieces of furniture in the examination room, for example, an examination table, a bank of cabinets, and some seating, the cat may dart from one location to another as it seeks cover (Figure 20-6, A). Once the cat is settled in a secluded location, there will be a sense of threat if practice staff then have to remove or chase the cat out from the safe haven. It can be better in this situation to have a cat stay in its carrier to prevent escalation of arousal from perceived confrontation and the resulting fear.

If the feline examination room is well designed, with resting and hiding places carefully planned to maximize comfort and security, then it is possible to offer a cat the opportunity to explore, which can help to reduce the cat's anxiety by allowing it to gather information at its own pace, thereby evoking less fearful behaviors. (Figure 20-6, B). It is hugely beneficial to design feline examination rooms to provide locations that accommodate a cat's need for a safe resting area, while still allowing the veterinary staff access to the cat. Providing seating for clients that allows an exam to be conducted while their cat is on their lap, or beside them, can significantly reduce stress for both the client and the cat (Figure 20-7). Cats often prefer to settle into places that have sides, even low sides, such as those on many feline weighing scales, and these locations can offer a significant degree of comfort (Figure 20-8). The bottom half of a hard-sided carrier

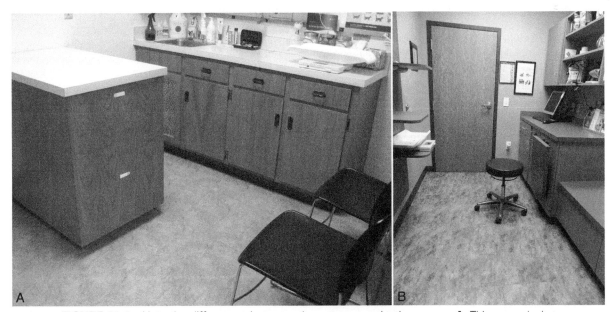

FIGURE 20-6 Note the differences between these two examination rooms. **A,** This room design offers potential hiding places beneath the chairs but also has poorly accessible cover and can encourage darting, so it is best to keep the cat in the bottom half of the carrier or in an area that is more confined and easily accessible. **B,** This room has no obvious places to hide, so the cat can be allowed to wander around because it cannot get stuck in areas that are inaccessible to staff.

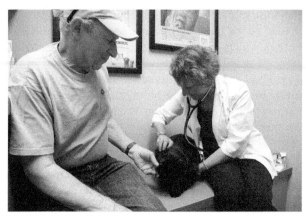

FIGURE 20-7 Cats that choose to sit next to their owners are often comforted, thus reducing stress for both client and cat.

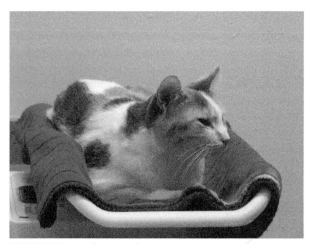

FIGURE 20-8 Cats prefer to rest in places where they have a sense of being protected. Many will prefer to sit on the consulting room scales with elevated sides to hide within rather than be on an examination table. (From Rodan, I: *Understanding the Cat and Feline-Friendly Handling.* IN Little, SE: *The Cat*, Elsevier, St. Louis, 2012)

also functions as a secure resting place (Figure 20-9). A large, empty litter box or a low storage container lined with towels or fleece can be equally effective (Figure 20-10). The resting place should be created and positioned in such a way that veterinary staff can readily access the cat and perform an adequate clinical examination. When using mobile resting places, such as weighing scales, the cat can be moved within the container when the veterinarian needs to gain access to another part of the cat's body and this is far less stressful than moving the cat itself. If an examination is taking place on the exam table, a cat will usually prefer this type of sided surface to a flat one. Again, the bottom half of many hard-sided carriers, or containers with low sides, function well to provide this type of secure resting place. If the carrier bottom or tray is placed in the lap of either the client or the veterinarian, care must be taken to ensure that it remains steady, because cats feel more secure if they can remain level on a stable surface (Figure 20-11).

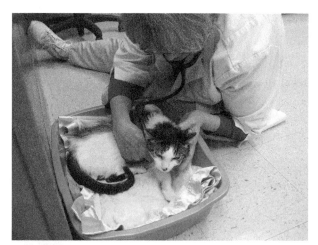

FIGURE 20-10 Large empty litter boxes with edges are helpful, especially for cats that are not brought to the veterinarian in a carrier.

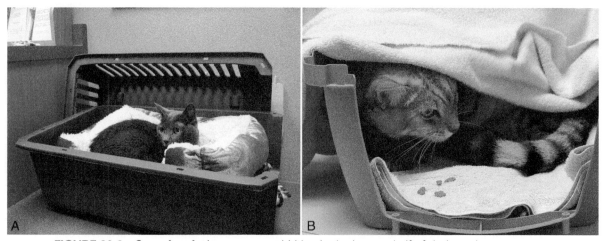

FIGURE 20-9 Cats often feel more secure hidden in the bottom half of their carrier.

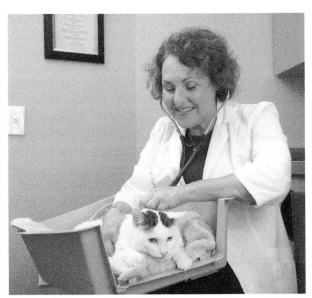

FIGURE 20-11   Holding the bottom half of the carrier on a lap with the cat facing away is an excellent handling procedure as long as the carrier is stable. (From Rodan, I: *Understanding the Cat and Feline-Friendly Handling.* IN Little, SE: *The Cat*, Elsevier, St. Louis, 2012)

Maximizing Comfort

An important principle to follow is to give the cat a sense of control by allowing it to be examined in a location of its choosing and in a position that is as comfortable as possible. Pursuing an examination by forcing a cat to be in a particular location or heavily restraining it will result in escalating its fear. A handling plan should be prepared that takes into account the characteristics of the examination space, as well as the demeanor of both the cat and the client. It is also important to incorporate sensory cues that could impart calming or comforting information, such as items with scents from home. Each case will require a different approach and it may be beneficial for the veterinarian(s) involved to have a strategy in mind, and to organize personnel, equipment, and supplies in such a way as to minimize the cat's stress. Many cats do best if all handling is done in one sitting so that they can then be allowed to retire to a safe, secure place, such as the carrier, while client discussion and education occur. However, some cats are rapidly aroused emotionally and these individuals may do better when the visit is broken into steps. It is important to observe the body language of the cat and to take a break at the earliest signs of increasing arousal rather than wait until the cat is in a highly stressed state. Notes from prior visits will be very helpful in guiding the handling experience. If this information is not available, be sure to include the results of the current visit in the cat's medical record in order to improve the feline experience at future visits.

It may be necessary to instruct the client to keep the cat inside the carrier when they enter the examination room, since the most important first step for the veterinarian or technician/nurse is to assess the body language and facial signals of the cat while it is still in the carrier. During this time, focus should be on the client and during the initial conversation overt observation of the cat, especially in the form of staring, must be avoided. When looking at the cat, slowly blink your eyes and turn your head slightly to the side. If the cat responds with a slow blink, it is an indication of decreased arousal.[8] Determine if it is appropriate to allow the cat to come out of the carrier and if the cat is comfortable doing so. A cat that appears fear-aggressive or fractious dictates a different course of action than one that is inhibited or one that wants to explore. Consideration must be given to the layout of the examination room before making a decision about allowing the cat to roam freely when it comes out of the carrier. The sensory input from the examination room may increase anxiety in some cats; therefore, it is essential to continually monitor the cat's body language to help guide decisions about choosing the best course of action for that cat.

If a cat is exploring the examination room while a history is being taken, providing treats, catnip, or distracting toys can be helpful to make the cat feel more secure or can redirect the cat's attention if fearful body language is detected. Cats that are more comfortable exploring the examination room tend to settle down after several minutes in the location where they feel the safest. Often this will be in one of the spaces with sides that have been provided (e.g., carrier or scale) or with the client.

Some cats will be comfortable on a lap. Not having a person towering over them and being more on their level is less intimidating. If the cat is calm, it can face the family member; if the cat is anxious, it can hide its head under bedding or a towel. Furthermore, allowing cats to lean against the person's arm or body will often make them feel more secure and prevent any sensation of a potential to fall. The examination can proceed with the cat on the client's lap, positioned where it feels safest. By sitting next to the client the veterinarian can also talk to them about the cat and their concerns, which allows them to feel part of their pet's healthcare team.

If a cat is more comfortable staying in the carrier, allow it to do so if possible. Cats that inhibit in response to their anxiety often choose to stay in their carrier. These cats strongly prefer to engage in covert behavior, and strategies need to be employed that can give them as much of a sense of being hidden as possible. Allowing them to stay in tray-like, sided resting places (such as the bottom half of a carrier) is important, but being surrounded by cover often provides them with more of a sense of security. Draping a towel over the bottom half of a carrier while the top is being removed maintains their sense of safety. Some may want to see out, and some will want to stay completely covered. Moving the towel to expose only the part of the cat that needs to be observed and palpated allows the cat to retain its sense of being hidden while making it easy for the veterinarian to carry out the necessary examination (Figure 20-12).

When cats are exhibiting extreme behavioral responses to their negative emotions during transport or in the examination room it may be appropriate to consider the use of anxiolytic medications such as gabapentin or alprazolam. Alprazolam is a short-acting anxiolytic that may also limit the memory of a fearful event and can be helpful for cats that show mild to moderate signs of anxiety related to the veterinary visit.

Gabapentin is another medication that has been used by the North American authors and other veterinarians to prevent anxiety prior to veterinary practice visits and has been extremely helpful. Administering gabapentin at 10 mg/kg up to 100 mg per cat (some veterinarians

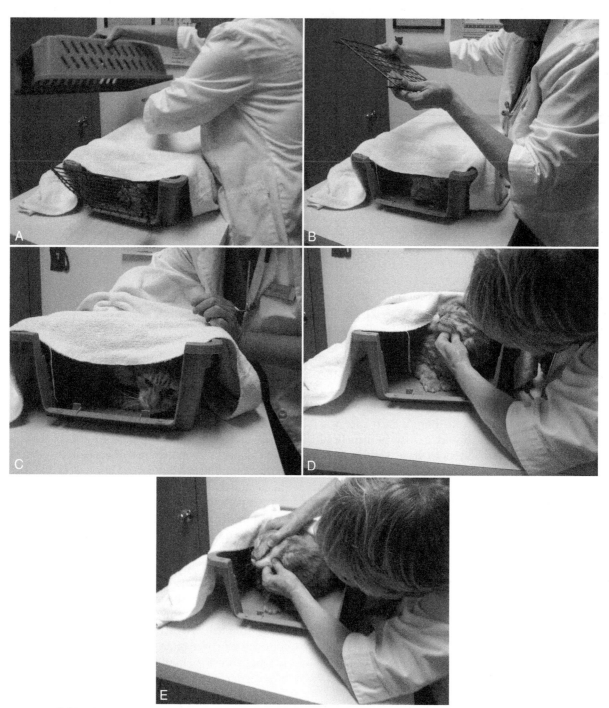

FIGURE 20-12 This series of pictures shows the sequence of taking the carrier top off while draping a towel over the cat. The towel is moved as needed to examine different parts of the cat. This is a very useful technique for cats that refuse to leave the safety of their carrier.

use up to 150 mg) can reduce cats' anxiety and fear-associated aggression. Many cats may also experience some degree of transient sedation. Gabapentin has a high safety margin. Excellent results have been obtained using 100 mg per cat administered 90 minutes to 3 hours prior to the visit. Results are more predictable when administered on an empty stomach or if mixed into a small amount of canned food or a treat. It can be a good option for cats that previously would have required heavier sedation or have not had an effective response to alprazolam. It is the drug of choice for the American authors. A more detailed discussion of pharmacologic options is provided in Chapter 19.

Ideally medication should be seen as a short-term solution and behavioral work to habituate the cat to the veterinary environment is required for a more long-term approach. Some cats may become more relaxed after carrier training and repeated less stressful real or "mock" visits to the practice. As a result they may change their reactions to such an extent that they no longer need medication.

If preventative measures have not been employed and a cat arrives at the practice in a state of high emotional arousal and already displaying repulsion (aggressive) behaviors, it may be helpful to give the cat the opportunity to remain in the carrier for several minutes in a quiet room. Some cats will calm but others may become further stimulated by the sensory signals in the consulting room and their repulsion responses may escalate. In these cases when simple handling techniques are impossible to implement safely, it may be necessary to consider the use of handling aids. Various toweling techniques have been described for mildly fear-aggressive cats. Sometimes a sense of pressure over the cat's body can act to minimize its aggressive responses. A product designed with this in mind is the Thunder-Shirt (ThunderWorks, Durham, N.C.). Opinion is divided on this approach, and use of the ThunderShirt is far more common in the United States than in the UK. As described in Chapter 22, clients can explore the use of this device but it is essential to determine whether the cat is amenable to having the device put on and it should not be used if it totally immobilizes the cat. Rigid muzzles can be helpful, as they can distract a cat's attention and keep staff safe while they handle a moderately fractious cat. However, it is not appropriate to try to use a muzzle when the cat is in a high state of arousal and already showing signs of lunging and biting. Rigid muzzles do not fit tightly on the cat's face, and they have an opening at the end where a cat can breathe comfortably. The only points of pressure are on several spots at the back of the muzzle. Many feline practitioners consider these muzzles preferable to a close-fitting device as they are less confining and can still give the cat a sense of control in that it can see out of the end if desired (Figure 20-13). The handler must be able to assess feline body language accurately to determine whether the cat's struggling abates and whether the cat's body tone and postural signals indicate diminished arousal. There are other techniques and devices available to aid in handling, but it is essential that the handler remain focused on the goal of decreasing the cat's fear. Whichever method is used, handlers must be able to assess whether they are truly diminishing the cat's fear by augmenting coping mechanisms or simply creating an inhibited or freezing response. When aids are used, the aim should be to decrease the cat's level of arousal, reactivity, and anxiety, and not simply to restrain the cat in order to

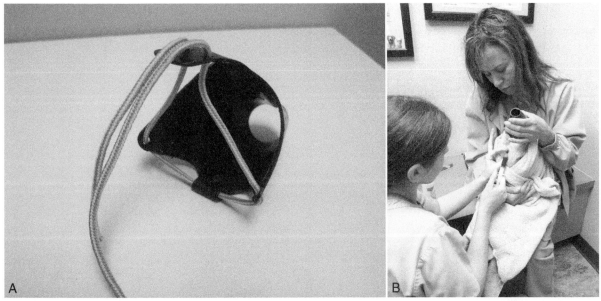

FIGURE 20-13   Rigid muzzles can be more comfortable than soft muzzles for cats and can help reduce fear and increase human safety.

complete a task. If the cat is restrained but still in a negative emotional state, it would be more effective to use appropriate chemical restraint (see Chapter 22).

THE CONSULTATION

Once steps have been taken to minimize the cat's stress as much as possible, the examination can be performed. The practitioner should continue to make efforts to reduce triggers that are likely to lead to a further negative emotional state while the examination and procedures are carried out. The goals of handling during examinations are to prevent fear and pain in the cat while remaining able to perform a comprehensive physical examination and educate the client.

The order of the examination procedures should be tailored to make it easier for feline patients that are fearful or in pain; instead of using a consistent order of starting at the head and working to the tail, veterinarians need to be flexible and first examine the nonpainful areas and those that do not arouse the cat as much. Distraction of anxious cats by engaging them in an alternative behavior that induces a positive emotional state, such as playing with an interactive toy, eating treats, or rubbing on catnip, can be beneficial (Figures 20-14). If a toy is used, it may be necessary to move it rapidly and unpredictably to increase the cat's interest, but it is important to avoid inducing high arousal even when it is positively motivated. It is possible to calm some cats and divert their attention from the procedures being performed by gently handling areas where cats naturally prefer to be touched. For example, gently petting the cat behind the ears, rubbing under its chin, or massaging its forehead between the ears and eyes (Figure 20-15). Patting or scratching over other areas of the body should be avoided, as many cats may become more aroused. In most situations, the examiner can handle the cat alone; this is preferable because the less fear and arousal, the more compliant it will actually be. Clients are often keen to reassure their pet and may engage in more intense handling, which is counterproductive.

To minimize discomfort, examinations should be performed with the cat on soft padding, such as folded towels or blankets, and not on a hard surface. A cat experiencing pain may be tense and resist examination in an attempt to protect itself. Sometimes a cat that has been designated fear-aggressive is really in pain. Veterinary visits will be much calmer once that pain has been

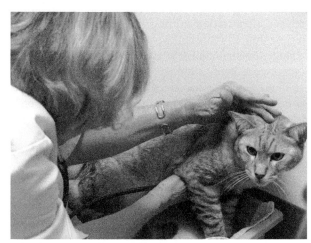

FIGURE 20-15 Cats prefer to be petted or touched on the head and neck, such as gently massaging the forehead between the ears and eyes.

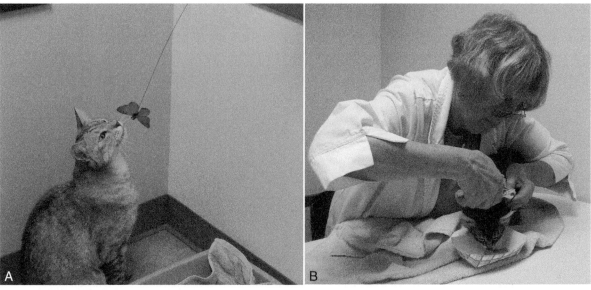

FIGURES 20-14 Distracting kittens and cats with toys and treats can help prevent or reduce fear.

addressed. Gentle handling and analgesia will facilitate the examination and keep the patient as comfortable as possible.[1,2] Refer to Chapter 21 for more information on preventing pain during veterinary visits.

The phrase "move slow to move fast" is especially helpful when discussing cat handling. All interactions need to be performed in a measured fashion and rapid and unexpected interventions should be avoided. For example, when extending a cat's leg for an examination or positioning its head to evaluate its mouth, these actions should be carried out slowly. The cat should be aware of your intention to interact and this can be achieved by placing a hand or finger on the part of the body about to be handled. Slow and gentle stroking of the skin as preparation for some form of intervention can be helpful, for example before lifting a lip to evaluate teeth and gums or picking up the skin to give a subcutaneous injection. When moving over the body to examine the rear quarters, underside, or feet, it is important to recognize that touching these areas can be poorly tolerated. The evaluation will be more successful if light, steady pressure is applied across the area in the direction of hair growth. Letting go and touching again can increase reactivity. Moving slowly is also safer for the staff. Rapid hand motion can trigger a fear-aggressive lunge or bite or induce a sequence of predatory motivated play.

It is important to evaluate the cat's body language and posture in order to assess what steps may be taken to maintain a more positive emotional state. The tactile component of the veterinary exam is very important and muscle condition scoring and lymph node and abdominal palpation can be done in a very unobtrusive way. Cardiac auscultation can be achieved by slipping the stethoscope to the sternal region without exposing the body. Many cats will be more comfortable staying under a cover for the entirety of the visit, regardless of where they have chosen to settle. If a cat so prefers, allow it to feel "invisible" by returning to the carrier or remaining hidden elsewhere during client discussion and education.

Getting a rectal temperature often causes the cat stress. In addition, stress-associated hyperthermia in a cat that does not have fever is common.[12] Many veterinarians evaluate body temperature only when it is indicated by the history and clinical signs. Others choose to use aural instead of rectal thermometers if circumstances permit. Regardless of technique, it is important to prevent stress or discomfort for the cat.

HANDLING FOR SPECIMEN COLLECTION AND PROCEDURES

The objective while handling for specimen collection is to minimize the cat's fear as well as limit the amount of resistance encountered in the process. Although it is difficult to avoid fear entirely, just as it is for humans during medical procedures, use of gentle handling instead of more heavy-handed methods reduces fear. Gentle handling can result in relaxation of muscle tension which can be physically monitored as a measure of the success of the handling technique. The examiner needs to assess the anxiety level of a patient throughout any procedure and should use visual, auditory, and tactile information from the cat to get a true picture of its emotional state.

It is beneficial to perform as much of the examination and procedures as possible in the examination room. Moving a cat to another part of the veterinary practice will elicit fear for several reasons. Changing locations generates fear in itself and, in the treatment areas of the veterinary practice, there will also be other noises and activities, as well as the presence or proximity of other animals that have the potential to heighten a cat's anxiety. Ideally, as few moves as possible should occur during the visit to the veterinary practice. Clients are often grateful and less anxious themselves when they are able to watch procedures such as blood pressure measurements, venipunctures, and cystocentesis in the examination room. When clients see staff members at work, they can develop a better appreciation of the level of care a veterinary practice provides and of the value of the services they are receiving. Clients who are not comfortable watching are often grateful to be given the opportunity to leave the examination room and feel more comfortable leaving the room themselves than watching a staff member remove their cat to the treatment area.

The requirement for analgesia should be assessed prior to commencing a procedure and this assessment should take into account the pain potential from the procedure itself and also from any unusual or uncomfortable positions in which the cat has to be placed. For example, anal gland expression can be quite painful for many cats. Using buprenorphine can greatly increase the cat's comfort during this procedure (see Chapter 21 for more information on handling the cat in pain).

In order to make the experience as positive as possible for the cat it is important to be as efficient as possible and all of the necessary supplies should be ready and available before procedures such as sample collection begin. Extra staffing with two people holding and a third collecting may be necessary to diminish the stress of the handling process; however, many cats can be cuddled in a blanket and thus require only one holder (Figure 20-16). It is important to be flexible and strive to perform procedures in such a way that the cat is most relaxed. Procedures such as blood draws or blood pressure measurement can often be performed while the cat stays in the soft bedding from the carrier that carries a familiar scent. It may help to speak softly and minimize environmental issues that

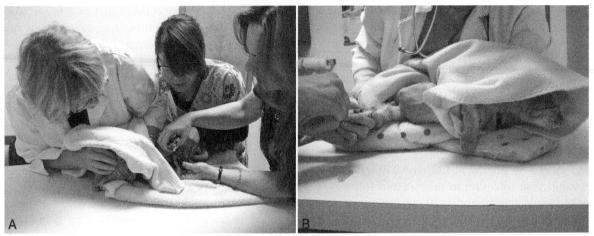

FIGURE 20-16   Although some cats need two people cradling them and one to collect the samples, many cats can be cuddled in their blanket to make them comfortable with only one holder.

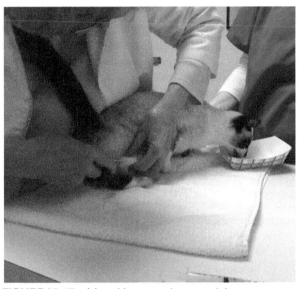

FIGURE 20-17   Many kittens and some adult cats can easily be distracted with food or treats when receiving injections.

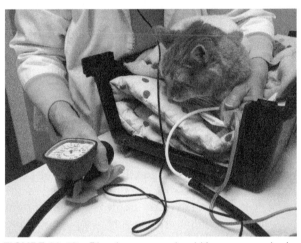

FIGURE 20-18   Blood pressure should be measured prior to other diagnostic testing. Many cats allow their blood pressure to be measured while in the bottom half of their carrier.

will exacerbate the cat's startle and anxiety responses. If it is possible, distraction with a toy or food can also be used. Some kittens will allow injections while eating and will not notice the needle (Figure 20-17). Needles can be blunted after going into a vial or, as with many vaccines, two vials. The use of a new needle can reduce the cat's discomfort on injection.

Many cats will tolerate minimally invasive procedures such as blood pressure measurement, aural examinations, or subcutaneous injections while on the client's lap. To avoid the risk of injury to clients, veterinary staff must use their professional judgment to determine if it is appropriate to perform tasks in this position. It is beneficial to have a veterinary practice policy that follows state or regional ordinances, in addition to providing staff with information about how to discuss this option

with clients, reviewing risks and benefits. A signed release may be in order as well.

Blood pressure measurements are an essential part of the veterinary exam of older patients and it is advisable to become adept at taking these in multiple locations in an examination room and at multiple locations on a cat. The blood pressure measurement should be performed either at the beginning of the examination or at least before any other procedures occur. Allow a cat to acclimate to the environment in its preferred location for at least 5 to 10 minutes.[13] Establishing a veterinary practice policy for blood pressure measurement is advisable so that all staff members know the appropriate sequence of the examination to minimize stress on the cat and thus obtain a more accurate reading (Figure 20-18). Determine if the cat will be less anxious if given a minute or two to get used to the presence of the cuff on its leg. Some cats do better with this than others, and some will be less stressed if the cuff is applied immediately and the pressure is assessed. The end of the cuff can then be attached to the tubing of the inflating device when the cat appears as comfortable as possible. Regardless of the method used, multiple readings are recommended. Inflating the cuff prior to taking readings can make the initial reading less startling to the cat.

Cats accept venipuncture much better when they are allowed to be in a comfortable position in which they have some sense of control rather than when they are scruffed or held tightly against their will. One successful approach involves using a cradling technique that allows the cat to drape itself across a handler's forearm so that the handler can gently keep the cat's upper foot flexed toward its body while holding off the saphenous vein in the lower rear leg (Figure 20-19, A and B). Many cats gain more comfort if the front half of their body in the cradling technique is allowed to be in a sternal position, even allowing some weight to be borne on the front feet. Although a forceful full-body restraint usually results in struggle, some cats will benefit from a slight sense of pressure over their body. When the holder snuggles a cat up to their body, they provide support for the cat's back. Light pressure from a towel or the torso of the holder as they lean over the cat can have a calming effect without causing the cat to panic from too much restraint. It is common to require only one person to hold a cat in this manner and a second to draw the blood sample. Some cats, however, especially large cats or ones experiencing pain, can benefit when one handler is positioned in the front and another at the back end. This can allow the cat to assume a more comfortable position with its front while struggling less with the veterinarian's attempts to access its vein. Some veterinarians have developed a technique of drawing blood from a jugular venipuncture single handedly but even in

these cases it can be helpful for another person to act as a back stop to prevent the cat from reversing (Figure 20-20). Gently extending a cat's front leg while allowing it to sit comfortably in a sternal posture is also used. Many cats need only light cradling of the head while the holder is stroking it between the eyes, on top of the head, or at the base of the skull.

With all positioning for procedures, the cat's limbs must be kept in normal alignment with the least resistance possible. It is important to be mindful of the cat's normal anatomy and range-of-motion limitations. Care should be taken not to hold the cat's limbs rotated in such a way that the cat will be injured.

Evaluation of a sterile urine sample is a critical part of a thorough diagnostic plan for a cat, and it is important to be confident in collecting a sample in a low-stress manner. Cystocentesis can be performed using similar holding strategies. Some cats will tolerate cystocentesis while standing or partially sitting sternally. Obese cats can present a challenge to palpating and stabilizing a bladder for the procedure and may require ultrasound for the bladder to be visualized. In most cats, however, their bladder is readily palpated in a variety of positions, including the standing position.

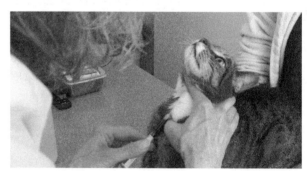

FIGURE 20-20 Some veterinarians and veterinary technicians are able to collect a blood sample from a jugular vein without any assistance. (Courtesy J. Brunt)

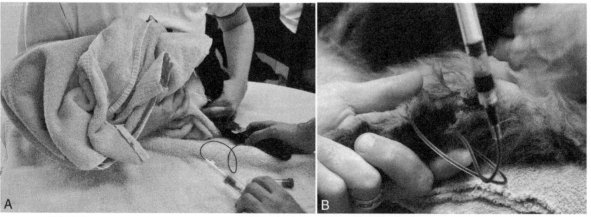

FIGURE 20-19 This cradling technique facilitates venipuncture from the medial saphenous vein. (A, Courtesy M. Brown)

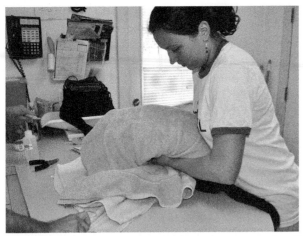

FIGURE 20-21 Many cats feel safer and stop struggling if wrapped in a "burrito" hold. (Courtesy M. Brown)

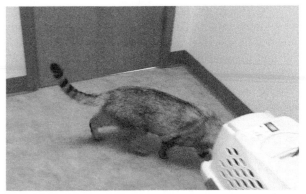

FIGURE 20-22 Most cats readily return to their carrier as soon as the examination and other procedures are completed. It is important to let them return to this safety and not force them to be present while discussions are being held with the client.

Whereas most cats can be handled successfully with the techniques described above, some, of course, cannot. Veterinary practice staff must be able to identify which cats can be appropriately handled using additional low restraint techniques without creating an excessive amount of stress, and which cats will need pharmacological intervention. If a cat decreases the amount of resistance and struggle when additional low-level restraint techniques are employed, this can be an acceptable approach. For example some cats allow procedures to be performed when wrapped in a towel, or "burritoed" (Figure 20-21), while others can be distracted by limiting the line of sight with the rigid muzzles described above. While using either or both of these techniques, gentle rocking and low-volume repetitive calming sounds may help to induce palpable relaxation, but some cats may become more anxious so it is important that the holder carefully monitors whether the technique is helpful.

If the cat is struggling and resisting in such a way that these techniques are unsuccessful, it is advisable to stop trying to work with the cat. An alternative plan involving the use of chemical restraint can be considered. The more negative experience a cat continues to have, the greater its anxiety and resistance will be the next time it is brought back to the veterinary practice. It is better to use medications that will not only sedate but also have some amnestic action. Discussion of how to approach a fear-aggressive cat is found in Chapter 22.

As soon as the handler is finished with procedures that require handling, the cat should be allowed to return to a safe place. Often this place will be the carrier. Many clients are surprised by how readily their cat returns to the security of the carrier, especially if they have not instituted carrier training at home and getting their cat into the carrier there has been a challenge (Figure 20-22). Any discussion and client education can be completed while the cat is in the security of the carrier. At the conclusion of the visit, the veterinarian should assess how the visit went, and make notes in the cat's record of what worked well and what did not in terms of managing the patient's stress and anxiety.

EXTENDING THE PRINCIPLES THROUGHOUT THE VETERINARY PRACTICE

All of the above-described principles apply to handling the cat not only in the consulting room but also while hospitalized or left at the veterinary practice for outpatient procedures. Blocking the cat's line of sight with other animals is imperative, as is controlling its exposure to odor, loud noises, and barking dogs. If housing is adapted to meet a cat's needs it will make it easier to carry out appropriate feline-friendly handling. It is important to identify environmental and social triggers which will challenge feline coping skills and modify them in order to prevent a cat's emotional state from escalating into full fear aggression. When a cat is not able to use avoidance or inhibition behavioral responses to its negative emotional state, it will have no option but to employ repulsion techniques.

Discussion of appropriate veterinary practice design can be found elsewhere in this textbook (see Chapters 9, 10, and 11). The optimal situation is to have purpose-built premises that meet cat-friendly requirements. However, many practices are dealing with existing premises and in this situation, it is possible to be creative in strategies that can maximize low-stress characteristics in the environment. Some cats may be more comfortable if left in their carriers or at least in the bottom of the carrier when placed in a cage. Covering the door of the cage to block the cat's line of sight and provide the cat with a sense of being hidden is often helpful (Figure 20-23). Providing a hiding place and a perch in a cage gives a cat the choice of elevation or hiding as potential coping strategies. It is possible to do this in any cage by using items such as cardboard boxes or plastic bins with soft bedding or by using specifically designed equipment like the Feline Fort from Cats Protection in the UK (Figure 20-24). (See Chapter 11 for more information.) Encouraging clients to bring towels or articles of clothing from home can help to increase olfactory familiarity in the cage, and the scent profile

of the veterinary practice can be further enhanced by the use of synthetic pheromones (see Chapter 18).

Take care not to approach a cat directly and abruptly when it is inside a cage. Approach from the side of a cat's line of sight, and, if possible, allow it to sniff at a hand before opening the cage door (Figure 20-25). Applying the slow-blink "winky eye" maneuver described previously can also help to reduce the cat's sense of threat while being approached.

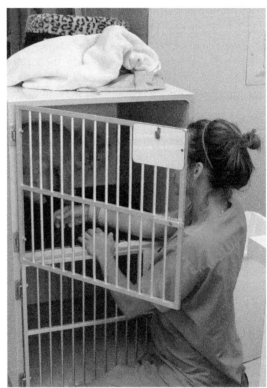

FIGURE 20-25 Be passive when approaching a cat in a cage and allow the cat to gather scent information from the extended stationary arm. The aim is for the cat to choose to move toward the front of the cage and to avoid grabbing at the cat or forcibly removing it. (From Rodan, I: *Understanding the Cat and Feline-Friendly Handling.* IN Little, SE: The Cat, Elsevier, St. Louis, 2012)

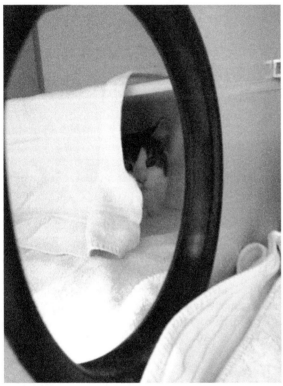

FIGURE 20-23 Providing cover for a caged cat increases security. They often choose to peep out and watch what is happening.

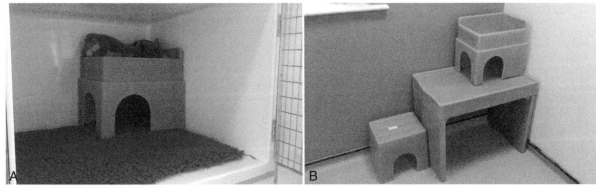

FIGURE 20-24 **A,** The Feline Fort provides both hiding place and perch, giving the cat a choice of elevation or hiding while caged. **B,** The whole Feline Fort provides excellent exercise space as well as hiding places and perches. (Courtesy H. Rooney)

Moving a cat from a ward or treatment area into a quiet examination room for exams and procedures is preferable to doing them in a busy location in the veterinary practice, even though it involves a change of location for the cat. Placing the cat in its carrier before it is moved and covering the carrier with a towel if the cat is frightened will reduce patient arousal and potential staff injury.

GOING HOME INSTRUCTIONS

When a feline patient is returning to a multicat household, it is important to remember that the cat or cats that have remained at home can be overwhelmed by the scent of the veterinary practice on their returning housemate. As smell is a critical part of a cat's ability to recognize its world, a resident cat may no longer recognize a returning cat, and thus hostility between the cats is not unexpected. To prevent this, clients should be advised to separate the returning cat in a safe room that has many olfactory sources, such as an owner's bedroom or office, so that it can lose the scent of the veterinary practice and reestablish the scent of the home before being reintroduced to the other household cats. Using a synthetic feline pheromone concurrently is also advised (see Chapter 18). If a problem with intercat aggression has previously occurred after separation for veterinary visits or hospitalizations, encourage the cats' owners to start pheromone use prior to bringing the cat home. Some clients with two cats in a household find it preferable to bring both cats to the practice at the same time to reduce the likelihood of conflict.

CONCLUSION

Within existing veterinary practices, it can be difficult to make the changes necessary to provide feline-friendly consultations, and it is important to recognize potential obstacles so that they can be overcome.

The physical layout of the workspace must be taken into account when deciding how to approach the cat. If changes that would enable cats to be free-roaming in the consulting room are not possible, it is better to focus on making the cat less stressed while retaining it in a more confined location.

Availability of staff to provide sufficient people to hold cats appropriately for procedures, such as venipuncture, can seem prohibitive in some practices, but it is important to have a third person available to assist if cats are to be comfortable during these interventions and struggling is to be minimized. Training front desk staff in low restraint feline handling can give more flexibility in terms of overcoming this obstacle. Developing skills in the area of feline-friendly handling takes patience, and learning to "move slow to move fast" can be difficult. It may initially feel that feline consultations will take too long using this approach, but in the long run less time will be wasted by using these techniques. Employing more heavy handed restraint not only is inappropriate from a feline welfare perspective but also runs the risk of injury to staff and clients. When such methods fail, they also leave the cat in an agitated and aroused state, which makes the use of chemical restraint less effective and necessitates a further delay while the medication takes effect.

Developing a cat-friendly practice is a challenge, and everyone in the veterinary practice needs to be committed to making the change and feel fully invested in the benefits of adopting different handling strategies. When multiple key team members lead by example, keeping a cat-friendly program going will be more successful and better sustained.

REFERENCES

1. Volk KO, Felsted KE, Thomas JG, Siren CW. Executive summary of the Bayer veterinary care usage study. *J Am Vet Med Assoc.* 2011;238:1275–1282.
2. Lue TW, Pantenburg DP, Crawford PM. Impact of the owner-pet and client-veterinarian bond on the care that pets receive. *J Am Vet Med Assoc.* 2008;232:531–540.
3. Employee injury trends at veterinary practices. *AVMA PLIT safety bulletin.* 2007;15(3), Summer.
4. *Bayer Veterinary Care Usage Study III: Feline Findings;* 2012. BayerBCI_BVCUS_III_Feline_Findings_2013.pdf Accessed February 2, 2015.
5. Notari L. Stress in Veterinary Behavioural Medicine. In: Horwitz D, Mills DS, eds. *BSAVA Manual of Canine and Feline Behavioural Medicine.* ed 2. Gloucester, UK: British Small Animal Veterinary Association (BSAVA); 2010:136–145.
6. Heath S. Feline Aggression. In: Horwitz D, Mills D, Health S, eds. *BSAVA Manual of Canine and Feline Behavioural Medicine.* ed 1. Gloucester, UK: British Small Animal Veterinary Association (BSAVA); 2002:216–228.
7. McMillan FD. Development of a mental wellness program for animals. *J Am Vet Med Assoc.* 2002;220:965–972.
8. Griffin B, Hume KR. Recognition and Management of Stress in Housed Cats. In: August JR, editor: *Consultations in Feline Internal Medicine.* vol 5, St Louis: Elsevier; 2006, 717–734.
9. Carlstead K, Brown JL, Strawn W. Behavioral and physiological correlates of stress in laboratory cats. *Appl Anim Behav Sci.* 1993;38:143–158.
10. Rand JS, Kinnaird E, Baglioni A, et al. Acute stress hyperglycemia in cats is associated with struggling and increased concentrations of lactate and norepinephrine. *J Vet Intern Med.* 2002;16:123–132.
11. Pageat P, Gaultier E. Current research in canine and feline pheromones. *Vet Clin North Am Small Anim Pract.* 2003;33:187–211.
12. Quimby JM, Smith ML, Lunn KF. Evaluation of the effects of hospital visit stress on physiologic parameters in the cat. *J Feline Med Surg.* 2011;13:733–737.
13. Belew A, Barlett T, Brown SA. Evaluation of the white-coat effects in cats. *J Vet Intern Med.* 1999;13:134–142.

Handling the Cat that is in Pain

Ilona Rodan and Sarah Heath

INTRODUCTION

Advances in veterinary medicine have resulted in an increased feline life expectancy with many cats living into their late teens or even early twenties.[1] Pain can occur at any age, but chronic pain is more prevalent in senior patients, with increased incidence and progression of painful conditions such as degenerative joint disease (DJD) and periodontal disease.

Regardless of the duration of a painful experience, cats are unable to rationalize the pain or recognize that it may not be a permanent state. From a welfare perspective, appropriate handling of the cat in pain is an important veterinary responsibility. Awareness of the occurrence of painful conditions, together with an ability to recognize pain and an emphasis on gentle handling of all cats in a comfortable practice environment, is a necessary component of veterinary consultations and will help to improve patient comfort, case outcomes, and human safety.

PAIN AND THE EMOTIONAL FACTOR

Pain is defined as an unpleasant sensory and emotional experience, with pain negatively impacting both physical and emotional health.[2,3] Emotions such as fear and anxiety often occur in association with physical pain.[3] Therefore, regardless of species, "Pain is not just *what* you feel, but *how* it makes you feel."[4]

Both acute and chronic stress can lead to an abnormally heightened sensitivity to pain.[5] Because stress can exacerbate pain,[6,7] providing appropriate handling and nursing care, designed to give the cat a sense of control and to minimize stress through consistency in the environment, is an important component of pain management and prevention.

RECOGNIZING FELINE PAIN

The subtle nature of the feline response to pain makes it difficult to detect. While canine patients may demonstrate their pain through obvious changes in mobility or in vocalization, the feline patient is more likely to withdraw or avoid contact. However, withdrawal or avoidance can also occur in association with fear, stress, or non-painful medical conditions, thus making a definitive diagnosis of pain even more challenging. Another consideration is that the experience of pain is individual; thus, a stimulus that is very painful for one cat might be only mildly painful for another.

The intermittent nature of some painful conditions makes it difficult for owners to recognize pain within the home environment when the cat is usually comfortable and active, but might occasionally withdraw from its normal behaviors. These subtle and individual signs combined with intermittent flare-ups, often lead owners to believe that the cat is simply "having a bad day" and that there is no reason for real concern. Only when a flare-up persists, does the owner realize that the cat needs medical attention. Indeed, recognizing the significance of pain in its early stages can be difficult for veterinary professionals as well. Reasons include the subtle signs of pain in the feline species and specific features of the veterinary practice environment that make recognizing pain in cats a challenge. The primary feline behavioral response to physical pain and negative emotional states is avoidance, which can lead to passive withdrawal or active fleeing. In a veterinary context, the use of avoidance (fleeing) is limited and even actively discouraged. As a result, the cat may enter into a state of inhibition (freezing) or begin to display signs of aggression. The similarity in behavioral manifestations makes differentiating between cats that are in a negative emotional state (e.g., fear or anxiety) and cats that are in physical pain difficult. This is further complicated by the fact that many cats at the practice are simultaneously experiencing both negative emotion and physical pain.

Physiological parameters offer limited assistance in differentiating between pain and emotional distress, because changes such as dilatation of pupils or increased heart rate, respiratory rate, body temperature, and blood pressure occur in response to pain, fear, and a range of physical illnesses.[8]

Despite these challenges to recognizing pain in cats, it is a veterinary responsibility to minimize it both in terms of the experience and the effects. Fortunately, many measures can be taken to achieve these goals while handling feline patients. Comprehensive information about pain in cats is found in Chapters 14, 15, and 16. The principles described in Chapter 20 to prevent fear when handling feline patients are equally relevant when interacting with the cat that is in pain. The purpose of this chapter is to provide guidance on how to recognize and anticipate pain and to describe techniques that can prevent exacerbation while handling the cat during the veterinary appointment.

RECOGNIZING PAINFUL PROCEDURES AND CONDITIONS

An important way to institute effective pain management and prevention within the practice is to recognize the potential for pain when carrying out routine veterinary procedures (Box 21-1). Using preemptive analgesia based on the actual or potential pain level associated with a procedure is an important welfare consideration. For example, topical analgesia is appropriate for intravenous catheter placement but systemic analgesia is needed for thoracocentesis. For procedures that might induce severe pain, combining sedation or anesthesia with analgesia is appropriate; surgical and dental procedures require a combination of analgesia and anesthesia.

It is also important to consider the potential for detecting painful conditions during both preventive care visits and consultations for cats that are showing clinical signs of disease. The most common causes of chronic pain in cats are DJD, feline idiopathic cystitis, trauma, and neoplasia.[9] Diseases of the oral cavity are also common, and advanced periodontal disease, resorptive lesions, fractured teeth with pulp exposure, stomatitis, and other dental conditions can cause unrecognized

pain, especially because appetite is often not affected. A list of clinical conditions that can cause pain in cats can be found in Box 21-2 and it should be remembered that senior patients often have concurrent conditions.

A cat presented to the veterinary practice for a non-painful condition may also be suffering from an unrelated painful condition that is not being adequately addressed. Providing analgesia during the consultation will increase patient comfort and facilitate examination and any necessary procedures or testing. Increasing client awareness will also ensure that the cat receives appropriate ongoing analgesia.

RECOGNIZING PAIN THROUGH BEHAVIORAL CHANGES

Physical pain and negative emotional states are associated with altered behavior and can also contribute to the onset of unwanted or unacceptable behaviors such as house soiling or aggression (Boxes 21-3 and 21-4).[9-14] Some pain-related behavioral changes may be noticed only during a veterinary visit. For example, palpation of a painful area can lead to the cat guarding the area by tensing, turning toward the palpated area, or, in an otherwise calm cat, behaving aggressively. However, most pain-related behavioral changes are best identified within the home environment. The client is therefore an important member of the cat's healthcare team. Clients often recognize pain in their own cat more accurately than veterinarians because they know their cat's normal behaviors and thus often recognize behavioral changes more readily. This is especially true in cats with DJD.[9-11,13,15] Unfortunately, clients notice the behavioral changes, but frequently associate them with "old age" rather than with pain or illness.[1,16] This misunderstanding can lead a client to accept the changes as

---

BOX 21-1	Examples of Procedures that Cause Pain in Cats

Medical Procedures
Abdominocentesis
Anal sac expression
Bandaging
Chest tube placement
Drains and drainage procedures
Ear cleaning
Feeding tube placement
Restraint and forceful handling procedures
    Examination
    Laboratory sample collection
    Handling for radiographic and ultrasound procedures

Handling: Even gentle handling on hard surfaces can increase existing pain
Intravenous catheterization
Manual extraction of stool
Thoracocentesis
Urinary catheterization

Surgical Procedures
Castration
Ovariohysterectomy
Growth removal
Onychectomy (declaw)
All other surgical procedures

Adapted from the AAHA/AAFP Pain Management Guidelines and the New Jersey Veterinary Medical Association Guidelines for Preventing, Recognizing, and Treating Pain in the Hospital Setting.

BOX 21-2   Physical Conditions that Cause Pain in Cats

Dermatological
Abscesses
Burns
Cellulitis
Severe chin acne
Clipper burns
Inflamed skin
Lacerations
Otitis (ear inflammation, from ear mites, yeast, or
   bacterial infections)
Pruritus (itchy and/or inflamed skin)
Shearing or degloving injuries
Urine scalding
Wounds

Gastrointestinal
Anal sac impaction
Constipation
Diarrhea with tenesmus or frequency
Foreign body
Hemorrhagic gastroenteritis
Inflammatory bowel disease (usually)
Megacolon
Pancreatitis
Peritonitis
Obstipation
Obstruction
Vomiting

Musculoskeletal
Degenerative joint disease (DJD)
Dislocations
Fractures
Immune-mediated polyarthritis
Intervertebral disc disease
Ligament pull or rupture
Muscle soreness
Spondylosis

Ophthalmological
Corneal ulcers and other corneal diseases
Glaucoma
Uveitis

Cardiopulmonary
Congestive heart failure
Pulmonary edema
Pleural effusion
Cerebrovascular accident
Thromboembolism
Pleuritis

Oral Cavity
Feline oral resorptive lesions ("neck" lesions)
Periodontal disease
Oral ulcers
Oral tumors
Stomatitis
Tooth abscesses
Tooth fractures

Urogenital
Acute renal failure
Enlarged kidneys (capsular swelling), regardless of cause
Ureteroliths
All conditions that cause straining and frequent
urination
   Feline idiopathic cystitis
   Crystalluria
   Uroliths
   Transitional cell carcinoma
   Lower urinary tract infections
Urinary obstruction
Kittening
Urine scalding
Vaginitis

Neoplastic
Most cancers are painful

Neurogenic
Diabetic neuropathy
Intervertebral disc disease
Central nervous system disease
Peripheral nerve disease

Adapted from the AAHA/AAFP Pain Management Guidelines and the New Jersey Veterinary Medical Association Guidelines for Preventing, Recognizing, and Treating Pain in the Hospital Setting.

inevitable, rather than as signs that require veterinary intervention. For this reason, client education is essential to train them to recognize the importance of subtle, and perhaps seemingly insignificant changes and to report to the veterinary practice as soon as possible to maximize the potential benefit of veterinary intervention. Client involvement is also important in understanding the efficacy of pain control[12,16] (see handout titled **Does My Cat**

Hurt?). Interestingly, one study demonstrated that owners of cats with feline DJD placed more importance on non-physical outcomes (60%), such as comfort during resting and grooming rather than physical outcomes such as mobility, as indicators of quality of life for a cat with DJD.[10] Therefore, it is important to ask clients about changes in both non-physical and physical aspects of behavior in their pet.

BOX 21-3 Changes in Normal Behaviors Associated with Pain

- Appetite
  - Decrease or increase interest in food
- Elimination
  - Changes in how stool or urine is passed (e.g., stand vs. squat to urinate)
  - Change in location where elimination occurs (e.g., not using the box in the basement due to difficult access)
- Vocalization
  - Yowling
  - Increase or decrease in volume
  - Not meowing for treats or food as usual
  - Increase or decrease in purring: Purring can occur in cats trying to comfort themselves
- Mobility
  - Changes in ability to get into and out of the litter box

- Grooming
  - Overgrooming in one or more areas
  - Not grooming, with or without matting
- Sleeping more
- Sleeping less
  - Unable to get comfortable
  - Restless
- Activity
  - Decrease or increase
- Play
  - Decrease
- Social interaction
  - Changes in interactions with people or other pets
  - Decrease in interaction - associated with withdrawal and hiding
  - Increase in interaction – appearing to be clingy
  - Hostile interactions and irritability

BOX 21-4 Unwanted or Unacceptable Behaviors Associated with Pain

- House soiling
  - Urine and/or feces outside the litter box
- Aggression
  - Non-specific irritability
  - Specific behavior directed toward humans
  - Specific behavior directed toward another pet or pets

The Significance of DJD for Patient Handling

DJD is a common cause of chronic pain in cats, but is frequently unrecognized and underdiagnosed.[11,12,17]. The common signs seen in dogs, such as limping, usually do not occur in feline patients because DJD in cats is usually bilateral. Far more noticeable symptoms are stiffness upon awakening and hesitation to jump up or down, as if trying to determine whether the goal is worth the effort (and potential pain). Other less specific changes include a cat's frequent readjustments when lying down (indicating difficulty in finding a comfortable position), no longer spending time with the owner, and matted fur (indicating difficulty with self-grooming). Because behavioral changes are commonly associated with physically painful conditions (see Boxes 21-3 and 21-4), asking the client questions about the cat's behavior can help with detecting DJD (Box 21-5).

As the frequency of feline DJD has only recently been recognized, the condition is often unrecognized and untreated. To safeguard the welfare of the cat, it is essential to understand the prevalence of this condition and to know the most common disease locations in order to prevent pain during handling.

Feline DJD occurs in both the spine and the appendages. Spinal or axial DJD is more frequently found between thoracic vertebrae T7 and T10, but the lumbar vertebrae are more severely affected.[21] Lumbar spondylosis was previously considered an incidental finding, but it can be very painful and could therefore be of clinical as well as welfare significance. There is potential for pain exacerbation and further injury if cats with spinal pain, regardless of etiology, are held or picked up by the scruff, or if other painful manipulations occur through inappropriate handling.

The more commonly affected appendicular joints are the elbows, hips, knees, and hocks. In contrast to axial DJD, appendicular DJD occurs equally throughout the different age ranges, with the youngest age group starting at 6 months of age.[17] However, the disease is progressive and both prevalence and pain burden dramatically increase at 10 years of age.[10] Although the condition may be more advanced in senior cats, many cats of all ages are uncomfortable when their legs are handled during examination or diagnostic testing, because of DJD. Therefore, it is important that the cat be allowed to remain in positions that it chooses for comfort, rather than the forced positions associated with some forms of handling. The cat's legs should not be held tightly and pulled to extend them, but rather should be held in a less extreme, more comfortable position (Figure 21-1, A–D). Analgesia or anesthesia may be required before evaluation to prevent induction or exacerbation of pain.

Radiographic evidence of DJD does not equate with pain. Cats with no supporting radiographic evidence of DJD may still exhibit decreased mobility and pain associated with the disorder. The pain of a previous

BOX 21-5   Behavioral Signs of DJD in Cats

- Interactions with others
  - Withdrawn or avoiding others
  - Hiding
  - More clingy or attention-seeking
  - Irritable when touched or handled
  - Hostile to other cats leading to intercat aggression
  - Hostile to people leading to cat-to-human aggression
- Sleep and rest
  - Increase or decrease
  - May feign sleep
  - Restless, trying to find a comfortable position
  - Lying in an unusual position (not curled up)
- Appetite
  - Increase or decrease
- Posture
  - Hunched
  - Head lowered
  - Stiff
  - Sitting or lying abnormally; not curled up normally when sleeping
  - Squinted eyes if acute pain
- Grooming
  - Decrease leading to matting
  - Increase leading to overgrooming of painful area and potential alopecia
- Litter box use
  - Change in position while eliminating (e.g., unable to squat as well as normal)
- Urine and/or fecal house soiling associated with inability to get into box
- Decrease in bowel movements and subsequent constipation
- Play
  - Overall reduction in play
  - Selective decrease in certain movements in play such as jumping
- Vocalization
  - Increase
  - Decrease in normal greeting and other pleasant vocalizations
  - Hissing if touched over painful area
  - Purring associated with pain
- Mobility
  - Slowing down ("getting old")
  - Not jumping as often or as high
  - Hesitant to jump up or down
  - Difficulty going up and/or down stairs
  - Stiff
  - Less active
  - Difficulty getting into or out of litter box
  - Sleeping in more easily accessible locations
  - Lameness (uncommon)
- Behavior problems secondary to DJD
  - Urine soiling
  - Fecal soiling
  - Cat-to-human aggression
  - Intercat aggression

musculoskeletal injury unknown to the client or excess body weight can also aggravate DJD pain.[18,19] Indeed DJD pain is an important issue in overweight cats, especially in the United States, where 58% of cats are overweight or obese.[20]

Concurrent medical conditions can be an issue with cats affected with DJD; one study found that 44% of cats with DJD showed signs of concurrent conditions, especially chronic kidney disease.[22] Therefore, discomfort from DJD must be taken into consideration when cats present with chronic kidney disease. More information on DJD is provided in Chapter 15.

THE HEALTHCARE TEAM'S APPROACH TO PAIN PREVENTION

The recognition, prevention, and treatment of pain—and consideration of the individuality of the condition—should be priorities in the veterinary practice as untreated pain is a serious welfare issue. Management and prevention of pain when handling cats demands a comprehensive approach from each member of the healthcare team. Veterinarians, technicians/nurses, veterinary assistants, and kennel assistants are all involved in handling feline patients and need to be educated to recognize the changes in behavior associated with pain and to use appropriate handling techniques to prevent exacerbation.[4] The veterinary team serves as the client's source of reliable information for pain prevention; early detection[7] and client education through appropriate literature and client educational meetings can be a valuable part of the practice protocol for pain management. Client service representatives or receptionists can be trained to help clients recognize when their cat might be in pain and when veterinary care is indicated between routine visits (see Mini Case Example). This approach can be extremely beneficial for promoting early intervention.

Mini Case Example

Mrs. Jones and Buddy are closely bonded, and have been coming regularly to the veterinary practice for 12 years. Buddy has always been a healthy cat, but recently he

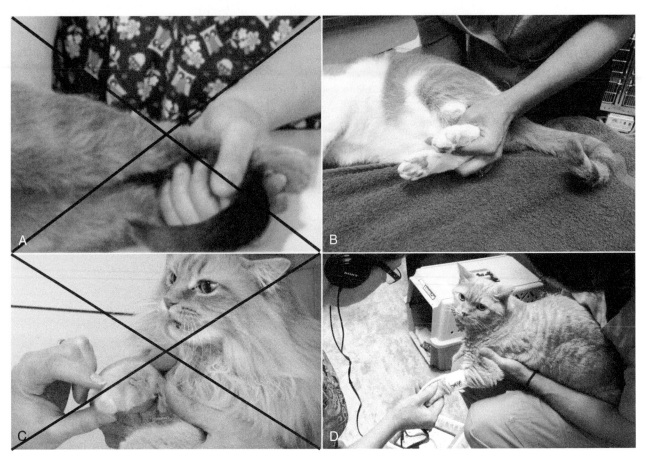

FIGURE 21-1   **A,** The cat's legs should not be held tightly or greatly extended, and the tail should never be held along with the hind limbs. Such holds can exacerbate both axial and appendicular degenerative joint disease (DJD). **B,** Restraining the cat's legs by placing one or two fingers between the hind limbs at the hock level without pulling on the legs to extend them is a more comfortable hold for the cat. Note that the tail is left in the position preferred by the patient. **C,** Standing in front of a cat and touching its toes to pull the leg forward can lead to pain, fear, and aggression and should be avoided. **D,** Gently placing a hand caudal to the forelimb at the level of the humerus and slowly moving the leg forward is a comfortable and non-threatening handling method to obtain blood pressure measurements.

stopped sleeping on the bed with Mrs. Jones, as he has done since he was a kitten, and started to miss the litter box occasionally. She was distressed and wanted to find out what was wrong.

A member of the Client Services team advised Mrs. Jones that Buddy's behavioral changes could possibly be a sign of a painful health issue, and she scheduled an appointment with the veterinarian. On examination, degenerative joint disease was found in Buddy's lumbar vertebrae and in his knees. Other problems were ruled out; medication was started for DJD; a follow-up plan was established; more litter boxes were placed in different locations; and Mrs. Jones purchased a set of steps so Buddy could climb up to the bed. When he was rechecked in 2 weeks, his behavior was back to normal and Mrs. Jones was very happy and grateful.

Handling techniques such as scruffing, firmly holding the cat down, or tightly grasping its legs while fully extending them can all exacerbate physical pain and potentially induce negative emotional states such as fear and anxiety. Educating all staff members about appropriate handling techniques is critical. Use of Feliway helps to increase positive emotion through signaling familiarity and security. Cats need to feel safe in the practice environment and be given the ability to choose their position and location for examination to prevent or reduce fear and subsequent increased arousal.

PREPARING THE PRACTICE FOR THE CAT IN PAIN

Comfortable Surfaces

Most veterinary practices have either stainless steel or laminate examination tables. Placing soft bedding or

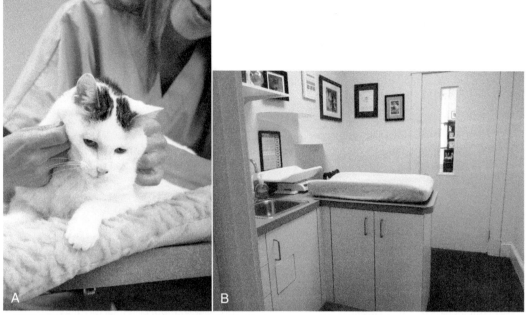

FIGURE 21-2   **A,** A very soft, padded "fluffy" helps to prevent pain for this cat with severe degenerative joint disease. **B,** Baby-changing padding provides a soft surface for the cat and has sides around it to make the cat feel more secure. (**B,** Courtesy J Bunt)

towels—preferably using familiar or favored items from home—on the table or providing soft, thick padded surfaces (Figure 21-2), protects the cat from the discomfort of such cold, hard surfaces. The padding is especially important with older, arthritic, or underweight cats. The cushioning must be non-slip. Placing a non-slip pad, drawer liners, or similar materials cut to size underneath bedding or towels will prevent slipping (Figure 21-3, A and B). Laundering padded surfaces, toweling, or bedding between patients eliminates the scent of other animals and reduces the possibility of cross infection.

During the consultation, most cats prefer to stay in their carrier or on a favored cat bed or bedding from home that contains their scent and is familiar (Figure 21-4, A and B). The cat may remain in the bottom half of the carrier for most or all of the examination, preventing uncomfortable handling and positioning. Even laboratory samples can be collected while the cat is still in the carrier or cat bed. A very helpful method is to place the cat on the lap of the handler, with a towel or the bottom half of the carrier beneath the cat (Figure 21-5). By using their body to keep the cat in position, the handler can readily detect if the cat's body tenses, whether from fear or pain. If the cat tenses or turns toward the examiner only during palpation of certain areas, such as the knees or abdomen, it is likely that pain is being felt in these locations.

The Cat and the Carrier

Client education about carrier training is important to prevent pain. For more information, see Chapters

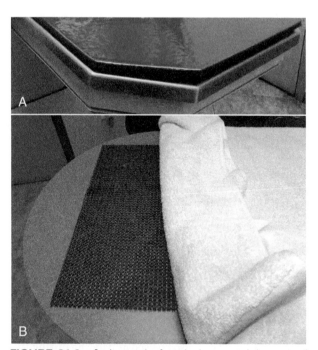

FIGURE 21-3   **A,** Instead of replacing a stainless steel table, fit an easy-to-clean pad to the table. This surface is warmer and more comfortable than a hard, cold stainless steel table for patients, and prevents slippage. **B,** This drawer liner material prevents the towel from slipping, which increases comfort and reduces patient fear.

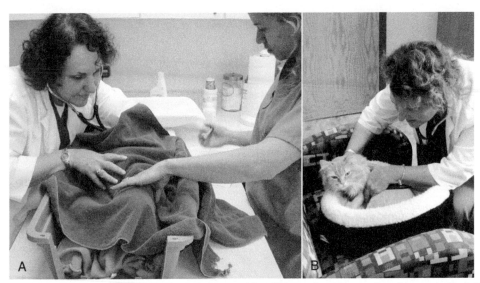

FIGURE 21-4 **A,** This cat is aggressive due to either pain or fear. Removing the top half of the carrier and replacing it with a towel lets the cat remain hidden, reducing potential for further aggression. The cat's head is turned away so that the cat does not see what is happening during the exam. Note the technician's hand position keeps the cat's head in place without potential for injury. **B,** This cat was brought to the practice in its own cat bed placed inside the carrier. Using this cat bed keeps the cat more comfortable and facilitates examination.

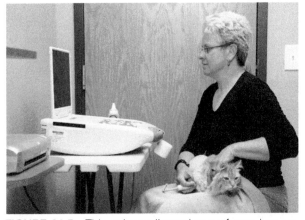

FIGURE 21-5 This echocardiographer performs her procedures with the cat on her lap. Even the most fearful cat will remain on the examiner's lap if looking away from the unfamiliar person.

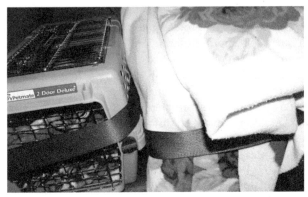

FIGURE 21-6 Putting a seat belt around the carrier prevents jostling and increases safety. Fearful cats should have a towel or blanket placed over the carrier to prevent visual motion.

9 and 20. Inform the owner that holding the carrier where the top and bottom meet, rather than by the handle, will produce a much smoother "ride" that enables the cat to remain in a position of choice and thus reduces fear and pain. Placing familiar bedding in the carrier will increase the cat's comfort and sense of security (the bedding can also be used as padding during the examination). Finally, securing the carrier in the vehicle with a seat belt increases safety and prevents the carrier from being jostled during travel (Figure 21-6).

The cat should never be dumped from or shoved into the carrier (Figure 21-7, A–C), because this can cause pain and fear. Instead, the cat should be given the choice

to remain in the carrier or to come out on its own while the history is being taken. This approach gives the cat time to acclimate to the examination room. Some cats will exit the carrier on their own, especially when enticed with treats (Figure 21-8). If the cat is still inside the carrier after the history has been obtained, removal of the top half of the carrier permits the cat to remain in the bottom half during as much of the visit as possible.

Examining the cat within a soft-sided carrier can be more difficult, but some models have both top and side openings that permit examination and procedures within the carrier (Figure 21-9). Clients with cats that prefer soft-sided carriers should be encouraged to use these models.

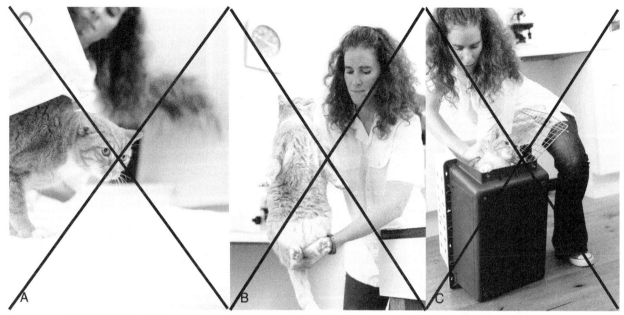

FIGURE 21-7   A, Dumping a cat out of a carrier can be frightening, and painful if the cat has degenerative joint disease or other discomfort with its limbs. Note the fear the cat expresses with its ears. **B** and **C,** Scruffing the cat, stretching the body, or holding on to the hind legs to shove a cat back into the carrier can cause back and/or limb pain and must be avoided. (Copyright © iStock.com)

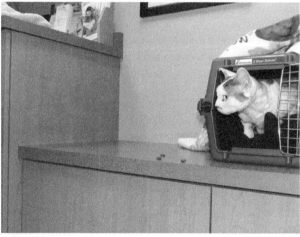

FIGURE 21-8   This cat is being enticed out of the carrier with treats during history-taking.

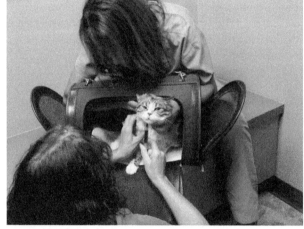

FIGURE 21-9   This soft-sided carrier with three openings, including the top that can be lifted up, is easy to use during an examination and when performing procedures.

RECOGNIZING AND PREVENTING PAIN DURING THE VETERINARY APPOINTMENT

The History

Asking open-ended questions and listening without interruption results in more comprehensive history-taking and provides information about client concerns that may be missed if only specific questions are asked.[23] This approach also improves communication and bonding with the client. For pain assessment, open-ended questions are critical for identifying relevant behavioral changes. Starting the history with the question, "What changes in behavior or attitude have you noticed?" both indicates the importance of changes in the cat's behavior and encourages the client to describe their most pressing concerns, which often include behavior. After the initial answer, a follow-up question such as "What else have you noticed?" will often elicit additional telling details.

More specific follow-up questions are appropriate when they are guided by the responses to the open-ended questions. For example, if a client notes that the cat is "slowing down" or "getting old," it is important to ask them why they think so. A cat that once raced up or down stairs may now climb the steps stiffly and slowly. A cat that loved to jump onto the bed or a window perch may now look at the desired place from the floor, but hesitate to jump. The client may describe that the cat starts to jump, hesitates, and then retries. Other signs include stiffness upon wakening, legs that tremble or shake, being "down" in hocks or carpi, or decreased overall mobility. Any changes - a loss of normal behaviors, development of new behaviors, or behavior problems – are significant and should be documented.

The Initial Observations

Taking the history gives the cat the 5 to 10 minutes it needs to acclimate to a new room.[24,25] Examination from a distance can occur at the same time with the veterinarian assessing the cat's quality of respiration, body posture, and (if possible) gait. A hunched posture, squinting eyes, and increased respiration are often associated with acute pain. If possible, the cat can be enticed to walk, but it is important not to force it to do so. Evidence of stiffness while walking or other gait abnormalities, muscle atrophy over limbs (from the reduced use of the affected legs), or difficulty with jumping or sitting is often associated with pain due to DJD or other musculoskeletal problems.

If the cat initially chooses to stay in the carrier, it is best to assess the gait at the end of the appointment, following both examination and diagnostic testing. Placing the cat on the floor as far from the carrier as possible usually provides a good opportunity to assess gait, because most cats will immediately head toward their familiar carrier. If the exam room is small or if the cat slinks rather than walks it is not appropriate to take cats into another room or a hallway in the practice to assess gait. While this may be a common approach with canine patients it is likely to induce fear and cause the cat to either totally inhibit or try to escape. If a cat that is attempting to flee is then chased it is probable that the defense response will change to repulsion and aggressive behavior will be displayed. Instead ask the client to take some videos of the cat's movements at home. Most smart phones can take videos, so costly equipment is not needed. Many veterinary software programs can incorporate patient-provided pictures and videos in the veterinary practice's medical records that make it easier to monitor changes at subsequent appointments. Reviewing the records from previous examinations can help to identify new problems, such as the previously well-fleshed cat that has become muscle-wasted.

Hands-On Examination

If at all possible, the cat should be allowed to remain on a stable and comfortable surface that has been chosen, rather than be moved from location to location. This approach provides the cat with a sense of control and both increases the cat's security and comfort and prevents fear and pain. Familiar bedding further increases the cat's sense of security and may prevent tensing due to fear. Most cats prefer a concealed place, such as the bottom half of a carrier, a cat bed with high sides, a small scale, or a lap (Figure 21-10). More confident cats may prefer a shelf, bench, or the floor. Unfortunately, some veterinary professionals still prefer to assess the entire patient by holding the cat in the air (Figure 21-11) or allowing only the back feet to contact the exam table (Figure 21-12). These positions are frightening and often uncomfortable for the cat and should be avoided.

The order of the examination should be tailored to the individual cat, postponing potentially painful or stressful segments until the end. Obtaining heart and respiratory rates and blood pressure readings before the cat experiences pain improves the accuracy of these results. If pain is noted at any time before or during the physical examination, immediately stop the examination and administer analgesia. Transmucosal or intramuscular buprenorphine is an excellent analgesic in this situation. The examination can continue with the non-painful areas and diagnostic samples can be collected before further assessment of painful areas.

Gait, posture, a visible wound, and the patient's history can all help to identify painful areas. For example, if the history includes vomiting or diarrhea, reserve abdominal palpation until the end of the examination; if the client thinks the cat is "slowing down," reserve examining the limbs until the end of the examination. If the history does not indicate any discomfort it may be preferable to perform the oral examination last because the signs of oral pain are less obvious but its presence is common.

Examination of the Head and Neck

Because dental disease is one of the most common painful conditions of cats, the oral cavity should be routinely evaluated in a manner that is most comfortable for the cat. Evaluation either from behind or from the side prevents fear and possible fear-associated aggression (Figure 21-13). Many veterinarians tend to pull on the fur to open the lower jaw (Figure 21-14), but this practice causes discomfort even if the cat has no oral pain, and can make it more difficult to assess the oral cavity.

In several situations, sedation or anesthesia are appropriate before performing a more thorough evaluation of the oral cavity. For example, it is not appropriate to probe the teeth and gums while the cat is awake. If the cat has any gingivitis localized to one or more teeth, a resorptive lesion or some other dental health problem is very likely, so anesthesia and dental radiographs are indicated. Further, if there is concern about an oral tumor, a foreign body, or another

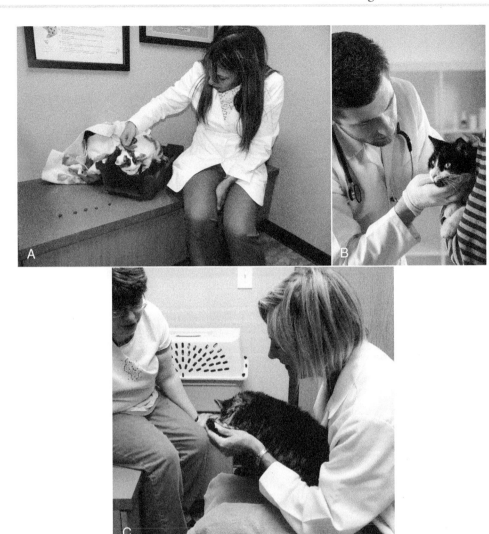

FIGURE 21-10   **A,** Allowing the cat to remain in its familiar carrier and on bedding from home increases security for the cat. The sides of the carrier provide a hiding place so that the cat feels protected. **B,** Providing soft toweling or a tall cat bed turned on its side for the cat to lie in allows the cat to be comfortable while evaluating the face. **C,** Holding the cat in the lap provides easy access for palpation and enables the holder to surround the cat to prevent escape and to detect any tensing, which is often associated with pain. (**A, C,** Courtesy D. Echelberry and M. Miller; **B,** Copyright © iStock.com)

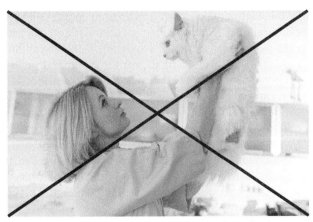

FIGURE 21-11   Holding up the cat in the air to obtain a general assessment can frighten the patient. Note that the cat's ears are back. This position can also be uncomfortable for the cat's back and forelimbs. (Copyright © iStock.com)

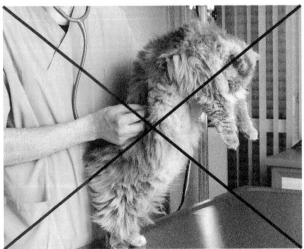

FIGURE 21-12   Raising the front half of the body does not give the cat any control and can be frightening and painful. Back and hind limb pain may occur with this type of hold, and the back legs can easily slip on the stainless steel table. (Copyright © iStock.com)

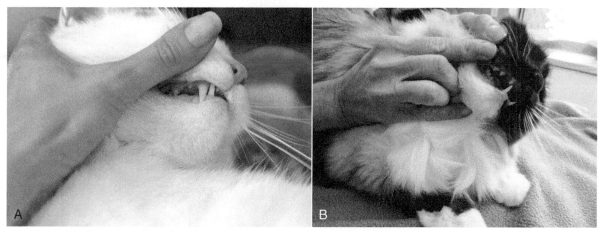

FIGURE 21-13   These handlers both approach the cat from the side to evaluate the oral cavity, thereby preventing fear caused by approaching the cat from the front. Instead of pulling on the cat's fur, they gently manipulate its lips to perform a thorough dental examination. (**A,** Copyright © iStock.com)

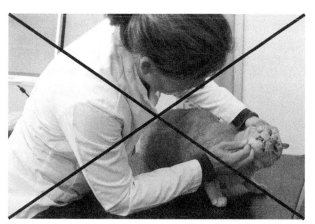

FIGURE 21-14   Pulling the fur to open the cat's mouth is painful. This method should be avoided. (Copyright © iStock.com)

painful condition, evaluation of the oral cavity with the cat under sedation or anesthesia will prevent pain and provide a better assessment. All examinations should include evaluation of the tongue, the palate, and the rest of the oral cavity to enable early detection of abnor-malities.

With the exception of the retinal exam, which should be left until the end of the consultation, examination of the head, neck, and ears should be carried out from the side or from behind (Figure 21-15, *A–C*). Some veterinarians can even perform the retinal exam from behind (Figure 21-15, *D*). If conjunctivitis, corneal ulcers, or any other eye irritation or trauma is present, a topical analgesic should be delivered into the eyes, preferably from behind (Figure 21-15, *E*).

Palpation of Limbs and Back

Palpation of the back and limbs should be performed to identify painful axial and appendicular DJD, respectively. Starting with mild pressure and a small range of

motion, and increasing only if there is no immediate sign of pain, can prevent aggravation (Figure 21-16). Axial pain is more severe over the lumbar or lumbosacral regions.[4] Muscle wasting may be noticed along the spine, but this can be seen with medical conditions not associated with pain and therefore should be evaluated in the light of all other clinical information. Thickening of the elbow or knee joints is not uncommon in cats with DJD, and crepitus, effusion within the joint capsule, and decreased range of motion can also be found so palpation must be performed carefully.[21,26]

A cat in pain may be tense and resist examination to protect itself. Recognizing that pain can be a factor in aggressive behavior and treating that pain appropriately helps to keep the patient comfortable and facilitates the exam and other necessary procedures. It also helps to make the veterinary visit much calmer and more pleasant for all involved.

LABORATORY SAMPLE COLLECTION

Collecting laboratory samples and performing blood pressure evaluation, venipuncture, and cystocentesis in the examination room, rather than transferring the cat to another location, often reduces fear and can prevent pain from fear-based struggling. Gently wrapping the cat in a towel or small blanket in order to allow the perception of hiding is also beneficial. Sample collection can often be performed with the cat remaining in the bottom half of the carrier. The cat should be allowed to remain in a natural position, without grasping its legs tightly or pulling to extend the legs or stretch the body. Usually, only one technician or assistant is needed to hold the cat, but occasionally two holders will prevent struggling and discomfort. Speaking softly to the cat or distracting it with food, treats, or toys can be helpful. Most cats that need more than two people to hold them

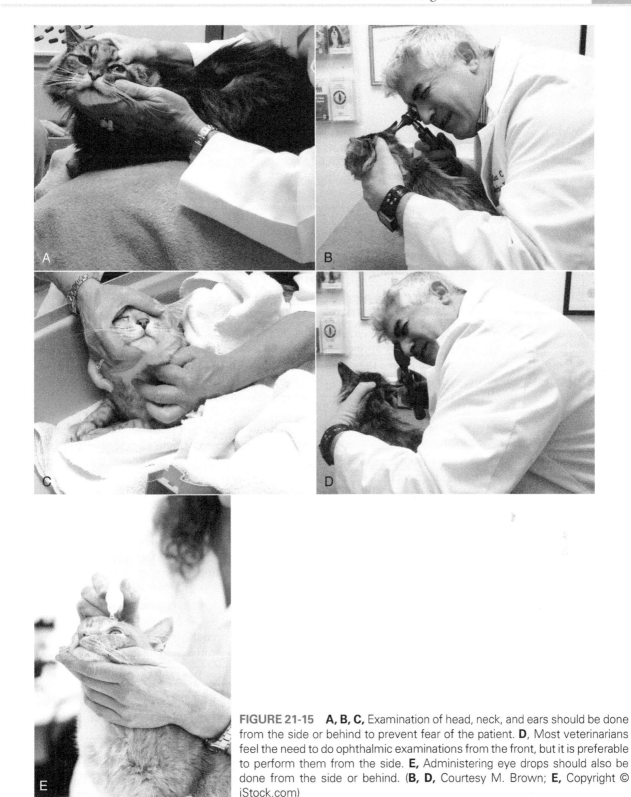

FIGURE 21-15   **A, B, C,** Examination of head, neck, and ears should be done from the side or behind to prevent fear of the patient. **D,** Most veterinarians feel the need to do ophthalmic examinations from the front, but it is preferable to perform them from the side. **E,** Administering eye drops should also be done from the side or behind. (**B, D,** Courtesy M. Brown; **E,** Copyright © iStock.com)

are in pain or fearful and benefit from analgesia, sedation, and/or anesthesia.

Keeping the cat in the consulting room offers another advantage of relieving the client's concerns about potential pain and distress for their pet from sample collections and work "done in the back" and out of sight. The evaluations and sample collections are also excellent opportunities for client education, and increase the clients' perception of value and bonding to the practice. If the client would prefer not to watch,

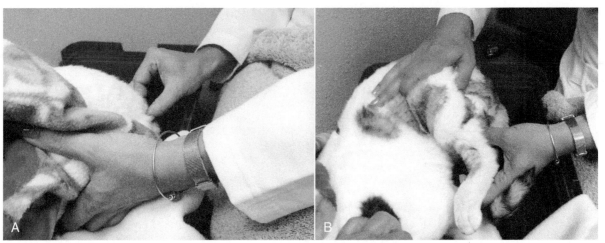

FIGURE 21-16 Palpation of the back and limbs should be done with mild pressure which can increase in firmness if there is no patient reaction. Testing range-of-motion of appendicular joints and assessing for thickness will also help to detect pain.

they can wait in the reception area, but the cat remains in a room to which it has acclimated. After all procedures are completed, the cat should be allowed to return to its carrier if it chooses while the client is informed about necessary treatments and future veterinary visits.

Blood Pressure Measurement

Measuring the blood pressure from a front leg is usually easiest for all involved. The cat should remain in a comfortable position, whether in a lap, sitting, or in the bottom half of the carrier and can be distracted with treats, catnip, or petting (Figure 21-17, A and B). The leg should never be moved by pulling on the foot, because this can lead to fear, pain, and potential aggression. Instead the forelimb is moved by gently pushing the caudal humerus forward. When DJD or other musculoskeletal disease is present it is preferable to perform the blood pressure measurement on an unaffected leg (Figure 21-17, C). If a hind limb is used, the leg is moved backward by gently pressing the femur back. The tail vein is the best possible option for blood pressure measurement in cats with DJD in all four limbs (Figure 21-17, D) although the measurement may not be as accurate. In order to avoid "white coat hypertension," blood pressure measurements should be taken after the history—either prior to or after the examination—and before other diagnostic tests, while the patient is as relaxed and calm as possible. The environment should be quiet and away from other animals, and client presence is important in preventing white-coat hypertension.[27]

Venipuncture

Venipuncture is most commonly performed in the cat from the cephalic, the medial saphenous, or the jugular vein. Each has its own benefits, and cats often prefer one position over the others. This preference can be influenced by the presence of pain and the cat's medical record should note the preferred position for future visits.

Obtaining blood from the cephalic vein often allows the cat to sit in the most comfortable position. Using a butterfly catheter allows the syringe and hands to be positioned further from the cat and prevents pressure issues so that the leg does not need to be pumped to get sufficient blood (Figure 21-18, A). Collecting blood from the medial saphenous prevents the cat from visualizing what is occurring (Figure 21-18, B–D) which can be stressful for some cats. Collection from the jugular vein is an important technique because a large sample can be taken more quickly. This is especially helpful in frail or smaller cats, those that are resistant to being restrained, and those with uncomfortable limbs. The cat should be positioned comfortably on its sternum or laterally. If the cat is on its sternum, the front legs should not be pulled down over a table edge, but rather kept on the same level as the rest of the body (Figure 21-19, A). For cats that need the front legs to be held during jugular collection, a gentle hold using the hands to prevent squeezing the legs together helps to prevent pain (Figure 21-19, B). If the cat is held in a lateral position, the head should be gently tilted up and front legs moved slightly back, preferably using a towel.

Cystocentesis

Cystocentesis is the preferred method of urine collection but it can cause some problems for cats which are experiencing pain. Samples are usually collected with the cat held in lateral recumbency with the hind legs pulled back to better localize the bladder. This positioning often leads to discomfort and struggling in cats with DJD. Other excellent techniques that can prevent discomfort include having the cat in a standing position (Figure 21-20, A), lying on the back without pulling back the hind limbs (Figure 21-20, B), or lying in lateral

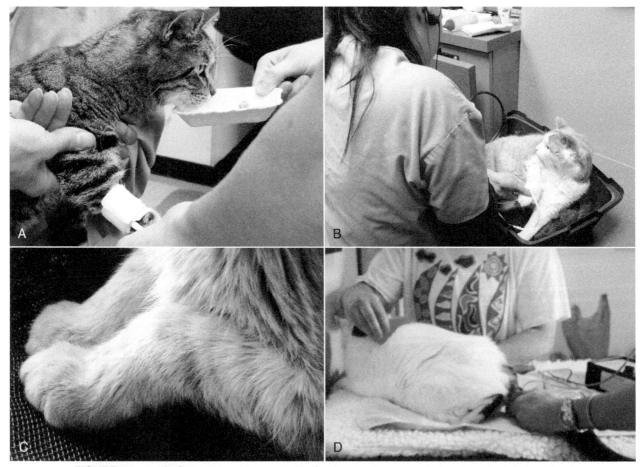

FIGURE 21-17   A, Cats that are interested in food or treats can easily be distracted during blood pressure measurement. **B,** Allowing the patient to remain in the bottom half of the carrier increases security and comfort for the cat, and can offer an easy location to assess blood pressure. **C,** Cats with severe DJD often have visible deformities in the limbs. Another limb should be used instead of this painful leg. **D,** DJD is usually a bilateral disease, and it is not uncommon for cats to have pain associated with DJD in all four limbs. The most accurate—and least painful—blood pressure measurement location in these cats may be on the tail.

recumbency without excessive hind limb extension (Figures 21-20, *C* and *D*).

Cats with feline idiopathic cystitis or other painful bladder conditions require the administration of appropriate analgesia before sample collection. Buprenorphine given either transmucosally or intramuscularly will prevent frequent attempts to void, thus allowing the bladder to fill and a sample to be collected. For cats with feline idiopathic cystitis, it may be preferable to allow the cat to void into a clean litter box or into one that contains non-absorbable sand or other litter to allow urine to pool in the litter box.

Radiographs and Abdominal Ultrasound

Radiography and abdominal ultrasound are performed in cats because of a medical concern and the use of analgesia to keep the cat comfortable is therefore advised. Pulling on a cat's legs to stretch the body to the full extent for radiography can be especially painful for cats with DJD, and anesthesia or heavy sedation with analgesia should be provided. (In some countries and regions in the United States the use of anesthesia or heavy sedation is compulsory for radiography in order to prevent the use of manual restraint). A cat that needs radiographs of the thorax or abdomen may also have DJD pain, and in these patients the analgesic helps with both the presenting and secondary conditions. The U.S. author's practice has a standard operating procedure that cats must receive analgesia before any radiographs are obtained and most cats also need analgesia for abdominal ultrasound.

ANALGESIC TRIAL AS A DIAGNOSTIC TOOL

Any procedure that causes pain to a person has the potential to cause pain to a cat. However, while people can be informed that a procedure (e.g., a needle stick for a blood draw) will cause only brief pain, that information cannot be communicated to a feline patient. If the

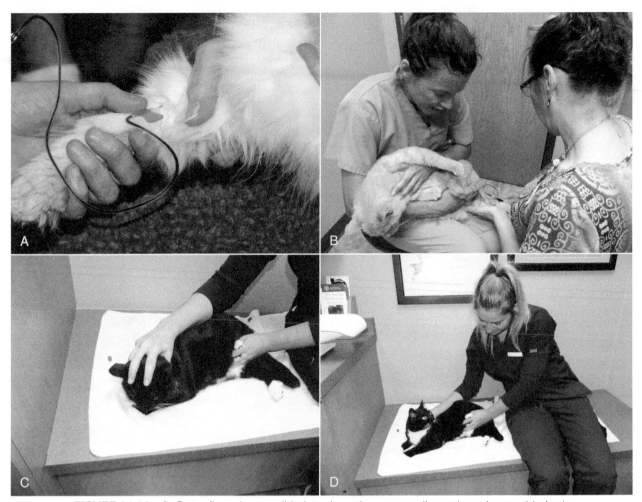

FIGURE 21-18   A, Butterfly catheters slide into the vein more easily, and can be used in both cephalic and medial saphenous veins. As with any sample collection, allowing the cat to remain in a comfortable position can maintain safety for holders and collectors. **B–D,** Three different handling options for medial saphenous collection.

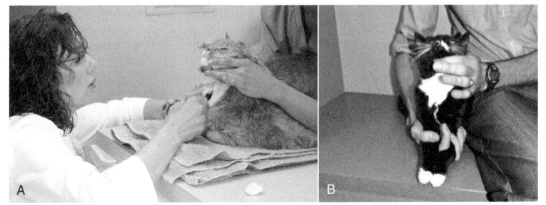

FIGURE 21-19   A, In this position for collecting a blood sample from the jugular vein, note how the front legs remain on the table and in the position that the cat prefers. This position does not interfere with the collection. **B,** If the front feet must be held, use one hand, placing fingers between the feet to prevent them from being squeezed together. Wrapping the hand loosely around the legs will prevent the patient from struggling.

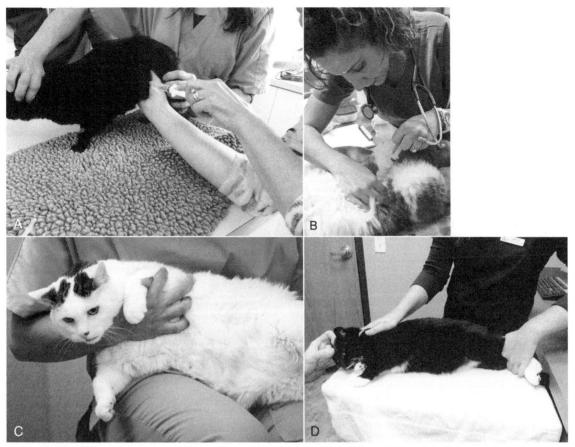

FIGURE 21-20   A, This arthritic cat is standing in a normal position with head angled away from the collector. The urine is collected without pulling on any limbs. **B,** The cat can be placed on its back, leaving the hind limbs in a frog-leg position so that they do not need to be extended for cystocentesis. **C,** Cystocentesis can be performed without pulling the hind limbs back, but rather by allowing them to be in a loosely held and relaxed position to facilitate cystocentesis. **D,** Note how the legs are gently pulled back and the second and third digits of the handler's hand gently keep the head in place for an excellent cystocentesis hold. Having someone distract the cat by gently massaging the head also helps comfort the cat. (**B,** Copyright © iStock.com)

patient has pertinent history which increases the likelihood that pain will be significant for that individual, analgesia should be given prior to the examination. If there is no history, the exam should proceed cautiously and analgesia should be administered as soon as suspicion of pain arises (based on body posture, reaction to palpation, change in normal disposition, or aggression) or before any pain-inducing procedures are performed.

If pain is suspected, based on the patient's history or on observation from a distance, it is preferable to auscultate the heart and lungs before analgesia is administered. Examination of the painful areas or performance of the pain-inducing procedure should be delayed until the analgesia has had time to reach maximum effect. For a procedure causing short-term pain, such as a rectal examination with anal gland expression, transmucosal buprenorphine or sedation can greatly relieve the discomfort, especially for a cat with a concurrent health issue, such as DJD. Buprenorphine becomes active

within 30 minutes, with peak effect at 90 minutes, whether delivered transmucosally or intravenously.[28,29] In a busy veterinary practice with other patients waiting, it may be appropriate to let the client know that other patients will be seen while the pain relief takes effect, and offer the client the option to wait or to leave the cat at the veterinary practice, so the client can return to work or run errands.

The use of analgesia is often necessary and appropriate before diagnosis of a condition is conclusive. For example, diagnosing both acute and chronic pancreatitis takes time, but early analgesia is important if pancreatitis is suspected.

Use of analgesia in these prophylactic ways needs to be discussed with the client prior to administration, but the majority of clients will be reassured to know that the veterinarian cares about their pet's comfort and it would be unusual for a recommendation to use analgesia in this way to be rejected.

A lack of outward evidence of pain does not mean that the cat is not experiencing pain and its negative consequences,[30,31] especially because pain is individualized.[32] If the patient's usual disposition is not known, comparing pre- and post-analgesic administration observations can often confirm whether the cat was in pain. This knowledge can be an important diagnostic tool, especially with an aggressive cat, and can help to distinguish pain from fear.[30,31] A positive response to analgesia is relatively easy to interpret, but when there is no response to analgesia it is possible that the dose or the type of medication is not sufficient or appropriate to control the pain. Multimodal analgesia or the use of another type of analgesia (e.g., for neuropathic pain) may be necessary. For further information, see Chapters 14, 15, and 16.

PREVENTING PAIN AT FUTURE VETERINARY VISITS

Because fear and stress can exacerbate pain, it is often beneficial to prescribe medication that the client can administer at home before veterinary visits. The aim of this medication is to prevent or reduce fear, anxiety, and pain during the visit. The U.S. author has found that gabapentin works well in cats both as an anxiolytic and an analgesic. The author uses 10 mg/kg up to 100 mg of gabapentin/cat administered to the cat approximately 1.5 to 3 hours before departing for the veterinary visit, by mixing the powder from the capsule into canned food or baby food.

Clients with cats with chronic and intermittent breakthrough pain can be provided with buprenorphine for when other analgesic treatment is not sufficient. Recommending that the buprenorphine be given transmucosally to these cats prior to veterinary visits will prevent pain during the visits. Even if a patient has pain which is well-controlled at home, manipulations and procedures that are necessary during veterinary examination may indicate administration of buprenorphine prior to the veterinary visit. The U.S. author recommends giving the cat transmucosal buprenorphine approximately 90 minutes before departure (time to peak effect) to reduce the discomfort of the travel and the veterinary visit.

Carrier training should be encouraged and educational materials provided to support the client in training their cat to the carrier. See Chapter 9 for training information. At the veterinary practice, prominent computerized "pop-ups" or notes in the medical record can be used to ensure that every member of the veterinary team is aware of the most comfortable positions for the individual cat for examination and the best location(s) to measure blood pressure and collect lab samples (e.g., the preferred vein for blood draws and the preferred position for cystocentesis).

CONCLUSION

The ability to recognize signs of feline pain coupled with an awareness of potentially painful procedures and conditions increases awareness of the need to use handling techniques that prevent pain and to use analgesia when it is indicated. Both of these approaches will improve patient comfort and job satisfaction and safety for all veterinary team members. Having a more comfortable cat also enhances the safety and value of the visit for cat owners, and increases the likelihood that they will return for future visits.

REFERENCES

1. Gunn-Moore D. Considering older cats. *J Small Anim Pract.* 2006;47:430–431.
2. International Association for the Study of Pain. *IASP Taxonomy: Pain.* http://www.iasp-pain.org/Taxonomy?navItemNumber=576#Pain, Accessed February 15, 2015.
3. McMillan FD. Quality of life in animals. Forum. *J Am Vet Med Assoc.* 2000;216:1904–1910.
4. Reid J, Scott M, Nolan A, Wiseman-Orr L. Pain assessment in animals. *In Pract.* 2013;35:51–56.
5. Imbe H, Iwai-Liao Y, Senba E. Stress-induced hyperalgesia: animal models and putative mechanisms. *Front Biosci.* 2006;11:2179–2192.
6. Khasar SG, Burkham J, Dina OA, et al. Stress induces a switch of intracellular signaling in sensory neurons in a model of generalized pain. *J Neurosci.* 2008;28: 5721–5730.
7. Stella J, Croney C, Buffington CAT. Effects of stressors on the behavior and physiology of domestic cats. *Appl Anim Behav Sci.* 2013;143:157–163.
8. Quimby JM, Smith ML, Lunn KF. Evaluation of the effects of hospital visit stress on physiologic parameters in the cat. *J Feline Med Surg.* 2011;13:733–737.
9. Robertson SA, Lascelles BDX. Long-term pain in cats: how much do we know about this important welfare issue? *J Feline Med Surg.* 2010;12:188–199.
10. Benito J, Gruen ME, Thomson A, et al. Owner-assessed indices of quality of life in cats and the relationship to the presence of degenerative joint disease. *J Feline Med Surg.* 2012;14:863–870.
11. Bennett D, Zainal Ariffin SM, Johnston P. Osteoarthritis in the cat: 1. How common is it and how easy to recognise? *J Feline Med Surg.* 2012;14:65–75.
12. Sparkes AH, Heiene R, Lascelles BD. ISFM and AAFP consensus guidelines: long-term use of NSAIDs in cats. *J Feline Med Surg.* 2010;12:521–538.
13. Lascelles BDX, Hansen BD, Thomson A, et al. Evaluation of a digitally integrated accelerometer-based activity monitor for the measurement of activity in cats. *Vet Anaesth Analg.* 2008;35:173–183.
14. Taylor PM, Robertson SA. Pain management in cats: past, present and future. Part 1. The cat is unique. *J Feline Med Surg.* 2004;6:313–320.

15. Zamprogno H, Hansen BD, Bondell HD, et al. Item generation and design testing of a questionnaire to assess degenerative joint disease-associated pain in cats. *Am J Vet Res*. 2010;71:1417–1424.

16. Bennett D, Morton C. A study of owner observed behavioural and lifestyle changes in cats with musculoskeletal disease before and after analgesic therapy. *J Feline Med Surg*. 2009;11:997–1004.

17. Lascelles BDX, Henry 3rd. JB, Brown J, et al. Cross-sectional study of the prevalence of radiographic degenerative joint disease in domesticated cats. *Vet Surg*. 2010;39:535–544.

18. Epstein M, Rodan I, Griffenhagen G, et al. 2015 AAHA/AAFP pain management guidelines for dogs and cats. *J Fel Med Surg*. 2015;17:251–272. http://jfm.sagepub.com/content/17/3/251.full.pdf+html, Accessed March 16, 2015.

19. Epstein M, Rodan I, Griffenhagen G, et al. 2015 AAHA/AAFP pain management guidelines for dogs and cats. *J Am Anim Hosp Assoc*. 2015;51:67–84. https://www.aaha.org/professional/resources/pain_management.aspx#gsc.tab=0, Accessed March 16, 2015.

20. Association for Pet Obesity Prevention. *Obesity Facts & Risks*; 2013. http://www.petobesityprevention.org/?s=pet+obesity+facts, Accessed February 15, 2015.

21. Lascelles BDX, Robertson SA. DJD-associated pain in cats: what can we do to promote patient comfort? *J Feline Med Surg*. 2010;12:200–212.

22. Marino CL, Lascelles BDX, Vaden SL, et al. Prevalence and classification of chronic kidney disease in cats randomly selected from four age groups and in cats recruited for degenerative joint disease studies. *J Feline Med Surg*. 2014;16:465–472.

23. McArthur ML, Fitzgerald JR. Companion animal veterinarians' use of clinical communication skills. *Aust Vet J*. 2013;91:374–380.

24. Brown S, Atkins C, Bagley R, et al. Guidelines for the identification, evaluation, and management of systemic hypertension in dogs and cats. *J Vet Intern Med*. 2007;21:542–558.

25. Love L, Harvey R. Arterial blood pressure measurement: physiology, tools, and techniques. *Compendium*. 2006;28: 450–461.

26. Lascelles BDX, Dong YH, Marcellin-Little DJ, et al. Relationship of orthopedic examination, goniometric measurements, and radiographic signs of degenerative joint disease in cats. *BMC Vet Res*. 2012;8:10.

27. Gunn-Moore D, Moffat K, Christie LA, Head E. Cognitive dysfunction and the neurobiology of ageing in cats. *J Small Anim Pract*. 2007;48(October):546–553.

28. Robertson SA, Lascelles BDX, Taylor PM, et al. PK-PD modeling of buprenorphine in cats: intravenous and oral transmucosal administration. *J Vet Pharmacol Ther*. 2005;28:453–460.

29. Robertson SA, Taylor PM, Sear JW. Systemic uptake of buprenorphine by cats after oral mucosal administration. *Vet Rec*. 2003;152:675–678.

30. Hellyer P, Rodan I, Brunt J, et al. AAHA/AAFP pain management guidelines for dogs and cats. *J Feline Med Surg*. 2007;9: 466–480. http://www.catvets.com/guidelines/practice-guidelines/pain-management-guidelines, Accessed February 15, 2015.

31. Hellyer P, Rodan I, Brunt J, et al. AAHA/AAFP pain management guidelines for dogs and cats. *J Am Anim Hosp Assoc*. 2007;43:235–248. https://www.aaha.org/professional/resources/pain_management.aspx#gsc.tab=0 Accessed February 15, 2015.

32. Landau R. One size does not fit all: genetic variability of mu-opioid receptor and postoperative morphine consumption. *Anesthesiology*. 2006;105:235–237.

Handling the Challenging Cat

Sophia Yin

INTRODUCTION

For many veterinarians and technicians, handling the challenging or aggressive cat can be baffling. Challenging cats are not only stressed themselves but also cause stress and anxiety in staff and clients. Often these cats and clients arrive later than the scheduled appointment due to problems catching the cat at home and this can disrupt the veterinary practice timetable by delaying subsequent appointments. The emanating yowls or shrieks can frighten other patients and distress other clients. Once in the consulting room the challenging cat is usually very difficult to remove from the carrier and may even try to lunge at staff from its confines. It resists any attempts at handling or restraint. Fortunately, there are many easy and effective techniques that are readily available which can assist veterinary staff in dealing with these patients, ranging from environmental modification and towel-wrap procedures to sedation.

The first essential fact to realize is that while a cat may be hissing and attacking at one moment in time, it may have been much calmer during previous visits or even earlier during the current exam. The style of handling on previous occasions or even earlier in the day could have contributed to the deterioration of the cat's behavior. For example, persisting in interacting with a fearful cat that hides in the back of a cage can often result in the cat becoming aggressive by the end of the stay in the veterinary practice. Veterinarians and other staff are often time pressured and may be rushing to get treatments done, but this rush can end up making the cats less manageable.

One might argue that these cats were just prone to becoming aggressive and there is nothing that can be done. However, historically relaxed and well-behaved cats can become aggressive if they are handled forcefully when they are stressed. For instance, a cat that is automatically scruffed or handled in an insensitive manner is more likely to hiss and swat to protect itself even if it has previously been calm and relaxed in the veterinary practice.

While this chapter focuses on handling challenging cats, it is not about using a magic technique to wrangle the attacking cat. Most of the techniques focus on creating a comfortable, safe environment and then handling in a calm, skilled, and low stress manner so that the historically explosive cat remains calm. The emergency technique for the attacking cat is shown, too; however, the goal is that during a given visit, the cat arrives in a state where it is calm enough that it is not attacking and the environment and handling allows the cat to remain at the same arousal level or lower throughout its veterinary practice experience. Care is taken to avoid increasing the cat's agitation or arousal level and to try to provide a pleasant experience. Ideally, with each visit, the cat improves rather than becoming aggressive and increasingly difficult to handle.

Instead of providing a plan for just handling the already challenging cat, this chapter will briefly cover a few steps the client can take to bring these cats to the veterinary practice in a calmer state. Next, the chapter will follow the cat through the veterinary practice visit, providing tips and instructions on techniques, tools, and medications to keep the cat calm. And lastly, it will provide information about when the cat goes home as well as client follow-up instructions. The techniques and environmental suggestions will help not only with difficult cats, but also with cats that are not yet a problem.

PREPARING THE CHALLENGING CAT FOR A VETERINARY VISIT

Frequently cats arrive at the veterinary practice in an already heightened state of fear and arousal due to the ride in the carrier and car.[1] This predisposes them to displaying aggressive behavior. As a result it is essential that techniques for handling aggressive cats start before they arrive at the veterinary practice. While many of these strategies are covered in more depth in Chapter 9, an overview is provided here[2] and considers some important steps to a successful veterinary visit..

Step 1: Desensitize and Countercondition to the Carrier and Travel

Clients can and should prepare their cats for veterinary practice visits by training them that being in a carrier and going for rides in the car are positive experiences.

This can easily be trained through a combination of **desensitization** and **counterconditioning**. It is important to present the stimulus at low intensity and then systematically increase the stimulus level at a rate such that the cat shows little or no signs of anxiety.[3] In the case of the carrier, the quickest way to combine desensitization and counterconditioning is to feed the cat its regular meals in it. Start with the food just inside the door of the carrier and place a blanket or towel inside so that the floor is comfortable. The goal is that you start at a point where the cat will approach and eat the food with little or no hesitation and the food is as close to or as far inside the carrier as the cat will tolerate. If the cat is unwilling or very slow to put its head into the carrier, the process should start with the food bowl just outside. Once the cat is comfortable eating meals with the bowl at its start location, the next stage is to try to position the bowl further inside. Systematically move the bowl further into the carrier every one to several meals. Tastier treats can be placed inside to see if the cat will go in even further voluntarily. Leaving these treats in the carrier creates the opportunity for the cat to find them at other times of the day if it decides to explore or wander inside voluntarily. Generally, cats are readily going into their carrier by days 3 to 4, and most will do this earlier. Ideally, the cats are starting to sleep or nap in it on their own because they associate it with positive experiences. The next step is to close the door while they are eating and then open the door as soon as they are finished. The client can even progress to the step of picking up the carrier and walking with the cat inside it while the cat is comfortable and eating. Within a week, most cats willingly go into the carrier on their own or when they see their owner approach with their meal. Some even choose to sleep in it at night if it is located in a desirable resting spot (Figure 22-1).

If the cat has a history of being stressed by the car ride, the clients can also desensitize and countercondition the cat to this part of the veterinary visit

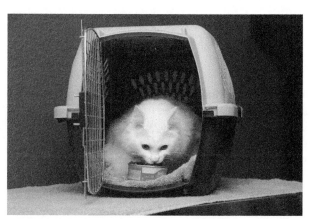

FIGURE 22-1 If a cat will settle in its carrier to eat it is a good sign that a positive association has been made with being inside the carrier. (Courtesy S. Yin)

experience.[3] This is more difficult to accomplish than the carrier training procedures but equally effective and straightforward. Start with a cat that is comfortable eating in the carrier and is also hungry and put the carrier in the car with the meal inside. If the cat is eating readily, then take a short drive around the block. The goal is that the ride takes less time than it takes for the cat to finish the meal and that the cat eats the meal rather than focusing on the motion of the car. End in a location where the cat feels comfortable, such as home, so that the car ride predicts traveling to a safe environment. Once the cat is comfortable for short rides and will readily eat the food without showing signs of stress such as vocalizing, hissing, or freezing in the carrier due to fear, then it is possible to extend the length of the car ride.

Step 2: Utilize Adjunctive Tools for Calming Cats

Once the cat is desensitized and counterconditioned at least to the carrier and hopefully to the car ride, it is ready for a veterinary visit.

Food can be helpful for creating positive associations with the veterinary environment but it can also help to ensure that the cat is motivated to eat its meal or treats during the potentially stressful veterinary visit by asking the client to withhold food prior to the visit. They can also bring treats that the cat is familiar with and has previously enjoyed.

Feliway pheromone spray can be applied to the towel that the cat will sit on during its car journey. Due to the alcohol carrier in the product, it is important for it to be sprayed at least 10 to 15 minutes before the cat will be on the towel. Alternatively, Feliway wipes can be used directly on the bedding within the carrier (see Chapter 18). Some cats act markedly calmer when exposed to this pheromone, and the results can occur within minutes. Catnip has also been shown to be calming in some cats but it can cause some cats to become more excited and this will not be beneficial in the context of a visit to the veterinary practice. These cats should not receive catnip prior to or during the veterinary practice visit.

A compression wrap, such as the ThunderShirt for cats, can be tried. It should be remembered that for some cats, the wrap may just immobilize them without decreasing their anxiety and, theoretically, this could potentially increase their anxiety. Indeed, many veterinary behaviorists do not recommend their use with cats for this reason. However, in some cats, the author has found that this wrap can be highly beneficial and the positive effects can be quick. In order to determine whether a compression wrap is decreasing anxiety, evaluate for changes in anxiety objectively and compare them to previous visits without the compression wrap.[4] Monitor heart rate for elevation, check for sweaty paws, and watch for behavioral signs of anxiety such as vocalization, urinating or defecating, hissing, and unwillingness to take treats when the cat should be hungry. Veterinary staff should also compare the amount of struggling during restraint or procedures compared to past behavior. Observations should continue even when the cat returns home. The owners should note the cat's demeanor when it arrives home compared to previous veterinary practice arrivals. Is the cat agitated, or does it act scared? Does the cat hide? How long does it take for the cat to settle into normal baseline behavior?

Step 3: Block Visual Access

Clients should be encouraged to use a towel to cover the carrier as needed during travel, during waiting, and during the appointment itself. This can help to decrease arousal by blocking visual access to people, animals, or environments that may scare the cat.

Step 4: Consider the Use of Sedatives and Fast-Acting Antianxiety Medications Prior to the Veterinary Visit (see Chapter 19)

The most common oral medications used in difficult cats are benzodiazepines (alprazolam, lorazepam, diazepam) and acepromazine. Acepromazine is a sedative but not an anxiolytic drug and is of questionable value in this context. It is important for staff to realize that a pet sedated with oral medications, especially pets on acepromazine without an anxiolytic such as a benzodiazepine, may become more sensitive to sounds and appear physically calm but still be highly reactive and lunge and swipe unexpectedly. Hence, such drugs can create a false sense of security in the veterinary practice staff and it is generally accepted that acepromazine is not a suitable drug for this purpose.

The effect of benzodiazepines is dose-dependent. Lower doses have a sedative effect while moderate doses have anxiolytic effects. Ataxia and profound sedation can occur.[5] Benzodiazepines can also cause disinhibition such that, theoretically, a cat that is fearful could, under the influence of benzodiazepines, become more likely to display fear as aggression.[5-7] Gabapentin has also been used in the United States as a short-acting anxiolytic prior to veterinary practice visits. For more information, see Chapter 20.

While oral sedatives or anxiolytics can be used in the anxious, potentially fear-aggressive cat, anecdotally they are not consistently effective. The Community Practice Department of the Ohio State University Veterinary Medical Center, which has a focus on low stress handling and a practice that welcomes difficult dogs and cats, rarely uses oral medications prior to veterinary visits with either species. They rely on creating a safe environment and preparing the patient, as described in Steps 1 to 3 here. If sedation is needed, they use injectable agents once the cat is in the veterinary practice (Cassandra-Cox, personal communication, July 2013).

If oral sedatives or anxiolytics are used prior to the visit, the dose and effect should be tested ahead of time over several test dosings. The client should be sent home with an information sheet listing the goal effects and side effects of the drugs or classification of drugs you generally recommend. The client should also receive an instruction sheet with the following information:

Drug name
Drug strength
Classification of the drug: The client can look at the drug information sheet you included and see which signs and adverse effects to watch for.
Dosing instructions: Include instructions on how you would like the client to increase or decrease the dose based on clinical signs of their cat.
Length of trials: State the number of test trials you want the client to perform.
Time of onset: Inform the client as to when the drug might take effect so that they can be watching for signs.
Character of effect: Describe any likely alterations in the cat's behavior—ability to ambulate, changes in time spent active, nature of their activity, as well as variations in signs of anxiety (vocalization).
Duration of effect: Inform the clients of the length of time that the drug is effective so that they know how long to monitor the cat for.

The effect of the drug on the day of the veterinary practice visit should also be documented and an evaluation made regarding whether to continue its use for future visits or not.

MINIMIZING STRESS ON ARRIVAL AT THE VETERINARY PRACTICE

Get the Cat into a Quiet Area Immediately

It is helpful to schedule the cat's examination during quiet times of day or to ensure that there is a clear, quiet pathway into the exam room. When the client arrives, ask them to bring the cat immediately into an exam room so that it can habituate to the practice environment. The room should be quiet. Acoustical panels can be installed to decrease the noise, and door seals can be used to decrease sound transmitted from noisy areas of the veterinary practice to exam rooms. A white noise machine can be played to dampen sudden sounds, or the *Through a Cat's Ear* DVD, which is bioacoustical music designed to calm cats, can be used. Keeping the room dimly lit at first, using a pheromone diffuser and providing comfortable surfaces such as towels on top of the exam tables can also increase the cat's comfort. Be sure to also have treats, such as canned cat food, squeeze cheese, or Greenies, to help provide a positive association if appropriate, as well as toys and catnip. Once cats are habituated to the area, they are more likely to feel comfortable enough to eat treats.

Preparing the Kennel Area

If the cat will be staying at the veterinary practice for any period of time and going into the hospitalization areas, it will be important to prepare a comfortable cage. The bottom should have a soft surface, such as a towel, and there should be a place to hide, such as a high-sided bed. It may be necessary to block visual access to other animals by placing a towel over part of the cage door.

If the cat can be fed, then you can also offer treats in a toy.

PERFORMING THE EXAMINATION AND PROCEDURES

By this stage of the visit, a number of factors that will help the cat to arrive in a calm state have been taken into account and the next step is to continue the positive trend into the clinical appointment.

The first moments of the examination create the clients' most lasting impression and the manner in which the cat is handled will have a significant influence on their perception of the practice.

Getting the Cat Out of the Carrier

Mini Case Example

Thor is a cat that has been treated at our practice for many years. He arrives in his carrier and begins lunging and hissing as soon as anyone approaches him. In the past, Thor has either been anesthetized in the carrier or it has taken 3 to 4 staff members to try to hold him down. It is not unusual for someone to be bitten or scratched. The goal was to change this experience.

After learning new handling techniques, we wanted to approach Thor differently. The veterinarian and one technician went into the room. With Thor's carrier moved so that Thor faced the wall and not us, the technician took off the top half of the carrier, while the veterinarian calmly slid a towel over the bottom half of the carrier so that Thor could still hide. The towel was then tucked around him and he was lifted out of the carrier. Thor did not struggle and the experience was much easier for everyone.

Often, if the carrier is placed on the floor or on an exam table with a soft surface, the cat will come out on its own. If it does not come out, it is better to open the top of the carrier rather than try to tilt it and shake the cat out (Figure 22-2). When lifting the top off, be sure to avoid dropping the door as this will scare the cat.

The examination can be performed in the carrier or on the table, wherever the cat is most comfortable. One way to determine how to proceed is to take the cat out of the carrier but allow it the freedom to retreat back inside. Remember that by keeping the cat calm, this helps to ensure that it does not become progressively more difficult to handle with each visit (Figure 22-3). Once it has been decided to carry out the examination on the consulting room table, it is preferable to place the carrier out of sight, as the frustration of not being able to

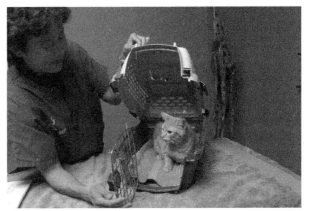

FIGURE 22-2 When removing a cat from its carrier it is important to be as passive as possible and where the design of the carrier allows, the top half of the carrier can be removed in a way that does not increase the cat's distress. This is preferable to trying to forcibly remove the cat from the carrier. (From Yin S: *Low stress handling, restraint and behavior modification of dogs & cats*, Davis, CA, 2009, CattleDog Publishing)

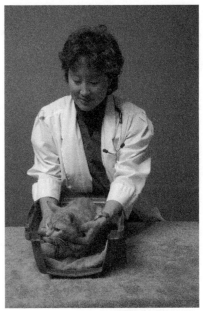

FIGURE 22-3 If the design of the cat carrier is suitable, then the clinical examination can be performed with the cat remaining in the carrier. (From Yin S: *Low stress handling, restraint and behavior modification of dogs & cats*, Davis, CA, 2009, CattleDog Publishing)

return to the carrier may keep levels of emotional arousal high.

Removing Difficult Cats from Carriers

Sometimes, veterinarians will encounter cats that are already at the point of swatting, hissing, and lunging at the beginning of the examination. In such cats, the method described in the case of Thor can be very successful.

Step 1: Start with one technician standing close to the front of the carrier and the other technician, who will do the toweling, near the rear (Figure 22-4, *A*). Undo the screws from the carrier and lift the top while keeping the front door in place so that the cat does not dart out. The towels should be thick and large (30 × 50 inch bath towels are a common size and thickness to use). If you think the cat is likely to try to bite or scratch, then one way to increase the thickness is to combine two towels together.

Step 2: Elevate the rear portion of the top of the carrier so that the towel can slide in and cover the cat (Figure 22-4, *B* and *C*). Note that it is important to do this in a room from which the cat cannot escape if it gets away from you.

Once the cat is covered, the top can be removed completely. At first, keep the front door in place until

the cat's head is covered with the towel. Tuck the towel around the sides of the cat. Then grasp the cat behind the front legs (Figure 22-4, *D*).

Lift the cat with the towel out of the carrier and onto a table (Figure 22-4, *E*). Many cats relax when you lift them in this manner in a towel (Figure 22-4, *F*). If they do not immediately relax, either allow the cat to remain in the bottom half of the carrier or use a different technique for getting them out of the carrier (refer to the emergency blanket wrap).

Towel-Wrap Techniques

In addition to using towels to cover cats as they are removed from their carriers, towels can also be used for wrapping techniques. It is important to know some

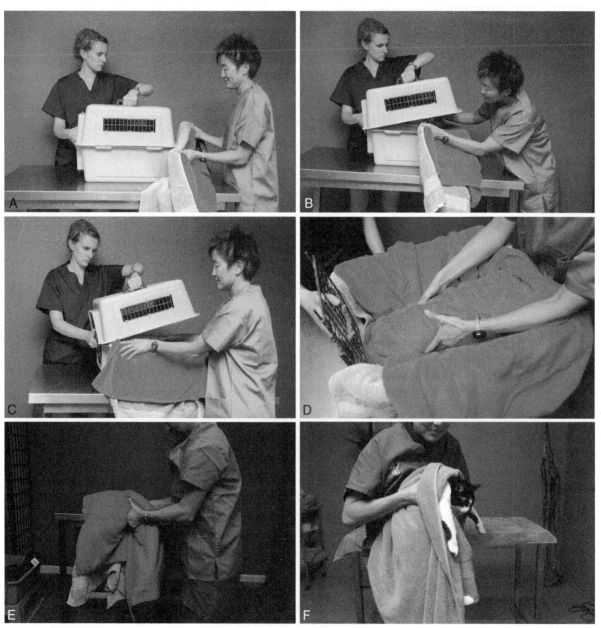

FIGURE 22-4 An example of removing a difficult cat from a carrier. (**A-E,** Courtesy S. Yin; **F,** From Yin S: *Low stress handling, restraint and behavior modification of dogs & cats*, Davis, CA, 2009, CattleDog Publishing)

basic principles about towel wraps and to know a variety of wraps so that there is a choice of options depending on the size, personality of the cat, and the actual procedure that will be performed. In this chapter, two specific wrap patterns are shown. For additional techniques and video instruction, refer to the references at the end of this chapter. Regardless of which wrap is used, here are a few rules to consider.[2]

Rule 1: Some cats like having their head covered. For these cats, simply covering the head with a towel may be sufficient. In other cases, you may need to perform a specific wrap that covers the head. Other cats dislike having their head covered. Choose whichever technique the individual cat is most comfortable with.

Rule 2: The purpose of the towel wrap is to keep the cat calm and secure, not to force the cat to hold still while it is straining to escape. In general, the aim is to place the wrap before the cat becomes agitated; however, some methods can be used in an emergency situation.

Rule 3: Wraps must be snug enough to control the cat and prevent squirming but loose enough so that the cat's breathing is not restricted. For wraps in which the head is covered, be sure to check the heart rate and respiration regularly.

Rule 4: The towel wraps can help prevent movement in all directions—forward, backward, up, down, left, right. Generally, the cat should be lying down when the wrap is started because if the cat is standing, it creates room between the cat's body and the towel.

Rule 5: These techniques look easy but they require skill and practice. It is best to practice on a stuffed animal first until the person feels comfortable with the routine, before using the technique on a calm cat.

Rule 6: If the client will be using these techniques, they should also have sessions where the cat sits on a towel and receives treats or its meal so that the cat maintains a positive association with the towel.

Two General Principles for Preventing Forward Movement Using Towels

There are many specific towel-wrapping techniques. It can be useful to learn a few of these, and it is also helpful to know how to use a towel to prevent a cat from moving forward without needing to scruff the cat and possibly cause the cat to become highly agitated. There are two basic methods for preventing forward movement. One method is to just pull the towel up and around the cat's neck and then hold the towel together behind the cat's head (Figure 22-5, *A–C*). Then you can scruff the towel to tighten it around the neck rather than scruffing the cat. This can be used loosely if your goal is to primarily stop forward motion. It can also be used as the beginning of a wrap that will be snug around the body. Note that you can start with the cat on top of the towel and just pull the forward edges around the front of the cat. Or you can start with having the entire towel in front of the cat.

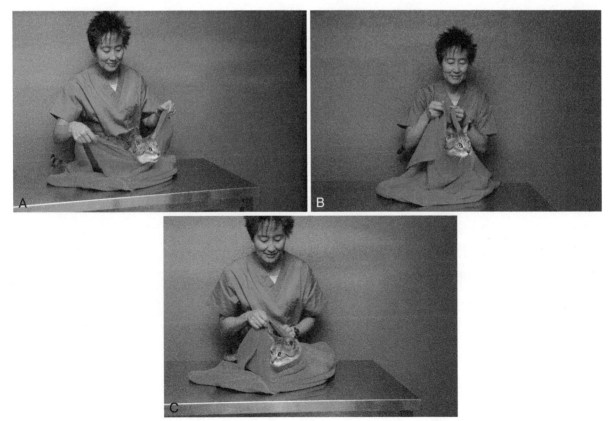

FIGURE 22-5 Towel-wrapping technique for preventing forward movement. (Courtesy S. Yin)

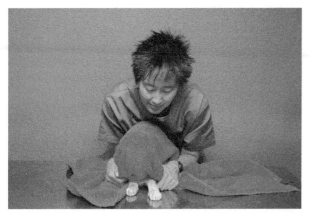

FIGURE 22-6 Keep the towel over the cat's head with your arms holding it down along the cat's side until the cat relaxes. (Courtesy S. Yin)

Another method for keeping a cat from darting forward is to fold the towel in over the cat's head and then tuck it in with your fingers so that the cat cannot lower its head to escape from under the towel. In the case where it is only to prevent forward movement but not part of another wrap pattern such as the emergency blanket wrap shown later on, the cat can have its paws sticking out. For this wrap to work, the cat should be lying down (Figure 22-6).

The Scarf Wrap

The scarf wrap permits examination of the rear end, hind legs and abdomen, as well as the head.

Start with the cat several inches from the front edge of the towel and equidistant from both sides. The cat's rear end should be against your body so that it cannot easily

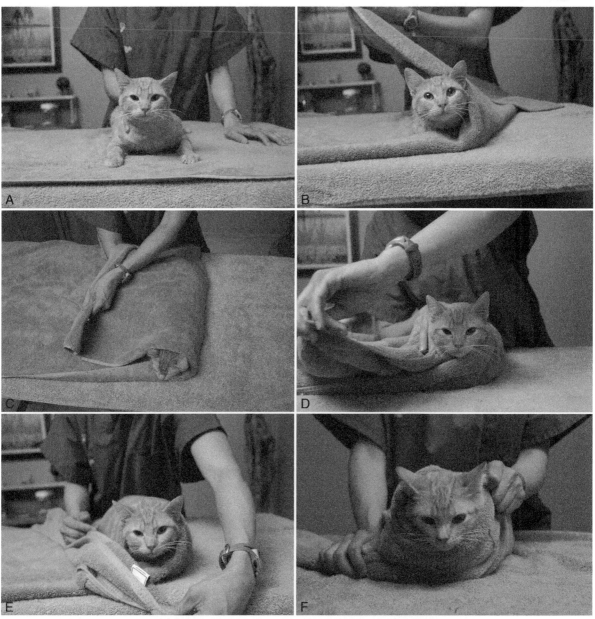

FIGURE 22-7 The scarf wrap. This wrap provides good access to the head for ear cleaning or examination as well as other procedures. (From Yin S: *Low stress handling, restraint and behavior modification of dogs & cats*, Davis, CA, 2009, CattleDog Publishing)

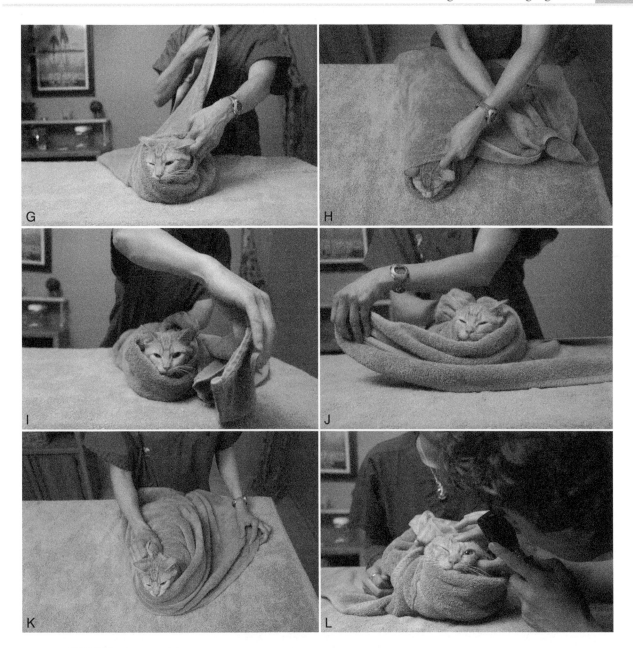

FIGURE 22-7, cont'd.

back up. Your hand should be behind the cat's head and your arm parallel to its back to encourage it to remain lying down and stationary (Figure 22-7, *A*). While holding the cat in place with one arm, use the other arm to grasp the forward edge of the towel and then wrap it around the cat's neck snugly, like a scarf (Figure 22-7, *B*). Continue until it is all the way around the neck (Figure 22-7, *C–F*). This is the first "scarf" portion of the wrap. Now make sure the back end of the wrap, the part that goes over the body, is snug too.

Once the towel is wrapped all the way around, take the other side and pull it over the cat (Figure 22-7, *G*). Make sure it is snug, especially around the back half of the cat as this is the loosest area (Figure 22-7, *H*). Now wrap this portion around the cat and under the neck like a scarf (Figure 22-7, *I* and *J*). Make sure it is

snug. Be sure to keep your hands away from the cat's mouth. Also, be sure to keep one arm on the cat running parallel to the spine so that the cat holds still while you are performing the wrap.

When the wrap is complete, you can scruff the towel instead of the cat in order to have good control. Keep the towel tight by scruffing the top of it (Figure 22-7, *K* and *L*). You can also make a trough with your arms on both sides of the towel.

A variation can be used where one of the front legs is left outside the wrap during the first stage of the scarf wrap, and it allows one to perform a cephalic venipuncture or otherwise examine and handle a front leg. To get more padding on one side of the head such as the side closest to the leg you may be examining, you can start with the cat toward the right or left edge of the towel.

The back of the cat can also be examined if you loosen the wrap on the backend.

As always, the goal is to use this wrap while the cat is still calm so that it can help to maintain a calm state.

The Emergency Blanket Wrap

This wrap can be used for emergency situations where there is a need to get cats that are fearful or even fear-aggressive out of a cage or to capture them if they are loose. Here's an overview of the wrap. More detailed instructions can be found elsewhere in the references at the end of the chapter.

Step 1: Start with a large, thick bath towel (30 × 50 inches). Hold your arms out parallel at shoulder width and with your fingers several inches from the end of

the towel. Then let the towel flop over your fingers (Figure 22-8, *A*). This is important, because you will need enough towel to wrap around the front of the cat's head; however, you don't want too much towel or you won't be able to wrap over the cat's head.

Step 2: For this wrap, it doesn't matter if the cat is facing you or facing away from you. When done correctly, the wrap only takes 2 seconds. In one move, with your arms parallel so that they will end up on each side of the cat, place the towel over the cat's head and then fold your fingers so that the towel folds over in the front (Figure 22-8, *B* and *C*). Remember that folding is what helps to keep the cat from darting forward. Your parallel arms should be on the table so that they tack the towel down.

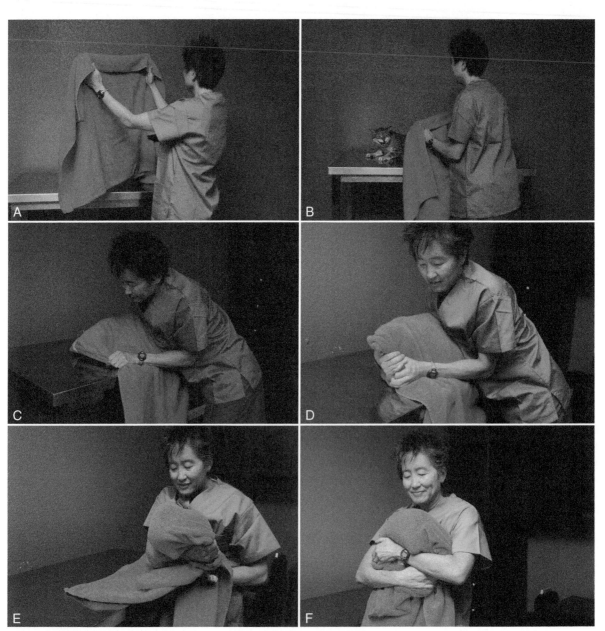

FIGURE 22-8 The emergency blanket wrap. (Courtesy S. Yin)

Next, pull your parallel arms together under the cat while simultaneously drawing the front of the towel closed with one or both hands (Figure 22-8, *D*). At the same time, pull the elbows closer to the body so that the cat is firmly pulled against your body. Now you have a cat that is encapsulated in the towel.

From here, pull the cat in towards the body (Figure 22-8, *E*).

The cat should be against your body, and the entire cat should be above your arms and encapsulated in the towel (Figure 22-8, *F*). From here the cat can be taken and put back into its carrier or cage. Cats often calm down quickly when captured and wrapped in this manner and if this wrap has been performed quickly (in a couple of seconds) and smoothly it is possible to put the cat on a padded exam room table and proceed with a procedure, such as a toenail trim or blood draw.

When the cat is placed onto the exam room table, it is important to cover the table with a towel so that the veterinarian or technician/nurse can adjust the towel based on the individual cat's needs. For instance, the front of the towel can be pulled around the cat's neck to prevent forward movement or a scarf wrap can be performed around the cat and around the towel that was used for the blanket wrap. Once you start the wrap, you can uncover the cat's head as needed.

The goal is that the cat feels relatively comfortable and safe in the wrap, and that is why he is cooperating. If there is any concern that the cat will start to struggle or become increasingly fearful, it is best to use IV or IM sedation.

Other tools for decreasing perception of visual and auditory stimuli can be used. For instance, cotton can be placed in the cat's ears to dampen sound (Cassandra-Cox, personal communication, July 2013). A calming cap can block vision, and a type of muzzle can protect from bites and block the cat's vision (Figure 22-9).

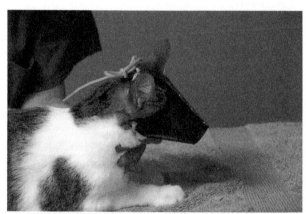

FIGURE 22-9 In the author's opinion, the cone muzzle provides good protection from being bitten and is easy to put on safely while avoiding a bite. (From Yin S: *Low stress handling, restraint and behavior modification of dogs & cats,* Davis, CA, 2009, CattleDog Publishing)

PSYCHOPHARMACOLOGIC MANAGEMENT

If it is thought that the measures already taken will not be sufficient to keep the cat calm and cooperative during the visit, injectable sedatives should be considered. In fact, sedatives should be used before the pet has a chance to become highly aroused or reactive, since they have a more consistent effect when used at this early stage. By preventing further fear, arousal, discomfort and psychological trauma, sedation may provide the best way to prevent the pet from having a highly negative experience.[1,6,7]

For the difficult cat, IM sedation can be used early in the visit and, in many cases, it will be administered immediately. When the client arrives with a challenging cat, it is helpful to take them directly into a comfortable room with the lights dimmed and with calming music, such as *Through a Cat's Ear*, played to help block out the veterinary practice sounds. A towel should be left on the carrier to decrease visual stimuli while the most appropriate personnel are selected. Ideally, three people are involved: one to hold the top of the carrier open and distract the cat, one to restrain the cat, and one to inject. Depending on the client and legal statutes in the area, the client may be asked to act as the distractor. Sedatives should be drawn up before entering the room and a Luer lock syringe used so that the needle does not get propulsed off the syringe during injection. Additionally, it is worth considering that a wider bore needle allows for faster injection as does a larger-sized syringe.

Once staff enter the room, care should be taken to speak only in a soft voice in order to avoid stimulating the cat. The client should lift the towel on the front of the carrier and distract the cat from the front while a technician approaches from the back of the carrier and opens it from the top. The handler slides a thick towel or set of towels (to increase thickness) over the cat and then restrains with the towel inside the carrier. The towels can be held snugly along the sides of the cat using both arms to tack the towel down and placing both hands around the shoulders and neck in a ring hold (Figure 22-10, *A*). The handler will have to lift one elbow up so that the injector can reach under the towel, palpate the vertebrae and give an IM injection in the epaxial muscles (Figure 22-10, *B*). This process of restraint and injection should take no more than several seconds. Then the towel should be left in the carrier with the cat and the lid replaced. The client and the cat can be left together in the quiet room until the cat is sedated (typically 15 minutes). The client should be instructed to be near the cat but to avoid physically interacting. Another possible method for sedating is to use a soft mesh carrier that is collapsible. The carrier can be covered with a towel, and the cat can be injected through the screen/mesh. Again, this process should only take several seconds.

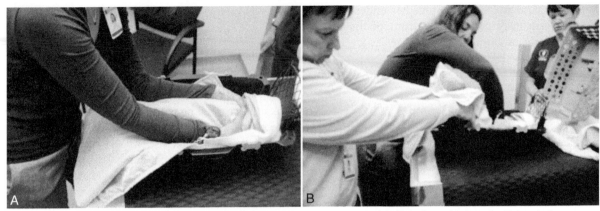

FIGURE 22-10 The Community Practice Department Team at the Ohio State University School of Veterinary Medicine sedates a challenging cat. **A,** A towel is kept over the top of the carrier to block visual stimuli. **B,** One person holds the carrier open, another restrains the cat, and a third gives the injection. The whole process takes just several seconds. (Courtesy S. Yin)

Drugs that can be reversed are most commonly used for sedation. The Community Practice Department of the Ohio State University Veterinary Medical Center, which has a strong focus on low stress handling, uses 20 to 30 mcg/kg dexmedetomidine with 0.2 to 0.4 mg/kg butorphanol IM (1/2 volume atipamezole IM is used for the reversal of dexmedetomidine). Dexmedetomidine is avoided in cardiac patients or those with heart murmurs and in geriatric or very sick patients (Cassandra, personal communication, July 2013).

The Ohio State University practice adds, if needed, 3 to 5 mg/kg of ketamine; however, adding the ketamine prolongs the recovery time such that the cat may not be able to leave the veterinary practice quickly.

An alternative to butorphanol is buprenorphine (0.02 mg/kg) IM.[6,8] Buprenorphine can also be given by oral transmucosal (OTM) delivery at 0.02 mg/kg using a 1-mL syringe. Given this way, it has a peak effect at 90 minutes,[9] with the effect starting in about 15 minutes.

MONITORING THE SEDATED CAT

Once the cat is sedated, it should be carefully monitored. The cat should be sleeping and unable to lie sternally. If the cat is not sedated enough, additional sedation may be used if appropriate. Once sedated, cotton can be placed in the ears and a calming cap and/or plastic muzzle can be placed over the eyes. The goal is to keep the external stimulus level low by blocking out sound and visual stimuli to avoid the cat becoming aroused and overcoming the sedation. During the examination, the technician should gently hold the cat in order to continuously evaluate muscle tension, respiration, heart rate, and other signs that indicate if the cat is reacting to the examination procedures. Often the most stimulating portion of the examination is when the cat is switched from one side to the other. If the cat becomes tense, gently hold the cat in place and give the cat 10 to 20 seconds to relax. Then reevaluate whether additional sedation is needed.

If venipuncture is being performed in an awake cat or even a lightly sedated one, and there is any suspicion that the cat may be sensitive to injections, it may be necessary to consider applying topical anesthetic (lidocaine/prilocaine) prior to venipuncture.

SENDING THE CHALLENGING CAT HOME

For difficult cats that have been sedated with a reversible agent, such as dexmedetomidine, reverse the sedation with atipamezole and then let the cat wake up in its familiar carrier in a quiet location and with the carrier covered. Once the patient has sufficiently recovered from sedation to go home, the client can receive the patient in a quiet room and be given home instructions. They should then be shown how to leave the practice using a quiet route which prevents them from having to go through a busy waiting room.

Clients should be advised that their cat may be sleepy and, if anxious, may display aggressive behavior toward people or other animals in the house. Hence, it may be best to place the cat in a quiet, comfortable location at home but away from other people and animals until it is fully recovered. The location will need a litter box, comfortable sleeping location, and water. Sometimes cats within the household may become aggressive to cats that have recently returned from the veterinary practice, most likely due to the foreign smells. Other times the cat that has had a potentially traumatic experience at the veterinary practice can, in a heightened state of anxiety or arousal, direct aggression toward the other household cats (see Chapter 26). If other cats reside in the household, towels with the mutual scent of all of the cats should be placed in the patient's room as well as in the sleeping area of the other household cats. The patient should be slowly reintroduced to other cats in the household in order to decrease the risk of social conflict. It is helpful for owners to record the behavior of the cat at home and note whether it shows aggression to people or other pets, as well as the length of time it takes for it to display its usual behavior patterns. If the cats in the household were compatible prior to the veterinary experience it may be appropriate to use Feliway to assist with the re-introduction (see chapter 18).

SCHEDULING TECHNICIAN SESSIONS FOR DESENSITIZATION AND COUNTERCONDITIONING

Veterinary practice visits and healthcare can be greatly improved if the clients are interested in training their cats to associate handling procedures with positive experiences. Hence, if the staff recognize that the patient has particular difficulty with certain procedures, such as toenail trimming, hair clipping, grooming, or receiving oral medications, then they can provide clients with the option to participate in short "technician behavioral health sessions" or "nurse clinics."

In these sessions, the technician can go over a specific desensitization/counterconditioning (DS/CC) plan and practice the technique and timing; first, using a stuffed animal to demonstrate the pairing procedure with the food or other positive experience. Once the client demonstrates the correct timing and presentation of the reward, they can progress to using a real cat, such as a veterinary practice cat, or practice with the patient. These training sessions can run for about 10 to 20 minutes. Technicians can start with common procedures and then add on other more patient specific DS/CC procedures. Instructions for counterconditioning can be found in references listed at the end of this chapter.[2]

CHARTING/RECORDING INFORMATION IN THE RECORD

Once the visit is over, it is essential to chart the pet's behavior and response to the various low stress procedures used. This charting will be helpful in planning future visits and tailoring the approach to the individual cat. Points to consider include the following:

- Response to: treats (describe which type), toys (type), catnip, petting
- Cat's demeanor upon arrival: hiding, exploring, purring, hissing, avoidance
- Use of sedatives: if used, what type and dosage?
- Response to sedatives: the level may be ideal for toenail trimming but the dose may need to be increased if any painful procedure is being performed
- Other tools or aids used and the cat's response: Feliway, catnip, towels
- Heart rate relative to the last visit
- Behavior of the cat once it returns home: fearful (hides, hisses), agitated

CONCLUSION

While handling challenging cats may seem impossible at first, by implementing the approaches and techniques in this chapter, veterinary practices will prevent most cats from displaying overt aggression. While sedation may be needed in more difficult cats, the techniques described in this chapter should enable the majority of consultations to be carried out in a more time efficient manner. Most cats simply require the veterinary practice staff to consider all situations from a feline perspective and work to ensure that they are kept feeling both comfortable and safe. It is beneficial to learn a few specific towel wrap skills to assist in the handling of more challenging patients. The aim is to help pets to be healthier and happier while forging a positive relationship with both the patients and the clients.

REFERENCES

1. Rodan I, Sundahl E, Carney H, et al. American association of feline practitioners and international society of feline medicine: feline-friendly handling guidelines. *J Feline Med Surg*. 2011;13:364–375.
2. Yin S. *Low Stress Handling, Restraint and Behavior Modification of Dogs & Cats: Techniques for Developing Patients Who Love their Visits*, Davis. CattleDog Publishing; 2009.
3. Yin S. Preparing Pets for a Hospital Visit. In: *Low Stress Handling, Restraint and Behavior Modification of Dogs & Cats: Techniques for Developing Patients Who Love their Visits*, Davis. CattleDog Publishing; 2009:125–138.
4. Velenovsky J. *Effects of Compression Device on Cat Behavior and Biometrics for Veterinary Visit and Related Transportation*. Chicago, IL: Case study presented at: 2013 ACVB/AVSAB Veterinary Behavior Symposium; 2013, ACVB/AVSAB, pp. 61–62.

5. Overall K. Behavioral Pharmacology. In: Overall KL, ed. *Clinical Behavioral Medicine for Small Animals*. St Louis: Mosby; 1997:293–322.

6. Landsberg GM, Hunthausen W, Ackerman L. Reducing Stress and Managing Fear Aggression in Veterinary Clinics. In: *Behavior Problems of the Dog and Cat*. ed 3. Edinburgh: Saunders; 2013:367–375.

7. Moffat K. Addressing canine and feline aggression in the veterinary clinic. *Vet Clin North Am Small Anim Pract*. 2008;38:983–1003.

8. Santos LC, Ludders JW, Erb HN, et al. Sedative and cardiorespiratory effects of dexmedetomidine and buprenorphine administered to cats via oral transmucosal or intramuscular routes. *Vet Anaesth Analg*. 2010;37:417–424.

9. Robertson SA, Lascelles BDX, Taylor PM, Sear JW. PK-PD modeling of buprenorphine in cats: intravenous and oral transmucosal administration. *J Vet Pharmacol Ther*. 2005;28:453–460.

Approaching Problem Behavior at Home

Normal but Unwanted Behavior in Cats

Jacqueline M. Ley

INTRODUCTION

There are many aspects of feline behavior that people find appealing, such as sitting on one's lap, purring, and seeking affectionate interaction. However, there are other behaviors that owners find less desirable, and some of these are associated with normal behavioral responses that have developed as cats have evolved.

The ancestral environment of the cat was very different from the typical home environment they share with people today. In order to meet their nutritional requirements, cats needed to be able to locate, stalk, and hunt small species of rodents, birds, reptiles, amphibians, and even insects. Because many of their prey species were active early in the morning or late in the evening, the cat developed a pattern of activity, peaking at dawn and dusk. In addition to being predators, cats are also prey themselves for other species and they would avoid being caught and eaten by exhibiting cautious behavior when out hunting and using withdrawal and hiding responses to protect themselves. Knowledge of feline evolutionary history helps to better understand cats today, but some of the behaviors they perform are still difficult for people to accept. Hunting is one example of a normal feline behavior that can be very upsetting for some owners and others include unacceptable toileting behavior and inconvenient periods of high activity. Understanding normal cats and the biological history of their behavior can help owners understand why their cat does what it does as well as make it easier for owners to offer mutually acceptable alternatives for the cat.

CIRCADIAN RHYTHM BEHAVIOR

Many cats are active in the early morning and early evening, and a cat may be motivated to get outside to explore and hunt, to track down an in-season queen, or to defend its territory from incursions by other cats as a result. This can be annoying if owners do not have to be awake before first light or would like some quiet after a day at work. The time the cat becomes active may alter seasonally to reflect the changing day length or may become unacceptable due to a time change, such

as Daylight Saving Time, which can be additionally stressful for owners.

Cats may attempt to escape out of doors or windows, vocalize, prowl between windows and doors, or otherwise attempt to entice their owners to let them out. Or they may be playful, stalking, and ambushing owners and other household pets, tapping their faces to wake them, climbing on furniture and knocking items off counters and bedside tables, or generally just making a nuisance of themselves. Evening activity, especially in young cats, can also occur because the cat has been home all day with inadequate environmental enrichment and becomes active when the owner returns home.

Although unwanted activity levels can be related to normal behavior, it is always important to rule out potential medical causes, and the cat should be examined and undergo any tests needed to rule these out. Hyperthyroidism can cause restlessness and vocalizing; diabetes, inflammatory bowel diseases, and renal disease may be the cause of seeking to go outside to toilet. Cognitive decline may lead to sleep disturbances and nighttime waking in older cats (see Chapter 25).

Management

Management involves meeting the cat's needs during the day and having strategies in place to distract the cat and direct its energies into desirable activities early in the morning and in the evening. This can be done through an enriched environment such as having toys available and scheduling regular play sessions with the cat.

The cat should have access to a rotating variety of toys (Figure 23-1). Some should reward interaction by dispensing food. The food can be some or all of the cat's daily food requirements and may include some treats (Figure 23-2). When first introduced, the toys can be left in obvious places so the cat learns to play with them to extract the food. Once it is readily interacting with the toys, they can be hidden so the cat must seek them out. This will help satisfy the cat's need to explore and hunt so it will be more likely to rest in the evenings and in the early morning.

Larger objects, such as tunnels, cardboard boxes, and paper grocery bags, can satisfy the cat's need to explore and small toys, such as mixed texture mice,

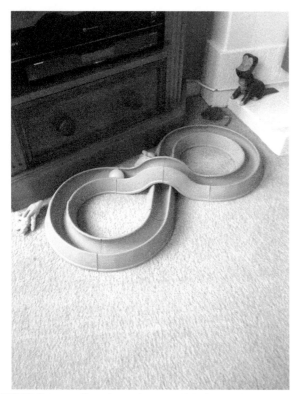

FIGURE 23-1 A variety of toys will help to stimulate the cat during the day and minimize unwanted activity at dawn and dusk. (Courtesy S. Heath)

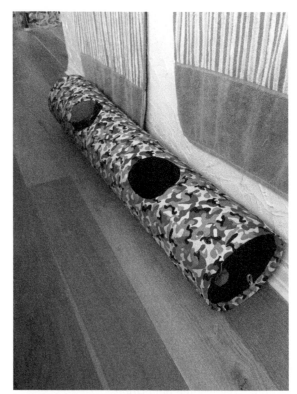

FIGURE 23-3 Tunnels can provide ideal places for cats to hide and they can be encouraged to explore them by hiding small toys or pieces of food inside. (Courtesy S. Heath)

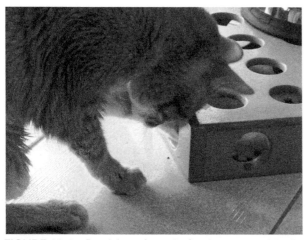

FIGURE 23-2 Provision of puzzle feeder toys which dispense part of the daily food ration can be very beneficial in terms of both physical and mental stimulation. (Courtesy I. Rodan)

can be hidden in them to further encourage investigation (Figure 23-3). Toys on strings must not be left with unattended cats as some may consume the string creating a gastrointestinal foreign body. Owners must also be warned not to leave toys that are suspended from door handles when cats, especially kittens, are alone as it is possible for them to get tangled in or even strangled by the string.

Owners need to schedule regular time for interaction in the form of play, petting, and grooming with their cat. The sessions do not need to be very long but do need to occur reliably at the same point in the owner's routine. Play sessions in particular can be shorter than many owners may think. Much of feline play that involves toys, or object play, motivates predatory behavior systems. Predatory behavior tends to occur in bouts of up to 30 minutes.[1] When a toy shares characteristics with prey, such as being small and furry, the cat may be motivated to explore and play with it but can quickly habituate to it. Changing the toy to a different one can motivate the cat to play again if the new toy is presented within 5 to 15 minutes of the previous toy.[2] It is important to educate owners to play in a manner which respects the shorter duration of normal feline play, which may be as short as 1 to 5 minutes, but if a cat becomes prematurely disinterested in a toy, it has been suggested that owners should change the toy or the game to keep their cat involved and playing.

SELF-CARE BEHAVIORS

Hunting/Predatory Behavior

Cats naturally hunt. Given enough practice and incentive, they can become very proficient at hunting. One

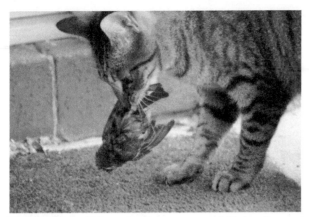

FIGURE 23-4 This cat has been successful in hunting and catching a juvenile sparrow.

study found that nearly half the prey animals were juvenile (Figure 23-4).[3] Hunting behavior by cats can be upsetting for owners, especially as cats may play with the injured prey before killing it. Hunting is also a source of conflict between cat owners and conservationists even though research suggests that landscape management is more important than predator management in preserving wildlife populations.[4]

Management

Predatory behavior by cats is best managed by confining cats either to the owner's house or to a purpose-built cat enclosure. Cat enclosures also protect the incumbent cat from dangers, such as cars, dogs, abscesses from fighting with other cats, feline infectious diseases, and the cat's own curiosity. Cat enclosures require resting places, food, water and toileting stations, and toys to provide enrichment when the cat is outside (Figure 23-5). Depending upon the style of enclosure manufacture, owners can build modular parks connected by tunnels

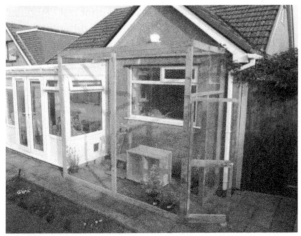

FIGURE 23-5 A cat pen can allow the cat to have access to fresh air and sensory stimulation while protecting local wildlife from predation.

TABLE 23-1	Antipredator Devices that are Marked to Stop Outdoor Cats from Killing Wildlife	
Device	**How it Works**	**Examples**
Bells	Attaches to the collar. Makes a sound when the cat moves and warns prey. May need more than one as some cats learn to silence a bell.	Numerous
Sonic devices	Attaches to collar or is part of the collar and makes a sound (some have lights too) when triggered by the sudden forward rush of cat's ambush	CatAlert Liberator Audio Visual cat collar
Lights	Various reflective and battery-operated lights that can be hung off or attached to the cat's collar. The flashing light startles the prey animals. Reflectors rely on ambient light. Battery-operated lights may need to be switched on to be effective.	Numerous
Antipounce bib	Large neoprene flap that hangs on collar in front of cat's chest and forelegs preventing the cat from getting its claws to the prey animal.	Catbib

and enclosed bridges or free form enclosures similar to large flight aviaries seen at zoos and wildlife parks.

Another option is to warn prey species of the presence of the cat, usually by attaching a device to its collar. Many devices have been invented and probably need to be trialed on an individual basis to see which are effective for an individual cat. There is evidence that collar-mounted devices can help reduce predatory behavior.[5,6] Table 23-1 lists some devices and how they work, and products available. It is important to consider the welfare of the cat when selecting one of these devices and to remember that predation is a normal feline behavior and the ability to engage in this behavior is a fundamental feline need. The aim of using a device is to make the hunt unsuccessful rather than to prevent the cat from physically engaging in the hunting process.

Toileting in Potted Plants

Combining cats and indoor or balcony plants can be difficult. Not only will some cats chew on plants (and care should be taken in selecting nonpoisonous plants), but also some cats use the pot as a toilet. This generally is not good for the health of the plant.

So why do they do it? In general, cats like a soft, loose substrate for toileting. If they are used to urinating or defecating outside, the pot plant may seem like a toilet more than the litter tray does. Some cats use a pot plant when their litter tray is dirty.

Management

There are two parts to managing this problem. One is making the litter trays attractive to the cat and the other part is to make the pot plants less attractive as a toilet option. Litter trays should be large and cleaned frequently, there should be more than one available, and these should be placed in different locations. A dirty litter tray is a bit like an unflushed toilet. No one wants to use them unless there are no other options and one is desperate. The choice of litter is also important. It should be light and easy for the cat to dig in, although some cats prefer no litter at all. Litter types, volumes or depth of litter, and litter tray types may need to be explored to see what the cat prefers. The number of litter trays and location may also need to be addressed (see Chapter 24 for full discussion). Cleaning should be frequent and should involve lots of hot water, gentle dish soap, and no deodorizers. Cats do not need their litter trays to smell lavender fresh.

Pot plants may need to be moved to make them less accessible to cats. The top of the pot can be lined with decorative pebbles, aluminum foil, or other materials as a deterrent for the cat. All plants in the house may need to be treated to prevent the cat from moving to a different plant, and it is essential that a suitable alternative toileting site is available.

Climbing Behavior

Most people do not consider that the cat evolved as a prey species as well as a predator and is therefore driven to look for places of potential safety. While owners can find their cat's desire to get up high frustrating, the cat finds it comforting to have access to locations from which they can survey their environment for potential prey and also for danger. Elevation is therefore practically useful but also serves as a coping mechanism to deal with potentially challenging situations and is an important behavior in moderating states of stress. Many cats like to get on furniture (Figure 23-6), on roofs, and/or trees. If owners and cats agree upon the cat's perching positions and the route taken to get there, then all is well. Problems occur when the position chosen by the cat is unacceptable to the owner, dangerous to the cat, or the route to get to the perch is unacceptable. Human concerns about hygiene may also occur when cats insist on sitting on kitchen work surfaces (Figure 23-7).

Management

Management involves blocking access to undesirable elevated locations from a human perspective while, at the same time, providing an acceptable (to the cat and human) alternative. Positioning cat towers near to previously accessed benches or shelves gives the cat an acceptable alternative indoors, and the cat can be moved there whenever it is found on the shelves (Figure 23-8).

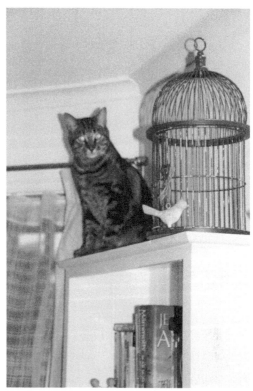

FIGURE 23-6   Cats like to gain access to high up vantage points. This is part of their natural behavior but can cause tension if the owner is not happy about the location or the route that the cat takes to access it. (Courtesy S. Heath)

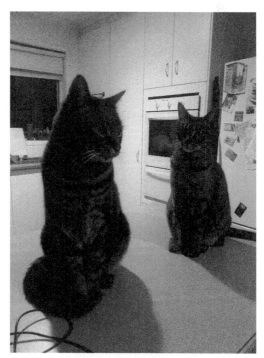

FIGURE 23-7   When cats insist on resting on kitchen work surfaces it can cause considerable tension with owners who are concerned about hygiene.

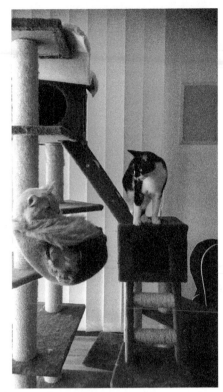

FIGURE 23-8 Cat towers can provide convenient ways for cats to access three dimensional space and rest in elevated sites that are acceptable to owners. In multicat households it may be necessary to provide towers in more than one location to prevent potential conflict over access to resting places. (Courtesy D. Jeffery)

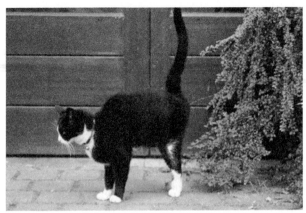

FIGURE 23-9 This cat is adopting the characteristic spraying posture while depositing a urine mark in the garden. (Courtesy A. Dossche)

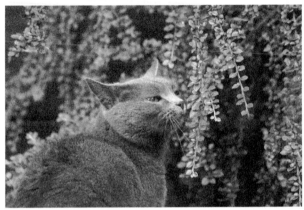

FIGURE 23-10 Cats show interest in the urine marks deposited by others within the shared outdoor territory. (Courtesy A. Dossche)

MARKING BEHAVIORS

Marking is a difficult behavior to manage. Unacceptable indoor marking is dealt with in Chapter 24. However, many owners find normal marking behavior in the outdoor environment unpleasant as well.

Marking is the act of leaving urine, either sprayed or deposited, or feces or other scents as a message for animals of the same species in the area that the marking individual is present.[7] Among animal species, there are many reasons to mark, such as territorial marking, advertising sexual receptiveness, and identifying individuals or group members.[7] Cats may use all of these motivations when marking. The information contained in the mark, along with information about how long ago the mark was made, allows cats that may spend time apart from other cats to be aware of social and spatial relationships.[8]

Marking with Urine

The most common way cats mark is by using urine,[8] and this behavior is referred to as spraying. It is commonly treated as a problem behavior in many texts of veterinary behavioral medicine and yet it is a normal communication behavior in a feline context (see Chapter 3). Little study has been done into the normal levels of marking by cats although some studies have reported it in confined, feral cats,[8] and free-living colonies of feral cats.[9]

The classic marking posture is that of a cat backed up to a vertical object with its tail vertical (Figure 23-9). As a small amount of urine is sprayed onto the surface, the cat's tail may quiver vertically and it may tread its back feet and half-close its eyes.[10] A squatting position may be used to mark horizontal surfaces and usually a smaller volume of urine is produced than if the cat is voiding for elimination.[11] Fresh sprayed urine marks elicit lots of attention in the form of repeated sniffing or Flehmen or gape responses (Figure 23-10).[12] Once the mark ages, the interest in the mark reduces, meaning that marks need to be renewed on a regular basis.

Males tend to mark more than females, with one study reporting 99% of all marks were performed by entire males.[8] Other studies have shown that neutering decreases the amount of spraying performed by both sexes.[13] Marking also varies with the time of the year, with more marking being seen during the breeding season (late winter to early spring),[8] which can be explained by the fact that the behavior has a role in sexual as well as social communication.

Urine marks are generally made in socially significant areas for cats.[11] These may be entrance and exit points to the house or a room or in the garden. The smell of cat urine is very strong and offensive to most people. Repeatedly having to clean urine deposits can be annoying for owners (especially if the deposits are not made by their own cat!), and marking behavior can be a cause of relinquishment and also tension between neighbors.

Management

A veterinary behavior consultation may be required to rule out abnormal levels of marking (see Chapter 24). If indoor marking is considered to be within normal levels in terms of location and frequency when stressors can be identified within the home environment but cannot for some reason be eliminated or managed, then it may be necessary to recommend changes to the home environment and possible antianxiety medication to preserve the human–animal bond. Rehoming to an alternative home environment may be beneficial.

If a low level of indoor urine marking is considered inevitable and the owners decide to live with it, then it can be managed in ways that will reduce damage to property and also make cleaning easier. Examples include providing an easily replaceable, disposable cover, such as plastic or foil, for the areas being marked which can be replaced each time it is soiled.

Feliway has been shown to have some efficacy in reducing spraying behavior[14] and if used diligently by owners, it may help. The diffuser device is generally considered to be the most useful form of the product for indoor marking problems, but the spray version can also be used on specifically targeted locations. It is important for owners to remember to use the spray on a regular basis (see Chapter 18). The cat may be observed to bunt the area after it is treated with Feliway.[11]

Reducing cat-related tension (either with other cats in the neighborhood or with cats in the same household) may also help reduce spraying. Owners of cats in highly populated areas may need to organize trapping of feral cats or discuss time-sharing of the neighborhood with other cat-owning neighbors. Owners with multiple cats may need to consider if some of their cats may be happier if there were fewer cats in their lives and the issue of rehoming should be discussed. If the cats are to remain within the same home, then separating cats, sometimes permanently, may be necessary.[11,15]

Marking with Feces

Cats may also use feces left in prominent areas as a signal for other cats, although the results of studies are variable as to the importance and frequency of fecal marking by cats.[8] One study found that cats were less likely to defecate in the core area of their home territories (the area they tended to use to sleep and raise kittens).[16] Feces may be left along pathways frequented by other cats or at the edge of home territories. This author knows of a cat that marked with feces on a clear skylight, which led to interesting shadows on the family room floor! The feces were replaced whenever they were removed or washed away after storms.

Marking by Clawing

Clawing has two main roles: it allows the cat to remove the blunted outer claw sheath from its front claws and it provides a means of advertising its presence to other cats and leaving messages to avoid more direct communication. The cat creates visual marks on vertical and/or horizontal surfaces.[8] Marking by scratching is performed by all adult cats in a group.[8] When trees or logs are marked this way, it is not a concern. However, a cat sharpening its claws can quickly ruin household furnishings and carpets. Often claw marks are put on prominent surfaces along well-defined thoroughfares.[8] This tendency guarantees that any damage to furnishings will be prominent and obvious to the owners and any visitors. In some households, clawing at furniture may be an effective attention-seeking device employed by the cat.

One study identified that cats over 12 months of age were likely to scratch and suggested that young, intact male cats were most likely to scratch at surfaces other than a scratching post.[17]

Management

Areas or items that are being damaged need to be protected. This may be by blocking access completely or by covering the area with materials that are likely to deter the cat from scratching. Cats appear to have preferences for trees with soft bark (Figure 23-11),[8] therefore materials that are hard or rough or feel uncomfortable could be used to cover objects being scratched. Feliway spray is licensed for helping to reduce scratching and is sprayed on the surfaces that the cat is clawing. The installation of a Feliway diffuser has also been suggested to be beneficial in terms of enhancing the feeling of security within the home and therefore reducing the motivation to mark.

Some cats can be encouraged to leave an area alone by the use of essential oils mixed with water and sprayed over the area. Citrus-based essential oils may be the most effective. Clients must patch test any surfaces before spraying more widely.

At the same time that the cat's preferred area is made less attractive, a new suitable scratching post must be

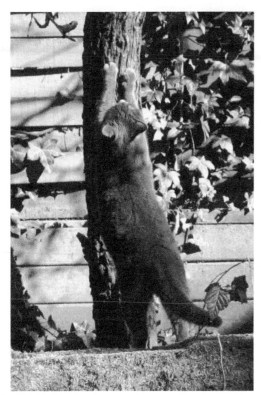

FIGURE 23-11 In the outdoor environment cats will select to scratch on surfaces such as soft bark. (Courtesy A. Dossche)

introduced and can be placed in the area. This gives the cat somewhere to direct its behavior. A survey of Italian cat owners found that cats that had a scratching post tended to use it.[17] The scratching post should be orientated in the direction the cat likes (vertical or horizontal, or somewhere in between), large enough to allow the cat to stretch out, sturdy enough to take the cat's weight, and located somewhere prominent (Figure 23-12).

FIGHTING

Cats will try to avoid physical confrontation and they have elaborate communication systems, which help them to minimize interactions with cats that are unfamiliar or incompatible (see Chapter 3). If fighting does occur, it is often related to territorial disputes and following confrontation. The cats will often use avoidance strategies to stay out of each other's way. Both within neighborhoods and within multicat households, the social system may become destabilized due to the maturation of kittens or the addition or loss of an adult cat. In feral situations, there may also be some degree of social instability during the breeding season. Much confrontational behavior between cats is passive in nature and involves posturing and positioning to send signals which are designed to reduce the risk of escalation to physical fighting. However, when aggression does

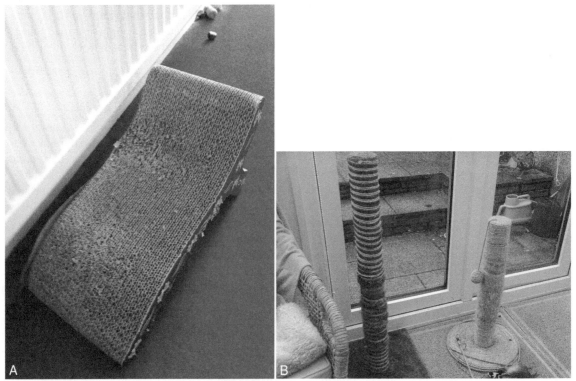

FIGURE 23-12 Scratching facilities come in many shapes and sizes and should be tailored for the individual cat's preferences. Some prefer horizontal surfaces **(A)** while others prefer a vertical surface **(B)**. (Courtesy S. Heath)

escalate, the absence of effective appeasement signaling in adult cats results in a high risk of serious wounds being sustained by both parties. Cats develop abscesses readily due to their sharp claws and teeth puncturing through the skin and introducing bacteria.[18] Many serious feline diseases, such as feline immunodeficiency virus and feline leukemia virus, are also spread through fighting.[19]

Management

The most important first step is to separate cats that are fighting (See Chapter 26). This is often easier to do if the aggression is occurring between neighborhood cats when it is possible to confine the cats to the owner's house and/or a cat enclosure. When conflict is occurring within a multicat household, total separation can be difficult to achieve and may be stressful for the owners as well as the cats. Whether within a household or a neighborhood, ongoing visual contact between the cats can lead to perpetuation of negative emotional states, and while physical conflict may be minimized, other unwanted behaviors, such as redirected (or frustration-related) aggression and marking, may persist. If the problems relate to cats in the neighborhood, the owner may need to consider blocking their cat's access to windows so they cannot see other cats, and it will also help to make the immediate vicinity of the house less pleasant for the invading cat. This can be done by scaring the cat off the property whenever possible; for example, spraying the hose in the direction of the cat, simply staring, or advancing toward it or yelling at it any time it is seen, but trying to avoid any interaction which will compromise the welfare of the other cat. Fences can be capped with devices to stop cats from going over and entering the property (e.g., Oscillot Cat Containment Solutions [for more information, visit http://oscillot.com.au/]). Fences can also be fitted with

devices such as plastic spikes, which can be positioned at intervals, making it impossible for the cat to lurk and rest on them while still allowing it to walk across the top of the fence (Figure 23-13). If the problematic cat is feral, it can be trapped and removed. If it is owned, then some delicate neighborly discussions may be needed. Time-share arrangements for allowing the cats out may be necessary to reduce feline tension. Any use of deterrents in the garden must take into account potentially detrimental effects on the resident cat if they have access to the garden, and it is essential that there is no risk of physical injury to any cat that enters the area.

When aggression is occurring between feline members of the same household, the recommendations are similar (see Chapter 26). Physical separation is required and it is not advisable to persist in forcing introductions when the cats are in a high state of arousal. If the fighting is due to introduction of a new cat, then it needs to be removed and confined for a while and then the reintroduction needs to be done slowly and gradually, starting with confining the new cat to one room for a week or longer then removing it to a new room and allowing the household cat(s) to explore the room. This way, the cats experience each other's scents and become used to the idea that a new cat is in the area. This can progress to allowing the cats to meet through a door that has a gap under it to allow scent exchange or one that is held ajar in such as a way as to allow scent contact but no physical interaction. Gradually, the level of contact can be increased under careful supervision.

When cats within the same household are socially incompatible, it is essential for owners to provide sufficient resources to ensure that all social groups have access to independent sets of resources. Time-share systems for access to communal areas of the house and to the owners may be necessary; in some situations, permanent separation will be required. In such cases,

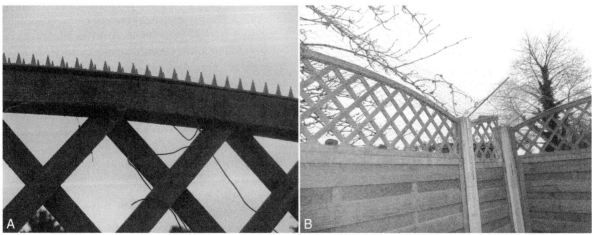

FIGURE 23-13 Owners can modify garden boundaries using a combination of plastic spikes **(A)** and fencing **(B)** to prevent other cats from entering the garden and resident cats from leaving. (Courtesy S. Heath)

owners need to consider the quality of life of all the cats involved and rehoming may be a necessary outcome.

REPRODUCTIVE BEHAVIOR

Cats come into season during the time of year when the days are lengthening. This is usually from late winter to early spring. Leading up to and during this time, male cats become more active and travel, looking for mates. Females are courted with enthusiastic vocalization, and potential rivals are banished in noisy fights—usually at nighttime. Castrating male cats will reduce the hormonal motivation for such behavior, but it is important for owners to realize that territorial behavior will not be entirely eliminated by neutering and some vocalization and confrontation can persist, particularly when neutering is carried out later in life.

Sexually active females may begin vocalizing or "calling" to advertise to males in the area that they are receptive. The vocalization can be very loud. During the breeding season, the queen has an estrous cycle every 21 days. Queens may have their first season as young as 4 months of age, and for many novice owners, the sudden odd and noisy behavior of their kitten can be confusing and distressing. Anecdotally, many think their cat is in pain. Spaying the queen stops sexual behaviors, such as calling, which is the primary concern for cat owners in relation to female sexual behavior.

When owners of breeding queens do not wish to use medication to manage their cats during periods when they do not wish to breed, ovulation can be induced by allowing mating with a vasectomized male cat.[20] In some cases, using a thermometer in the vagina can also induce ovulation and cause the calling behavior to stop until the next cycle.[20]

PLAY BEHAVIOR

Play behavior in cats is often seen as being charming and amusing but not when the cat is directing its claws and teeth at the owner. Play provides an important outlet for the practice of important life skills, such as predation and self-protection,[21] and when cats are encouraged to play with their owner's hands or feet as little kittens, the behavior will often continue into early adulthood.[22] As a result, it is common for owners to complain that their cats will ambush them and will strike at their legs or other body parts, biting and clawing and then leaping away. Kittens may grab a petting hand with their forepaws, bite the hand, and rake with their hind claws, and if owners do not respond appropriately, this behavior can become problematic due to the real risk of human injury.

Management

Prevention of unwanted play-motivated interactions is better than a cure, so new kitten owners need to be counseled to use toys to play games with their kittens from the beginning. Toys that encourage hunting and striking at a distance from the human are ideal. These can include fishing-rod style toys, self-propelling toys, and kitten-sized stuffed toys. Predatory play behavior is directed toward the toy, and if the kitten attempts to engage with human hands or feet, the owner can be advised to stay still and go limp while a toy is introduced to redirect the kitten's attention. It is important to allow the kitten to grab hold of the toy and mimic the kill so owners should be advised against the use of the laser pointer unless it alights on a tangible object that the kitten can grab hold of.

Unfortunately, most owners seek help after encouraging their kittens to play with human hands and feet, and many have started to use punitive interactions in their attempts to stop the cat from hurting them. These may include spray bottles or air horns. Such tools can induce fear and can also damage the relationship between the cat and the owner. After all, the cat is only doing what it has been previously encouraged to do and the introduction of punishment into this context will create confusion. Unwanted play behavior needs to be dealt with using distraction and redirection, and owners need to learn to read their cat's body language so that they can identify when it is getting in position for an ambush. It may be helpful to apply a bell to the cat's collar so that the owners have some warning as to the whereabouts of the cat when they are walking around the house. Common ambush sites can also be identified and the environment can be altered to remove potential hiding spots. If necessary owners can wear protective clothing around their arms and legs to ensure that they can resist the temptation to react. The owner should approach any persistent ambush locations carefully and call the cat out to them as they approach. The cat can then be rewarded for coming out with a toy or other acceptable game.

When the problematic behavior is seen in the context of being petted, it is important for owners to ensure that all interactions with the cat reward calm, quiet behavior and that handling ceases as soon as the cat becomes aroused. The owner needs to watch for body language signals of increasing arousal, such as the cat's pupils dilating, ears going back, body tensing, tail swishing faster, and body posture changing to potential attack positions. The owner should stop petting and providing any attention to the cat at the first sign of arousal. If the cat settles then petting and attention can resume. If the cat fails to settle then the owner can use a toy to direct the arousal toward a more suitable outlet (see Chapter 27).

CATS AND COMPUTER AND ELECTRONIC EQUIPMENT

Many cats lie on computers and other electronic equipment, including computer keyboards (Figure 23-14)

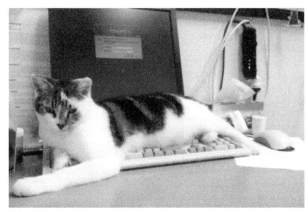

FIGURE 23-14   Many cats sit or lie in inconvenient places. Here a young veterinary practice cat is lying on the keyboard of the consultation room computer.

and printers, and this can be very problematic for some owners. It may be that the equipment is warm and therefore attractive to the cat or the cat may use its position to solicit attention from the owner in the same way as when it sits on newspapers, homework, and books. Bonded cats spend time in close proximity to the cats within their social group,[23] and if they have formed a social bond with humans, they will tend to remain in close proximity to the humans.

Management

Management requires providing an acceptable lounging place for the cat and protecting equipment. Covers for computers, keyboards, and printers can minimize damage to these devices, and then the most important approach is to provide an alternative desirable place for the cat to rest that is close to the owner. Some authors have advocated using positive punishment techniques, such as motion-detection devices attached to sprays or other noisemakers, or using electrified mats that deliver an electric shock when the cat jumps on them. These may seem simple and logical approaches to owners but they run the risk of inducing negative emotional states, such as fear and anxiety in the cats, which may lead to more problematic behaviors and

therefore should be avoided. Punitive interaction is an unnecessary way of responding to what is a normal and, for most owners, desirable display of a social bond between the cat and its owner. After all, we keep pets to form a bond with them and to be able to be in close contact with them so punishing them for displaying this behavior may damage the bond between the owner and the cat.

If the cat is using its position to solicit attention from the owner, it can be taught an alternative behavior that will reliably result in it receiving attention. For example, the cat can learn that going to a place near the owner, which can be made more obvious by the placing of a mat or cushion as a marker, and sitting there will result in human attention. The use of a portable marker enables the owner to move it to wherever they are working or relaxing and they can reinforce the positive association by encouraging the cat onto the marker with treats and attention. If they also ignore the cat when it leaves the marker, the cat will learn that if it desires interaction with the owner, being on the marker will reliably allow it to get that attention.

CONCLUSION

Cats are fascinating animals that can form affectionate bonds with people. Like all significant relationships in life, loved ones are not perfect and sometimes do things that their families may not like but have to learn to live with. This courtesy needs to be extended to the feline members of the family. By understanding their behavior from a biological and ethological perspective, cat owners can learn to accept some of the less desirable features of feline behavior or find ways in which cats can be encouraged into more acceptable alternative ways of displaying them.

ADDITIONAL RESOURCES

Information on products available from Oscillot Cat Containment Solutions can be found at: http://oscillot.com.au/

REFERENCES

1. Turner DC, Meister O. Hunting Behaviour of the Domestic Cat. In: Turner DC, Bateson P, eds. *Domestic Cat: The Biology of its Behaviour*. Cambridge, UK: Cambridge University Press; 1988:111–121.
2. Hall SL, Bradshaw JWS, Robinson IH. Object play in adult domestic cats: the roles of habituation and disinhibition. *Appl Anim Behav Sci*. 2002;79:263–271.
3. Kays RW, DeWan AA. Ecological impact of inside/outside house cats around a suburban nature preserve. *Anim Conserv*. 2004;7:273–283.
4. Schneider MF. Habitat loss, fragmentation and predator impact: spatial implications for prey conservation. *J Appl Ecol*. 2001;38:720–735.
5. Nelson SH, Evans AD, Bradbury RB. The efficacy of collar-mounted devices in reducing the rate of predation of wildlife by domestic cats. *Appl Anim Behav Sci*. 2005;94:273–285.
6. Calver M, Thomas S, Bradley S, McCutcheon H. Reducing the rate of predation on wildlife by pet cats: the efficacy and practicability of collar-mounted pounce protectors. *Biol Conserv*. 2007;137:341–348.

7. Ralls K. Mammalian scent marking. *Science*. 1971;171: 443–449.

8. Feldman HN. Methods of scent marking in the domestic cat. *Can J Zool*. 1994;72:1093–1099.

9. Natoli E, Baggio A, Pontier D. Male and female agonistic and affiliative relationships in a social group of farm cats (Felis catus L.). *Behav Processes*. 2001;53:137–143.

10. Dards JL. Home ranges of feral cats in Portsmouth dockyard. *Carnivore Genetics Newsletter*. 1978;253:357–370.

11. Neilson JC. Feline house soiling: elimination and marking behaviors. *Vet Clin North Am*. 2003;33:287–301.

12. de Boer J. The age of olfactory cues functioning in chemo-communication among male domestic cats. *Behav Processes*. 1977;2:209–225.

13. Hart BL, Cooper L. Factors related to urine spraying and fighting in prepubertally gonadectomized male and female cats. *J Am Vet Med Assoc*. 1984;184:1255–1258.

14. Mills DS, White JC. Long-term follow up of the effect of a pheromone therapy on feline spraying behaviour. *Vet Rec*. 2000;147:746–747.

15. Overall KL. Clinical Behavioural Medicine for Small Animals. St Louis: Mosby; 1997.

16. Ishida Y, Shimuzu M. Influence of social rank on defecating behaviors in feral cats. *J Ethol*. 1998;16:15–21.

17. Mengoli M, Mariti C, Cozzi A, et al. Scratching behaviour and its features: a questionnaire-based study in an Italian sample of domestic cats. *J Feline Med Surg*. 2013;15: 886–892.

18. Souza MJ, New JC. Feline Zoonotic Diseases and Prevention of Transmission. In: Little SE, ed. *The Cat: Clinical Medicine and Management*. St Louis: Saunders; 2012:1090.

19. Kennedy M, Little SE. Infectious Diseases: Viral Diseases. In: Little SE, ed. *The Cat: Clinical Medicine and Management*. St Louis: Saunders; 2012:1049, 1056.

20. Little SL. Female Reproduction. In: Little SE, ed. *The Cat: Clinical Medicine and Management*. St Louis: Saunders; 2012:1200.

21. Bateson P. Behavioural Development in the Cat. In: Turner DC, Bateson P, eds. *The domestic cat: the biology of its behaviour*. Cambridge, UK: Cambridge University Press; 2000.

22. Horwitz DF, Nielson JC. Blackwell's Five Minute Veterinary Consult Clinical Companion: Canine and Feline Behavior. Ames, Iowa: Blackwell Publishing; 2007, pp. 141–147.

23. Curtis TM, Knowles RJ, Crowell-Davis SL. Influence of familiarity and relatedness on proximity and allogrooming in domestic cats (Felis catus). *Am J Vet Res*. 2003;64: 1151–1154.

House Soiling Problems

Kersti Seksel

INTRODUCTION

House soiling problems, including marking and elimination motivated events, account for a significant percentage of reported behavioral problems in cats. One study found that 36.8% of all pet cats exhibited house soiling problems and 12.3% sprayed urine.[1] Blackshaw reported that 33% of behavior referrals to The University of Queensland involved house soiling.[2] Of these, 35% involved urine spraying, 19% involved urination, 31% involved defecation, and 16% involved both urination and defecation.

In one study of feline behavior cases that were referred to three behavioral practices in the United States, Canada, and Australia, 58% of 225 cats had a primary complaint of house soiling, with 70% of the cats eliminating (or not using the litter box or tray), 30% exhibiting markings, and 13% exhibiting both behaviors.[3] House soiling is also one of the main reasons for feline relinquishment.[4]

Behavior is determined by three main factors: genetic predisposition, learning from previous experiences, and the environment. The genetic or inherited component predisposes an animal to behave in a certain way and influences the behaviors that are expressed at any given time. Cats learn from every interaction they have with people, other cats, dogs, or the environment. Therefore, all previous experiences, good or bad, are influential. The socialization period occurs between 2 and 7 to 9 weeks of age and is a particularly important and impressionable time in terms of learning. In addition, the environment or current situation which a cat is in at any particular time will influence the behavior that is exhibited.

Once medical problems have been ruled out, elimination in locations that are unacceptable to people is generally due to factors that lead to avoidance of the litter box, the litter, or the location (which may be intermittent or continuous) or to a preference for substrates or locations other than the litter box (which may be acquired through avoidance).

Marking, which is most commonly displayed in the form of urine spraying, may be caused by an underlying medical problem, territorial competition, anxiety-provoking situations, or arousing events, and it may be elicited by novel sights, sounds, or smells, especially from other cats. When changes in the environment lead to stress or anxiety, spraying might be considered to be an adaptive behavior for maintenance of social organization.

Both males and females, neutered and intact, may present with house soiling, and it has been reported in all breeds and across all age groups. Elimination in unacceptable locations should be differentiated from urine-marking, as the underlying cause(s) are often different. Table 24-1 provides an overview of how to begin to differentiate between spraying and periuria but no one feature can be used as a definitive diagnostic tool, and a comprehensive history is needed in every case.

Treatment of behavior problems involves three key areas: environmental management, behavioral modification, and, in some cases, use of medication and other supportive therapies, such as pheromonatherapy.

BEHAVIORAL HISTORY

It is useful to ask clients to complete a behavioral questionnaire in order to aid the collection of a vast amount of information. Some behaviorists prefer to send the questionnaire to the clients ahead of the consultation so that they have time to think about the answers to the questions.

The questions asked should include information on the following, and each question may need to be explored in more depth.

- What is the nature of the problem (i.e., are there deposits of urine or feces, or both)?
- If the deposits are of urine, is it deposited on vertical surfaces or horizontal surfaces, or both?
- What percentage of the urine and/or fecal deposits is outside the box (i.e., does the cat also use its litter box)?
- Information about the litter box: size, covered or uncovered, litter type, number of boxes, frequency of cleaning, use of liners.
- A map of the home with the location of the food and water stations and resting areas as well as locations of

TABLE 24-1 **Features of Spraying and Periuria**

	Spraying	Periuria
Position	Stand, squat	Usually squat
Amount of urine	Small quantity	Large quantity
Location of urine	Usually vertical surfaces	Horizontal surfaces
Scratching after	Rarely	Often
Reason	Emotional—for example, territorial, agonistic, or hormonal/sexual	Physiological—elimination of waste

Adapted from Seksel and Lindeman, 1998.[5]

the litter boxes. Location of the urine and/or fecal deposits should also be indicated and, where possible, the chronological sequence of discovery of those deposits should be noted.

- Is there a substrate preference for the urine and/or fecal deposits?
- Are there substrates or areas in which the urine and/or fecal deposits do not occur?
- Frequency of house soiling (e.g., daily, weekly, etc.).
- When did the house soiling issues start?
- Has it increased or decreased since it was first noticed?
- When does soiling occur? (e.g., when the owners are home or out, mornings, or evenings, etc.)
- What is the daily routine of the cat and its owners, and does this correlate in any way to the house soiling?
- Was there any change in routine at the time of onset?
- How many other cats live in the household, and how do they behave toward each other? Are there agonistic interactions between cats (either active or passive)?
- Previous treatment and outcomes.

A videotape of a day in the life of the cat(s) can provide more valuable information. If not possible, asking the clients to provide pictures of the household will often complement the information in the questionnaire and help the veterinarian to better identify underlying problems (Figure 24-1).

In all cases of house soiling, one of the most useful approaches to history-taking is to ask the clients to provide a plan of the house which indicates the locations of the urine and/or fecal deposits and also provides information about the household environment, particularly from a feline perspective. In Figure 24-2 a house plan has been provided by the owner of a spraying cat. The peripheral distribution of the urine deposits in the dining room, lounge, and kitchen supports the potential for an external stressor, such as a neighborhood cat, triggering the behavior. In addition, the inappropriate location of the litter box next to the cat flap

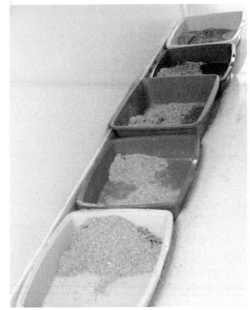

FIGURE 24-1 Requesting videos or photographs can detect problems that may not otherwise be identified. Five litter boxes may be sufficient for this environment, but when all the boxes are lined up in the same location, it is equivalent to one box for a cat. In this case, the photo also reveals serious problems related to an inadequate amount of litter in the trays as well as the limited size and depth of the trays and issues of inadequate frequency of cleaning. It is really not surprising in situations like this that the cats choose alternative sites in which to eliminate. (Courtesy I. Rodan)

may be contributing to the resident cat's sense of insecurity, and the positioning of the water and food bowls next to each other in the same room as the litter box may be adding yet more emotional pressure.

CLINICAL EXAMINATION

House soiling can be precipitated by medical problems. In a retrospective study of cats with problematic elimination, 60% of the cats had a history of feline urologic syndrome (FUS) or feline lower urinary tract disease (FLUTD).[5] Over recent years, there has been a great deal of interest in the interplay between stress and the incidence of feline idiopathic cystitis (FIC), and research has confirmed that FIC is a very important differential in cases of feline house soiling.[6-8] Elimination in unacceptable locations can also be a sign of any medical problem that causes increased volume of urine or feces, increased discomfort during elimination, decreased control, or problems that affect mentation, temperament, or cortical control (Figure 24-3). On the other hand, systemic illnesses which might lead to alterations in behavior could contribute to marking by altering hormonal states or increasing anxiety. Assessment should therefore begin with a physical examination and blood and urine tests to rule out any medical problems.

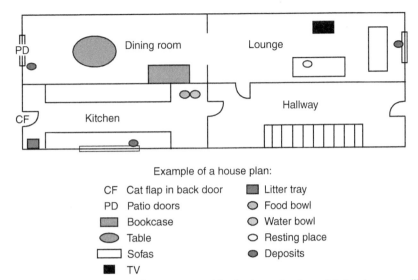

FIGURE 24-2   A house plan is an important tool in the investigation of feline house soiling problems. (Courtesy S. Heath)

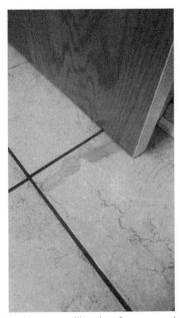

FIGURE 24-3   House soiling is often associated with an underlying medical problem. If there is blood in the urine deposits, it is important to investigate possible medical causes. (Courtesy E. Wiley)

Currently, no single specific diagnostic test or marker will confirm FIC, which may be obstructive or non obstructive in its presentation and can also present as a chronic, often recurring, disease. According to Westropp and Buffington, cats are diagnosed with FIC when they have one or several episodes of FLUTD and a thorough diagnostic workup finds no single etiology (i.e., no stones, urinary tract infection, tumor, or other physiologic causation).[6]

Evidence of masculinization, such as penile barbs or odorous urine, might be indicative of a hormonal disorder.

DIFFERENTIAL DIAGNOSIS

The major diagnostic categories for house soiling include medical differentials, location preference, substrate preference, litter aversion, location aversion, and marking behavior. When the cat eliminates on vertical surfaces, the diagnosis is usually urine marking. The problem arises when a cat that is depositing urine on horizontal surfaces might also be spraying. Differentiating between the different motivations for the house soiling may be helped by obtaining information about the locations and surfaces used (i.e., are they similar to those that would be used for spraying), the volume of urine (usually small amounts when marking), whether the deposits occur in response to specific stressors, whether the cat is in pain leading to increased frequency of voiding, and whether the cat is also using its litter.

ELIMINATION IN UNACCEPTABLE LOCATIONS

When this problem was first described, the terminology used for cats that did not use the litter box for urination was *inappropriate elimination or toileting*. It has recently been suggested that it should more correctly be termed *elimination in unacceptable locations,* or peri-uria, as the urination or defecation itself is not inappropriate, it is the location that is unacceptable to owners.

Clinical Signs

Elimination in unacceptable locations most commonly involves urination and/or defecation outside the litter box but it may also include cases where cats that previously toileted in an outdoor location start to deposit urine and/or feces within the home. If the elimination is changed in amount or frequency, as well as location it may be associated with medical conditions and these should certainly be ruled out. It more commonly involves the cat passing normal amounts of urine or feces and is associated with the elimination of waste. In most cases, the cat squats to produce a normal quantity of urine or feces. Cats usually eliminate on a horizontal surface and often scratch to cover the waste product afterwards. The unacceptable behavior may be a normal response to environmental factors, such as an unclean litter box or an inability to get into the litter box if the sides are too high or access to the litter box is prevented by a closed door or other obscuring factors. Likewise elimination in unacceptable locations may occur in response to an inability to access outdoor latrine sites due to confinement or inter-cat tension in the neighborhood.

Predisposing Factors

There are three main predisposing factors for elimination in unacceptable locations: a medical condition, litter box issues, and/or anxiety disorders.

Disease

Many diseases can contribute to the cat not using a litter box. FIC or other causes of FLUTD (e.g., bladder calculi), diarrhea, constipation, stress-related disorders, and any of the causes of polyuria have been reported to be involved.[9]

Litter Box Issues

Litter box issues can be divided into two main categories: aversion to substrate and/or to location of the litter box, and preference for another substrate and/or location.

Litter Box Aversion

Aversion to the litter box may develop for many reasons. Cats can develop an aversion to the litter box if they associate the box with something unpleasant such as being caught by the owner in order to be medicated, groomed, or transported to the vet or being frightened by another household pet while using the tray.

They may also develop an aversion due to specific features of the box such as type of litter provided, the depth of the litter, the cleanliness of the litter box, the size of the litter box, the litter box type, or the location of the litter box (Figure 24-4).

Many new litter materials, such as corn, pine, newspaper, and crystals, and litters with strong deodorizers, have been marketed on the basis of human preferences rather than feline preferences and the majority of cats prefer sand litters without deodorizers (Figure 24-5).

Many commercial litter boxes are too small for cats, not allowing them to turn around and scratch as they normally would (Figure 24-6) and this can be a significant factor in encouraging a cat to seek out an alternative location.

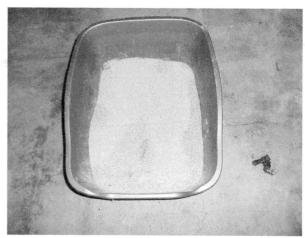

FIGURE 24-4 When a cat is soiling next to the litter box, it is important to consider why the tray may be aversive to the cat. In this case, the tray is wet and there is not enough clean free space in the tray to defecate. The lack of litter depth may also be an issue in this case.

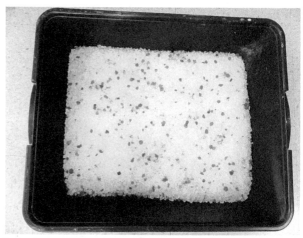

FIGURE 24-5 Many litter types, such as crystals with deodorizers, are developed and marketed for human preference rather than that of cats. Many cats will find alternative places rather than use these types of litter. (Courtesy I. Rodan)

Cleanliness is an important factor in selection of toileting sites and the cat may find the litter box aversive if it is unclean, if a heavily scented litter is used, or if the cleaning products used to clean the litter box are too pungent. Additionally, if another cat has used the litter box recently or if a dog is waiting by the litter box, for example, to eat the waste product, the cat may prefer to use another location to eliminate (Figure 24-7).

Cats that experience pain while urinating or defecating (e.g., due to constipation, arthritic pain or, lower urinary tract pain) may also develop an aversion to using the litter box and cats that do not like the feel of large or sharp pieces of litter between their toes (Figure 24-8) or

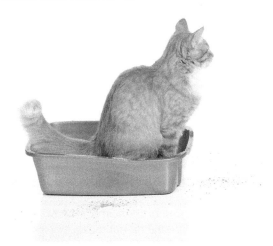

FIGURE 24-6 Many commercial litter boxes are too small for adult cats. Litter boxes should be big enough for the cat to enter, turn around, scratch, and eliminate. (Copyright © iStock.com)

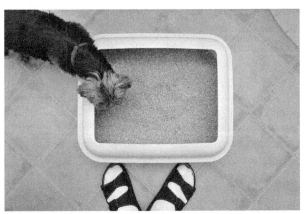

FIGURE 24-7 Many dogs like to eat cat feces because of the high protein content in the cat food, making these appealing to them. If a dog is loitering around the litter box, the cat is likely to choose another location. (Copyright © iStock.com)

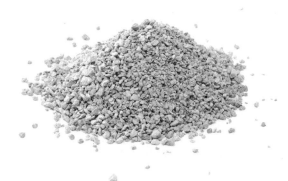

FIGURE 24-8 Some litters are uncomfortable for a cat's feet. This is a clumping litter with very large pieces, making it more likely to clump between toes, especially in long-haired and polyuric cats (e.g., diabetic cats and cats receiving subcutaneous fluids). Discomfort from getting pieces of litter between toes or the pressure of the rocks on sensitive feet can lead to house soiling. (Copyright © iStock.com)

have so much hair growing there that the litter gets caught in it, leading to discomfort, may also seek an alternative toileting location.

The positioning of the litter facilities is a crucial factor in determining their usage, and in multicat households there can be problems relating to the distribution of the boxes in relation to the numbers of social groups of cats in the household. When all of the litter boxes are placed side by side in the same location there can be issues of access for some cats; for example a confident cat may sit blocking the path to the boxes and, as a result, a more timid cat may eliminate in another area to avoid potential confrontation (see Figure 24-1). The selection of a location for the litter box may be based more on what is convenient for the owner than on the preference of the cat; for example, when litter boxes are placed in basements near equipment that is noisy or that intermittently vibrates, such as a washer, dryer, water softener, or furnace, the cat may look elsewhere for a suitable toileting area.

Preference for Alternative Substrate and/or Locations

Preferences for alternative substrates and locations can also develop for many reasons. In some cases, it is because the cat has developed an aversion to the litter box type, the litter, or the location and has eliminated in an alternative location or on a different substrate, which it learns to prefer. For example, if the litter box is located in a very busy location, the cat may seek a more private area in which to eliminate. Once found, this may quickly develop into a preferred option. Similarly, if cats are offered litter substrates that do not appeal to them, they may eliminate on soft materials, bedding, carpets, or even empty bathtubs and find these more attractive in the future (Figure 24-9).

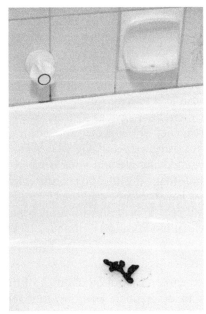

FIGURE 24-9 Some cats will use the empty bathtub to eliminate. (Courtesy J. Ley)

Anxiety-Related Problems

Anxiety is caused in part by a problem with how the brain functions, and it is a medical problem just as diabetes is caused by a problem with how the pancreas functions. Information is conveyed between different parts of the brain via neurotransmitters and there is a vast array of these chemical messengers that have varying effects on emotional responses. These messengers bind to neuroreceptors, and therefore emotional responses can be affected either by varying concentrations of neurotransmitters, such as low levels of serotonin or noradrenaline, or by problems related to the number or function of the neuroreceptors. These emotional responses may then lead to physiological reactions in other parts of the brain and body. For example, the bowel and skin may be affected and this may lead to gastrointestinal or dermatological problems. In the brain, this may lead to difficulty remembering new information. The result is that anxious animals can find it difficult to learn new things. They may also have issues of pruritus or gastric sensitivity.

Cats with anxiety disorders or fearful cats may eliminate when they are frightened or may not go to the litter box as they are too frightened to move to that area.

Although separation-related anxiety is not well described in cats, this condition may also lead to elimination problems, which are usually seen when the owner is absent. The cat may choose to eliminate on the objects associated with the owner, such as clothes, bedding, briefcases, and shoes. In the author's experience it is usually seen after separations greater than 12 hours; however, it may also occur immediately after the owner returns.

Differential Diagnoses

Medical conditions, such as FIC, other causes of FLUTD, and any of the multiple causes of polyuria have been implicated as factors that may contribute to problems of urine elimination. Likewise, diarrhea, constipation, hyperthyroidism, or other gastrointestinal problems can lead to fecal soiling. However, these cats often use their litter box as well as other locations, and the frequency of the waste products or the consistency of the waste products is altered (see Figure 24-10). Once the underlying medical issue is resolved, the cat may continue to use the litter box consistently, but preferences may have become established for other locations and this will need to be dealt with using behavioral and environmental modification techniques.

Treatment

As outlined earlier, careful questioning of the client is important to differentiate marking from elimination in unacceptable locations. A questionnaire that the client may complete prior to the consultation is an effective way to make sure that as many differentials as possible are considered. The clients should also be asked to provide a map of the house (see Figure 24-2) with the location of litter boxes, food, water, and resting stations as well as any deposits that the client has considered to be in an unacceptable location, as this can add valuable information.

Treatment of elimination-related house soiling problems involves three key areas: dealing with potential disease and addressing litter facilities and emotional motivations. The combined use of environmental management, behavior modification, and, where applicable, medication and additional therapies, such as pheromonatherapy, will offer the best chance of resolution.

Disease

In addition to a complete behavioral history, a thorough physical examination is needed and complete blood count and chemistry profile with electrolytes, urinalysis, and radiography, or other imaging procedures may also be required to exclude medical causes. Since urine and fecal soiling may occur with hyperthyroid disease, thyroid testing should occur in cats 7 years and older or in younger cats if there is reason for suspicion. Urine culture should be performed if the soiling is urine-related. If an underlying physical disorder is identified, appropriate medical treatment should be instituted alongside the necessary behavioral and environmental modification.

Addressing Litter Facilities

Dealing with the litter box related factors in cases of elimination in unacceptable locations involves two main areas:

- increasing the attractiveness of the area the owner wants the cat to use; and
- decreasing the attractiveness of the area that the cat wants to use.

Appropriate cleaning is a very important part of reducing the attraction of previously soiled locations by removing not only the physical stain of the deposits but also the odor. The soiled areas should be cleaned with non ammonia-based products, such as enzymatic clothes-washing powders which break down the protein component of the deposit. A 10% solution is usually recommended. The subsequent use of an alcohol to remove the fat component of urinary deposits is also recommended but it is important to ask clients to test an area to ensure the colorfastness of their carpets or furnishings before using this on a large scale. There are a number of commercially available neutralizers such as Animal Odour Eliminator, Bac to Nature, Anti Icky Poo, or Urine Off, which can be effective in removing the odor when used after cleaning the area with water, but results can vary.

Increasing the attraction of the appropriate toileting site is achieved through environmental management to help make the litter box more attractive to the cat.

Litter and litter box preference tests, done one at a time, provide an opportunity to find the litter type and box type as well as the location that best meets the individual cat's needs. Cats are very good at showing their preferences so using a diary to record when and how often the cat uses each litter box, with each litter type and in which location, can provide valuable information to get the cat back into the litter box. In the author's experience providing three locations and three litter types for a period of 2 weeks each and then swapping is a technique that is a good starting point.

There are a number of important features of the litter facilities that should be addressed.

1. Cleanliness

Cats do not like dirty litter boxes, and it is therefore very important to institute an appropriate and regular cleaning regime. A routine of daily scooping and cleaning the tray out completely once a week is recommended for non clumping litter. This regime is also recommended for clumping litter in the UK and Australia, but in the United States (or North America) a complete change of clumping litter only once every 2 to 3 weeks is considered adequate. This may be due to a difference in litter products in the different countries. However, it is important to top up boxes with clumping litter after daily scooping to ensure an adequate depth of litter is maintained. The cleaning regime must also be modified dependent on the number of boxes, the feline preference for specific boxes, and the presence of relevant medical conditions. For example, if a cat has diabetes mellitus or diarrhea, more frequent cleaning is needed (Figure 24-10), and if the cats in the household prefer one location, more frequent scooping and changing may also be needed (Figure 24-11).

Changing the products used to clean the litter box can also help to attract cats, especially if disinfectants or bleaches have been used in the past. These products can be extremely pungent and therefore offensive to the feline sense of smell. Using soapy water or hot water only and allowing the litter box to dry in direct sunlight (or air dry when direct sunlight is not available) is recommended.

2. Number and location

Increasing the number of litter boxes, especially in multicat households, is essential. A good rule of thumb is one litter box per cat group or family and one extra. However, the number of trays is not the only consideration, and it is essential that the trays are placed in different locations (different rooms) that are easily accessible at all times and that provide the opportunity for cats from different social groups to eliminate in separate and visually protected locations. The litter box

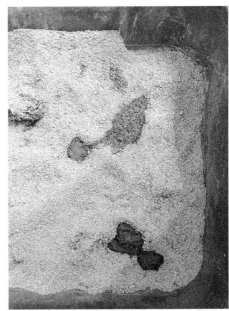

FIGURE 24-10   This cat developed diarrhea following a diet change. This litter box was cleaned less than 12 hours ago but it is important to alter cleaning regimes to take into account changes in the cat's health, and in cases like this, cleaning frequency will need to be substantially increased in the short term. (Courtesy I. Rodan)

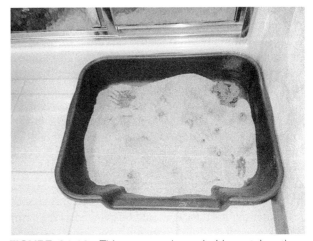

FIGURE 24-11   This two-cat household contains three large litter boxes in different locations around the home. However, both of the cats prefer this litter box, possibly because of its location. This is what the box looked like prior to scooping after a 24-hour period and it illustrates the importance of owners adjusting the frequency of cleaning to take into account the increased usage. It is also important to consider why the other two litter box locations are not considered suitable by the cats. Note that this is a large litter box designed for dogs up to 35 pounds. Each of the two cats weigh between 7 and 10 pounds. (Courtesy I. Rodan)

distribution should be such that if all of the cats in the household decided to eliminate at the same time they would be able to access a latrine without running the gauntlet of an unfamiliar or incompatible cat. Once the trays have been distributed, the frequency of use should be noted as this will help owners decide which locations are preferred by the cats and which locations are less attractive to them.

If the cat is eliminating in very specific locations, placing a litter box over the area being used by the cat can help to direct it back to using the litter box. Then, once the litter box is being used consistently, it can very gradually be moved to another location. This may mean moving the box in increments as small as 5 cm daily.

To decrease the attractiveness of the area the cat prefers to use, it can be helpful to change the function of the unacceptable elimination location. However, these ideas will only be useful if the cat has one or two areas that are used for elimination.

Most cats will prefer not to eliminate in their feeding, resting, or play areas so the function of the previously soiled locations can be altered by providing food, bedding, and play activity.

Confining the cat to a small area in order to reestablish its toileting association with a suitable litter box and litter material has been suggested, but it is important to ensure that the area offered provides for all of the cats other behavioral needs. The cat is gradually allowed access to larger areas as it uses the litter box consistently. This approach may be helpful in some cases, but if it is a multicat household, the act of confinement and therefore separation from the other cats may help the problem resolve initially but once the cats are reintroduced, the problem may recur. In such cases, the elimination issues may be an indication of tension between the cats, which needs to be further investigated.

Making the unacceptable locations less accessible by covering the area with thick plastic, aluminum foil or double sided sticky tape has been recommended by some authors but the most important aim is to provide an alternative toileting site which is attractive to the cat and fulfils its basic toileting requirements. Any devices that aim to make the unacceptable locations unpleasant or frightening for the cat should be avoided as they run the risk of contributing to negative emotional reactions from the cat, which could further complicate the behavioral issues.

3. Box size and type

Some cats prefer a larger area, and the provision of larger boxes might be a first consideration.[10] The provision of a litter box that is large enough for the cat (at least 1½ times the length of the cat from the tip of the nose to the base of the tail) can be beneficial. Seedling trays or storage boxes can make good alternatives to

cat litter boxes (Figures 24-12 and 24-13) as commercial litter boxes are often not large enough.

Some cats prefer privacy when they eliminate, so covering the litter box to make it more private for the cat may be helpful. Placing a cardboard box, with appropriate openings over the litter box, has been reported to be useful, and if it is found that the cat has a preference for being enclosed, a hooded litter box may be used (Figure 24-14). However, it is important to inform owners that the scent is usually stronger in covered boxes, and these boxes, including the covers, will require a more frequent cleaning regime.

4. Litter type

Providing the cat with alternative types of litter, such as clumping litters, sand, or soil, will help determine the cat's preference for substrate. Sometimes a combination of substrates is effective.

Work by Borchelt has shown that texture and granularity or coarseness affect the cat's preference for litter material.[11] Cats prefer finely textured litter that is not

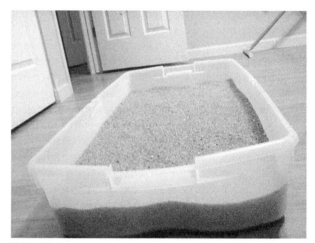

FIGURE 24-12 Large storage containers can make excellent litter boxes. (Courtesy K. Mundschenk)

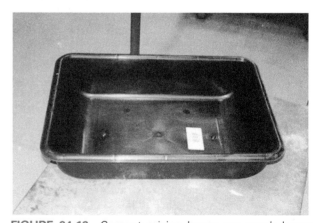

FIGURE 24-13 Cement mixing boxes are much larger than commercial litter boxes and may make good litter boxes. (Courtesy K. Mundschenk)

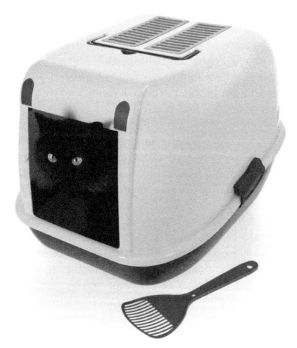

FIGURE 24-14 Some cats prefer covered litter boxes. The scent of elimination deposits is stronger in a covered box, which means these boxes often need increased frequency of cleaning, and the lid should also be cleaned. (Copyright © iStock.com)

too heavy, or a substrate of fine sand consistency (compare Figures 24-8 and 24-12).

One study indicated that there might be a correlation between time spent digging and litter preference[12] and this may offer a means of assessing litter preference.

Studies have shown that cats have preferences for clumping litter over clay, recycled paper, and a lightweight flushable litter with a pH indicator.[11,13,14] Litter additives have been developed to increase litter appeal but no controlled trial data has been published to support their use. Scented litters were found to be a risk factor for elimination in unacceptable locations in one study, while a more recent study found no association with elimination problems.[12] Therefore, it might be prudent to offer both scented and unscented litters in separate boxes and locations as in a preference test.

Removing the liners in litter boxes can also add to the attractiveness of the litter box.

For cats that prefer smooth surfaces like bathtubs and sinks, an empty litter box can be effective. If the cat persists in urinating or defecating in the bathtub, sometimes leaving a few inches of water in the bottom helps to stop this habit. However, the cat should always be provided with another litter box.

5. Litter depth
Varying the depth of litter can help to provide information about the cat's preferences. In relation to

defecation, sufficient depth has also been determined to be a factor, with a strong preference for defecation in deeper litter.[15] It is always important to consider individual preferences as some cats may prefer less litter. For example, some cats with long fur may prefer a shallower substrate because of their coat dragging in the litter.

Addressing Emotional Motivations

In some cases of elimination in unacceptable locations there is an interplay between the cat's emotional health and their toileting behavior. Extensive behavioral history-taking will be necessary to determine the origins of any negative emotional states such as fear or anxiety, and behavioral and environmental modifications should be employed to help increase self-confidence and improve positive emotional responses. Specific triggers for anxiety, such as tension between cats in the household or in the neighborhood, will need to be addressed. Medication may be needed for some cats that are anxious (see Chapter 19), and the treatment plan may also include the use of the synthetic pheromone, Feliway. Further details on the practical application of pheromone therapy are included in Chapter 18.

Elimination is a physiological response and is always appropriate for the individual even when the location is unacceptable for the humans with whom the cat lives. For this reason, punishment is never an appropriate response to this behavior. In addition, a punitive approach serves to further increase anxiety as well as impede learning of appropriate, nonanxious behavior and is therefore counterproductive in dealing with cases of elimination in unacceptable locations.

MARKING

The most common manifestation of unacceptable marking behavior in the home is urine spraying. Feces can also be used as a communication tool, and marking using fecal deposits is referred to as middening. However, defecation outside the litter box is only rarely seen as a marking behavior and is far less common than urine marking. Treatment is based on dealing with the underlying emotional motivation in the same way as when dealing with spraying cases and for this reason, the references to marking behavior in this chapter will be primarily related to urine marking.

During urine spraying, a cat usually backs up to a vertical surface or object and directs a stream of urine toward it. However, it can also occur in some cats voiding on horizontal surfaces. It is a response to hormonal motivation when it is used in a sexual context but can also be a behavioral response to an emotional state and may be motivated by territorial or agonistic situations (see Chapter 3). In multicat households indoor marking is commonly associated with overt or covert aggression. Due to the sexual role of urine marking, intact cats are reported to spray more than neutered cats, but emotionally motivated spraying occurs in males and females, both neutered and not. Male cats are generally considered to spray more than female cats, and in one study, the problem is reported in 12% of neutered males and 4% of spayed females,[16] while another study reported that 10% of castrated males and 5% of spayed females spray.[17] Spraying appears to be more common in multicat households, with a reported 100% chance of at least one cat spraying in a household with more than 10 cats.[18]

Commonly sprayed sites include prominent objects such as plants and furniture, boundaries and exits, and new objects in the home. Cats that spray generally still use their litter box for elimination of urine and feces. On rare occasions, cats that urinate or defecate on horizontal surfaces may also be marking.

Territorial, agonistic encounters and highly arousing environmental or social stimuli (e.g., the sight, sound, and/or smell of another cat within the household as well as outside) have been reported to be associated with spraying. Subtle changes in scent profiles within the home through the introduction of new furnishings or through the use of electrical items can also be associated with marking behavior, and the targeting of urine onto household items can be very distressing for owners and even dangerous. An example is when urine is deposited into plug sockets or onto electrical devices, such as toasters and kettles.

Triggers for anxiety-related marking problems may include significant changes in routine like moving to a new house and the introduction of a new spouse, new baby, or new cat, but may also be more subtle changes such as changes in the owners daily routine or reorganization of existing furniture within the home. Alterations in the neighborhood feline population may also be significant, and some authors report links between indoor marking and separation related behavior.

Clinical Signs

Cats that urine spray usually stand and deposit the urine onto vertical surfaces but they may also squat and leave deposits on horizontal surfaces. They usually produce only a small quantity of urine and rarely engage in any scratching or covering behavior afterwards.

Differential Diagnoses

It is reported that up to 30% of cats that present for spraying may have a concurrent medical condition,[19] and it is therefore important to consider possible medical differentials as a first line approach. The possibility of lower urinary tract disease, resulting in partial blockage of the urethra of the male cat and causing the cat to adopt a standing posture to urinate should always be considered as prompt medical attention is needed in these cases. The potential for other medical conditions such as impacted anal glands or conditions associated with the urogenital system, including urinary calculi, renal failure or cystitis, to be involved should also be considered. Feline idiopathic cystitis is an important differential when multiple small deposits of urine are found in the house.

Treatment/Management

After a complete behavioral history and a thorough physical examination, other tests including complete blood work and biochemistry, urinalysis, and radiography (or other imaging or diagnostic techniques) may be required to exclude medical causes. Medical problems need to be dealt with prior to, or at least concurrently with, any behavioral therapy that is instigated.

Owner education of normal cat behavior (see Chapters 3 and 23) is important, so that they understand that the behavior may not be completely eliminated but can usually be managed successfully.

The majority of owned cats in most countries are already neutered, but if the motivation for the marking behavior is hormonal then neutering the intact cat has been shown to be successful in most cases. Castration will reduce or eliminate spraying in up to 90% of intact males,[18] and therefore should be considered a sensible first approach in these cases.

The treatment/management approach for emotionally motivated indoor urine marking involves three key areas: environmental management, behavior modification, and, where necessary, medication, pheromones, and nutraceuticals.

Environmental Management

Indoor urine marking results from a loss of security within the household and a loss of perception of the home as a core territory for the cat. Environmental management aims to restore the core territory status of the home and increase the cat's perception of it as a safe place to be. If possible, specific anxiety-provoking stimuli should be removed or minimized, but this can often be difficult to achieve in practice. For example, it is not practicable to remove the next-door neighbor's cat, the new baby, or new spouse or entirely prevent other anxiety-provoking circumstances, such as moving.

However, it is possible to mitigate the effects of these stressors, and recommendations that have been beneficial include:

- Decreasing the number of cats in the household if possible. This can sometimes be achieved by separating the cats so they cannot see each other, but in some cases, rehoming should be considered and owners will need to be given appropriate counseling when considering this option.
- Decreasing physical access to windows and doors to decrease the sight, sound, and smell of cats outside

the house that may increase arousal. It may also help to limit visual access by the addition of temporary frosting to the surfaces of windows and glass doors.

- Changing the amount of time spent indoors or outdoors. If it is possible to give access to outdoors this may be beneficial, but all decisions should be made on a case-by-case basis. The decision must take into account the need for the cat to express normal behaviors and receive adequate mental and physical stimulation and also the need to protect the cat from potential confrontation from other cats in the neighborhood or harm from traffic. It may be beneficial to consider building a cat enclosure so the cat is still confined on the property as is required in some jurisdictions and favored by some owners due to risk from roads in built-up areas.

- Changing the function of sprayed areas by designating them to be core territory through the provision of food, bedding, and toys.

- Removing the scent of previous deposits which will decay and potentially induce the cat to overmark in order to keep its signal fresh. The areas should be cleaned effectively following the guidance given earlier in this chapter.

- Some cats will be content to spray inside the litter box itself, making the spraying behavior more acceptable to owners. Cats are more likely to do this in boxes that have high sides. This type of box is also effective for cats that tend to rise during elimination, which sometimes causes the urine to spill over the edge of the box (Figure 24-15).

Behavior Modification

Cats should always be rewarded for calm and relaxed behavior, and this should be done with quiet praise rather than with food or physical petting, which may increase arousal levels. Marking is a natural behavior

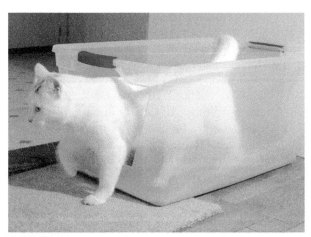

FIGURE 24-15 Providing a box with high sides but with easy access in and out of the box can be useful for "high risers" or cats that raise their hind ends as they urinate. (Courtesy D. Givin)

and is designed to reduce the risk of feline confrontation. Punishing cats that are marking indoors will therefore lead to confusion and increase negative emotional states of anxiety and fear. This will impede learning of appropriate, nonanxious behavior and is therefore counterproductive in managing these cases.

Medication/Pheromones and Nutraceuticals (see Chapters 18 and 19)

When medication is considered, the aim is to reduce the anxiety level of the cat by altering the neurochemical environment in conjunction with behavior modification and environmental management.

Potential side effects should be explained to the client prior to instigating any therapy, as most of the medications are not registered/licensed for use in cats. The use of signed consent forms is also important. Complete diagnostic testing should be carried out prior to medication, and all medication should be gradually withdrawn under veterinary supervision and never stopped suddenly.

The most commonly used medications are tricyclic antidepressants (TCAs), such as clomipramine, and selective serotonin reuptake inhibitors (SSRIs), such as fluoxetine. However, benzodiazepines, azapirones, and antihistamines have proven useful in some cases. Many of the studies on marking have been careful to avoid other concurrent therapy, which might alter the outcome. Therefore, with concurrent behavioral modification, environmental management, and using medication in conjunction with pheromones, an even greater level of improvement and lower recurrence might be achieved.

Clomipramine has been shown to reduce spraying and is licensed in Australia for this use.[5,20-22] In one study, 25 cats were treated with clomipramine at a dose of approximately 0.5 mg/kg daily for a minimum of 30 days. Twenty of the 25 cats had a 75% or greater reduction in spraying within 4 weeks and spraying resolved or improved to a level of 90% or greater in 17 of the cats.[20]

After 6 months, 15 cats remained on the medication, many on a lower dose, and five cats were successfully withdrawn.[20] Another study determined that a dose of 0.25 to 0.5 mg/kg was the optimum dose for initiation of clomipramine therapy.[21]

Amitriptyline has also been widely used at a dose rate of 0.5 mg/kg once daily but many veterinarians report difficulty with administration due to the bitterness of the medication.

Fluoxetine has been shown to be effective for treating spraying at a dose of 1 mg/kg once every 24 hours.[23] In a placebo controlled study of 17 cats, those treated with fluoxetine had a significant decrease in spraying by week 2 and continued to decrease through weeks 7 and 8. Two of the cats that did not improve to a level of 70% or greater were given an increased dose of 1.5 mg/kg in weeks 7 and 8. Recurrence after drug withdrawal was variable, with cats marking the greatest at baseline most likely to recur.[24] Generally, it is recommended to start at a dose of 0.5 mg/kg once every 24 hours and assess response.

Other SSRIs such as paroxetine (0.25 to 1 mg/kg every 24 hours) and sertraline (0.5 to 1 mg/kg every 24 hours) have also been used off-label with, anecdotally, some success.

Another study compared the efficacy of clomipramine at 0.5 mg/kg per day with fluoxetine at 1 mg/kg per day in cats treated for 16 weeks. Efficacy was similar with treatment of longer than 8 weeks, leading to increased efficacy. Recidivism occurred after abrupt drug withdrawal of fluoxetine in most cats but could be controlled if medication was reinstituted.[23]

Diazepam has been reported to be effective at reducing spraying by 75% or greater in 55% to 74% of cats.[24,25] In one study, higher success was achieved in neutered males (84% to 25%).[23] Dose rates of 0.5 mg/kg daily have been reported to be effective. However, diazepam has been associated with hepatotoxicity in some cats and its use has been superseded by the TCAs and SSRIs in recent years.[26,27]

Buspirone, although not widely used, has also been reported to be effective in reducing spraying in 55% of cats, with 33% resolved. The relapse rate after 8 weeks of treatment upon withdrawal was 53% compared with over 75% with diazepam.[25] Dose rate is reported as 0.5 to 1 mg/kg every 8 to 12 hours.[24]

Cyproheptadine has been reported as being effective for the control of urine marking, especially in male cats. However, in one study, clomipramine was found to be more effective than cyproheptadine.[28]

Although progestins have been shown to improve behavior in about 30% of marking cats (50% of neutered males and 10% of spayed females), their use is now considered to be inappropriate and outdated as the potential for adverse effects (immune suppression, mammary tumors, etc.) is high and they do not address the underlying cause of anxiety.

The synthetic analogue of feline facial pheromone, Feliway, has been reported to reduce urine spraying in 74% to 97% of cats; but in one study, only 33.3% of treated households had a complete resolution of the spraying.[29,30] A Feliway, diffuser has been found to be effective at reducing urine marking. When spraying is due to a recent change in the environment, such as the introduction of a new cat, renovations, or moving, Feliway could be considered as a stand-alone option.

It should be used for a minimum of 2 to 3 months. Feliway MultiCat is a newer product which is recommended for use in multicat households and when introducing a new cat into the household but is currently only available in the United States. More details about pheromone therapy can be found in Chapter 18.

In addition to medications and pheromone therapies, there are several nutraceutical products on the market containing active ingredients such as L-theanine, tryptophan, α-casozepine, which to date only have weak studies or anecdotal reports of their usefulness in spraying (see Chapter 19).

CONCLUSION

House soiling problems are a common source of enquiries to veterinary practices and raise significant welfare concerns for feline patients. They are also potentially distressing for clients and threaten the pet–owner bond. Differentiating between medical causes, elimination problems, and marking problems is the key to successfully managing these cases, and a combination of medical and behavioral history and examination will be needed in order to achieve this. Once an accurate diagnosis of the underlying cause has been made, the treatment and management of the case will involve a combined medical, environmental, and behavioral approach. Client education relating to normal feline behaviors will also be important.

ADDITIONAL RESOURCES

AAFP and ISFM Guidelines for Diagnosing and Solving - House-Soiling Behavior in Cats (2014), http://jfm.sagepub.com/content/16/7/579.full.pdf+html (Accessed March 22, 2015).

House-Soiling: Cat Owner Questionnaire, http://jfm.sagepub.com/content/suppl/2014/06/17/16.7.579.DC1/Cat_owner_questionnaire.pdf (Accessed March 22, 2015).

House-Soiling: Take-Home Instructions for Cat Owners, http://jfm.sagepub.com/content/suppl/2014/06/17/16.7.579.DC1/Take_home_instructions_for_cat_owners.pdf (Accessed March 22, 2015).

Feline House-Soiling: Useful Information for Cat Owners (client brochure), http://www.catvets.com/public/PDFs/ClientBrochures/HouseSoiling-WebView.pdf (Accessed March 22, 2015).

REFERENCES

1. Overall KL. *Clinical Behavioural Medicine for Small Animals.* St Louis: Mosby; 1997, pp. 5–8.
2. Blackshaw JK. Feline elimination problems. *Anthrozoös.* 1992;5:52–56.
3. Denenberg S, Landsberg GM, Horwitz D, Seksel K. A Comparison of Cases Referred to Behaviorists in Three Different Countries. In: Mills D, Levine E, Landsberg G, et al. *Current Issues and Research in Veterinary*

Behavioral Medicine. Ashland: Purdue University Press; 2005:56–62.

4. Salman MD, Hutchison J, Ruch-Gallie R, et al. Behavioral reasons for relinquishment of dogs and cats to 12 shelters. *J Appl Anim Welf*. 2000;2:93–106.

5. Seksel K, Lindeman MJ. Use of clomipramine in the treatment of anxiety-related and obsessive-compulsive disorders in cats. *Aust Vet J*. 1998;76(5):317–321.

6. Westropp JL, Buffington CA. Feline idiopathic cystitis: current understanding of pathophysiology and management. *Vet Clin North Am Small Anim Pract*. 2004;34:1043–1055.

7. Cameron ME, Casey RA, Bradshaw JW, et al. A study of environmental and behavioural factors that may be associated with feline idiopathic cystitis. *J Small Anim Pract*. 2004;45:144–147.

8. Buffington CA. Idiopathic cystitis in domestic cats: beyond the lower urinary tract. *J Vet Intern Med*. 2011;25:784–796.

9. Carney HC, Sadek TP, Curtis TM, et al. AAFP and ISFM guidelines for diagnosing and solving house-soiling behavior in cats. *J Feline Med Surg*. 2014;16:579–598.

10. Neilson JC. *Is Bigger Better? Litter Box Size Preference Test*. New Orleans: Proceedings of ACVB/AVSAB; 2008, pp. 46–49.

11. Borchelt PL. Cat elimination behavior problems. *Vet Clin North Am Small Anim Pract*. 1991;21:257–264.

12. Sung W, Crowell-Davis SL. Elimination behavior patterns of domestic cats (Felis catus) with and without elimination behavior problems. *Am J Vet Res*. 2006;67:1500–1504.

13. Neilson JC. Pearl vs. Clumping Litter Preference in a Population of Shelter Cats. In: *Proceedings of AVSAB*; 2001:14.

14. Smith K, Dreschel NA. A comparison of cat preferences for litterbox substrates. *Newsletter of the American Veterinary Society of Animal Behavior*. 2008;30(2):6–7.

15. Mills DS, Munster C. *Litter Depth Preference in the Domestic Cat*. Caloundra, Australia: Proceedings of the 4th International Veterinary Behaviour Meeting; 2003, pp. 201–202.

16. Hart BL. Behavioral and pharmacologic approaches to problem urination in cats. *Vet Clin North Am Small Anim Pract*. 1996;26:651–658.

17. Hart BL, Cooper L. Factors related to urine spraying and fighting in prepubertally gonadectomized cats. *J Am Vet Med Assoc*. 1984;184:1255–1258.

18. Pryor PA, Hart BL, Bain MJ, et al. Causes of urine marking in cats and effects of environmental management on frequency of marking. *J Am Vet Med Assoc*. 2001;219:1709–1713.

19. Frank DF, Erb HN, Houpt KA. Urine spraying in cats: presence of concurrent disease and effects of a pheromone treatment. *J Appl Anim Behav Sci*. 1999;61:263–272.

20. Landsberg G, Wilson AL. Effects of clomipramine on cats presented for urine marking. *J Am Anim Hosp Assoc*. 2005;41:3–11.

21. King JN, Steffan J, Heath SE, et al. Determination of the dosage of clomipramine for the treatment of urine spraying in cats. *J Am Vet Med Assoc*. 2004;225:881–887.

22. Hart BL, Cliff KD, Tynes VV, Bergman L. Control of urine marking by use of long-term treatment with fluoxetine or clomipramine in cats. *J Am Vet Med Assoc*. 2005;226:378–382.

23. Pryor PA, Hart BL, Cliff KD, et al. Effects of a selective serotonin reuptake inhibitor on urine spraying behavior in cats. *J Am Vet Med Assoc*. 2001;219:1557–1561.

24. Hart BL, Eckstein RA, Powell KL, et al. Effectiveness of buspirone on urine spraying and inappropriate urination in cats. *J Am Vet Med Assoc*. 1993;203:254–258.

25. Marder A. Psychotropic drugs and behavioral therapy. *Vet Clin North Am Small Anim Pract*. 1991;21:329–342.

26. Center SA, Elston TH, Rowland PH, et al. Fulminant hepatic failure associated with oral administration of diazepam in 11 cats. *J Am Vet Med Assoc*. 1996;209(3):618–625.

27. Park FM. Successful treatment of hepatic failure secondary to diazepam administration in a cat. *J Feline Med Surg*. 2012;14(2):158–160.

28. Kroll T, Houpt KA. A Comparison of Cyproheptadine and Clomipramine for the Treatment of Spraying Cats. In: *Proceedings of the 3rd International Conference on Veterinarian Behavioural Medicine, Herts, UK*; 2001:184–185.

29. Ogata N, Takeuchi Y. Clinical trial of a feline pheromone analogue for feline urine marking. *J Vet Med Sci*. 2001;63:157–161.

30. Mills DS, Mills CB. Evaluation of a novel method for delivering a synthetic analogue of feline facial pheromone to control urine spraying by cats. *Vet Record*. 2001;149:197–199.

31. Tynes VV, Hart BL, Pryor PA, et al: Evaluation of the role of lower urinary tract disease.

Behavior Problems of the Senior Cat

Gary M. Landsberg and Sagi Denenberg

INTRODUCTION

As a result of advances in veterinary medicine and feline nutrition, along with responsible and caring pet ownership, domestic cats are living longer than ever before. The average lifespan of cats has increased by approximately 15% over the last 20 years, and senior cats now account for approximately 30% of the feline populaion.[1,2] The senior years can be a challenging period for both the owner and the cat. Hyperthyroidism, renal failure, sensory impairment, a decline in immune function, and an increase in painful conditions, such as degenerative joint disease (DJD), become increasingly more common with age. For many of these health problems, the first and sometimes only sign is a change in behavior. In addition, coping abilities decline and increases in anxiety and irritability and alterations in social interactions begin to occur. While changes in the pet's environment or medical issues may cause or contribute to these changes, cognitive dysfunction syndrome (CDS) may also be responsible for many of the behavioral changes that arise in senior pets.

Early recognition and reporting of behavioral signs provide the best possibility for effective management, yet many clients do not discuss changes in behavior with their veterinarian.[3] This may be because the clients:
(1) do not know the difference between normal and abnormal aging;
(2) are unaware of the importance of prompt reporting;
(3) do not know that treatment options might be available;
(4) think that euthanasia might be recommended.[4]

Primary veterinarians must be proactive in asking about behavioral changes, in educating pet owners about the value of early detection, and in describing treatment options that are available to treat or slow the progress of many of the health, behavior, and welfare issues of senior pets.

ASSESSING SENIOR CATS DURING VETERINARY VISITS

When a senior cat is presented for each healthcare visit, the use of a detailed questionnaire can be useful to detect subtle behavioral changes and to allow the clinician to focus on the client's concerns (Table 25-1). The findings of the physical exam and laboratory screening tests, together with the knowledge of all of the cat's medical and behavioral signs, provide the information needed to make a diagnosis and implement treatment strategies. Many of the diseases of senior cats can cause or contribute to behavioral changes (Table 25-2). While cognitive dysfunction may be the cause of many of these changes, ruling out other medical conditions is the first step. Painful conditions, endocrinopathies, renal and hepatic disease, neurologic disorders, and sensory decline might contribute to the confusion, irritability, and aggression of the pet. Endocrinopathies, renal or hepatic disease, musculoskeletal disease, and urinary tract disease can lead to house soiling. Dermatologic conditions including hypersensitivity reactions, neuropathic pain, and neurologic disease and myopathies can lead to excessive grooming or hyperesthesia, while any disease affecting the central nervous system (CNS) can lead to changes in mentation, mood, and cognition (see Table 25-2). In addition, since nutrient digestibility and absorption may be affected by age, underlying deficiencies may also account for some of the physical and behavioral signs.[5]

CATEGORIES OF BEHAVIOR PROBLEMS IN SENIOR CATS

The behavior problems of senior cats can be categorized into:
(1) more serious behavior concerns presented to the veterinarian by the client because of their effects on the client's health and welfare or the welfare of the cat
(2) behavior changes associated with aging that may not be of sufficient concern to the client to mention to the veterinarian without prompting.

In the latter category are many of the early cases of feline cognitive dysfunction for which prevalence increases with age, but reporting is likely to be low (Box 25-1).[6–8]

TABLE 25-1 Feline Cognitive Screening Questionnaire*		
Pet's Name: **Age:** **Date:**		
	When did signs begin?	**Score**

A: DISORIENTATION—AWARENESS—SPATIAL ORIENTATION
Gets stuck or cannot get around objects
Stares blankly at walls or floor
Cannot find/leaves dropped food
Goes into wrong side of door; walks into door/walls
Aimless vocalization

B: ALTERED SOCIAL INTERACTIONS
Decreased interest in petting/avoids contact
Decreased greeting behavior
In need of constant contact, overdependent, "clingy"
Altered relationship with other household pets—less social
Altered relationship with other household pets—fear/anxiety
Aggression
• to family members __ ; unfamiliar people__
• to family pets__ ; unfamiliar pets ___
• Other:

C: RESPONSE TO STIMULI
Decreased response to auditory stimuli (sounds)
Increased response, fear, phobia to auditory stimuli
Decreased response to visual stimuli (sights)
Increased response, fear, phobia to visual stimuli
Decreased responsiveness to food/odor

D: SLEEP-WAKE CYCLES; REVERSED DAY/NIGHT SCHEDULE
Restless sleep/waking at nights
Increased daytime sleep

E: ACTIVITY INCREASED/REPETITIVE/ANXIETY
Pacing/wanders aimlessly
Increased vocalization
Excessive grooming

F: ACTIVITY—APATHY/DEPRESSED
Decreased interest in food/treats
Decreased exploration/activity
Decreased interest in social interactions/play
Decreased self-care

G: LEARNING AND MEMORY—WORK, TASKS
Decreased ability to perform task
Decreased responsiveness to cues and tricks
Inability/slow to learn new tasks (retrain)

H: LEARNING AND MEMORY—HOUSE SOILING
Indoor elimination at sites previously trained
Forgets the location of litter box

*To be used by veterinarians and staff for screening feline patients.
Modified from Landsberg G, Hunthausen W, Ackerman L: Behavior problems of the dog and cat, ed 3. St Louis, 2013, Saunders.
Key: 0=none 1=mild 2=moderate 3=severe.

Behavior Complaints Presented to Veterinarians by Clients

Compiling evidence from three different behavior referral practices of 83 cats, the most common problems were house soiling (both vertical and horizontal, urine and stool) accounting for 73%; inter-cat aggression, 10%; aggression to people, 10%; excessive vocalization and restlessness, each with 6%; and overgrooming, 4%.[6,7,9] In a survey of three behavior referral centers (St Louis in the United States, Sydney in Australia, and Toronto in Canada), it is found that among senior cats, 53% presented with house soiling, 17% with aggression problems, 17% with anxiety (including excessive vocalization and night waking), and 7% with repetitive behaviors. An important consideration is that the cases in each of these surveys were seen prior to the increased awareness of CDS in cats. To further evaluate the extent of these more serious client concerns, a search has been conducted on the Veterinary Information Network (VIN) for "senior cat behavior problems" and

TABLE 25-2 Medical Causes of Behavioral Signs	
Medical Condition	**Examples of Behavioral Signs**
Neurologic:	
Central (intracranial/extracranial), particularly if affecting forebrain, e.g., tumor, CDS, limbic/ temporal, and hypothalamic; REM sleep disorders	Altered awareness, response to stimuli, loss of learned behaviors, house soiling, disorientation, confusion, altered activity levels, temporal disorientation, vocalization, change in temperament (fear, anxiety), altered appetite, altered sleep cycles, interrupted sleep, aggression
Seizures (partial): temporal lobe epilepsy	Repetitive behaviors, self-traumatic disorders, alterations in temperament (e.g., intermittent states of fear or aggression), tremors, shaking, interrupted sleep, hyperesthesia
Peripheral neuropathy	Self-mutilation, irritability/aggression, circling, hyperesthesia
Sensory dysfunction	Altered response to stimuli, confusion, disorientation, irritability/ aggression, vocalization, house soiling, altered sleep cycles
Endocrine:	
Hyperthyroidism	Irritability, aggression, urine marking, decreased or increased activity, night waking
Diabetes mellitus	Altered emotional state, irritability/aggression, anxiety, lethargy, house soiling, altered appetite
Functional ovarian and testicular tumors (Increased androgen-induced behaviors)	Males: aggression, roaming, marking, sexual attraction, mounting Females: nesting or possessive aggression of objects
Metabolic/organ dysfunction:	
Hepatic (including hepatoencephalopathy)	Irritability, aggression, altered sleep cycle, mental dullness, decreased activity, restlessness, confusion, pica, changes in appetite
Renal	House soiling, excessive drinking, apathy, irritability, excessive vocalization, irritability
Urogenital	House soiling (urine), polydypsia, waking at night
Gastrointestinal	Licking, polyphagia, pica, fecal house soiling, unsettled sleep, restlessness
Pain	Altered response to stimuli, decreased activity, restless/unsettled, vocalization, house soiling, aggression/irritability, self-trauma, waking at night
Dermatologic	Psychogenic alopecia, hyperesthesia, other self-trauma (chewing/biting/ sucking/scratching)

CDS, Cognitive dysfunction syndrome; *REM*, rapid eye movement.

BOX 25-1 What Is Feline Cognitive Dysfunction Syndrome (CDS)?

CDS is a neurodegenerative disorder of senior cats that is characterized by gradual cognitive decline and increasing brain pathology. Initial studies into brain aging in dogs identified a number of clinical and pathological changes that model the early stages of human Alzheimer disease (AD). More recently, there is evidence that this same condition is seen in cats and may parallel the changes in the aging human with respect to brain pathology, altered social relationships, and a decline in learning and memory. The diagnosis is based on a constellation of clinical signs that were first described in dogs using the acronym DISHA, or (1) Disorientation (2) altered Interactions with people or other pets, (3) altered Sleep-wake cycles, (4) House soiling, and (5) Altered activity levels.[6,7] This also encompasses a decrease in awareness or response to stimuli. In addition, fear and anxiety also appear to be associated with cognitive decline.[6,7] A similar spectrum of clinical signs have also been described in cats.[6-8] Once signs are identified, the diagnosis of CDS is made by excluding all other possible medical causes of the signs. (See Table 25-2).

"feline senility," and the most recent 100 posts pertaining to cats over 11 years have been selected. Forty-three of these cats were waking their owners and vocalizing at night, 31 had increased vocalization throughout the day, 22 showed signs of house soiling (4 spraying), 17 had signs of disorientation (wandering, pacing, staring, being unsettled), 2 were "clingy"/constantly seeking attention, and 1 case presented for inter-cat aggression and repetitive licking. The most common medical considerations were hyperthyroidism, chronic kidney disease, cardiac disease, hypertension, sensory decline (hearing, vision), and DJD. The most frequently reported environmental factors were the death of a companion cat, moving, a new baby, or a new cat in the home.

Behavior Changes Discovered by Proactive Screening

In a survey of 154 senior cats between the ages of 11 and 21 years, using a behavior questionnaire provided during routine healthcare visits, owners were asked to report any behavior changes.[6,8] Behavior signs were reported in 67 of the cats. Nineteen of these cats were diagnosed with underlying health problems (e.g. renal, thyroid). These medical issues may not have been the cause of the behavioral signs but after excluding these cats, 48 (36%) were diagnosed as having changes consistent with CDS. Older cats were more commonly affected and had more signs per cat. Fifty percent of cats over 15 years and 28% of cats aged 11 to 14 years were affected. In cats 11 to 14 years of age, the most common change was an alteration in social interactions, whereas in older cats, excessive vocalization and changes in activity were the most common signs.[6,8]

DIAGNOSIS AND TREATMENT OF SENIOR CAT BEHAVIOR PROBLEMS

Senior cat behavior problems are diagnosed in a similar manner to younger cats; however, the increased probability of a medical condition in a senior pet necessitates that the practitioner place a strong focus on ruling these out first. In fact, feline CDS is diagnosed by exclusion of other medical and behavioral causes.

Treatment of behavior problems in the senior cat can be more difficult and less successful than in younger cats, given the limitations imposed by sensory decline, organ health, endocrinopathies, pain, mobility problems, and CDS. Furthermore, the choice and dose of medications for senior cats may need to be altered due to preexisting medical conditions and increased potential for adverse effects, such as with drugs that sedate or have anticholinergic effects. Thus, behavior modification, environmental management, and drug therapy will need to be integrated to meet the needs of each individual senior cat to achieve maximal improvement.

Since many of the behavior problems of the senior pet can be seen in pets of any age, they have been discussed in other chapters throughout this text. Therefore, the following discussion will focus on some of the specific concerns that may need to be addressed in the senior pet.

Excessive Vocalization

Vocalization becomes a problem for cat owners when it occurs at unacceptable times (e.g., during the night, or when a baby is sleeping) or is particularly loud or long. (For night waking, see below.) The clinician should ask questions about the onset of the problem, its frequency, the time of the day it occurs, its duration, the type and pitch of the sound, and other changes in health or behavior. In addition, the history should look into any triggers (e.g., outdoor animals, feeding times, threatening situations, owners' absence), whether there were any known health or household issues that coincided with the onset of the problem, and the owner's response to the vocalization. Any form of attention might reinforce the behavior, while punishment, even if it reduces the behavior for the moment, only increases the cat's anxiety and does not address the underlying

cause. Painful medical conditions (e.g., DJD, gastrointestinal, urogenital, oral/dental, neuropathic, neoplasia), metabolic disorders (e.g., chronic renal disease with uremia), CNS disease including cognitive dysfunction and sensory decline, and hunger or thirst might lead to increased vocalization. Vocalization may indicate anxiety, which in the older pet could be due to health issues (discussed above), an increased sensitivity to changes in the environment, and an increased dependence on the owner to maintain comfort and security—all of which might lead to distress vocalization when the cat is separated from the owner.

Treatment

Once causes of the vocalization are identified, appropriate management can be initiated. Assuming medical issues have been addressed, the clients will next need to ensure that the cat has ready access to all of its resources, and that all of its needs, including the appropriate provision of food, drink, litter, play, exploration, rest and social interactions, are effectively met at all times and not only when the cat is actively vocalizing. In fact, if the stimuli and situations inciting vocalization can be identified, the cat can be engaged in enriching activities (play, food, toys, reward training, exploration) as an alternative to vocalization. The clients should be advised to reward calm and quiet behaviors and to passively ignore (neither reinforce nor punish) vocalization. Therefore, provided all of the cats' needs are effectively met, it might be necessary to house the cat in an area where vocalization does not disturb the owners and neither rewards nor punishment need to be given. Confinement might also serve as time out (negative punishment), provided that confinement is immediate as vocalization begins and the cat is released when quiet. Depending on the cause, medication including analgesics, anxiolytics, or products that help to induce or maintain sleep (such as a prebedtime benzodiazepine or melatonin) may be indicated.

Night Waking

Cats are described as crepuscular animals (dusk and dawn activity pattern) related to their food acquisition needs (predation) and the activity of prey.[10] Most domestic cats adjust to their owners' activity patterns. However, some cats become more active at nighttime when the owner is trying to sleep. These cats may wake the owner for attention or food. On the other hand, it may be that the cat wakes for some other reason and the behavior is reinforced by the owners who try to calm the cat by giving food or attention. While younger cats may also wake their owners at night, the problem is most common in senior cats because of CDS and the many other health issues that might be contributing factors. When presented with a case of night waking, the clinician should consider disease conditions that cause pain, discomfort, confusion, or unsettled sleep including DJD, gastrointestinal disease, kidney or liver disease, endocrine disorders such as hyperthyroidism, and hypertension. Any disease process that might increase hunger or thirst or increase urine or stool frequency could also contribute to night waking. A decline in sensory function, especially hearing or vision, may further alter the cat's awareness, activity, response to stimuli, and schedule, including when and where it sleeps. Since commonly presenting complaints of CDS are altered sleep–wake cycles and activity patterns, this is an important diagnostic consideration if other medical conditions have been ruled out. Conversely, finding another medical condition does not exclude the possibility of concurrent CDS. A diagnosis is made by thorough evaluation of the history, physical exam, blood pressure, neurologic evaluation, pain assessment, relevant laboratory testing, and all other medical and behavioral signs. It is important to be thorough in investigating whether there are other concurrent signs that might increase the index of suspicion of other medical or behavioral causes, such as decrease in activity, altered mobility, increased anxiety or avoidance, an increase in seeking attention, changes in appetite or in litter box usage, and increased vocalization. Changes in the household or daily routine, including limiting access to outdoors or to locations in the home, decreasing daytime activity, changing the feeding routine, and altering relationships between household pets, might lead to decreased quantity, quality, or length of nighttime sleep. It is also important to consider that factors that might initiate nighttime activity may not be the same as those that maintain it. Once the cat's schedule has been altered, it may be difficult to reverse as the cat sleeps more through the day. In addition, waking at night might lead to feeding and giving attention, which might reinforce the behavior, or owner responses, such as anger, frustration, or punishment, which might increase the cat's anxiety.[10] If perceived rewards are given intermittently, the problem becomes increasingly harder to resolve through extinction (removing rewards).

Treatment

Nighttime waking becomes increasingly difficult to improve the longer it has persisted. The first step is to identify and resolve underlying medical problems. However, some problems cannot be successfully resolved and health might continue to decline (e.g., sensory function, renal failure, neoplasia), improvement might be limited (e.g., gastrointestinal disorders, DJD), or the drugs used to improve the problem may in themselves have side effects (e.g., steroids). Therefore, both medical and behavioral approaches along with realistic expectations for what can be achieved may all be required to achieve a level of improvement that is satisfactory to the owners.[11]

Behavioral management should begin with investigating the possible cause of the problem to ensure that the inciting factors have been effectively addressed. Therefore, a cat that is waking at night for food may require ad lib access to food so that it can feed whenever it is motivated to do so. Where ad lib feeding is not possible, alterations in feeding patterns such as providing more frequent small meals throughout the day as well as a pre-bedtime meal and an early morning meal, a change in diet formulation, type, or amount (e.g., protein level, canned versus dry, nutrient composition), or even nighttime feeding from an automated feeder may be beneficial.[6] If night waking is triggered by relationship issues with other cats or a change in the household or daily routine, addressing the underlying issues may help improve the nighttime sleep. Make sure that the home and schedule promotes nighttime sleep by providing the cat with an easily accessible and comfortable resting place (and rewarding its use), clean litter, increased stimulation throughout the day (e.g., toys, training, and attention), and perhaps increased access to the outdoors if appropriate for the cat and the home. Cats with CDS may also require cognitive therapeutics.

House Soiling

House soiling is the most commonly reported behavior problem in cats of any age. This includes both unacceptable elimination of either urine or stools due to aversions (e.g., location, substrate, box) and preferences (e.g., locations, substrates), a medical condition (e.g., feline idiopathic cystitis, DJD), and marking behavior, which includes the spraying of urine usually on vertical surfaces, arising out of situations of anxiety or heightened arousal.

The first step in the senior cat is to perform a full physical exam including relevant laboratory testing, such as complete blood count, biochemistry levels, evaluation of thyroid and blood pressure, and urinalysis. Diagnostic imaging may also be indicated. An increase in frequency or volume, painful elimination, incontinence, or altered mobility might indicate a primary medical cause. However, even if the medical problem is identified and treated, some cats will persist due to learned avoidance, new preferences, or other concurrent health issues. For further details on house soiling, see Chapter 24. In a previously trained cat without any evidence of medical disease, the possibility of CDS should be considered. Cats with CDS are more likely to soil indiscriminately and therefore, in cases where the cat is soiling in selected locations or avoiding specific locations or surfaces, CDS is a less likely diagnosis. Although less common in senior cats, marking may also be reported. Underlying medical problems might include a retained testicle or extratesticular tissue that has developed into a functional tumor leading to marking behavior, and disease processes that might contribute to an increased irritability (e.g., hyperthyroidism).[12] Diagnosis and treatment of urine marking requires the same approach in cats of any age (see Chapter 24).

Treatment

The first step in the treatment of soiling is to manage the environment to increase the appeal of the litter area and decrease the appeal of and the access to the soiled areas. Treatment options that might prove particularly useful for the senior cat would include adding more litter boxes, including in the areas where the cat is soiling; providing easier access to the litter location and the box itself (e.g., lower entry side, providing a ramp); improving lighting or providing a nightlight in the area; and providing more frequent cleaning. In cats that are visually impaired, familiar odor cues (e.g., litter attractant, aromatherapy) or pheromones might help the cat to better navigate to the area and perhaps increase the appeal of the area. Inciting factors should be identified so that stimuli might be avoided or conflicts addressed. Once the needs of the senior cat are addressed, behavior modification and medications might also be needed as has been discussed in relevant sections throughout the text. However, there may be limitations on both the behavior modification and medications used, depending on the physical and health limitations of the pet.

Anxiety

Senior cats have reduced ability or perhaps even an inability to cope with changes to their routine, household, or environment. In addition, medical conditions (as discussed above) can limit the cat's ability to engage in desirable activities, leave the cat weak or irritable, or may cause an increase in avoidance. Anxiety might be increased by sensory and motor impairments that alter the cat's ability to recognize or respond to stimuli or impede its ability to avoid. Preexisting anxieties can be exacerbated over the years and new anxieties can develop. Feline CDS is a complicating factor since the pet's ability to learn, adapt, and remember is affected. Owners will also influence anxiety with inconsistent responses (resulting in unpredictability and lack of control), for example when they respond with frustration or anger, inadvertently reward undesirable behavior, or use punishment to deter undesirable behavior (which can be particularly stressful to the older cat). As with younger cats, senior cats can develop anxiety in a variety of situations (e.g., noise, new people or pets in the home or property, household changes), but their health and age can leave them more sensitive to change.

Treatment

Management of anxiety in senior cats is generally similar to that of younger cats. However, owners may require more time, repetitions, consistency, and patience to achieve the desired goals. The focus should be on the desired rewarding and training, on nonanxious behaviors, and on acceptable activities, such as social interaction and play. In many cases, medications such as buspirone, fluoxetine, or benzodiazepines may need to be considered.[7,11] Selection will need to be based on both the problem and the health of the pet. Natural supplements such as feline facial F3 pheromones, α-casozepine, L-theanine, or the feline Calm diet may be helpful alone or in combination with medication. Cognitive therapeutics may also reduce the anxiety associated with cognitive dysfunction. (Adjunctive therapeutics and cognitive drugs and supplements are discussed below.)

Repetitive Behaviors

Senior cats may be presented with pacing, excessive grooming, or excessive licking. Some behaviors may appear to be more frequent or intense at night, although this may be simply due to owner awareness. Pain including neuropathic pain, disease processes affecting the CNS, gastrointestinal disorders, and dermatologic conditions are among the many medical conditions that can contribute to the development of these behaviors. Increased pacing and restlessness, especially during nighttime, might also be a sign of CDS.

Treatment

If the problem persists once medical factors have been ruled out or diagnosed and treated, the focus should move to resolving the underlying environmental or behavioral stressors. Of course if CDS is a component of the problem, this too should be concurrently addressed. Keeping a diary in order to determine the daily routine and identifying situations, times, and inciting factors for the behavior might provide an opportunity to avoid these situations or stimuli or keep the pet preemptively occupied in alternative desirable behaviors. Increasing enrichment in the form of feeding toys, opportunities to explore and social activities including play and training, and helping the cat in finding a comfortable and secure area for rest should decrease underlying stressors. Owners must avoid rewarding the behaviors, such as by giving the cat treats or by playing to stop the behavior. Punishment must also cease as it increases anxiety and conflict. Using a command–reward sequence, the owner might be able to engage the pet in an acceptable and incompatible behavior (e.g., "come," "high-five," "let's play"). The behavior might be interrupted without rewarding with a hand clap or a very gentle pull on a leash, which has been left attached to a harness as long as the owner does not engage with the cat during this action and immediately engages the cat in an alternative desirable behavior. In many cases, medications and/or natural supplements might be required (as discussed in Chapter 19).

Aggression

Senior cats can develop aggression for similar reasons to younger cats. Therefore, the first issue would be to identify any changes to the household or incidents that were coincident to the onset of aggression (see Chapters 26 and 27). Health issues can have a direct role in contributing to increased pain, irritability, altered mobility, sensory decline (e.g., vision, hearing), or cognitive dysfunction that might alter the cat's behavior, such as displaying aggression, in situations where it might previously have been more passive. In addition, medical factors such as a decline in sensory or motor function may alter the cat's ability to effectively communicate with other cats or people. Some senior cats might show worsening of existing aggression.

Treatment

Management of aggression should first focus on ensuring safety. All triggers should be identified and avoided by preventing situations in which aggression might arise. Providing more resources to reduce conflicts (e.g., hides, litter boxes, perches) or separating the cat from other cats or people to whom it might display aggression may be necessary. Of utmost importance in the treatment of the senior cat is providing realistic expectations of what might be achieved when one considers the cat's health and the household. Medical treatment for underlying health problems and CDS, as well as behavioral drugs or supplements, may help the cat achieve an acceptable level of improvement or control. However, even if medical problems are successfully controlled, reestablishing a harmonious relationship, including the implementation of desensitization and counterconditioning, may be difficult or impractical especially in a senior cat. The diagnosis and treatment of aggression is discussed in greater detail in Chapters 26 and 27.

COGNITIVE DYSFUNCTION SYNDROME

A neurodegenerative disorder of senior cats, cognitive dysfunction syndrome (CDS) is characterized by a process of cognitive decline due to age-related pathology that includes cerebral atrophy, neuronal loss, ventricular enlargement, lesions associated with the deposition of amyloid, and compromised cerebrovascular blood flow.[6–8,11,13–17] Although much of the work published on the clinical syndrome in cats has been extrapolated from humans and dogs, there is an increasing body of data that supports the use of similar diagnostic criteria in cats[6–8,11] (see Table 25-1).

Characteristic patterns of neuropathology have been reported to develop in parallel to the development of clinical signs. The development of β-amyloid deposits in cats have been reported from 10 years of age onward, which appears to correlate with the age of onset of clinical signs as well as reflexive learning deficits

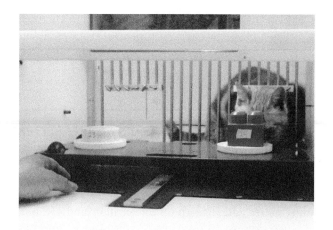

FIGURE 25-1   Feline cognitive testing apparatus. (Courtesy G. Landsberg, Cancog Technologies)

and impairments in motor function.[6–8,16–18] However, functional changes in the neurons of the caudate nucleus that impair ability to process information have been reported at as young as 6 years of age.[19] In addition, as demonstrated in dogs, neuropsychological test performance in cats declines with age (Figure 25-1).[6,7,11,13,20,21]

When presented with a senior cat with signs that may be attributed to CDS, the diagnosis is made by excluding any other factors that might be the cause of the behavioral signs. This involves an extensive history to determine if there are any other concurrent signs, physical and neurological exams, sensory and pain assessments, and any laboratory diagnostics that might be indicated to rule out possible medical causes. On the other hand, since these are senior cats, the finding of a medical problem does not rule out the possibility of concurrent cognitive dysfunction.

Laboratory Studies

Compared with dogs, there are far fewer scientific studies that have evaluated learning and memory performance with respect to senior cats. One study found deficits in eye-blink conditioning in cats 10 years of age or greater compared with cats 1 to 3 years of age; similar findings are also seen in aged humans and patients with Alzheimer disease (AD).[18,22] In another study, using a hole board task, it is found that there is no difference in learning between cats less than 3 years of age and those age 3.1 to 8 years and age 8 to 15 years, although working memory and reference memory errors increased with age.[23] However, the population may have been skewed in that only the cats that passed the initial screening criteria were enrolled in the study, leading to the removal of a greater number of senior cats. Most recently, a battery of cognitive assessment tests have been developed by CanCog Technologies (cancog.com); these tests are based on cognitive tasks that were originally developed for cognitive assessment of dogs.[20,24,25] In the initial acquisition task, the tester baits one of the food wells with canned food and then covers the well with an object. Once the cat learns to displace the object to get the food, the cat must then learn under which of two objects the food is hidden (i.e., a discrimination task) (see Figure 25-1). Each object is baited with food to prevent the animal from identifying the correct object by smell. The next test is a reversal task where the cat must learn that the food is now under the previously incorrect object. This test of executive function is affected by increasing age. Similar age effects have been found in cats in the spatial memory task (delayed nonmatching to position) and in the reversal phase of a positional discrimination (egocentric) task.[13,20,24,25]

Pathological Data

Recent advances in senior cats have identified changes in the brains of aging cats that parallel those seen in aged dogs and, to some extent, humans with early AD.[6-8,11,14-17,26-29] Most notably, cats have been shown to develop β-amyloid pathology, which has been described as a partial model for human AD, with diffuse plaques seen primarily in the deep cortical areas of the frontal and parietal lobes, as well as vascular amyloid deposition, in cats over 10 years of age.[26-29] Frequency and quantity of β-amyloid and intensity of staining increase with age.[16,17,26-29] Within the neurons, immunoreactive tau deposits have also been identified.[16,27] However, neuritic plaques and mature neurofibrillary tangles, which are present in humans, have not been identified in the cat.[16,26,27] While a correlation between β-amyloid deposition and CDS in dogs has been identified, the relationship in cats is unclear.[16,26-31]

There have also been other types of age-related pathology that are reported in cats and are similar to those reported in dogs, including neuronal loss, a decrease in grey and white matter, enlargement of the lateral ventricles, widening of the sulci, a decline in neuronal function, and small multifocal lesions in the pyriform lobe, with increasing age.[6-8,15,32,33] Finally, there is evidence of changes in cerebellar function with aging, which could contribute to a decline in motor function in senior cats.[6,8,14]

In a study using both light and electron microscopy of aged cats, marked cholinergic atrophy was found in the tegmental nuclei of aged cats.[34] These changes would likely contribute to age-related changes in rapid eye movement (REM) sleep and a decline in cognitive ability.[34,35] This likely corresponds to the decline in cholinergic activity in canine cognitive dysfunction syndrome.[36-38] These findings, together with recent studies in humans, appear to indicate that use of anticholinergic drugs in seniors might increase the risk of cognitive impairment.[39]

Increased oxidative damage and decreased mitochondrial function, leading to reduced cerebral metabolism, have been identified as contributing factors in neurodegenerative disorders such as AD and cognitive dysfunction in dogs and likely also in cats.[8,40-43] With increasing age, mitochondrial function declines, leading to an increased production and decreased clearance of free radicals (reactive oxygen species), which further damage mitochondria.[40-42] In dogs, mitochondria function can be improved with an antioxidant diet, independent of the effects of enrichment.[43]

Another factor that might contribute to or exacerbate the signs of cognitive dysfunction is cerebrovascular compromise, including β-amyloid accumulation together with microhemorrhage and infarcts within the periventricular cerebral blood vessels.[16,26-28] Cerebrovascular circulation may be further compromised in the senior cat by disease processes that lead to decreased cardiac output, hypertension, anemia, and alterations in blood viscosity and platelet hypercoagulability.[6-8,11,13,42] Neurons are particularly susceptible to hypoxic damage.

Management of Cognitive Dysfunction in Cats

Until recently, most therapeutic options used for the treatment of CDS in cats have been products and drugs that have been developed and evaluated primarily in dogs. While there are products labeled for use in cats, very few have any evidence to support their efficacy. Products that have demonstrated efficacy in dogs must be used with caution and close monitoring in cats due to differences in drug metabolism and toxicity. When treating cognitive dysfunction, the more advanced the signs, the more difficult it may be to achieve significant improvement; however, preventive strategies and early intervention with behavioral enrichment and cognitive supplements may provide the greatest benefit since neuropathology is less extensive.[13,21,43-52]

Drug Therapy

Currently, there are two drugs approved for cognitive dysfunction in dogs but none for cats. Thus the potential benefits must be weighed against possible risks.

Selegiline is categorized as a selective irreversible inhibitor of monoamine oxidase B (MAOB), although its mode of action in dogs is not entirely clear. It is licensed for the treatment of clinical signs of canine CDS in North America. Selegiline has demonstrated an improvement in the clinical signs of CDS and an improvement in working memory in a laboratory model.[53,54] Although feline use is off-label, beneficial effects in cats with signs of CDS in relation to disorientation, vocalization, and decreased interest in affection have been reported at a dose of 0.5 to 1 mg/kg per day.[6,8,42,55] In one study, no toxicity was seen at a dose up to 10 mg/kg.[56] Selegiline should not be used concurrently with drugs that might enhance serotonin transmission; such drugs include selective serotonin reuptake inhibitors (SSRIs), such as fluoxetine, and tricyclic antidepressants (TCAs), such as clomipramine, tramadol, buspirone, and most narcotics. In fact, in dogs, a withdrawal time of at least 2 weeks is suggested between use of SSRI or TCA and initiating selegiline therapy—a practice which would also be prudent in cats.

Propentofylline is a xanthine derivative which may improve microcirculation to increase oxygenation to the brain and the periphery. It is licensed for use in dogs in some countries (although not in North America) for signs of senility including mental dullness, lethargy, and tiredness when no other underlying medical cause is identified.[57,58] In cats, there are anecdotal reports of efficacy at 12.5 mg orally taken twice daily.[6,8,42]

Based on evidence of cholinergic decline in aging cats and on findings in both dogs and humans, it seems prudent to avoid the use of anticholinergic drugs wherever possible in senior cats.[34,36–39] In fact, drugs or natural products that might enhance cholinergic transmission or increase availability of acetylcholine might have the potential for beneficial effects in feline CDS; however, both efficacy and safety have not been established.

Natural Supplements and Dietary Management

Considering the lack of availability of pharmacologic options for the treatment of feline cognitive dysfunction, the use of natural supplements that are labeled and tested in cats might be the first preference. In addition, the therapeutic strategy for most cognitive supplements is to reduce the risk factors that contribute to brain aging and cognitive decline rather than specifically treating clinical signs. However, it is likely that no single ingredient can help in maintaining brain health or in slowing cognitive decline and that an integrative approach is required to achieve brain health; for example, with a Mediterranean diet or a diet fortified with a mixture of antioxidants including fruits, vegetables, and polyunsaturated fatty acids (PUFAs), the risk of Alzheimer's disease might be reduced.[40,49–52] Thus, the components of diets and supplements for brain aging in pets have focused on a mixture of components that might reduce the effects of oxidative stress; improve mitochondrial function, neuronal health, and neuronal signaling; supplement ingredients to improve age-related deficiencies; and provide alternative sources of energy for the aging brain cells.[5,6,8,13,21,41–44,46–48,59,60]

Currently there are two diet formulations available for dogs that might slow the progress or improve signs of CDS. One diet (Canine b/d, Hills Pet Nutrition, Topeka, Kan.) has been formulated with a focus on improving antioxidant defenses and to reduce the effects of oxidative damage. After 2 years, the combination of diet and environmental enrichment provided greater improvement than the diet or enrichment alone.[46–48] Another diet (Purina One Vibrant Maturity 7+) uses botanic oils containing medium chain triglycerides to provide ketone bodies as an alternative source of energy for aging neurons and to increase PUFA levels in the brain.[61,62] However, a dietary approach to the prevention or treatment of cognitive dysfunction must consider the specific needs of the target species, since nutritional requirements and nutrient metabolism differ considerably; in fact, α-lipoic acid is much more toxic in cats than dogs.[63]

Recently, Nestlé Purina Research has published data on a nutritional strategy for middle-aged and old cats using a diet supplemented with fish oil, ascorbic acid, B vitamins, antioxidants, and arginine. The ingredient mix was developed with the intent of slowing brain atrophy and eliminating risk factors associated with brain aging. The use of fish oil containing docosahexaenoic acid (DHA) and eicosapentaenoic acid (EPA) was intended to correct potential age-related deficiencies in fatty acids and aid in preventing damage from reactive oxygen species and for their potential antiinflammatory effects. Arginine might enhance nitric oxide synthesis to improve circulation and lower blood pressure.[13,64] B vitamins were added to correct potential deficiencies and reduce the risk of high homocysteine.[13,65] Antioxidants were enhanced to help protect against oxidative damage. In this trial, the cats fed with the test diet showed significantly better performance on egocentric learning, discrimination and reversal learning, and acquisition of a spatial memory task than those fed with controlled diet.[13]

In another 30-day placebo-controlled study of 44 cats, the treatment group received a diet developed by Hills Pet Nutrition, supplemented with a combination of ingredients that were designed to decrease production and increase clearance of free radicals and reduce oxidative stress which include tocopherols, L-carnitine, vitamin C, β-carotene, DHA, cysteine, and methionine. Cats on the test diet had significantly improved activity levels, compared with when the cat was 8 years of age.[66]

In another trial assessing the effect of a diet fortified with antioxidants and other nutritional supplements, 90 healthy cats aged 7 to 17 years were fed with a controlled diet, a diet with antioxidants (vitamin B and β-carotene), or a diet supplemented with antioxidants, dried chicory root (a prebiotic), and a mix of omega-3 and 6 fatty acids. After 5 years, cats fed with diet with the antioxidants, chicory root, and fatty acids lived longer and had an improved health status compared with cats fed with controlled diet.[67]

Novifit (Virbac Animal health) is a natural supplement containing S-adenosyl-L-methionine (SAMe), which is labeled for use in both cats and dogs for CDS. SAMe may help to maintain cell membrane fluidity and receptor function, regulate neurotransmitter levels, and increase production of glutathione, which may decrease oxidative stress.[21] In addition, SAMe levels may be deficient in human patients with AD.[21,68] Improvement in clinical signs of cognitive dysfunction in dogs has been demonstrated in a placebo-controlled trial.[69] In reversal learning in aged cats, there was a non significant reduction in errors in the treatment group compared with the control group. However, when the cats were divided into top- and bottom-half performers, the top-half performers had significantly less reversal learning errors consistent with improved executive function. This suggests that Novifit improves an age-related decline in executive function that is less beneficial in cats that are most affected.[21]

Two other ingredient blends labeled for use in cats contain phosphatidylserine, an important building block of cell membranes that is purported to facilitate neuronal signal transduction and enhance cholinergic transmission.[70,71] One of these products, Senilife (CEVA Animal Health), has been demonstrated to improve cognition in both a laboratory model and clinical studies in dogs.[60,70] In addition to the phosphatidylserine, the supplement contains *Ginkgo biloba,* vitamin E, and resveratrol for their potential antioxidant effects as well as vitamin B6 (pyridoxine), which may have neuroprotective effects.[65,72] Although it is labeled for use in cats, no efficacy studies have been published. The second product, Activait (Vet Plus Ltd), which contains phosphatidylserine, omega-3 fatty acids, vitamins E and C, L-carnitine, α-lipoic acid, coenzyme Q, and selenium, has also demonstrated significant improvement over placebo in improving social interactions, disorientation, and house soiling in dogs with CDS.[59] A feline version which does not contain α-lipoic acid is also marketed, but its efficacy has not yet been evaluated.[8]

Another supplement for senior cats, Cholodin-Fel (MVP Labs) contains choline, phosphatidylcholine, methionine, inositol, vitamin E, zinc, selenium, taurine, and B vitamins. In one preliminary study, 9 of 21 aged cats showed improvement in confusion and appetite.[73]

Adjunctive Therapy

Independent of, or concurrent with, the treatment of cognitive dysfunction in senior cats, there may be a need for additional medications to treat specific clinical presentations. Of course, treatment for underlying medical problems and a behavioral plan should also be implemented concurrent with or prior to beginning behavior medications. The contraindications when using selegiline for the treatment of CDS have been outlined above. In addition, consideration must be given to other potential contraindications and adverse effects, both with respect to the individual and with senior pets in general. For example, every effort should be made to avoid drugs that might have anticholinergic effects. Thus, a selective serotonin reuptake inhibitor, such as fluoxetine, would

be preferable to paroxetine or TCAs, such as clomipramine. As buspirone has minimal side effects and does not cause sedation, it might be a good option for senior cats with mild to moderate anxiety. Lorazepam, oxazepam, and clonazepam have no active intermediate metabolites and might therefore be safer in senior cats or those with compromised hepatic function. Together with or as an alternative to drug therapy some of the natural therapeutics may also be a consideration in the reduction of anxiety or perhaps in reducing the effects of environmental stressors, including Feliway (feline F3 facial pheromone, CEVA Animal Health), Anxitane (L-theanine, Virbac Animal Health), Zylkene (α-casozepine, Vetoquinol), Royal Canin Calm Feline (which is supplemented with α-casozepine, tryptophan, and B vitamins), or melatonin. For more details on individual products, see Chapter 19).

Behavioral and Environmental Management

Studies in dogs have demonstrated that not only can there be improvement in quality of life through mental stimulation and environmental enrichment, but there might also be improvement in both the behavioral signs and the physical changes associated with brain aging, or their declines might be slowed.[43,45-47] This is consistent with studies in which education, brain exercise, and physical exercise have been found to delay the onset of dementia in humans. In dogs, the greatest cognitive improvement was achieved by the combined effects of enrichment and supplementation. Neuronal loss in the hippocampus was slowed by enrichment. Mitochondrial function was improved by diet but not enrichment, while the strongest effect on β-amyloid pathology was with the combined effect of antioxidant therapy and enrichment.[43,45,74]

Although the effects of enrichment on brain aging in cats has not yet been evaluated, providing both mental and physical stimulations is important in maintaining both behavioral and physical health.[75] However, at the same time, aged cats may have limitations in their mobility, sensory function, or cognitive function, or they may have other medical health issues (e.g., renal, diabetes) that limit their ability or desire to engage in a full range of normal daily activities. Therefore, the challenge with the senior pet is to maintain enrichment by making environmental modifications and by providing alternative outlets and enrichment that are age and health appropriate. Keeping the environment as stable as possible is important in order to help maintain predictability and reduce anxiety, thereby allowing the cat to better adjust to change. First, be certain that all of the cat's basic needs for feeding, elimination, sleep, and security, as well as its social requirements, are being adequately met. While it is best to minimize change, if problems arise, there may be a need to move one or more of these to an area that is more readily accessible

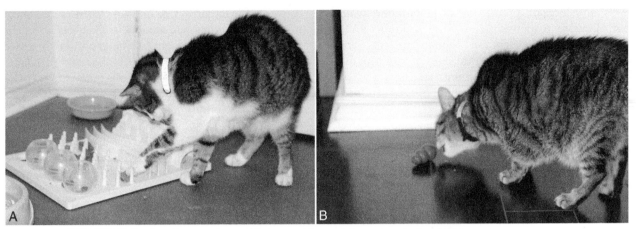

FIGURE 25-2   Feeding puzzles and toys used for enrichment and stimulation.

or more appealing. For example, with sensory decline, reduced mobility, or disease processes such as chronic kidney disease that increase urinary frequency, adjustments may need to be made to the cat's litter and sleeping or play areas to help the cat and the owner to better cope with these issues. Heights of perching and resting sites may need to be lowered or intermediate levels may need to be added to facilitate climbing activities. Moving the litter box to require less climbing and adding better lighting or a ramp or lower sides for easier entry and exit may be useful and it may be appropriate to add a larger box or more boxes in more locations. In addition, while novelty items such as new feeding toys and objects to explore (e.g., paper bags) may further enrich the environment, change may also be a stressor, particularly for older animals. Therefore, make change slowly. Give the cat choices that are acceptable to the family and the household, and allow the cat to have control to make its own selections as to what it prefers (e.g., sleeping sites, perches, litter boxes, food, toys).[76,77] Reward behaviors you want the cat to repeat and prevent those that are unacceptable. Other potential stressors, such as animals or people (especially children), should be controlled, so aged cats can have a quiet and secure household that allows them to engage when and with whom they want. Avoid positive punishment of any type. Within the limitations outlined above, it is important to work to find ways to maintain or increase stimulation of the body and the brain by encouraging social play, more frequent

use of rewards (toys, treats) to improve communication, and train what is desirable. Provide some of the cat's food in puzzles and toys (Figure 25-2) or with games of search and find, and offer new items to explore (e.g., paper bags) and practical places to climb and perch. Begin with basic enrichment and, if successful, gradually increase complexity as long as the cat continues to remain interested and motivated.

If there are changes to the family or household to which the cat does not readily adapt or if it can no longer cope successfully because of its physical or mental health, it may be best to place the cat in a separate room or portion of the home so that it can settle. When confining the cat, be certain to provide all of its needs appropriately distributed within the area (e.g., food, water, litter box, social interactions). It may then be possible to allow the cat back into some of the parts or the entire home for times of the day when the cat is settled or when the stress-evoking stimuli are not present. However, in some cats, long-term confinement may be best for the cat and the family, with slow and gradual efforts made for some level of positive reintroductions if practical. Specific details of enrichment and gradual reintroduction are discussed in Chapters 6 and 8. At all times, the quality of life of the cat must be the paramount consideration, and when the time comes, it is important to compassionately assist the owners with the process of making a decision about euthanasia.

REFERENCES

1. Broussard JD, Peterson ME, Fox PR. Changes in clinical and laboratory findings in cats with hyperthyroidism from 1983 to 1993. *J Am Vet Med Assoc.* 1995;206:302–305.
2. Venn A. Diets for geriatric patients. *Vet Times.* May 1992.
3. Hill's Pet Nutrition. *US marketing research summary: Omnibus study on aging pets.* Topeka: Hill's Pet Nutrition; 2000.
4. Stewart M. Reasons for contemplating euthanasia. *Companion animal death: A practical and comprehensive guide for veterinary practice.* Oxford: Butterworth-Heinemann; 1999.
5. Fahey Jr. GC, Barry KA, Swanson KS. Age-related changes in nutrient utilization by companion animals. *Annu Rev Nutr.* 2008;28:425–445.

6. Landsberg GM, Denenberg S, Araujo JA. Cognitive dysfunction in cats: A syndrome we used to dismiss as "old age". *J Feline Med Surg*. 2010;12:837–848.

7. Landsberg GM, Hunthausen W, Ackerman L. The effect of aging on behavior in senior pets. In: *Behavior problems of the dog and cat*. ed 3. St Louis: Saunders; 2013:211–235.

8. Gunn-Moore D, Moffat K, Christie LA, et al. Cognitive dysfunction and the neurobiology of ageing in cats. *J Small Anim Pract*. 2007;48:546–553.

9. Chapman BL, Voith VL. Geriatric behavior problems not always related to age. *DVM*. 1987;18(3):32–39.

10. Fitzgerald BM, Turner DC. Hunting behaviour of domestic cats and their impact on prey population. In: Turner DC, Bateson P, eds. *The domestic cat: The biology of its behaviour*. ed 2. Cambridge, UK: Cambridge University Press; 2000:166–171.

11. Landsberg GM, DePorter T, Araujo JA. Management of anxiety, sleeplessness, and cognitive dysfunction in the senior pet. *Vet Clin N Am Small Anim Pract*. 2011;41:565–590.

12. Doxee AL, Yager JA, Best SJ, et al. Extratesticular interstitial cell and Sertoli cell tumors in previously neutered dogs and cats: A report of 17 cases. *Can Vet J*. 2006;47:763–766.

13. Pan Y, Araujo JA, Burrows J, et al. Cognitive enhancement in middle-aged and old cats with dietary supplementation with a nutrient blend containing fish oil, B vitamins, antioxidants, and arginine. *Br J Nutr*. 2012;110(1):40–49.

14. Zhang C, Hua T, Zhu Z, et al. Age-related changes of structures in cerebellar cortex of cat. *J Biosci*. 2006;31:55–60.

15. Dobson H, de Rivera C. *Aging and imaging based neuropathology in the cat*. Presented at Proc 2011 ACVB/AVSAB Veterinary Behavior Symposium, 2011, pp. 59–60.

16. Gunn-Moore DA, McVee J, Bradshaw JM, et al. Ageing changes in cat brains demonstrated by β-amyloid and AT8-immunoreactive phosphorylated tau deposits. *J Feline Med Surg*. 2006;8:234–242.

17. Takeuchi Y, Uetsuka K, Muruyama M, et al. Complimentary distributions of amyloid-β and neprilysin in the brains of dogs and cats. *Vet Pathol*. 2008;45:455–466.

18. Harrison J, Buchwald J. Eyeblink conditioning deficits in the old cat. *Neurobiol Aging*. 1983;4:45–51.

19. Levine MS, Lloyd RL, Hull CD, et al. Neurophysiological alterations in caudate neurons in aged cats. *Brain Res*. 1987;401:213–230.

20. Milgram NW. Neuropsychological function and aging in the cat. In: *Proceedings of the 15th Annual Conference on Canine Cognition and Aging*; 2010, Laguna Beach.

21. Araujo JA, Faubert ML, Brooks ML, et al. Novifit (NoviSAMe) tablets improve executive function in aged dogs and cats: Implications for treatment of cognitive dysfunction syndrome. *Int J Appl Res Vet Med*. 2012;10:91–98.

22. Solomon PR, Beal MF, Pendlebury MW. Age-related disruption of classical conditioning: A models systems approach to memory disorders. *Neurobiol Aging*. 1988;9:535–546.

23. McCune S, Stevenson J, Fretwell L, et al. Aging does not significantly affect performance in a spatial learning task in the domestic cat (Felis silvestris catus). *Appl Anim Behav Sci*. 2008;3:345–356.

24. Christie LA, Studzinski CM, Araujo JA, et al. Age-dependent spatial learning deficits: Characterization of egocentric and allocentric spatial learning in the beagle dog. *Prog Neuropharmacol Biol Psychiatry*. 2005;29:361–369.

25. Head E, Mehta R, Hartley J, et al. Spatial learning and memory as a function of age in the dog. *Behav Neurosci*. 1995;109:851–858.

26. Cummings BJ, Satou T, Head E, et al. Diffuse plaques contain C-terminal A beta 42 and not A beta 40: Evidence from cats and dogs. *Neurobiol Aging*. 1996;17:653–659.

27. Head E, Moffat K, Das P, et al. Beta-amyloid deposition and tau phosphorylation in clinically characterized aged cats. *Neurobiol Aging*. 2005;26:749–763.

28. Nakamura S, Nakayama H, Kiatipattanasakul W, et al. Senile plaques in very aged cats. *Acta Neuropathol*. 1996;91:437–439.

29. Brellou G, Vlemmas I, Lekkas S, et al. Immunohistochemical investigation of amyloid beta protein (Abeta) in the brain of aged cats. *Histol Histopathol*. 2005;20:725–731.

30. Colle MA, Hauw JJ, Crespau F, et al. Vascular and parenchymal beta-amyloid deposition in the aging dog: Correlation with behavior. *Neurobiol Aging*. 2000;21:695–704.

31. Cummings BJ, Head E, Afagh AJ, et al. Beta-amyloid accumulation correlates with cognitive dysfunction in the aged canine. *Neurobiol Learn Mem*. 1996;66:11–23.

32. Tapp PD, Siwak CT, Gao FQ, et al. Frontal lobe volume, function, and beta-amyloid pathology in a canine model of aging. *J Neurosci*. 2004;24:8205–8213.

33. Borras D, Ferrer I, Pumarola M. Age related changes in the brain of the dog. *Vet Pathol*. 1999;36:202–211.

34. Zhang JH, Sampogna S, Morales FR, et al. Age-related changes in cholinergic neurons in the laterodorsal and the pedunculo-pontine tegmental nuclei of cats: A combined light and electron microscopic study. *Brain Res*. 2005;1052:47–55.

35. Chase MH. Sleep patterns in old cats. In: Chase MH, ed. *Sleep disorders: basic and clinical research*. New York: Spectrum Publications; 1983:445–448.

36. Araujo JA, Nobrega JN, Raymond R, et al. Aged dogs demonstrate both increased sensitivity to scopolamine and decreased muscarinic receptor density. *Pharmacol Biochem Behav*. 2011;98:203–209.

37. Araujo JA, Studzinski CM, Milgram NW. Further evidence for the cholinergic hypothesis of aging and dementia from the canine model of aging. *Prog Psychopharmacol Biol Psychiatr*. 2005;29:411–422.

38. Pugliese M, Cangitano C, Ceccariglia S, et al. Canine cognitive dysfunction and the cerebellum: Acetylcholinesterase reduction, neuronal and glial changes. *Brain Res*. 2007;1139:85–94.

39. Cai X, Campbell N, Khan B, et al. Long-term anticholinergic use and the aging brain. *Alzheimers Dement*. 2013;9:377–385.

40. Sullivan PG, Brown MR. Mitochondrial aging and dysfunction in Alzheimer's disease. *Prog Neuropsychopharmacol Biol Psychiatry*. 2005;29:407–410.

41. Head E, Liu J, Hagen TM, et al. Oxidative damage increases with age in a canine model of human brain aging. *J Neurochem*. 2002;82:375–381.

42. Overall K. Assessing brain aging in cats. *DVM Newsmagazine*. October 2010;41(10):6S–9S.

43. Head E, Nukala VN, Fenoglio KA, et al. Effects of age, dietary, and behavioral enrichment on brain mitochondria in a canine model of human aging. *Exp Neurol*. 2009;220:171–176.

44. Pan YL. Enhancing brain function in senior dogs: A new nutritional approach. *Top Companion Anim Med*. 2011;26:10–16.

45. Siwak-Tapp CT, Head E, Muggenburg BA, et al. Region specific neuron loss in the aged canine hippocampus is reduced by enrichment. *Neurobiol Aging*. 2008;29:39–50.

46. Head E. Combining an antioxidant-fortified diet with behavioral enrichment leads to cognitive improvement and reduced brain pathology in aging canines: Strategies for healthy aging. *Ann NY Acad Sci*. 2007;1114:398–406.

47. Milgram NW, Head E, Zicker SC, et al. Long-term treatment with antioxidants and a program of behavioral

enrichment reduces age-dependent impairment in discrimination and reversal learning in beagle dogs. *Exp Gerontol.* 2004;39:753–765.

48. Araujo JA, Studzinski CM, Head E, et al. Assessment of nutritional interventions for modification of age-associated cognitive decline using a canine model of human aging. *Age (Dordr).* 2005;27:27–37.

49. Scarmeas N, Stern Y, Tang MX, et al. Mediterranean diet and risk for Alzheimer's disease. *Ann Neurol.* 2006;59:912–921.

50. Joseph JA, Shukitt-Hale B, Willis DM. Grape juice, berries, and walnuts affect brain aging and behavior. *J Nutr.* 2009;189:1813S–1817S.

51. Donini LM, De Felice MR, Cannella C. Nutritional status determinants and cognition in the elderly. *Arch Gerontol Geriatr.* 2007;44:143–153.

52. Kidd PM. Neurodegeneration from mitochondrial insufficiency: Nutrients stem cells, growth factors, and prospects for brain rebuilding through integrative management. *Altern Med Rev.* 2005;10:268–293.

53. Ruehl WW, Bruyette D, DePaoli DS, et al. Canine cognitive dysfunction as a model for human age-related cognitive decline, dementia, and Alzheimer's disease: Clinical presentation, cognitive testing, pathology, and response to 1-deprenyl therapy. *Prog Brain Res.* 1995;106:217–225.

54. Campbell S, Trettien A, Kozan B. A non-comparative open-label study evaluating the effect of selegiline hydrochloride in a clinical setting. *Vet Ther.* 2001;2:24–39.

55. Landsberg G. Therapeutic options for cognitive decline in senior pets. *J Am Anim Hosp Assoc.* 2006;42:407–413.

56. Ruehl WW, Griffin D, Bouchard G, et al. Effects of l-deprenyl in cats in a one-month dose escalation study. *Vet Pathol.* 1996;33:621.

57. Vivitonin® MSD Animal Health [Product Insert]. August 2010. http://www.msd-animal-health.co.nz/binaries/Vivitonin_website_label_Aug_10__tcm51-37350.pdf.

58. Parkinson FE, Rudophi KA, Fredholm BB. Propentofylline: A nucleoside transport inhibitor with neuroprotective effects in cerebral ischemia. *Gen Pharmacol.* 1994;25:1053–1058.

59. Heath SE, Barabas S, Craze PG. Nutritional supplementation in cases of canine cognitive dysfunction: A clinical trial. *Appl Anim Behav Sci.* 2007;105:274–283.

60. Osella MC, Re G, Odore R, et al. Canine cognitive dysfunction syndrome: Prevalence, clinical signs and treatment with a neuroprotective nutraceutical. *Appl Anim Behav Sci.* 2007;105:297–310.

61. Pan Y, Larson B, Araujo JA, et al. Dietary supplementation with medium-chain TAG has long-lasting cognition-enhancing effects in aged dogs. *Br J Nutr.* 2010;103:1746–1754.

62. Taha AY, Henderson ST, Burnham WM. Dietary enrichment with medium chain-triglycerides (AC-1203) elevates polyunsaturated fatty acids in the parietal cortex of aged dogs:

Implications for treating age-related cognitive decline. *Neurochem Res.* 2009;34:1619–1625.

63. Hill AS, Werner JA, Rogers QR, et al. Lipoic acid is 10 times more toxic in cats than reported in humans, dogs or rats. *J Anim Physiol Anim Nutr.* 2004;88:150–156.

64. Dong JY, Qin LQ, Zhang Z, et al. Effect of oral L-arginine supplementation on blood pressure: A meta-analysis of randomized, double-blind, placebo-controlled trials. *Am Heart J.* 2011;162:959–965.

65. Selhub J, Troen A, Rosenberg IH. B vitamins and the aging brain. *Nutr Rev.* 2010;68(2):112S–118S.

66. Houpt KA, Levine E, Landsberg GM, et al. Antioxidant fortified food improves owner perceived behavior in the aging cat. Prague: Proceedings of the ESFM Feline Conference; 2007.

67. Cupp CJ, Jean Philippe C, Kerr WW, et al. Effect of nutritional interventions on longevity of senior cats. *Int J App Res Med.* 2006;4:34–50.

68. Panza F, Frisardi V, Capurso C, et al. Polyunsaturated fatty acids and S-adenosylmethionine supplementation in predementia syndrome and Alzheimer's disease. *Scientific World J.* 2009;9:373–389.

69. Rème CA, Dramard V, Kern L, et al. Effect of S-adenosylmethionine tablets on the reduction of age-related mental decline in dogs: A double-blind placebo-controlled trial. *Vet Ther.* 2008;9:69–82.

70. Araujo JA, Landsberg GM, Milgram NW, et al. Improvement of short-term memory performance in aged beagles by a nutraceutical supplement containing phosphatidylserine, Ginkgo biloba, vitamin E and pyridoxine. *Can Vet J.* 2008;49:379–385.

71. Tasakiris S, Deconstantinos G. Phosphatidylserine and calmodulin effects on Ca21-stimulated ATPase and acetylcholinesterase activities in the dog brain synaptosomal plasma membranes. *Int J Biochem.* 1985;17:1117–1119.

72. Dakshinamurti K, Sharma SK, Geiger JD. Neuroprotective aspects of pyridoxine. *Biochim Biophys Acta.* 2003;1647:225–229.

73. Messonier SP. Cognitive disorder (senility). In: *The natural health bible for dogs and cats.* Roseville: Prima Publishing; 2001:56–57.

74. Pop V, Head A, Hill MA, et al. Synergistic effects of long-term antioxidant diet and behavioral enrichment on beta-amyloid load and non-amyloidogenic processing in aged canines. *J Neurosci.* 2010;30:9131–9139.

75. Buffington CA, Westropp JL, Chew DJ, et al. Clinical evaluation of multimodal environmental modification (MEMO) in the management of cats with idiopathic cystitis. *J Feline Med Surg.* 2006;8(4):261–268.

76. McMillan FD. Maximizing quality of life in ill animals. *J Am Anim Hosp Assoc.* 2003;39:227–235.

77. Hetts S, Heinke ML, Estep DQ. Behavioral wellness concepts for general practice. *J Am Vet Med Assoc.* 2004;225:506–513.

Intercat Conflict

Sarah Heath

INTRODUCTION

As the cat increases in popularity as a companion animal, the number of households owning cats is increasing and the number of homes with multiple cats is also on the rise. Considering natural feline behavior, one can understand why these changes are potentially stressful for the domestic cat and why issues of intercat conflict can be problematic within households and neighborhoods. These issues have serious welfare implications for the cats concerned and if they are not addressed can result in one of four outcomes. First, the cats may remain in the same household or neighborhood with resulting ongoing chronic stress and the behavioral and physical consequences that it brings (see Chapter 12). While the welfare of the cat is the primary concern for the veterinarian, it is also important to remember that there may be stress for the owner. There can be significant emotional effects from living in a household where ongoing feline conflict is an issue, or in a neighborhood where human disputes are associated with intercat conflict. Second, the cat(s) may be rehomed, and studies have shown that intercat conflict is a significant factor in relinquishment and return of domestic cats to rescue centers in the United Kingdom. A study in 2009 of 6089 cats that were relinquished and returned to 11 rescue facilities in the United Kingdom over a 12-month period found that 7% were relinquished for behavioral reasons and the most common reason within that group was aggression between cats in the household.[1] In the United States there is a similar situation, with the second most common behavior problem to result in surrender being a newly adopted cat not getting along with the already existing cats in the household.[2] Relinquishment was found to be associated with the number of pets in the household, as well as the introduction of new cats to the home environment.[2] The third possible outcome in a case of intercat conflict in a household is putting one of the cats permanently outside. This can have serious welfare implications for the cat as it is a domestic pet and not well equipped to live a feral lifestyle. The fourth outcome is that owners request euthanasia of their pet with all of the human emotional consequences that this is associated with.

INCIDENCE OF INTERCAT CONFLICT

It is difficult to gain access to reliable data on the incidence of intercat conflict in domestic environments because the level of reporting is poor and many owners tolerate tension between their cats without seeking professional help. The Association of Pet Behaviour Counsellors (APBC) in the United Kingdom published a report in 2012 and stated that 35% of cats seen by their members during that year presented with aggression problems, most often toward other cats (26%) with the majority of that aggression (25%) being directed toward unknown cats.[3] The data in the review are derived from clinical cases that have been referred to a selection of members of the association; therefore they represent a limited and somewhat biased population. However, data from other countries suggest that intercat conflict is a significant problem for cat owners around the world. A review of 736 cats presented to the Animal Behavior Clinic at Cornell University between 1991 and 2001 showed that 25% of cases were diagnosed with problems of intercat aggression,[4] and in a study carried out at the Barcelona School of Veterinary Medicine reviewing 336 feline behavior cases presented to the Animal Behavior Clinic between 1998 and 2006, 30% were reported to involve issues of aggression between cats.[5]

THE ROLE OF FELINE SOCIAL BEHAVIOR

The incidence and nature of aggressive responses in cats is strongly related to their natural behavioral responses and to their social and communication systems in the wild. Although the traditional image of the cat as a solitary creature is not entirely accurate, it is important to remember that much of feline behavior is based on individual survival and many of the fundamental behaviors, such as feeding, hunting, resting, and eliminating, are performed in a solitary context with no social significance (see Chapter 4). Feline society is based on cooperative groups of females who are related to one another and live together in a mutually beneficial environment, which supports the successful rearing of kittens. Males are usually excluded from these social groupings and live their lives as solitary individuals who only venture into the main social context at times of breeding. The size of feline social groups is largely determined by resource availability,[6] with areas of abundant resources being able to sustain relatively large colonies and areas where food is widely dispersed housing smaller social groupings or even truly solitary felines. Where groups do exist, they tend to be insular in nature, and while levels of hostility within the groups are low, intrusion by others is poorly tolerated. Overt hostility is one possible consequence but physical aggression carries with it the risk of injury, and for a species where pack structure and hierarchy does not exist[7] and ultimate survival is an individual responsibility, it makes sense to avoid situations which could result in a decreased ability to take care of oneself. For this reason overt aggression is minimized by the use of elaborate distance maintaining behaviors which are designed to keep strangers at bay and discourage social interaction with individuals outside of the social group. These signals include postural and vocal communication, marking behaviors, such as urine spraying, and elaborate use of eye contact and facial communication including ear positions (see Chapter 3).

Where outsiders do successfully integrate into existing social groupings the process is extremely gradual and the newcomer will spend time at the periphery of the colony before becoming slowly integrated over a number of weeks.[8]

In order to maintain the integrity of the social group it is important to have reliable means of identification of fellow members. Affiliative behaviors, such as grooming and rubbing of social partners, referred to as allogrooming and allorubbing, are used to cement relationships and to exchange scent signals (Figures 26-1 and 26-2). The mixing of scents results in the formation of a group social odor which reassures individuals that the social group is stable and enables them to relax in close proximity to one another. When tension does occur, the cat has a range of subtle body postures and facial expressions, which can be used to avoid physical conflict and, for a solitary hunter, this is important in order to prevent injury and consequent threat to the individual's survival[9] (Figure 26-3). In addition, a range of vocalizations can be used to further increase the success of communication and in a feline context, repulsion is usually the last resort in terms of behavioral defense strategies. However, because the presence of a social group is not essential for survival, reconciliation behaviors are limited within a feline context and a tendency to disperse rather than to work at maintaining relationships results in a certain level of fragility within feline society.

THE PRESSURES OF THE DOMESTIC ENVIRONMENT

When considering the features of normal feline social behavior and contrasting them with the demands of a domestic environment, it becomes apparent that humans unintentionally place social demands on domestic cats which are at odds with their own natural behavior. The increasing popularity of the cat is leading to an increase in the number of households owning more than one cat. As a result, cats often find themselves living in groups of unrelated individuals, being made to share important resources, and being denied the opportunity to hide or retreat from situations of potential conflict. They may also be living in neighborhoods with large feline populations and find interaction with their feline neighbors something of a challenge (Figure 26-4).

THE MEDICAL CONSEQUENCES OF FELINE TENSION

Over recent years there has been increasing interest in the potential for feline stress to be involved in the etiology of commonly presented feline medical problems, such as feline idiopathic cystitis. Intercat tension has been identified by several authors as one of the possible factors in this complex medical condition,[10] and recommendation of environmental modification, as part of the medical approach to these cases, is now accepted as best practice.[11] Feline idiopathic cystitis is not the only medical condition influenced by chronic stress, and the interplay between emotional state and physical illness highlights the need for behavioral medicine to be an integral part of feline veterinary practice. Intercat conflict can be a significant factor to consider when working to prevent and treat feline medical conditions. An important duty of the veterinary profession is to safeguard the welfare of the cats in their care, and a consideration of behavioral health is an essential aspect of this (see Chapters 2 and 12).

PREVENTION OF INTERCAT CONFLICT

Maximizing social skills by raising kittens in a way that prepares them for life in a domestic environment is a key part of the prevention strategy. Between the ages of 2 and 7 weeks, adequate and appropriate socialization with other cats will help the development of appropriate feline communication skills and help to decrease the risk of intercat conflict issues later in life (see Chapter 7). As a result of the natural social behavior of cats, socialization alone will not give any guarantee of a harmonious feline household. Selecting potential housemates from a feline perspective and restricting numbers of cats within the household to socially

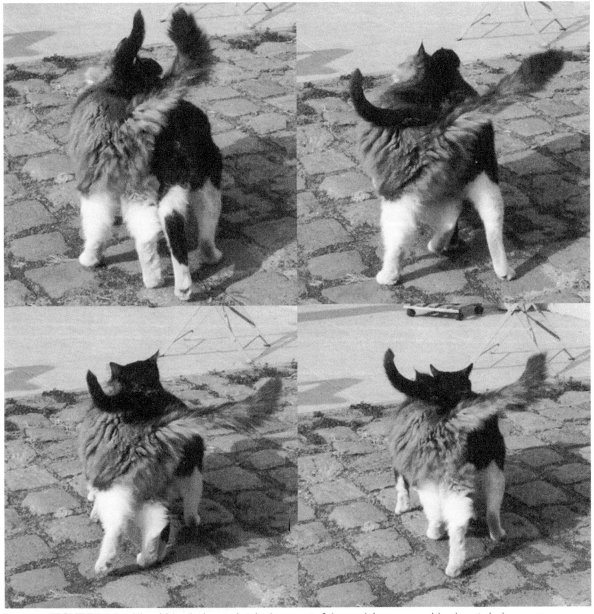

FIGURE 26-1 Allorubbing helps maintain the scent of the social group resulting in cats being more secure together. (Courtesy A. Dossche)

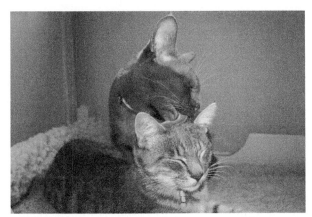

FIGURE 26-2 Cats that are in the same social group can be seen to groom one another, especially around the head and neck, in a behavior referred to as allogrooming. (Courtesy S. Ellis)

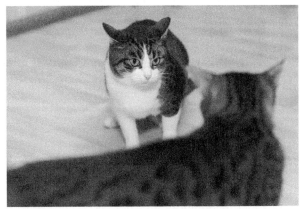

FIGURE 26-3 A combination of postural and facial expressions is used to prevent escalation to physical altercations. (Copyright © iStock.com)

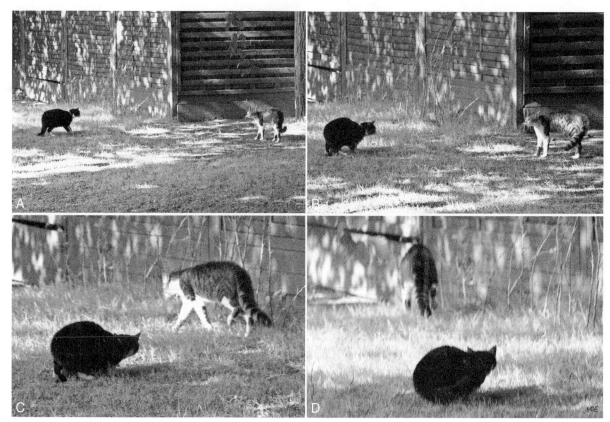

FIGURE 26-4 The increased population of outdoor cats in some neighborhoods can lead to intercat conflict over territory. Note how the body and facial posturing is used to communicate between the cats and to prevent physical confrontation. (Courtesy A. Dossche)

compatible levels will be essential (see Chapter 6). One study compared the behavior of unrelated pairs of cats from the same household while confined in a cattery with pairs of littermates in the same context. It showed that the littermates spent more time in physical contact with one another, groomed one another more often (Figure 26-5), and were more likely to feed close to one another than unrelated cats.[12] The most likely explanation for this difference is that ties are established between individual cats during the socialization period (2 to 7 weeks) and persist throughout life if the cats continue to live together. Advising clients to take on littermates or to introduce future housemates as early as possible is therefore beneficial.

When owners introduce a new cat to an already established feline household, one important aspect of prevention of intercat conflict is the introduction process. A study of feline households following the adoption of a cat from a local animal shelter in the United States showed that half of them reported fighting (defined as scratching and/or biting) between cats when the new individual was introduced and approximately half of the people introduced the cats by putting them together immediately.[13]

Whether the multicat household is established from scratch or expanded through introduction, it is

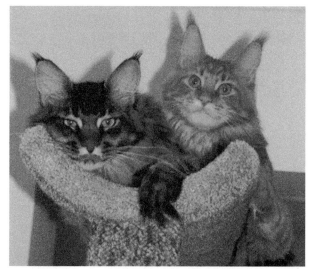

FIGURE 26-5 These sibling cats can frequently be found in close contact whereas cats that are not in the same social group would be unlikely to choose to share a resting place. (Courtesy D. Givin)

important to ensure that all cats have free and immediate access to their essential resources without running the gauntlet of other cats.[14] Several feeding, drinking and toileting sites will need to be distributed around

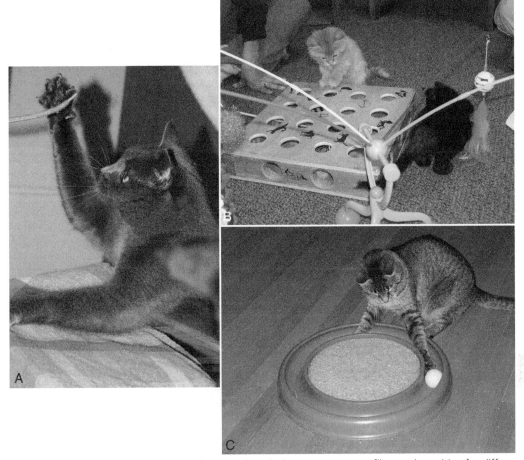

FIGURE 26-6   Providing a variety of play options helps to prevent conflict, and provides for different styles of play in a multicat household. (**B,** Courtesy I. Rodan. **C,** Courtesy M. Baily)

the home to enable cats to have a real choice of location for these activities (see Chapter 8). Toileting sites may also need to be created in the garden, although this may have more relevance to potential intercat conflict within the neighborhood. Outdoor latrines may take the form of hooded trays positioned close to the house to offer security or sunken latrines in the yard which offer a reliable round the year site for toileting (see Chapter 8).

Provision of appropriate play opportunities is an important part of creating a harmonious feline household and it is useful to assess the play styles of each individual cat to ensure that all are catered for (Figure 26-6). Discrepancy between play styles can lead to tension between cats, for example when a highly motivated cat practices predatory style play with the tail of one of its housemates. This discrepancy can be associated with age differences and a playful young kitten can be stressful for an unrelated older cat (Figure 26-7).

In order to prevent aggression problems between cats in the neighborhood, it would be ideal if owners could consider the present local cat population density and

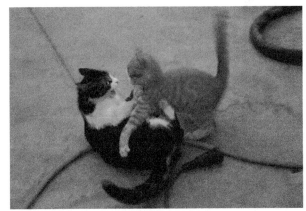

FIGURE 26-7   A very playful kitten can interact inappropriately with older unrelated cats, leading to stress and potential conflict. (Courtesy A. Dossche)

whether it can cope with the addition of another cat before attempting to introduce one. However, this is unlikely to happen because every household bases its decision to acquire a cat on personal factors rather than any consideration of the neighborhood as a whole. Steps

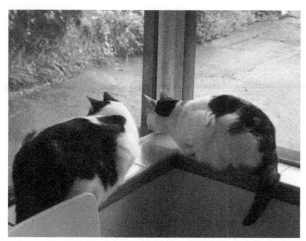

FIGURE 26-8 Visual intrusion from other cats in the neighborhood can be an important factor in intercat conflict. (Courtesy A. Dossche)

can be taken to reduce the risk of intercat conflict developing and these would include providing a secure demarcation between outdoor and indoor territory, such as a microchip operated cat flap, and making access to the outside world predictable. Limiting visual intrusion into the home from cats outside is also beneficial (Figure 26-8), and providing high up resting places within the garden from which cats can observe their territory in safety should also be considered. In situations of severe overpopulation in the neighborhood, the provision of accessible outdoor latrines may also be helpful (see Chapter 8).

INTRODUCTION OF A NEW CAT INTO A FELINE HOUSEHOLD

Before introducing a new cat it is important to assess the likelihood that resident cats will accept it. Any existing feline stress within the household should be addressed, but unfortunately veterinary practices are rarely contacted for advice prior to the acquisition of a new cat and the chance to give appropriate advice at that stage is often lost. Ethologically insensitive, direct introduction of cats carries a strong risk of fighting and long-term intolerance between cats.[13] Even when overt physical conflict does not occur, the increase in feline tension can lead to a situation where any further stressors, such as the addition of further cats to the neighborhood, will unmask the problem and lead to overt signs of intercat aggression and other behavioral problems such as marking (see Chapter 24). If advice is sought at an early stage and clients have decided that the introduction of another cat is appropriate, then the process by which that introduction is achieved is of the utmost importance (see Chapter 1 for more information on preadoption counseling).

It should always be assumed that the newcomer will be in a separate social group to the existing cats and therefore, it should initially be housed in its own core territory. This may be one room or an area within the house depending on the size of the home. Within this territory the newcomer should be provided with all the necessary resources such as a litter box, food, water, and a variety of resting and hiding places that are appropriately distributed. In the United States, a new product based on feline appeasing pheromone (Feliway Multi-Cat) has recently been suggested as a potentially useful addition to the feline introduction process, especially for fearful cats (see Chapter 18). Installing an F3 diffuser (Feliway, CEVA Animal Health) will increase the sense of familiarity and security, and should be provided for the newcomer and for the resident cats in their respective areas of the house. The resident cats should also be given several feediing stations, places to drink, and additional places to hide in their safe zone. Feliway Multi-Cat can be used in conjunction with Feliway but it is not currently available in all countries.

It is important to give enough time for the new cat to become fully confident in their own part of the home and to be eating, resting, and approaching humans comfortably. The timescale is entirely dependent on the individual cat and the total time for the introduction process may vary from a couple of weeks to a couple of months. There is no shortcut if harmony is to be achieved. Patience is essential, as rushing the introduction at any stage increases the risk of tension developing.

The next stage of the introduction process involves the transfer of scent between the newcomer and the resident cats. This can be done indirectly through the use of cloths that are used to collect odors from the face and flank of each cat on a daily basis. When the owner interacts with the cats, to greet, feed, or play with them, they can present the cloth from one of the other cats. If there are multiple cats in the household, then the resident cats should be presented with the new cat's smell, and the new cat with odors from different cats in the group. The cloths should be passively presented and the cats given time to investigate the scent at their leisure. It is important not to force contact as the cat may become fearful and negative associations with the other cat(s) may be formed.

With repeated presentation of the cloths, the cats should ultimately ignore the odor or may react positively to it. The next stage is to use the same cloth to gather scents from all of the cats (resident and newcomer) and to introduce this combined scent not only through direct exposure but also by rubbing it onto objects that cats regularly rub against, including the owner's legs. Once all cats are accepting this new odor and are either ignoring it or actively rubbing against the cloth and other objects that have been marked with it, then it is time to allow the new cat the opportunity to explore and utilize the rest of the house, while the other cats are excluded or shut in an inaccessible room. This allows the new cat to learn all of the hiding and escape places so that it does not feel vulnerable when the other cats are eventually introduced. Once the new cat is using the resources in the home confidently, then it is time to move on to very well managed face to face introductions.

When introductions begin, the cats need to be able to see each other without any risk of physical interaction, and this can be achieved using a glass door or mesh screen. Mesh barriers are best, as they allow some diffusion of body odors that are involved in identification, but if these are not available a part open door, for example securely fixed open with a hook at the top of the door, may be used (Figure 26-9). It should be open just enough for the cats to be able to see each other but not get through. It is also useful to rub the door or screen with the odor from the cats so that there is maximum chance of recognition of scent. On either side of the screen the cats can engage in their normal daily activities which help to increase their positive emotional state, such as playing, resting, and feeding. It is important to continue mixing odors between the cats and applying their "group odor" to the owner and common marking places in the house. Owners should also continue with F3 diffusers and other environmental modifications which make the territories on either side of the door

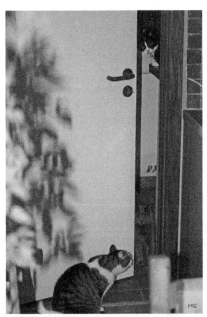

FIGURE 26-9   A partially open door can be used to assist in intercat introductions. The door should be kept secured with a hook at the top of the door and the gap should be small enough to prevent either cat from physically entering the safe territory of the other(s). This picture illustrates the concept, but the door is open too far and would allow potential physical interaction between the cats which would not be considered until later in an introduction process. (Courtesy A. Dossche)

as safe and secure for each of the cats as possible. Where available, the use of Feliway MultiCat diffusers may also be considered. Once the cats are showing no aggressive or fearful behavior at the screen or partially open door they can be allowed to meet face to face, but this introduction should be as passive as possible with no direct attempts being made to get the cats to interact with one another. Coexistence is the aim of the introduction rather than deep and meaningful friendship.

INVESTIGATING CASES OF INTERCAT CONFLICT

Even when prevention factors are considered and cat introductions are well managed, it is possible for issues of intercat conflict to arise. When this happens veterinary practices may be informed directly, as clients seek help to resolve obvious conflict, but they may also discover these issues indirectly when treating the cats for medical conditions (see Chapter 12). The majority of cases of intercat conflict which are presented to the primary veterinarian involve cats within the same household, but when serious intercat conflict occurs within neighborhoods, human tension can run high and there can be intense pressure to find a solution.

CLASSIFICATION OF AGGRESSION

The term "aggression" can be used to refer to a number of different behavioral responses, ranging from hissing and spitting to infliction of physical injury. Aggression should be considered a perfectly normal feature of the feline behavioral repertoire and the term "aggressive" should not be used to define a cat's personality. The natural feline predatory sequence contains "aggressive" elements and these are learnt and perfected through play. Social conflict may also be manifested in normal and appropriate "aggressive" displays, which are designed to diffuse tension and avoid physical confrontation. Within the context of problem behavior, it is therefore essential to determine the motivation for aggressive behavior and to identify elements of normal feline behavior, such as predation, play, or social related aggression (Figure 26-10).

There have been various schemes for categorizing feline aggression. The first question to consider is whether the aggression is normally motivated or not. Normal aggression is contextually appropriate and usually relatively well controlled and predictable, so it carries a good prognosis as long as the cat's behavioral needs can be met within the domestic environment. Abnormal aggression can result from physical illness or inappropriate learning.

From a clinician's perspective, the most helpful approach to categorization is to define aggression in terms of its immediate target, its motivation, and

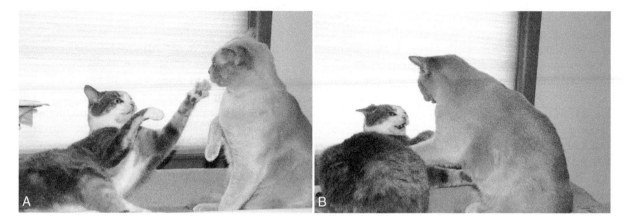

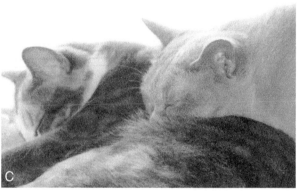

FIGURE 26-10   "Aggressive" displays may be seen between cats that are members of the same social group either in the context of play (**A** and **B**) or in justified confrontations. **C,** After these encounters these cats sleep together, indicating that they share a positive social relationship. (Courtesy J. Hynum)

its offensive, defensive, or frustration-related nature. Owners may find it helpful to attach labels according to the circumstance or context of the aggression, but it is the underlying motivation that will determine the treatment approach.

DETERMINING THE MOTIVATION

The motivation for the aggression in any particular case should be determined through a combination of observation and history-taking. The list of possible differentials is similar to that relating to aggression toward people (see Chapter 27) and includes fear, anxiety, and frustration-related aggression as well as inappropriate play. It is important for clients to accurately interpret interactions between the cats, and accurate description of body language, facial expression, and vocalization before, during, and after "aggressive" incidents will help to achieve this. Many clients may find it difficult to accurately describe their cat's signals and video footage of interactions between the cats can therefore be a very useful tool in the diagnostic process. In this technological age it is far easier to ask clients to submit footage taken with smartphone or tablet devices. Clearly it is not acceptable to stage aggressive events for the purpose

of making a diagnosis especially where there is a serious risk of injury.

Passive conflict manifested by staring, posturing, and keeping distance from one another can easily be overlooked, and when these signs are not recognized the ensuing physical confrontation can sometimes appear unprovoked and intense (Figure 26-11). This misperception can lead to cats being labeled as "evil"

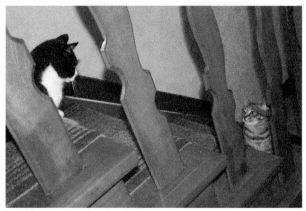

FIGURE 26-11   Passive stand offs, episodes of staring, and a tendency to avoid proximity should not be overlooked in multicat households. (Courtesy A. Dossche)

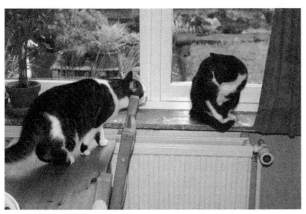

FIGURE 26-12   Learning to recognize passive signaling of tension between cats can help to prevent escalation to more physical altercations. (Courtesy A. Dossche)

and "malevolent," and in intercat encounters it can contribute to the mistaken belief that some cats are more "dominant" than others. The truth is that cats are not hierarchical creatures and their social interactions are not based on any system of dominance or submission. Instead they act as independent units who need to establish appropriate social signaling to facilitate cohabitation.[15] The use of avoidance behavior and withdrawal responses is related to the protection of their own survival rather than deference to the other party. Studies in the United Kingdom and the United States have suggested that owners find it extremely difficult to identify intercat tension based on passive signals. Active aggressive behavior including hissing, dashing, swiping paws, and chasing cats out of the room are readily recognized, but owners are less able to identify tension based on passive stand-offs such as staring (Figure 26-12).

AGGRESSION BETWEEN CATS IN THE SAME HOUSEHOLD

Immediate Response

If a client contacts the practice with reports of overt fighting between cats in the household, it is important to give immediate advice in order to prevent injury and avoid escalation. Fights need to be broken up before they result in injury, but owners must be careful not to get injured.

Where possible, intervention should be used as early as possible in the sequence of aggression, for instance, to terminate threatening eye contact. When used too late in the sequence, when the cats show great body tension and are preparing to strike, intervention may escalate emotional arousal and actually trigger an aggressive attack. Picking cats up while they are in the midst of a fight can result in very damaging redirected aggression toward the person and therefore, when separating the cats, it is

necessary to use indirect means (noise to distract or a physical barrier placed between the cats) rather than direct human intervention. It is important to remember that fear, anxiety, and frustration are driving forces for aggressive behavior and anything that increases tension will probably favor fighting. Use of punishment, in the form of rattle cans or water pistols, in order to diffuse aggressive encounters between cats, is therefore not recommended. A better method of distracting the cats is to try to trigger predatory behavior that is directed toward a toy. Everyday toys may not provide sufficient distraction, but something unusual like a laser pointer or a bird flight toy may be used to break the cats' concentration and lure them away from each other into a game. If a laser pointer is used, it is important for it to settle on a toy or object once the cat has been moved away from the other cat. Sudden disappearance of the light point without alighting on a tangible object runs the risk of inducing frustration.

Once the cats are separated, they should be placed in their own territory with a complete set of suitably distributed resources (food, water, a selection of toys and resting places, and a litter box). It is futile to try to reconcile cats from a position of conflict because there is no mechanism in their natural behavioral repertoire to achieve this. Isolation of individuals or of different social groups is therefore the first step, and this is particularly important when there is a significant risk of injury or where previous attempts at reconciliation have been unsuccessful. Once a detailed investigation of the underlying causes of the conflict has been carried out and necessary modifications to the physical environment have been made, the prospect of reintroduction, following the same principles as when introducing a new cat, can be considered.

Investigation

In any case of intercat conflict it is important to monitor the frequency and intensity of conflict behavior. It can be useful for owners to keep a diary in order to ensure that an accurate assessment of the extent of the problem can be made.

Reports of intercat conflict in previously harmonious feline households should alert veterinary practices to the possibility of medical influences such as pain or debilitating disease, and a clinical examination should be carried out as soon as possible (Figure 26-13). Other triggers for the onset of overt manifestation of feline tension include inappropriate introduction procedure with a new cat and temporary isolation of individual cats leading to loss of group odor and failed recognition when they return. Social pressure, due to an excessive population density or incompatible groupings of cats, may have been present for some time and outward signs may have been triggered by another change in the household or the neighborhood, for example the

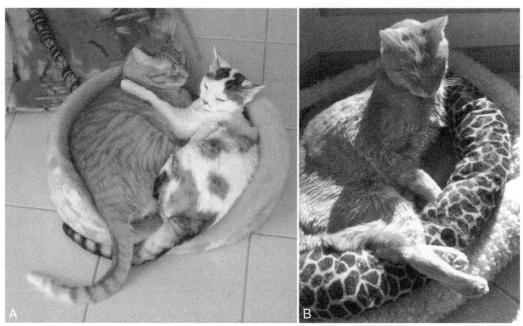

FIGURE 26-13 These cats showed affiliative behaviors for years **(A)** until the older cat developed multiple health conditions including severe degenerative joint disease. He then started to hiss at the younger cat any time he approached as a result of the pain and only wanted to rest alone **(B)**. (Courtesy I. Rodan)

introduction of a new person, alteration of furniture, or acquisition of a new cat by a neighbor.

Potential emotional motivations for aggressive displays include fear, frustration, predatory behavior, or play. Often conflict problems in multicat households will relate to a combination of these causes and accurate and comprehensive history-taking is an essential part of reaching a diagnosis.

Redirected (frustration-related) aggression is common, especially when aggressive displays toward cats outside the house are thwarted (Figure 26-14), and the cat turns its attention to an easier target within the house, such as another cat. Feline play often involves rehearsal

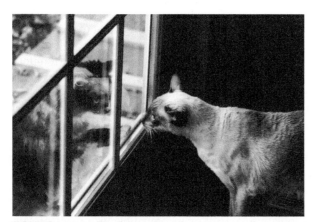

FIGURE 26-14 The frustration of seeing an unfamiliar cat outdoors can lead to the indoor cat redirecting its aggression toward another household cat or person. (Copyright © iStock.com)

of predatory behavior, which is appropriate when it is directed toward inanimate objects. However, other cats in the household can become mock-predatory targets and predatory play is a common motivation underlying apparent aggression in multicat households, particularly where there are varying ages and breeds (see Figure 26-7).

In order to deal with intercat conflict cases, it is important to fully understand the nature of the cats' relationships with each other and the way that they make use of their domestic territory. A plan of the home and garden indicating the location of feeding places, latrines, resting places, and any other resources the cats make use of is an important tool in the diagnostic process (Figure 26-15). The plan should also include information about resting places, clearly identifiable passage tracks through the territory for each cat, and preferred entry and exit points either between the indoor and outdoor territory or between rooms in the house. Common locations of feline conflict should be marked and if there are any other unwanted behaviors occurring, such as marking or unacceptable elimination, these should also be indicated on the plan.

Determining the existing social groups within the household is essential and the relationship between the cats can be determined by looking at the pattern of allorubbing, allogrooming, and other affiliative behaviors, such as tail-up greetings between individual cats. Within the household there are often a number of smaller social groups and some cats may be entirely solitary. There may also be "socially mobile" individuals who show affiliative behavior toward and are accepted by members of all of the groups. These cats may be instrumental in preventing

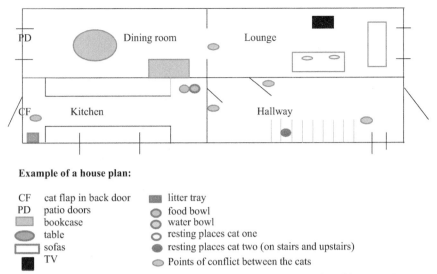

Example of a house plan:

CF   cat flap in back door
PD   patio doors
     bookcase
     table
     sofas
     TV

     litter tray
     food bowl
     water bowl
     resting places cat one
     resting places cat two (on stairs and upstairs)
     Points of conflict between the cats

FIGURE 26-15   A house plan is an important tool in investigation of multicat tension.

outbreaks of aggression. As well as looking for affiliative behaviors which indicate the existence of social harmony, it is important for owners to identify passive "aggressive" behaviors between the cats, such as chasing and staring, that indicate social conflict between factions or group members. It can be helpful for owners to observe the cats closely over a 7-day period and to record the interactions on a behavioral map. Behavioral interactions are dynamic and important information could be missed if the cats are only observed on 1 or 2 days. The maps can become very complex and it can help for owners to use pens of differing colors to record different behavioral interactions, such as grooming and rubbing. Arrows are drawn between the cats when interactions take place and when the interactions are repeated another arrow is added so that the overall width of the arrow at the end of the 7-day period of recording is indicative of the frequency of the affiliative interactions between the individuals. Separate maps for affiliative and conflictual behaviors may also be needed to avoid confusion and make it easier to identify the social groupings from the information provided (Figure 26-16).

AIMS OF INTERVENTION

The ultimate aim of behavioral intervention is to produce a fully functioning cat group in which there is maximal affiliative behavior and minimal aggression. However, owners do need to be realistic and also respectful of natural feline behavior. In many cases the environment will need to be permanently modified to meet the cats' needs. This may mean giving the cats access to more space, a larger number and diversity of resources, and possibly indoor–outdoor access if the cats are currently kept inside. For some owners, provision for the natural behavioral needs of all of the cats may not be possible, and in this situation part of the

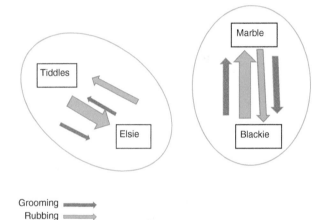

Grooming
Rubbing

FIGURE 26-16   Behavioral maps can be used to illustrate both affiliative and conflictual behavior patterns between cats. In this very simple version of an affiliative behavior map two distinct social groups can be identified.

solution may be to sensitively reduce the overall cat population by identifying and rehoming incompatible individuals. In this case the resolution is to produce several functioning cat groups that live separately and while it may not be the outcome that the owner originally wanted, it may be the best solution in terms of the welfare of the cats. Some owners are fortunate enough to be able to provide two or more separate "homes" for their cats within their own property and this may also be an acceptable outcome. Guiding owners into the right decision for the cats requires an in-depth analysis and understanding of the social dynamics of the group and how it accesses resources. A good solution that improves the welfare of all the cats should never be regarded as a failure, even if the cats are unable to continue living with the current owner.

One significant problem in cases of intercat aggression in the household is when the owners are engaging in animal hoarding. An *animal hoarder* is defined as the someone who accumulates a large number of animals and who: 1) fails to provide minimal standards of nutrition, sanitation, and veterinary care; 2) fails to act on the deteriorating condition of the animals (including disease, starvation, or death) and the environment (severe overcrowding, extremely unsanitary conditions); and often, 3) is unaware of the negative effects of the collection on their own health and well-being and on that of other family members.[16] Suspected animal hoarders should be carefully and sensitively counseled, and if unwilling to sensibly rehome and depopulate, they should be reported to local authorities. Animal hoarders or collectors should not be supported in their attempts to keep excessively large populations of cats.

MANAGING INTERCAT CONFLICT WITHIN THE HOME

In order to maximize the possibility of restoring harmony or at least tolerance within a feline household, it is important to consider the basic factors that encourage cats to spontaneously form groups in feral or wild situations. In addition to any innate (genetic or acquired) tendency toward sociability in the individuals making up the group, there will also need to be an excess of resources (food, resting places, latrines, water), the opportunity for free and immediate access to available survival resources, and sufficient space (including three-dimensional space) to avoid unnecessary physical interactions.

The first step to treating intercat aggression is determining the number and composition of social groups. Identifying any particular instigators of aggressive interactions is important and if it is possible to give other cats in the household prior warning of the approach of these individuals, for example through the use of bells on collars, this can help to improve the success of avoidance behaviors in reducing conflict. Unfortunately this is not always successful as some cats can alter their body posture and move in such a way as to prevent the bell from ringing.

In order to establish separate and distinct core territories, each social group within a household should be provided with its own collection of resources. When the cats no longer have to queue for access to resources in close proximity to cats from opposing factions, this will allow the cats to live in greater isolation from each other. Giving them the option to spend less time together will enable the possibility of positive passive encounters, without the complication of competition for food or space (Figure 26-17). The security of the core territory can be further advanced by the installation of an F3 synthetic pheromone diffuser device and the use of the new Feliway MultiCat product may be appropriate where it is available.

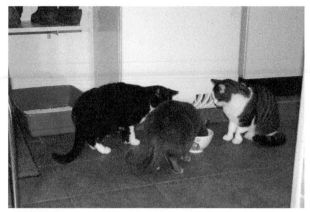

FIGURE 26-17 When cats from differing social groups are expected to share feeding time and location, it can contribute to intercat tension within the household. (Courtesy A. Dossche)

Increasing access to space is critical. The cat's primary means of controlling its interaction with other cats is to maintain distance from them. In the relatively small rooms that are typical of many homes it may be very difficult for a cat to feel safe because it is always forced into closer than desirable proximity to other cats. This tends to favor repulsion-style defensive behavior, because escape and avoidance are not possible. Fortunately, cats are able to make greater use of three-dimensional space than humans and dogs, so giving them high perches in the form of shelves or cat furniture (Figure 26-18) will enable the cats to reengage in avoidance and distance-maintaining behaviors. There are numerous designs of cat trees available and selection should be made with regard to the composition of the feline household. In multicat households with problems of tension between the cats, it is best to select trees with tunnels rather than boxes to prevent problems of ambushing and to ensure that the tree has a selection of comfortable resting places or hammocks as well as observational platforms. More than one tree

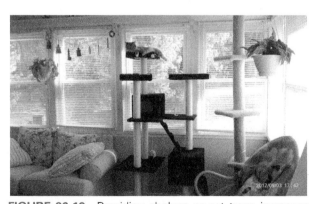

FIGURE 26-18 Providing shelves or cat trees increases vertical space, enabling cats to maintain distance from each other. (Courtesy P. Putnam)

may be necessary, depending on the number of social groups within the household, to avoid problems of cats elevating to reduce stress and finding themselves in closer proximity to incompatible cats because the only elevation sites are on the one cat tree.

Cardboard boxes and other low-down hiding places provide an excellent escape route for cats that are regularly chased aggressively or during play (Figure 26-19). This enables cats to take refuge without having to run too far, and removes some of the reinforcement for chasing by other cats. However, it may be beneficial to open up the cardboard box into a tunnel so that there is no risk of a cat getting trapped and intimidated when it has chosen to retreat. If the motivation for chasing is predatory play then the owner should also provide other play opportunities for the instigator as an outlet for this motivation, such as play with a fishing-rod style toy and a changing supply of small, easily moved, brightly colored toys (Figure 26-20).

While it is important to ensure that cats have plenty of space to retreat to, it is also important to minimize the risk of vantage points becoming established from which more confident cats can intimidate other cats while they are accessing resources or moving from space to space. Examples of areas in which control over feline movement may become an issue include cat flaps, doorways, and corridors and if essential resources, such as latrines or feeding stations, are positioned close to these areas, the potential for stress is increased.

In order to maximize available space for the cats, it may be possible to consider use of the outdoor

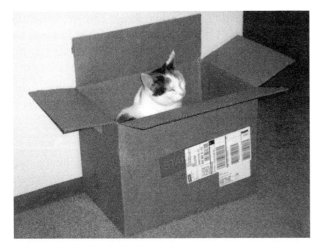

FIGURE 26-19 A cardboard box or other safe place with high sides provides refuge. The box may also be laid on its side and opened up at both ends to form a hiding tunnel which also allows for easy escape in case of problems related to ambushing between cats.

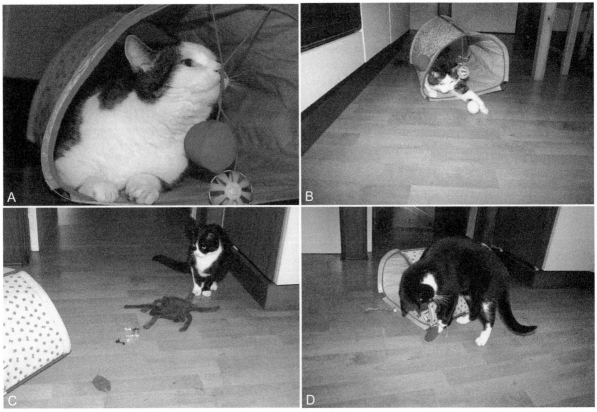

FIGURE 26-20 It is important to provide lots of opportunity for appropriate play by providing a range of toys that are rotated regularly to help to maintain interest. (Courtesy A. Dossche)

environment. The provision of more resources, such as resting places, perches, and latrines, within the expanded territory can significantly reduce tension. Access to sheds and outbuildings can be used to increase available sheltered space, as can providing sheltered perches. Some owners are reluctant to give cats access to the outdoors, and in some countries cats are not permitted to roam free. In these cases a secure outdoor run may be a viable option to increase space.

In addition to considering the physical environment, it is helpful to pay attention to the olfactory environment. Repeated face and flank marking of objects in the central section of the cats' territory, combined with allorubbing and allogrooming (rubbing and grooming of social partners) creates a strong sense of security and identity. This can be lost when factions of cats or individuals dissociate from one another. A decrease in exchange of social information via this olfactory route may happen when people are not present to transfer odors between cats (for example when they go on holiday), or when a "socially mobile" cat within the group has been lost, perhaps through going missing for a period of days or being away in the veterinary practice due to an illness. Alterations in scent profiles within the home can also occur when a house is redecorated, stripping odor marks from the environment. The use of F3 diffusers (Feliway, CEVA Animal Health) can simulate the effect of dense facial and flank marking within an environment, while the cats reestablish their own marks and exchange odors that identify them. The pheromone F4 (Felifriend, CEVA Animal Health) ought to be very useful for treating intercat aggression within the household, but unfortunately its effects are not always reliable. F4 signals indicate familiarity, but with cats that have already had a number of aggressive encounters, there may be a dissonance between the memory of the visual appearance of the aggressor cat and the chemical "familiarity" signal. This has been seen to trigger apparent panic and intense behavioral responses. F4 is therefore not recommended for treating intercat aggression within the household, but may be useful in countries where it is available for reducing fear of unfamiliar people and other animals when they are first encountered. The use of the new Feliway MultiCat product may also be beneficial but this is only available in the United States at the time of writing (see Chapter 18).

In some cases where owner interaction is highly valued by the cats, it may be necessary to consider the role of human company as a resource and to alter the level of owner involvement in providing access to other vital resources such as food or access to outside. Cases where this may be an issue include those where cats are fed regimented meals and cannot gain access to food in any other way or where cats are actively let in and out of the house by the owner at human determined times. If the cats are unable to gain access to food or go in and out of the house when the owner is not present they may tend to congregate around the owner when they return, which places them in close proximity to each other at a time when they are most desperate to get access to a vital resource such as food or outdoor access. Where possible, free access to food in bowls or activity feeders that always contain some food and are merely topped up by the owner at random will enable the cats to maintain distance from one another, but it is important to consider the risk of obesity and manage feeding accordingly (see Chapter 13). Likewise, cat-doors which can be microchip-protected for better safety may be better than a "human operated" back-door.

The prognosis for cases of intercat conflict within the household is not only dependent on the feline factors, such as sociability of individuals within the group and the ability of the physical home environment to support the intended cat population. Human factors also play a significant role, and owner compliance with environmental modifications and with continued maintenance of the conditions that enable the group to coexist (provision of sufficient resource stations and so on) is crucial, combined with realistic owner expectation of the end result.

Successful resolution of aggression is most likely if individuals recognize each other as part of the same social group. This can sometimes be achieved by swapping odors between the cats and possibly by isolating factions or individuals so that a complete reintroduction is carried out, as if the cats were being brought into the house for the first time (see earlier section on introducing new cats). Owners do need to be aware that if there was no relationship between the cats prior to the onset of the problematic behavior it is unlikely that one will form, and therefore the best outcome that they can expect is one of mutual toleration. In these situations it is important to consider the potential for chronic tension to develop and to assess whether a lack of overt aggression is associated with true toleration or with a change of behavioral strategy to one of passive conflict. When social behavior, even at the level of toleration, cannot be maintained or where passive conflict is occurring rather than toleration, the welfare of the feline household needs to be considered. The use of pharmacological or nutraceutical intervention to reduce negative emotional states and facilitate social integration may be considered but this should be used alongside the environmental modifications outlined in this chapter and not seen as a substitute for them. If conflict continues despite such modifications or social behavior, even at the level of toleration, cannot be maintained without pharmacological or nutraceutical intervention, clients should be advised to consider rehoming of one or more of the cats.

AGGRESSION TO OTHER CATS IN THE NEIGHBORHOOD

Identifying Intercat Tension Within a Neighborhood

When cat owners are dealing with repetitive physical injury to their pets as a result of intercat conflict within a neighborhood, the problem will be readily identified (Figure 26-21). However, wounds and abscesses are not the only consequence of tension between neighboring cats and other potential outcomes such as the onset of problems of house soiling, obesity, and intercat aggression within households must also be considered. These behavioral changes are related to the reduction of access to outdoor territory caused by passive tension between neighboring cats (Figure 26-22). This tension can lead to an inability to access outdoor latrines or to engage in high energy–consuming activity within the outdoor environment. Where "despotic" neighbors are breaking and entering and when there is simply a challengingly high feline population density, some cats will be more likely to stay within the home thereby putting tension on fragile feline relationships with the household.

Aggression to other cats in the neighborhood is more likely when the local population is destabilized by introduction of a newcomer, when there is one or more entire tomcat in the local population, or when a feline despot is resident in the neighborhood. Conflict is also at a peak

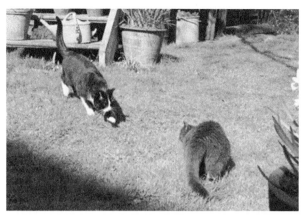

FIGURE 26-22   Tension between cats in the neighborhood can result in a reduction in ability to move freely in the outdoor environment. (Courtesy A. Dossche)

when entire queens are beginning to call and territorial areas are disputed.

Understanding and Managing Intercat Conflict in Neighborhoods

In order to understand and deal with issues of intercat conflict within neighborhoods, cat owners need to have an awareness of the principles of feline territory and look at the situation from a feline perspective. The acquisition of pet cats is usually based on decisions that are made purely on the basis of what is right for the immediate family, but when cats live in highly populated urban areas, the arrival of a new cat impacts neighboring feline households as well. Ideally cat owners need to be aware of the local feline population density before introducing more cats to an area, and part of the process of responsible rehoming should involve questions asked about the neighborhood that a cat is going to live in as well as the household. If a cat comes with a history of intercat tension in a previous home, and particularly a history of actively breaking and entering into neighboring properties, it is not appropriate to rehome it to an area with a dense feline population, but sadly information about the cat's behavior in a previous home may not be available. Similar consideration should be made when taking on a young kitten, and paying attention to the territorial requirements of the resident cats in the neighborhood as well as the newcomer is the key to making the integration process as smooth as possible.

The feline territory is divided into three zones. The central core territory needs to be safe and secure, but the home range may be traversed by other cats as they go between different parts of their own territory. The larger hunting range is also shared by cats in the local vicinity. The sharing of access to territory means that time share systems are important in avoiding conflict. Conflict is most likely in the home range when cat densities are high. Dawn and dusk are high risk times in

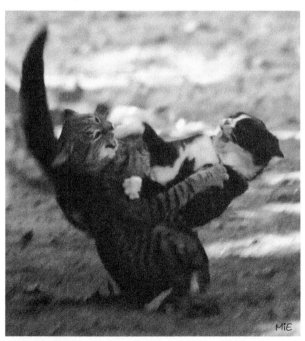

FIGURE 26-21   Intercat tension within neighborhoods is more readily identified when there is overt aggression. (Courtesy A. Dossche)

terms of aggression and this may be due to the fact that prey is most active at these times, and there is increased competition for this important resource, or simply a consequence of the increased chance of feline encounters because more cats are out and about at these times. Territorial area closely corresponds to the availability of survival resources, and the defense of territory is therefore linked to the defense of resources. Provision of a surfeit of resources within the neighborhood is therefore one of the keys to a reduction in territorial behavior and potential aggression.

Invasion of core territories and threat to resources within homes not only leads to a potential for conflict between the neighboring cats but also threatens the stability of the feline population within the house. The balance between resource availability and social cohesion is a delicate one and if another cat is entering the home and stealing essential resources, such as food and resting places, the relationships between cats within the invaded home will be pressurized.

Most cats engage in defense of their existing territory but there are some individuals for whom the occupation of additional territory, actively displacing others from their territory or monopolizing resources, is a goal. This so called "despotic" behavior is characterized by regular and repeated attempts to take over the territory of other cats, including their core territory or home range, and increases the potential for intercat conflict. These individuals may enter the homes of other cats to attack or intimidate them, or to leave urine marks, often leading to misdiagnosis of intercat aggression or indoor marking problems within the homes they are targeting.

Entire male cats are more likely to be despotic as they search for enough territory to allow them access to intact females. The majority of domestic cats are neutered and intercat aggression within neighborhoods is consequently reduced but, in situations where two entire males live in close proximity, the risk of overt aggression is greatly increased. In such situations the aggression can be very serious because reproductive, and hence genetic and evolutionary, success is at stake. Neutering before 12 months of age has been shown to decrease fighting by as much as 88%, which suggests that in the case of male to male intercat aggression hormonal influences are perhaps more significant than learning. Intact male cats that are the cause of aggression should be neutered, but prevention is always preferable to cure and it is therefore advisable for all cats to be neutered at the earliest opportunity. The current thinking supports the practice of neutering females at 4 months of age or earlier to minimize the risk of unwanted feline pregnancies. When entire unowned male strays or feral cats are present within a community, a program of trapping, neutering, and relocating may be recommended. Some of these cats may even make good pets once they have been castrated. If the intact male belongs to a local resident they must be contacted for permission to have the animal neutered. The surgery may be sponsored by a local charity or shelter organization if the owner is unable to pay. In a minority of cases, the owner may be unwilling to have the cat neutered. If there are no good grounds for this refusal it may be symptomatic of a general lack of care, which may enable the cat to be removed on welfare grounds.

Aggression between entire males and females is rare, although it may occur if the female is not ready or willing to mate. The mating process is a very noisy event and it is not uncommon for inexperienced owners to misinterpret this as an episode of aggression. When owners report that entire cats are acting in a hostile manner toward one another it is therefore important to consider the differential of normal mating behavior.

There is no exclusive correlation between reproductive status and despotism. Breed differences in territorial behavior should be taken into consideration. Hybrid cats may pose a particular challenge in this respect and owners should research this before bringing new cats into established feline neighborhoods. The behavior of despotic cats is often a source of tension between human and feline neighbors throughout the potentially very large area that the despot attempts to control.

If a "despotic cat" is identified within a community, it is important for the local cat owners to work together. The owners of the "despot" should temporarily keep the cat indoors while preparations are made to limit the problem and neighboring owners should ensure that any entry and exit points in their houses are as safe and secure as possible. This may involve investing in microchip protected cat flaps and also ensuring that the area around the entry and exit points is as visually protected as possible. In many cases it is possible to limit aggression by "time-sharing" access to outdoors, thereby allowing cats outside at times that prevent them coming into contact with each other.

In addition to time share systems, there are other ways in which neighboring cat owners can cooperate in order to minimize feline tension. Providing places in the garden for resident cats to claw mark, such as trees, fence posts, and sheds, and ensuring the availability of buffer zones for urine marking between adjacent properties can be beneficial. Increasing the cats' access to height in their respective gardens by creating perches in trees and on walls or fences that look away from the house gives cats a chance to defend their own territory while preventing other cats from using the perches to spy on the cat's house. Provision of outdoor latrines (such as sunken tray or sand pits) in protected locations toward the periphery of the gardens can reduce competition for appropriate latrine sites and it can also be beneficial for all local cat owners to adopt activity feeding and other environmental enrichments within their own homes that are known to encourage cats to spend time in their respective core territories.

Human cooperation is obviously essential if these approaches are to work, and cat owners may consider setting up a local "cat club" of people living in the neighborhood so that they can swap ideas about improving gardens and homes to suit the cats better.

CONCLUSIONS

Cats are social creatures but their social behavior differs greatly from that of people and dogs. They will naturally live in small groups of related individuals and avoid contact with other felines. It is therefore understandable that cats can find it stressful to live in a domestic environment. By paying attention to natural feline behaviors and modifying the environments accordingly, it is possible to offer ethological solutions and to manage multicat households and neighborhoods in a way that effectively minimizes stress and offers practical solutions for cases of intercat conflict. It is also important to minimize the risk of intercat tension by choosing cats that are likely to be sociable and then introducing them in the right way. Limiting the number of cats within households to ethologically sensible levels is also important and client education is vital if this is to be achieved. When issues of social incompatibility arise, it is important to accept that in some cases rehoming a cat or indeed some cats may be essential to provide the whole group with better welfare. When problems arise between cats in the neighborhood, the prognosis is guarded because there is limited opportunity to manage the potential for future introductions. Every change or increase in population brings further competition and instability. Successful management of a local overpopulation problem therefore depends upon active participation by all cat owners.

REFERENCES

1. Casey RA, Vandenbussche S, Bradshaw JWS, Roberts MA. Reasons for relinquishment and return of domestic cats (*Felis silvestris catus*) to rescue shelters in the UK. *Anthrozoos.* 2009;22:347–358.
2. Salman MD, Hutchison J, Ruch-Gallie R. Behavioral reasons for relinquishment of dogs and cats to 12 shelters. *J Appl Anim Welf Sci.* 2000;3:93–106.
3. Millsopp S, Westgarth C, Barclay R, Ward M: APBC Annual Report 2012. http://www.apbc.org.uk/system/files/apbc_annual_report_2012.pdf.
4. Bamberger M, Houpt KA. Signalment factors, comorbidity, and trends in behavior diagnoses in cats: 736 cases (1991–2001). *J Am Vet Med Assoc.* 2006;229:1602–1606.
5. Amat M, Ruiz de la Torre JL, Fatjo J, et al. Potential risk factors associated with feline behaviour problems. *Appl Anim Behav Sci.* 2009;121:134–139.
6. Liberg O, Sandell M, Pontier D, Natoli E. Density, spatial organization and reproductive tactics in the domestic cat and other felids. In: Turner DC, Bateson P, eds. *The domestic cat: the biology of its behaviour.* ed 2. Cambridge, UK: Cambridge University Press; 2000:119–148.
7. Bradshaw JWS, Lovett RE. Do domestic cats form hierarchies? *British Small Animal Veterinary Association Congress Scientific Proceedings*; 2003, BSAVA Birmingham, UK p. 104.
8. McDonald DW, Yamaguchi N, Kerby G. Group-living in the domestic cat: its sociobiology and epidemiology. In: Turner DC, Bateson P, eds. *The domestic cat: the biology of its behaviour.* Cambridge, UK: Cambridge University Press; 2000:95–118.
9. Bradshaw JWS, Hall SL. Affiliative behaviour of related and unrelated pairs of cats in catteries: a preliminary report. *Appl Anim Behav Sci.* 1999;63:251–255.
10. Cameron ME, Casey RA, Bradshaw JWS, et al. A study of environmental and behavioural factors that may be associated with feline idiopathic cystitis. *J Small Anim Pract.* 2004;45:144–147.
11. Buffington CAT, Westropp JL, Chew DJ, Bolus RR. Clinical evaluation of multimodal environmental modification (MEMO) in the management of cats with idiopathic cystitis. *J Feline Med Surg.* 2006;8:261–268.
12. Bradshaw JWS. *The behaviour of the domestic cat.* Wallingford, UK: CAB International; 1992.
13. Levine E, Perry P, Scarlett J, Houpt K. Inter cat aggression in households following the introduction of a new cat. *Appl Anim Behav Sci.* 2005;90:325–226.
14. Rochlitz I. A review of housing requirements of domestic cats (Felis silvestris catus) kept in the home. *Appl Anim Behav Sci.* 2005;93:97–109.
15. Bradshaw JWS. *Cat sense: the feline enigma revealed.* London, UK: Penguin; 2013.
16. Frost RO, Steketee G, Williams L. Hoarding: a community health problem. *Health Soc Care Community.* 2000;8:229–234.

Human-Directed Aggression in Cats

Rachel Casey

INTRODUCTION

Aggressive behavior toward owners is one of the most common reasons for referral to a specialist behavior center; the author's unpublished data suggests around 13% of the feline caseload.[1] The types of aggressive behaviors which result in injury (i.e., biting and scratching) are usually those for which cat owners seek advice from their veterinarian. However, agonistic behaviors in cats also include hissing, spitting, lashing out, "ambushing" (running up to an owner and grabbing them, often scratching or biting), and holding on with forelimbs while "scraping" with hind legs. Importantly, though, aggression is not a diagnosis *per se*. Just as limping might be a sign of an orthopedic condition, which requires a clinical workup, observing aggressive behavior in a cat is a sign of an underlying problem needing further investigation. There is, therefore, not a "prescriptive" treatment program for aggressive behavior in cats. The appropriate course of action will vary with causal factors and situation for each individual case. The aim of this chapter is to explore the reasons why cats may commonly show signs of aggression toward people and consider some of the treatment tools, which may be useful in addressing such cases.

REASONS FOR HUMAN-DIRECTED AGGRESSIVE BEHAVIOR IN THE CAT

There are four main reasons for the occurrence of aggressive behavior in cats. These are: aggression occurring as a defensive response when cats feel threatened; a displaced play/predatory/attention-seeking response, which can include signs of aggression; aggression as a response to frustration; and aggression which arises as a result of disease processes. These causes of aggressive behavior are described separately in the sections below.

Aggression Occurring as a Defensive Response

This is probably the most common reason for aggressive behaviors to develop. As with all species, aggression is one of a range of "options" used by cats in response to a perceived threat (Figure 27-1). Cats will perceive people as a threat if they have had limited socialization experience of people and/or a negative experience of handling. Although cats are predators, they are a small species and vulnerable to attack from both larger predators and other cats. Their preferred strategy in the face of threat is, therefore, avoidance, such as to withdraw, hide, or climb. However, aggression is used as a defensive strategy when other options, such as running away, are not possible or successful. This might happen where owners pursue cats and try to interact with them or where cats are restricted and cannot get away; for example, in a veterinary practice cage. A cat, which is fearful of people, will generally try and withdraw to the back of the cage and may pull away or hunch up as much as possible to avoid contact (Figure 27-2). Where people continue to approach, the only option remaining for the cat is to lash out to keep the threat away (Figure 27-3).

One of the key misunderstandings about aggressive behavior in cats is the differentiation between apparently "defensive" aggression, where a cat lashes out while pulling away and showing other signs of fear or anxiety, and "offensive" aggression, where the cat may appear more confident, perhaps leaping toward an owner or lashing out from a work surface. Historically, these signs were regarded as being different in origin; however, they differ only in the phase of development of the behavior, based on the learning opportunities for each animal. It is probably easiest to understand this by considering the example of a fearful cat in a cage within the veterinary practice. A cat that is poorly socialized to people might start by backing away to the back of the cage or hiding under blankets or inside the litter tray. In most cases, veterinary practice staff will need to get the cat out for treatment, so they will reach in to try and get hold of the cat. Because pulling away is not successful, and other options, such as climbing, are not possible for the cat in this environment, the only remaining "strategy" for the cat is to show aggressive signs to keep the threat away. When a cat lashes out like this, most people will react by pulling their hand back, even if momentarily. This reaction reinforces the aggressive response of the cat, and with repetition, the cat will learn that aggression is an effective "strategy"

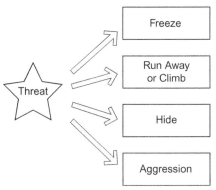

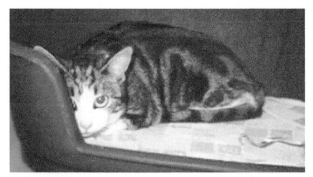

FIGURE 27-1 Cats have a number of behavioral responses to perceived threat, including aggression.

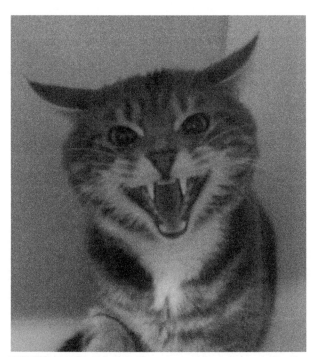

FIGURE 27-2   A cat that is anxious or fearful of people may initially retreat to the back of the cage, hunch up, cower, or try and hide.

FIGURE 27-3   Fearful cats may often show defensive aggression when enclosed in a pen as other avoidance strategies are not possible. (Courtesy K. Borgeat)

to keep people away in this situation. With this repetition, the cat will gradually become more confident in the expression of this behavior and will develop an expectation that aggression will be successful to avoid the threat in this context. Therefore, over repeated learning opportunities, cats may develop apparently "offensive" aggression, even launching at people. They will also learn the various events which predict the threatening situation and start to show aggression more rapidly when they first recognize predictive cues that threat is likely to occur. Cats, which "launch" at owners and appear to be very confident in behavior, can therefore still be motivated by fear, but they have become confident that their strategy is likely to be effective at removing the perceived threat.

Anxiety- or fear-based aggression can also develop if the owner is associated with other stimuli that a cat is worried by. A common example is where an owner has been handling another cat and then approaches his or her own cat. The scent of an unfamiliar cat, or even one from the same household which is not part of the same social group, can precipitate aggression toward the owner.

Aggression Occurring as a Misplaced Play/Predatory/Attention-Seeking Response

In some cases of aggression toward people, behavioral signs develop through inappropriate play or interaction with owners. Play behavior in kittens is important in the development of the motor responses needed for predatory behavior.[1] In a feral situation, this "practicing" is initially directed at inanimate objects but is later directed by the queen towards prey items that she brings back to the nest site.[2] The kittens, therefore, learn the appropriate conditioned cues that stimulate these behaviors (in other words, they learn what to direct predatory responses toward). In the domestic environment, owners are frequently tempted to play with their kittens by, for example, wiggling their fingers or moving their feet under a duvet. The kitten learns to direct these behaviors to bits of people because it is reinforced by the response of their owner—often laughing or moving around more to engage in play. While this is apparently harmless with a kitten, it can lead to inappropriate play/predatory aggression being directed toward hands or feet once the cat matures to an adult. Often, this progression occurs because as the kitten grows up and is less cute, they have to "work harder" in order to get a response from the owner; for example, grabbing feet as they come out from under the duvet when bouncing on the duvet is no longer reinforced by the owner's response. Cats may also start to "ambush" their owners as they walk past by rushing out from behind furniture and grabbing their feet or legs or swiping at them as they walk past. This type of behavior is often reinforced further by the response of the owner: shrieking, pulling arms away, or running about tend to reinforce the response just as movement and squealing of a prey item would encourage predatory responses.

Although this behavior starts as an appetitive (reinforced) response, it often becomes more complicated as owner responses change over time. Once people have a cat that bites or scratches, they often change their response to a more punitive one; for example, using a water spray, throwing cushions, or shouting at the cat. This change in response can commonly result in "emotional conflict" in the cat where mixed emotions are associated with performing the behavior. In such cases, cats will often still be motivated to start the behavioral sequence, because it has been strongly reinforced from a young age, but also be anxious about the consequences. This can lead to the behavior becoming more extreme; for example, the cat dashing out, biting hard, then running off and hiding again. Using punishment-based techniques for cats which show aggression as a displaced play/predatory response is, therefore, counterproductive.

Aggression Occurring as a Response to Frustration

Although less common, aggressive behaviors can also occur in cats as a result of frustration. This is sometimes called "redirected aggression" as it can be directed toward a target other than the source of frustration. Frustration arises where an expected outcome does not occur; an example might be when a cat, which normally runs outside and chases off other cats, only sees them through the window and is unable to get to them because the cat door is locked. In this situation, the frustration of being unable to do the expected behavior can result in aggression being directed at the owner or at another household pet purely because they happen to be in the wrong place at the wrong time. This behavior can occur more commonly in households where cats are always kept indoors due to the increased risk of frustration when seeing outdoor cats and being unable to access them. However, it is not exclusively a problem of indoor cats, and this is only one example of how frustration may be induced.

Aggression that Arises as a Result of Disease Processes

Aggression will occasionally arise entirely because of an internal disease process. In rare cases, such as partial seizures with a focus in the limbic region, cats can show aggression spontaneously without any environmental cues or precipitators. More commonly, physiological or pathological changes influence the threshold at which aggression due to anxiety or frustration occurs. For example, a cat, which is uncomfortable with being handled but has always tolerated it, may start to show aggression on being petted with the onset of hyperthyroidism or degenerative joint disease (for more information see Bradshaw et al [1] and Chapter 15).

PREVENTION

The most common types of aggression—those arising from anxiety and misplaced predatory/play responses—are easily preventable with appropriate early advice to kitten owners. It is a key role of the veterinary practice team to ensure that each client coming to the practice with a new kitten is given information on the simple rules summarized below.

Preventing Anxiety- and Fear-Based Aggression

The key to preventing aggression toward humans that is motivated by anxiety or fear is ensuring that kittens are adequately "socialized" to people. The socialization period for kittens is earlier than in puppies. It is thought to finish by around 7 weeks of age.[3] The responsibility for ensuring that kittens have adequate and appropriate basic socialization to humans therefore lies with breeders or fosterers of abandoned kittens. However, kittens' responses to people have been found to continue to be influenced by interaction until 4 months of age,[4] so continued careful handling by owners after homing is also important. Kittens should always associate handling with positive outcomes. To ensure that this is the case, it is best for owners to start by encouraging their kitten to approach them for interaction rather than going to the kitten to pick them up. Allowing a kitten to approach gives him or her a choice of whether to do so or not. If contact is enforced, it is more difficult to be sure that the kitten perceives the interaction as positive. Where kittens or young cats show signs of anxiety and do not approach, owners should be encouraged to follow a program of desensitization and counterconditioning (see next section) immediately. This program is easier to follow before cats display established avoidance responses, and this will ensure that aggressive responses to people do not develop.

It is important to be aware of the risk of inducing and reinforcing aggression responses in cats when they are housed in veterinary practice cages. This can be minimized by ensuring that cats have the opportunity to hide as an alternative avoidance response.[5,6] The use of cardboard boxes, strategically positioned towels, tall-sided or covered cat beds, or the Feline Fort (Cats Protection) or Hide and Perch box is recommended (Figure 27-4). Nervous cats should be encouraged to approach for handling rather than reaching in to get hold of them. Although this takes more patience in the short term, the long-term benefits of preventing aggression will be worthwhile both for staff safety and the welfare of the cats.

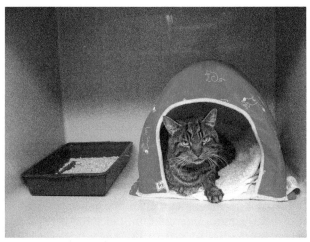

FIGURE 27-4 Giving cats the opportunity to hide can help reduce the risk of aggression developing. (Courtesy M. Cannon)

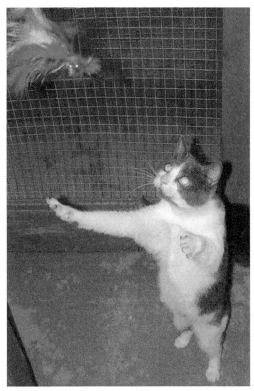

FIGURE 27-5 Owners should be encouraged to play using toys that are distant from the body, such as 'fishing rod' toys. (Courtesy E. Blackwell)

Preventing Aggression as a Misdirected Play/Predatory Response

One key piece of advice that veterinary practice staff should give all kitten owners is not to play with kittens with parts of the body, for example, by moving feet under the duvet. Kittens do need to play, but practice staff should encourage owners to play with toys, which are distant from the body; for example, "fishing rod" type toys (Figure 27-5). If owners have already started to play with their kittens with their hands or feet by the time of their first visit to the practice, they should be advised to stop reacting at all when their kitten jumps on hands or feet but to engage the kitten in appropriate forms of play at other times. If necessary owners should wear protective clothing in the form of gloves or shoes in order to make it possible to comply with this advice.

Preventing Frustration-Related Aggression

Cases of frustration-related aggression can be difficult to predict because they often arise due to "chance" circumstances. However, cats are less likely to become frustrated if they have some control over their environment. This can be achieved by ensuring that cats have plenty of outlets for their natural behaviors. Providing areas for hiding, climbing, and scratching and supplying puzzle feeders and plenty of opportunities to play will reduce the risk of cats becoming frustrated. It is important that these resources can be easily accessed by all cats in a multicat household; for example, by making sure they are available in the core area for each cat or social group of cats. It may also be beneficial to restrict access to windows and glass doors or keep blinds closed if the sight of cats or birds outside is a particular trigger for a frustration response.

DIFFERENTIATING TYPES OF AGGRESSION

Human-directed aggression can occur for a number of different reasons and the first challenge is to identify the main causal factors in each case. This should not only involve a detailed description of the behavior and the context in which it occurs, but also the history of development of the behavior. The situation in which the behavior was first shown will give important insights into the original motivation. Investigation should also include other factors, such as the behavior of the cat with owners and other people in contexts other than where the aggression occurs and the early life history of the cat, to establish the potential impact of socialization experience. Cats should also have a thorough medical examination and review of their medical history to establish whether any health factors may be contributing to the behavioral signs.

TREATMENT STRATEGIES

The treatment approaches used will vary with the cause of the behavior. The specific "tools" used in a behavior-modification program will also vary with the specific factors of the case. Tailoring treatment protocols to ensure they are practical and feasible for owners in their home situation is an important part of behavior modification. The main elements, which may be incorporated into behavior-modification programs for the most common causes of human-directed aggression, are suggested in the sections below.

Treatment for Anxiety- and Fear-Based Aggression

The primary aim of treatment for fear-related aggression is to teach the cat that being handled by people is no longer threatening but instead associated with a positive outcome. This is achieved with a program of desensitization and counterconditioning. The first stage is to ensure that the owner stops trying to approach their cat to interact. It is important for the cat to learn that the owner is no longer a potential threat before a positive association can be formed. The next stage is desensitization and counterconditioning. This is best carried out by allowing the cat to choose whether to approach the owner for a reward, since the subtle signs of anxiety can be difficult to read in cats. If the cat is given the choice whether or not to approach its owner, it is clear that the interaction is perceived as positive. Where owners approach their cat to interact, they may miss indications that their cat is worried and having problems progressing with the program.

In devising a desensitization and counterconditioning program for an anxious or fearful cat, the level of interaction which the cat *consistently* tolerates should be established first. For some cats, this may be when the person sits quietly reading on the far side of the room, while in others, it may be when the person strokes the cat once (Figure 27-6). Tolerance of interaction can be influenced by other factors (e.g., the presence of other

stressors), so it is common for cats to tolerate more contact on some occasions than others; for example, biting as soon as their owner puts a hand toward them or tolerating a number of strokes before biting. The starting level for desensitization should be less than the minimum interaction tolerated. For example, for a cat that turns and bites after between one and four strokes, the program should start with just rewarding approach, then for one short stroke, then two, and so on. As with any desensitization and counterconditioning program, the aim is to start interaction at a level that the cat tolerates and associate this with a positive outcome. This can be a food treat or play, depending on what the individual cat is more interested in. Once the cat consistently approaches to receive the reward, the level of contact can be gradually increased. For example, once a cat consistently runs up to an owner for a treat without any hesitation, the owner can start to put their hand toward the cat before dropping the treat, and then start gently touching the cat before giving the treat. At each stage, it is essential to progress very slowly and ensure that the cat consistently tolerates one stage before progressing to the next. The most common cause of failure for this type of program is owners trying to progress too fast. As soon as the cat becomes anxious about contact, the owner needs to stop and reduce the level of interaction to that previously tolerated. By building up in gradual stages, cats can learn to perceive close contact with people as consistently positive, and this removes their perceived need to show human-directed aggression.

Treating Aggression as a Misdirected Play/ Predatory Response

It is often found that by the time predatory/play/attention-getting aggression is presented to the veterinary practice team, cats have some degree of emotional conflict due to owners punishing them for their ambushing behavior. Nevertheless, the motivation for cats initiating this type of behavior is to achieve the perceived reward of owner response. The key to treating such cats is, therefore, to ensure that they have the opportunity to learn *both* that other behaviors are successful at achieving a response and that ambushing is no longer effective at doing so. In many of these cases, the cat's focus on people is exacerbated by limited opportunities to engage in other activities. Where this is the case, an important element of treatment is ensuring that the cat has plenty to do. Through imaginative enrichment of the environment, there are many ways in which cats' activity can be directed into behaviors, which are distant from the owner.[7] For example, feeding cats using puzzle feeders or hiding food in different places around the house will direct the cat's interest to another activity (Figure 27-7). Cats that show predatory/play/attention-getting aggression do so because they highly value social contact with people, so outlets for

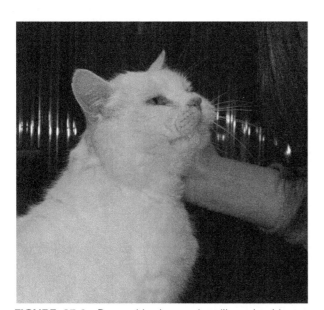

FIGURE 27-6 Desensitization to handling should start with a single stroke when the cat chooses to approach and is relaxed.

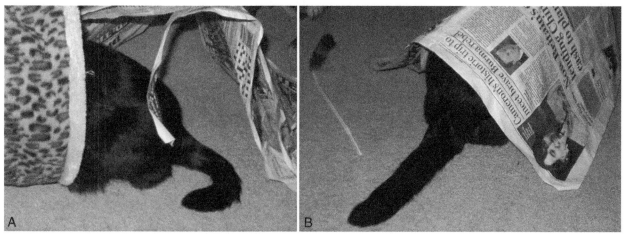

FIGURE 27-7   Aggression risk can be reduced by providing other forms of enrichment, such as hiding treats or encouraging independent play. (Courtesy J. Revell)

this interaction are required as well as more independent activities. Owners should be encouraged to have periods of interaction with their cat; for example, playing with toys which are distant from the body, such as 'fishing rod' type toys, or using a point of light or laser to direct the cat to a hidden food treat. (It is important to note that the use of a light or laser to encourage activity without a specific target, such as a toy or a treat, is not recommended due to the risk of inducing frustration). Talking to the cat during these games is likely to enhance the interactive experience for the cat. It is important, however, that the owner does not use this play as a "distraction" when their cat is attacking them or about to do so. Trying to engage the cat in other activities at this time is likely to reinforce the ambushing behavior. Instead, owners need to make sure they start playing with their cat when he or she is relaxed and not when they are starting a bout of "ambushing."

The more an owner can direct their cat into other activities, the less likely it is that "ambushes" will occur. However, the effect will not be immediate and they are likely to still occur at least for a short period and the owner needs to be prepared for this. It is clearly unrealistic to expect an owner to stand still and not react while their cats is biting or scratching at them, so it is important to emphasize to owners the importance of wearing something that will protect them in the short term, so that they can stand completely still and ignore this behavior. The type of protection will depend on the extent of the biting or scratching and the part of the body which is targeted. For example, a thick pair of socks and jeans or horse riding "chaps" could be used. It is essential that the owner wears suitable protection in all circumstances in which a bout of this type of aggression could occur. They also need to be clear that it is important to stand completely still and not react to the cat in any way during the behavior. Cats learn very quickly that this response

is no longer reinforced with attention and that other behaviors are. However, owners will need guiding through this first stage while their cat is learning these new "rules" of human interaction. Where some members of the household are particularly nervous of their cat, it is better for more confident family members to start the program, as learning an alternative behavior with one person will make the process easier for other family members.

It is important with this treatment approach that owners are not just instructed to ignore the behaviors. Such an approach is not going to be beneficial for two reasons. Firstly without careful guidance, most owners will be unwilling or unable to do this and secondly without directing cats into alternative responses, the act of ignoring the behavior is likely to result in an increased frequency and intensity of the behavior because of frustration. Engaging cats into other independent activities and giving them a new way of interacting with their owners that has a positive outcome is important in changing this behavior.

CONCLUSION

Aggressive behavior in cats is a behavioral sign rather than a diagnosis. Cats can start to show aggression toward people for a number of reasons. The most common are anxiety about contact with people resulting in a defensive response and aggression which arises from a misdirected play/predatory response due to inappropriate early play interactions with people. Less commonly, aggression can occur as a response to frustration or as a consequence of a medical disorder. The veterinary practice has a key role in preventing aggression in cats through advising breeders and owners on appropriate socialization and how to play with kittens. Where cases do develop, the treatment for aggressive behavior in cats is often very successful with tailored behavior-modification programs. It is unusual to require adjunctive pharmacological agents in such cases, but this may be necessary where the circumstances of a case make behavior-modification difficult to achieve. There is no evidence that any nonprescription or over-the-counter products have efficacy in the treatment of human-directed aggression in cats.

REFERENCES

1. Bradshaw JWS, Casey RA, Brown SL. *The behaviour of the domestic cat.* ed 2. Wallingford: CABI; 2012.
2. Kitchener A. The natural history of wild cats. London: Christopher Helm; 1991, p. 70.
3. Karsh EB, Tuner DC. The human-cat relationship. In: Turner DC, Bateson P, eds. *The domestic cat: the biology of its behaviour.* Cambridge: Cambridge University Press; 1988:159–178.
4. Lowe SE, Bradshaw JWS. Responses of pet cats to being held by an unfamiliar person. *Anthrozoös.* 2002;15:69–79.
5. Kly K, Casey RA. Provision of hiding enrichment for domestic cats *(Felis sylvestris catus)* in a rescue shelter environment: Effects on behavioural measures of stress and re-homing potential. *Animal Welfare.* 2007;16(3):375–383.
6. Casey RA: *You can't see me…the value of hiding enrichment for cats.* https://behaviourvet.wordpress.com/2013/10/12/you-cant-see-methe-value-of-hiding-enrichment-for-cats. Published October 12, 2013. Accessed October 21, 2013.
7. Ellis Sarah. Environmental enrichment: practical strategies for improving feline welfare. *J Feline Med Surg.* 2009;11(11):901–912.

Note: Page numbers followed by *f* indicate figures, *b* indicate boxes and *t* indicate tables.

Client Handouts

Advantages and Risks of Feline Spay or Castration Surgery

Debra Horwitz and Amy Pike

The information presented in this handout is intended to help you, the client, make an informed decision about neutering your pet. If you have any questions or would like more information about any of the points below, please feel free to ask your veterinarian or veterinary technician.

Advantages

- Roaming is generally reduced in both sexes. This also decreases the chances that your pet will be lost or hit by a moving vehicle during a roaming period.
- Sexual behavior by males, including that directed towards people, is reduced or eliminated.
- Females will not show "heat" (estrus) behavior and attract males.
- If aggression or urine marking/spraying is hormonally motivated, it may be eliminated.
- Animals will not suffer from infections of sexual organs, including sexually transmitted diseases. Infections of the uterus (pyometra) can be life threatening.
- Certain cancers may be less likely to occur in the absence of reproductive hormones from the ovaries and testicles. Testicular, ovarian, and uterine cancers are eliminated completely.
- Cat fights (and the wounds and abscesses associated with them) are reduced when cats are not sexually active.
- A neutered pet does not contribute to the growing pet overpopulation problem!

Risks

All surgeries have inherent risks, although complications are extremely rare in elective surgeries of healthy animals. However, the risks include:

- Abnormal reaction to anesthesia, even leading to death. However, each animal is monitored constantly throughout anesthesia using similar equipment to that used in human medicine.
- Bleeding. All surgeries are closely supervised so that the risk of bleeding is minimized.
- Stitches breaking or tearing out. This problem is kept to a minimum with suturing technique and owner compliance postsurgery to keep the animal quiet and inactive until full healing has occurred.
- Infections. Local infections (at the incision site) are often caused by licking or chewing at the incision. This can be prevented with special collars. Some cats may be upset by the collar and its removal can occur when supervised. Infections can be treated with antibiotics if they occur.
- Although some problem behaviors that are hormonally motivated may be completely diminished with neutering, others are likely to persist and need the intervention of your veterinarian or a veterinary behaviorist.

Advantages of Boarding Your Cat at a Veterinary Practice

Ilona Rodan

When your cat boards at our practice, we monitor your cat at least twice daily and provide the TLC you would want for him or her. If medication such as insulin or oral medication is needed, it will be administered as often as prescribed.

During periods of monitoring, a technician measures the amount of food and water consumed and assesses litter box habits and your cat's weight. Provision of affection, attention, play, or exercise can be offered to boarders in a larger room during quieter times (evenings, weekends, or mid-day) if they are willing to leave their condominium or suite. If any problems are noted at any time, the technician will inform the veterinarian who will examine your cat and identify what is needed. We will notify you and make recommendations, and follow the plan you choose.

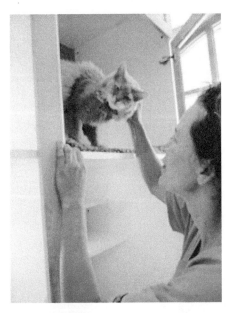

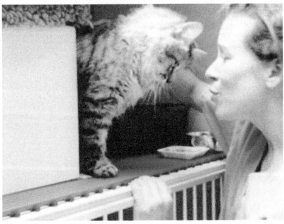

We welcome you to bring your cat's favorite bedding, small or interactive toys, and their favorite or special diets. If your cat has not boarded with us routinely, a veterinarian will meet with you to discuss your cat's needs and normal behaviors, and to examine and assess the health of your cat. Some clients request that necessary dental care or diagnostic tests are carried out while their cat is boarding, and we work to accommodate these requests.

Large Suites

Our suites are large enough for cats to climb and exercise, which is important for their welfare. Several have a view, others are full rooms, and hiding options are provided for cats that prefer to hide. For cats that stay for more than a few days or who we know are comfortable with a big room, we allow cats to go into large examination rooms during the quieter times of the day.

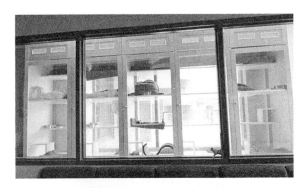

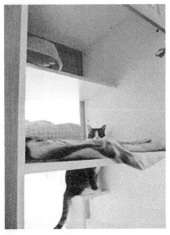

A Safe Place to Hide

Hiding places are important for cats as they like to be able to choose whether they want to be hidden or not. This is especially helpful for cats that may be more fearful when they are staying with us. A hiding place is necessary for most cats for the first day, but it is always available throughout their stay. Bringing your own cat's bed will help it feel more comfortable, but we have plenty available. If your cat prefers to stay in its carrier with the door open, that too is an option.

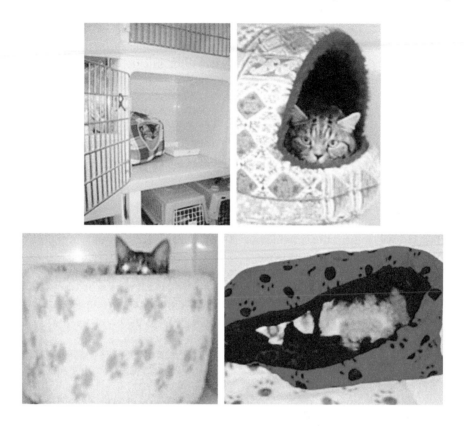

A Private Room

Cats that are shy or more active can have a private room based on availability.

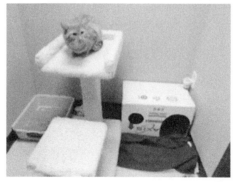

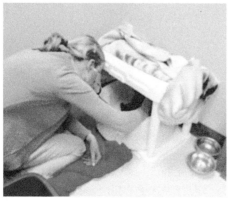

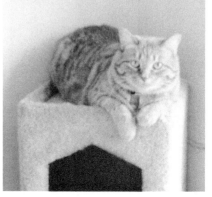

Personal Time

Many cats want attention or play time and our technicians are fond of the cats who board at the veterinary hospital. Staff often provide extra affection for boarders during lunch breaks and at quieter times in the day.

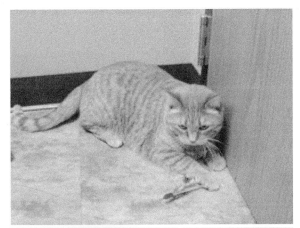

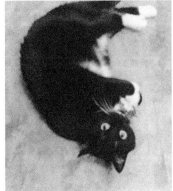

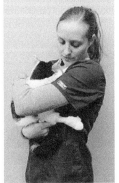

What if You Have Two or More Cats to Board?

Even cats that love each other want to have separate places to rest at least some of the time. We will provide the options for them to choose to rest either together or separately, and will monitor to see how they do together. Sometimes cats will prefer their own space when away from home and we will provide that if needed. The cats may also be separated for short periods to ensure that each cat is eating. If you have three to four cats, we can increase the size of any of the condominiums with a view, or provide a large room. Please let us know if your cats do not like each other at home, and we will provide separate suites.

Your Cat's Comfort and Safety Are Our Priority

Feel free to contact us to see how your cat is doing. Please let us know if you would like for us to send you pictures of your cat periodically. If you have any questions or would like to visit our boarding facilities prior to your time away, please contact us and we will be glad to help.

Cat-Friendly Medication Administration Techniques*

Iris Cloyd and Theresa DePorter

Administering medication to a cat can be a stressful event for both you and your cat. With proper preparation, training, and patience, giving medication to your cat can be easier and less stressful for everyone. The length of time that a cat requires medication can vary from just a few doses to life-long. Physical restraint and manual manipulation may not be unpleasant for all cats but will be for many and cause a strain on your relationship, decrease your cat's interactions with you, and create stress for both you and your cat. This handout discusses how to make giving medication a hands-free process or at the very least less stressful for both you and your cat.

How to Begin

If treatment allows the start date of the medication to be delayed, the cat can be preconditioned to the medication process. First identify what is a delectable food or treat for your cat. When utilizing food to administer medication, introduce the food item first on its own to determine if the cat will eat it willingly and to create an initial pleasant association with the food.

Once or twice daily give the cat only nonmedicated treats or food at the same time and place to mimic the recommended medication dosing schedule. This can help the cat develop a routine of pleasant and predictable associations with the food which should allow for easier administration of medication.

Overcoming Initial Suspicion of Novel Foods

For cats that are especially suspicious, introducing the medication in sets of three should help reduce the cat's concern. Begin by offering three small separate treat piles of the favored treats or food. Once the cat will eat all three piles without medication added, you can proceed to medicating the cat. All of the piles should be identical except for the pile in the middle; this one will contain the medication. Offer the cat the first nonmedicated treat, and immediately after it is ingested offer the second treat with the medication well hidden, followed by the third treat which is nonmedicated. Alternatively, a food trail using food of a paste consistency can be laid down requiring the cat to follow and eat each small bolus.

Placing Medication in Food or Treats

Soft foods such as canned cat food and meat-flavored baby food are ideal vehicles for pill placement. Crunchy peanut butter (assuming there are no peanut allergies in the home) makes discerning pills from the peanuts difficult and encourages the cat to ingest the pill without being able to separate the medication from the food. Pastes such as feline hairball remedies, cream cheese, and anchovy paste are all highly palatable and adhere nicely to tablets and capsules, making it more difficult to lick the food off of the pill while increasing the likelihood that the cat will ingest the pill when swallowing the paste.

Opening Capsules and Crushing Medication

Opening capsules and crushing tablets are also options before mixing them in food, but may create other problems. Always ask your veterinarian before opening any capsules or crushing pills. Some medications are time-released so opening the pill may alter how it is absorbed. For some medications, crushing the tablet may be acceptable but only if the medication is given immediately. Some pills or capsules contain a bitter substance that is difficult to mask in food, potentially causing an aversion to the food. If the medication can be added to the food, be sure to notice if the cat eats all of the food so that it consumes all of the medication.

Oral Suspensions

Oral suspensions can also be combined with food. It is best to combine like flavors together. For example, if the suspension has been compounded into a meat flavor it ideally should be combined with canned cat food, clam/oyster juice, or meat-flavored baby food (the latter which contains no onion or onion powder that can cause anemia in cats). Liquid medications that have a sweet flavoring such as bubble gum or cherry should be paired with small amounts of sweet food such as slightly melted ice cream or whipped cream. Other liquid combining agents may include cat milk, chicken broth without onion, and tomato juice.

Medicating when Masking in Food is not an Option

There may be urgent situations when delaying the starting time of the medication may not be possible and food may be contraindicated to give at the same time as the medication. This will require administration of the medication to your cat. Ideally you will want to practice these techniques prior to introducing medication. Start by gathering a pile of dry cat food kibbles, crunchy and

---

*This is a modified version of a handout authored by Melissa Spooner, LVT, VTS (Behavior), BS, KPA-CTP, Behavior Technician at Oakland Veterinary Referral Services, Bloomfield Hills, Mich.

403

soft cat treats, and a few slivers of real tuna or chicken. Use one hand to lightly but firmly cup the cat's head and upper jaw. The index finger on the second hand will open the cat's mouth by placing the finger at the mouth opening, just under the cat's nose but just above the lower incisors. While the other hand holds the cat's head in place, the index finger will be used to open the cat's mouth. Once the mouth is open, drop a piece of the very delicious food into that cat's mouth and release your hold. The cat may seem unsure and even puzzled after this first interaction but with several more repetitions the cat will quickly form a positive association with this process. Give a variety of preselected treats each time the cat is held to medicate and faux-medicated.

A practice schedule should look like this:

Round 1: chicken
Round 2: cheese
Round 3: hard cat treat (later the pill may be substituted for a hard treat)
Round 4: tuna

Utilizing a random and variable schedule of food type will keep the cat guessing what food comes next and help keep this exercise positive, pleasant, and fun. Avoid treats your cat dislikes but offer a variety to teach acceptance of novel foods. Once you have mastered the use of administering food treats this way, you can progress to introducing the medication as one of the "treats."

Did You Know? Fun Facts and Figures to Help Select a New Feline Family Member

Debra Horwitz and Amy Pike

- There are over 70 recognized breeds of cats, each one with its own set of unique behavioral characteristics and physical attributes.
- Breed association websites like The International Cat Association (www.tica.org), the Cat Fanciers Association (www.cfa.org), and the Governing Council of the Cat Fancy (www.gccfcats.org) provide detailed descriptions and pictures of each breed.
- Reputable breeders will allow you to visit their facility and meet both parents (if kept onsite) prior to purchasing a cat.
- There are many breed-specific rescue organizations that have cats available for adoption.
- The friendliness of a cat appears to be genetically linked to the friendliness of its father, whether or not the cat ever even interacted with its father.
- Urine marking/spraying (depositing urine on vertical surfaces) is a **normal** cat behavior.
- Studies have shown that approximately 10% of neutered males and 5% of spayed females will urine mark in the house.

- Male cats tend to be friendlier towards unfamiliar people and visitors to the home.
- Female cats tend to be more aggressive towards other cats.
- Siblings are the most likely to sleep together and groom each other—signs that the cats like each other.
- The following pairs of nonrelated cats are best together: male/male relationships, followed by male/female relationships, and lastly, female/female.
- There appear to be three basic feline personality types: active/aggressive, timid/nervous, and confident/easy-going.
- It is important to attempt to match the personality types currently in your household with that of the new member.
- In a multicat household it is important to provide sufficient resources for each cat in order to diminish the possibility for intercat aggression and behavioral problems.
- **Your veterinarian can help you choose the right feline for your family—just ask!**

Does My Cat Hurt?

Sheilah Robertson

Figuring out if your cat is in pain can take a bit of detective work because cats are good at hiding their pain. You know your cat better than anyone and even though the signs are sometimes subtle, you will catch them if you look closely.

Cats can hurt after surgery or if they have suffered an injury, and some diseases can cause pain; one example is herpes virus infection which can cause painful eye and mouth lesions; these are all examples of acute pain. Just remember: if it would be painful for you, it will be painful for your cat.

Does your cat seem uncomfortable? Be suspicious of pain if your cat keeps shifting positions and looks like it is trying to find a comfortable one.

Changes in your cat's behavior or attitude can be an indicator of pain. If your cat used to be playful and outgoing but starts to hide and does not want anything to do with you, something is wrong.

Other things to look for are changes in posture—if your cat is hunched or tucked up, it could have a sore belly.

A change in how your cat's face looks may give us some clues about its pain. Hanging its head, flattened ears, pulled back whiskers, a clenched mouth, and half shut eyes may indicate pain.

If a cat stops eating, something is wrong—but cats that are in pain may continue to eat.

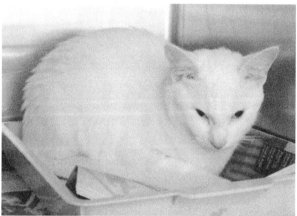

A cat showing facial signs of pain.

If you are worried that your cat might be in pain, call your veterinarian.

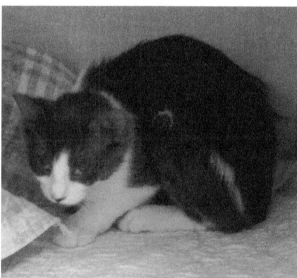

This cat is in pain after being spayed, showing signs of a hunched or tucked-up body posture and half-shut eyes.

Does My Cat Suffer From Chronic Pain?

Richard Gowan

As many people know from experience, age brings with it the inevitable onset of aches and pains and it is no different for our pets. Many pet owners regard their pets as slowing down, or showing their age, but in truth they are reacting to how their body feels and compensating behaviorally to these conditions. With advances in feline medicine, veterinarians now realize that many disease states are associated with chronic and often debilitating pain.

The following is a list of common diseases that affect cats and which are known to cause both acute and chronic pain:

- Dental disease, gingivitis, resorptive lesions or holes in teeth, and tooth infections: change in appetite may be seen, but many cats learn to eat in a manner that is more comfortable.
- Degenerative joint disease (also known as arthritis): mobility impairment with hesitation or slowing down when climbing steps and jumping to favored locations.
- Tumors: many cause direct pain as well as inflammatory and nerve pain.
- Cystitis or bladder inflammation: very common cause of discomfort and distress, and possibly house soiling.
- Skin and ear conditions: besides being irritating, many are uncomfortable.
- Gastroenteritis and pancreatitis: can be debilitating, and lead to nausea, decreased appetite, and weight loss.

Pain affects cats both physically and emotionally, as it does with us. The subtle changes seen with feline chronic pain are better recognized today than ever before. These changes manifest as changes in routine behaviors, the advent of a new abnormal behavior, or changes to appetite, mood, and interactivity. These changes are often slow in onset and therefore harder to notice. In some cases, the source of pain is easy to identify, such as a wound. However, many conditions require a thorough physical examination, and perhaps laboratory tests, x-rays, and/or ultrasound to help identify the source of the pain.

Changes to behavior and routine as a consequence of chronic pain in cats include:

- More secluded, more time spent sleeping
- Changed mood, unhappy, withdrawn
- Abnormal interactive patterns, sleep–wake pattern changes
- Aggression towards owners or other animals
- Aggression on manipulation or being touched in places
- Less inclination to play and interact physically
- Reduced appetite or weight loss
- Altered daily activity or routines
- Elimination disorders, missing litter box

It may be difficult for veterinarians and cat owners to truly assess the level and impact of pain experienced until the underlying cause is appropriately treated, the previously normal behaviors return, and mood changes and interactions improve. Cat owners are therefore instrumental in assessing their cat's improvement with treatment.

Cat owners are actually very perceptive, as routines and interactive rituals are part of being owned by a cat. When these patterns change acutely, it is easy to recognize these as abnormal. However, when they change over months and years as seen with chronic pain, the cat's behavioral changes and coping strategies may be missed. Preventive care programs in veterinary practices help detect these subtle changes, leading to earlier detection and pain management.

Does My Cat Suffer From Painful Arthritis?

Richard Gowan

As in humans, arthritis becomes increasingly common with age. Studies estimate that almost 90% of cats that are 12 years and older suffer from the disease. Arthritis, more accurately known as degenerative joint disease (DJD), is characterized by degradation and reduced function of cartilage within the joints. DJD results in reduced joint function and associated pain.

This pain usually results in altered mobility and changes in household routines and behaviors. The most common and recognizable signs that your cat is suffering from painful DJD are decreased ability or willingness to jump up and down. However, it is well known that it is difficult to recognize signs of illness and debility in pet cats, so careful home observation and regular veterinary visits are important tools in diagnosing DJD and keeping your cat comfortable. It is important to let your veterinarian know if there are any changes in normal activity, mobility, mood, or if there are any abnormal or new behaviors.

Mobility changes often associated with painful DJD include:

- Reduced height of jumping
- Reluctance to jump up or down
- Reluctance or difficulty climbing up and down stairs
- The use of intermediate points to access favorite high places
- Loss of cat-like grace and agility
- Reduced playing with toys or other animals
- Missing landing spots, especially jumping up
- Pulling themselves up onto couches and beds
- Consideration or hesitation before jumping down from a height
- Heavy landings when jumping down
- Changes to gait (e.g., more stiff and stilted gait)

Lameness is uncommon. If you suspect your cat is suffering from painful joints, then a thorough veterinary examination is the first piece of the puzzle. Cats 12 years and older are very likely to show x-ray changes of joint disease, but this does not necessarily correlate to pain. Thorough health screening may also be undertaken as part of senior feline healthcare programs. A mobility questionnaire can be invaluable in identifying key traits to monitor once therapy is instituted.

	Yes	Maybe	No
My cat is less willing to jump up or down			
My cat will only jump up or down from low heights			
My cat has difficulty climbing up or down steps			
Overall, my cat is less mobile than previously			
My cat doesn't seem as happy as usual			
My cat has accidents outside the litter box			
My cat spends less time grooming			
My cat is more reluctant to interact with me			
My cat plays less with other animals or toys			
My cat sleeps more and/or is less active			

Excessive Vocalization

Gary Landsberg and Sagi Denenberg

Management of Excessive or Unwanted Feline Vocalization

a) Medical problems including diseases that increase blood pressure, increase hunger, or cause pain can cause or contribute to excessive or unwanted vocalization. Gastrointestinal disorders, renal disease, and any disease of the nervous system including cognitive dysfunction are just a few examples of the problems that need to be ruled out. Therefore, the first step is to take your pet for a full physical examination, and any necessary diagnostic tests, such as blood and urine tests, blood pressure, and radiographs or ultrasound to rule out all possible medical causes. When a disease is diagnosed a treatment plan can then be instituted. Not all diseases can be resolved; for some the best that might be accomplished is to improve the symptoms (e.g., pain relief for arthritis or supplements for cognitive dysfunction). However, even if a medical problem is identified and treated some behavior problems such as vocalization might persist once they have been learned.

b) Once medical conditions have been ruled out or treated, attention must then be paid to the cat's behavior. The history you provide is critical in determining what can be changed to improve the problem. Helpful information will include details about the household, your cat's daily routine, and any social interactions as well as any situations that might be identified as stressful or anxiety evoking. It is important to address the basic feline behavioral needs and ensure that there are sufficient and appropriate resources including the right type, amount and frequency of food; availability of water; number, type and location of litter boxes; comfortable sleeping areas; increased opportunities for climbing, perching, or scratching; and increased play and social interactions your cat enjoys. It is also important to avoid interactions that the cat dislikes. (See handouts on enrichment)

c) Stressors (such as outside cats, loud noises, or anything the cat finds threatening or fear evoking) should be identified and, if possible, eliminated. If not possible, every effort should be made to avoid or minimize these stressors. For example, if outdoor cats or noises cause your cat anxiety consider blocking access to windows or rooms so that your cat cannot see or hear the sights or sounds, or using a white noise machine to reduce the impact of some of the sounds.

d) Since learning plays an important part in this behavior and anxiety or uncertainty can increase vocalization you should avoid punishing the vocalizing, which increases anxiety and runs the risk of making your cat scared of you. Punishment may also stop the behavior only when you are present. It is also important to avoid giving treats, toys, or affection to your cat while it is vocalizing as this might reward the behavior.

e) If the vocalization is in a senior cat or one that is ill, there may be a limitation as to what can be achieved, until the health issues can be effectively improved. Placing food, water, bedding, and litter boxes in more easily accessible places, providing lowered perching areas, a ramp to climb into the beds or litter boxes, or leaving some lighting on or scents along pathways, might help those cats who have mobility issues, arthritis, or a decline in sensory function to better navigate the home. This can reduce anxiety and attention seeking, which might be the cause of vocalization.

f) It is important to ensure regular enrichment throughout the day, to meet the needs of senior cats. Shorter, more frequent sessions may be more practical for some cats. Consider increasing reward training, play, food, toys, and novel items to explore. Stimulating your cat during daytime and evening hours might help it to sleep better and decrease attention seeking overnight. Providing more frequent small meals, including some placed inside feeding toys, can further help increase daytime stimulation and spread feeding throughout the day and evening which may be beneficial for some cats. You can also consider a timed feeder set to feed throughout the day, or even at night to decrease your importance as the source of food and reinforcement.

g) Establish a regular and predictable daily routine that includes all your cat's needs for sufficient enrichment, feeding, and rest. Knowing your cat's schedule and engaging with it before it seeks attention and while it is calm, can teach it that toys, affection, and meals are provided on a schedule and can avoid the risk of giving these things as rewards for undesirable behavior. Over time you can also gradually manipulate the schedule to keep your cat stimulated, active, and awake throughout the day and evening, and to keep it occupied in desirable activities and increase the likelihood that it will sleep through the night.

h) Finally and most importantly, do not reward any type of attention seeking behavior including vocalization. Provide for your cat's needs in advance. Ignore attention seeking until your cat is calm—walk away if necessary. Reward with play, toys, and treats (consider clicker training) when the cat is calm. If necessary find a sleeping area that is out of your bedroom so you can ignore your cat if it is active and vocal during the night.

Feline Orofacial Pain Syndrome (FOPS)

Clare Rusbridge

What Is Feline Orofacial Pain Syndrome (FOPS)?

FOPS is a disease characterized by face and tongue mutilation and other behavioral signs suggesting oral and facial discomfort (e.g., exaggerated licking and chewing movements). The apparent discomfort and/or mutilation are disproportionate to any possible causes for the pain (for example teething). Clinical signs may be triggered by tongue movement.

What Type of Cat Is Affected by FOPS?

FOPS is most common in the Burmese cat; however, the disease may be seen in any variety including Siamese, Tonkinese, Burmilla, and the domestic shorthair. Any age of cat can be affected. However, many affected cats will first show signs when erupting permanent teeth (i.e., teething).

What Are the Clinical Signs?

FOPS is characterized by face and tongue discomfort and affected cats are most commonly presented with exaggerated licking and chewing movements, with pawing at the mouth. In more severe cases, cats may mutilate their tongue and lips and may even require surgery to repair tongue tears. Typically, the discomfort seems to be worse on one side. The apparent discomfort is often episodic and bouts of pain can be triggered by tongue movement as with grooming, eating or drinking. Bouts of pain last between several minutes to several hours and are often preceded by a short period of behavior suggesting anxiety. Some cats are in more continuous discomfort, are at greater risk of mutilation, and may also be anorexic or unwilling to eat. Oral lesions, especially dental disease, and environmental stress can precipitate the condition.

What Causes FOPS?

FOPS has similarities to trigeminal neuralgia in humans and is a neuropathic pain disorder, that is, pain due to abnormal nervous system processing of pain messages. The trigeminal nerve conveys sensory information, such as pain and touch, about the face and mouth to the brain. It is suggested that affected cats have misfiring of this cranial nerve. In FOPS when the nerve fires, for example during teething or dental disease, it sends an inappropriately large message of pain. Conditions of neuropathic pain can be greatly influenced by environmental factors (imagine if you have a headache—it can be made worse by stress). The most common environmental factor that can trigger FOPS is stressful interaction with other cats, for example between house mates or neighborhood cats invading the home and garden territory. Visits, for example to cat shows, veterinary practices, and catteries, can also be a trigger.

How Is FOPS Diagnosed?

There is no definite diagnostic test for this disease and the diagnosis is made on the basis of the characteristic clinical signs, elimination of other explanations, and identification of contributory causes.

1. **Ruling out other causes of facial and oral pain.**
   a. *Medical examination.* Your veterinarian will examine your cat for other causes of mouth pain, in particular dental disease. Dental disease may cause the cat to be distressed. However, the difference between FOPS and more straightforward dental disease is that in FOPS, the response to the pain is inappropriate and characterized by mutilation. Your veterinarian may recommend other tests such as blood tests or x-rays.
   b. *Neurological examination.* Although FOPS is thought to be due to misfiring of the trigeminal nerve, tests to examine the function of this nerve will be normal. These tests include lightly touching the face, eyes, and lips to ascertain whether the cat can feel. The presence of neurological problems such as a failure to feel touch or close the mouth is not consistent with FOPS. Your veterinarian may recommend other tests to investigate the trigeminal nerve such as magnetic resonance imaging.

2. **Investigation and treating dental disease.**
   The majority of cases of FOPS are triggered by periodontal disease and it is essential that this is investigated and treated even if on causal inspection the cat only seems to have a little gingivitis (inflammation of the gums). Remember, in FOPS the trigeminal nerve sends out an inappropriate message and so even apparently minor dental disease should be treated. Cats are predisposed to feline oral resorptive lesions (FORLs) which may be hidden under plaque or the swollen gum. FORLs are characterized by loss of the tooth enamel and exposure of the sensitive pulp and are very painful. It is so important to identify and treat dental disease that your veterinarian is likely to recommend x-ray images of the teeth and may suggest referral to a veterinary dental specialist.

3. **Identifying environmental stress and triggers.**
   As environmental factors can influence this condition it is important to look for possible contributory factors, for example social stress. Identification of social incompatibility in a multicat household is a key step. Questions to consider are:
   a. Does the cat have its own **secure core territory** (i.e., own litter box, feeding area and private space)?
   b. Can the affected cat see another cat though a window?

c. Does another cat block access going in, out, or even within a territory?

d. Is there adequate provision of **privacy**?

e. Is the cat able use its **natural behavioral strategies** for coping with stress, such as hiding, elevation, and distancing?

How Is FOPS Treated?

The main aim of treating FOPS is to reduce the discomfort, limit the mutilation, and identify and treat or prevent the underlying triggers

1. **Preventing mutilation.** Until discomfort can be controlled, mutilation should be prevented by using an Elizabethan collar and/or paw bandaging. This is a pain disorder and merely preventing the cat from mutilation without attempting to prevent the discomfort is inappropriate.

2. Identify and treat **dental disease,** as above.

3. Identify and reduce **environmental stress,** as above. It is essential that there is appropriate distribution of the five essential feline resources: food, water, resting places, latrines, and points of entry and exit into the territory. The cat should also have a private area(s) and the ability to hide and elevate in order to control stress. Use of commercially available diffusers or sprays containing feline facial pheromone F3 can be useful.

4. **Reduce discomfort**. Your veterinarian will prescribe drugs to reduce discomfort. For mild cases these may include nonsteroidal anti-inflammatory drugs such as meloxicam and/or opioids such a buprenorphine. However, these common painkillers are not always effective for neuropathic pain and consequently your veterinarian may recommend unlicensed drugs that have been shown to be useful for this condition, for example phenobarbital, carbamazepine, gabapentin, or amitriptyline. These drugs are antiepileptic or antidepressants which reduce misfiring of nerves and consequently reduce pain.

What Are the Possible Side Effects of Phenobarbital and Similar Drugs?

Phenobarbital is the most common drug used to treat FOPS. Other antiepileptic drugs have similar adverse effects. It is important not to discontinue phenobarbital suddenly; the drug must be withdrawn slowly to prevent severe withdrawal signs including seizures.

Common Side Effects That Are Dose Dependent

1. **Sedation, poor coordination, and poor jumping ability.** This may be seen at the start of therapy and after increases in doses. Typically this effect wears off within 2 weeks. If it does not or is excessive, your veterinarian may advise that you reduce the dose or switch to another drug.

2. **Increase in thirst, urine volume, and urination frequency.**

3. **Increase in hunger**. Antiepileptic drugs send a message to the brain that the cat should eat despite there being no need for extra calories. Consequently there is a tendency for weight gain which can be challenging to avoid. Try feeding more of a reduced calorie food and presenting the food in ways to prolong mealtime, for example using a maze food bowl.

Rare but more serious side effects are liver damage or blood cell abnormalities.

What Is the Prognosis for FOPS?

Classically FOPS is an episodic condition, at least initially. The first episode may be seen at teething and the second may not be until the cat develops periodontal disease. After starting treatment the discomfort should lessen within 3 days and is usually absent or infrequent after 7 days of therapy. Attempts should be made to wean off medication after 4 weeks, especially if the predisposing causes have been treated or have resolved. For immature cats erupting permanent teeth, the discomfort will resolve when the permanent dentition is fully erupted. **Seek veterinarian advice before withdrawing—sudden discontinuation of phenobarbital can cause withdrawal seizures.** Unfortunately in a proportion of cats the signs of FOPS become continuous, that is there is no remission and long term therapy is required. In addition, pain can be more difficult to treat and sometime more than one drug is necessary to control the discomfort. Kittens that present with FOPS during teeth eruption are highly likely to re-present as older cats, therefore prophylactic dental healthcare, maintaining oral health, and preventing periodontal disease is advised. Environmental stress should also be limited. The numbers of cats within the household should be restricted to socially compatible levels and careful attention should paid if further cats are to be introduced.

Can I Breed My Cat or Its Relatives?

FOPS is thought to be inherited and an autosomal recessive inheritance would fit with the limited data that is available. An autosomal recessive inheritance would mean that both tom and queen of an affected cat either have or carry the condition. Because environmental factors such as dental disease and stress influence the disease, not every animal with an affected genotype will necessarily have clinical signs. In addition the signs of the disease might occur after the animal has been bred. This makes it particularly difficult for a pedigree cat breeder to select disease-free stock and it is hoped that ultimately the disease gene can be identified to enable easy screening. In the meantime breeders are advised not to breed any cat which has had signs of the disease even if the signs are not persistent. Breeding the tom and queen of affected cats is also not advised, especially the tom as his genetic influence can be so far reaching.

Help! My Cat Keeps Waking Me Up!

Ilona Rodan

No one likes to be woken during the night or too early in the morning, but cats may do this either to get fed or for attention. It's like Simon's Cat in "cat-man-do" at www.youtube.com/watch?v=w0ffwDYo00Q. Even if a cat has never woken you, you will want to watch this video!

It can be tempting to get up and feed or pet the cat, especially if this results in a temporary solution and allows you to get back into bed and have more sleep. However, your cat has received some positive reinforcement for being awake and active at that time and this can lead to perpetuation of the behavior and to a situation where you have days, weeks, months, or even years of interrupted sleep.

Fortunately, you can break this habit by not giving in or reinforcing it. Punishment will **not** work, but ignoring will! Here is how:

- If your cat meows or paws at you, pretend you are still asleep. If your cat is vocalizing and wandering or pacing, or if the sounds are loud and plaintive, contact your veterinarian because several medical conditions can lead to vocalizing, especially at night.
- Medical problems can be a source for cats waking people. Have a veterinarian knowledgeable about cats examine your pet and assess for problems that can cause cats to wake owners (e.g., hyperthyroid disease, high blood pressure).
- If your cat is deemed healthy, it may be time to wear earplugs to bed or to cover your head with the blankets.
- Do not have any interaction with your cat that could be misinterpreted by it as either reinforcement or punishment—do not give food, do not shout or push the cat off the bed.
- Keep consistently responding to your cat's behavior in this way for 2 weeks and in most cases the habit of waking you in the night will be broken.
- If your cat really needs food at night, you can use a timed feeder to open at a certain time of night so that you are not involved with the nighttime feeding.

Preventing Cats from Waking People

Unless your cat is sick, do not wake up to feed or give it attention.

- Play with your cat and then provide a feed just before bedtime so that you know your cat is not without attention or food.
- Establish a routine in the morning so that your cat does not associate you awakening with breakfast. For example, go for a run and then feed your cat, or shower and get ready for the day before feeding your cat.

If you still have problems, contact your veterinarian. If not, sweet dreams.

How to Pill Your Cat With Kindness: A Cat Friendly Approach to Medicating*

Iris Cloyd and Theresa DePorter

Pills can be tucked inside tasty soft treats or foods. But to avoid startling your cat with a new routine and a "hidden agenda," it is a good idea to try the following exercises before there is any need to medicate your cat at all. It does not take long—just a few minutes a day!

First, get your cat accustomed to accepting small soft treats at a specific time and place. Make a ritual of it. Cats differ in their preferences, so choose a food or treat that not only is delectable for your cat but also has pill-hiding potential for you. Options include: Pill Pockets, canned paté-style cat foods, cream cheese, meat-flavored baby foods, squeeze cheese, whipped cream, and yogurt. Consult your veterinarian if your cat has dietary restrictions. Canned foods can be warmed to enhance aromas. Many cats are suspicious of novel foods but may accept these foods after repeated invitations.

Most cats are amenable to having designated treat times—you may find that your cat has already trained you! Have at least two sessions a day, morning and evening if possible, each of several minutes' duration. Just be sure to give your cat quality attention and praise at this time. Stroke or engage your cat in some way if your cat enjoys these interactions.

Initially you will give the treats without anything hidden inside. Use tiny amounts so that you can offer four to six treats per session. And try different methods: some cats will accept a treat from your hand; others prefer that you place it on a dish. But it is suggested that you also try placing the treat on a pill gun, so your cat will become familiar with it in case you ever need to use it. (A pill gun is a product designed to administer a pill directly into a pet's mouth, with the pill gun holding the pill in place of your fingers.) At this stage, simply use the pill gun as you would a spoon—just a means of extending a treat out toward the cat. But let your cat come to it; do not force it on your cat. If the treat is tasty enough, some cats will grab the pill gun with their teeth!

After several sessions of your cat readily accepting treats when offered and, in fact, running to you at the designated times, try slipping one kibble of cat food into some of the treats. Use only enough of the treat to cover the kibble, to discourage the cat from eating around it. Most cats will detect the hard core inside, but after examining it, will not be concerned. Continue this method until your cat readily eats the kibble-filled treats without scrutinizing them.

If your cat is one who grabs the pill gun with its teeth, slip the treat-cloaked kibble into the end of the pill gun and gently push the plunger (to pop the pill into its mouth) as it chews at the pill gun. If your cat has a more leisurely licking style (and therefore might lick off the treat and leave the kibble behind), load the treat-cloaked kibble into the pill gun and add a more tasty treat on top. Then when your cat begins to lick the treat off the end of the pill gun, gently nudge the pill gun closer, and give the plunger a boost to pop the hidden kibble into her mouth. Don't forget the praise and positive attention!

These exercises are as much for you as they are for the cat. If your cat spits out the kibble, just be patient and work on improving your technique at the next session. The practice sessions should be stress-free for both of you. When your cat eagerly consumes a kibble hidden inside a treat, you can have confidence knowing that you can substitute a pill into the treat whenever needed.

When it is time for the real thing, first offer a treat without a pill, followed by the treat-cloaked pill.

If despite all your efforts, your cat refuses to accept pills, ask your veterinarian for other options. For medically urgent conditions, it may be helpful to try flavored liquid medications or transdermal formulations available from compounding pharmacies. However, it is important to note that some drugs (e.g., many anti-anxiety drugs used in behavioral therapy) are unstable and of uncertain efficacy when compounded. In these instances, try crushing the pills and mixing them with liquid from canned tuna or clams—many cats find these pungent juices appealing. Again, seek guidance from your veterinarian if needed. Ultimately, the goal is to use kind, gentle medication strategies which will be amenable to your cat long term and allow for optimum health and well-being.

---

*© 2015 Iris Cloyd and Theresa DePorter, Behavioral Medicine, Oakland Veterinary Referral Services.

Informed Consent for Psychotropic Drug Use for a Cat

Theresa DePorter

Cat's name: _____ Sex: _____ Age: _____ Weight: _____

Owner name: _____

Owner address: _____

Your veterinarian has recommended that your pet be treated with a medication that is not licensed for use in cats. This means that use of it in your cat is considered "extra label." This does not mean that the drug is dangerous to cats, just that cats were not the subjects tested for approved use. Many psychotropic drugs are used commonly and licensed for use in people but not labeled for use in pets.

This medication, _____, has been chosen for your cat because it has been deemed to have the potential to be efficacious. This is not a guarantee that the medication will be efficacious in treating your cat's problem.

Your cat has been evaluated and diagnosed with the following behavioral condition or concern:

_____
_____
_____
_____

As with all medications, the medication that your cat will be taking may have potential side effects. Although serious side effects are uncommon with psychotropic medications, your cat may experience side effects such as lethargy, sedation, or gastrointestinal signs. When experienced, they are usually transient, but if your cat experiences any of them, please call us so that we can make informed decisions about your pet's care. Overdoses of this medication may be harmful or fatal. Some rare paradoxical effects include insomnia, agitation, tremors, or increased anxiety.

Other side effects specific to this medication may include:

_____
_____
_____
_____

Drug interactions may occur. Please list below the medications or supplements your cat receives. Notify the veterinarian if you begin new medications or supplements for your cat while being given this medication.

_____
_____

Be careful about using other medications which may cause interactions with SSRIs; especially avoid common medications such as tramadol and metoclopramide. Natural supplements may also have significant effects when combined with psychotropic medications; this includes supplements such as melatonin, St John's wort or tryptophan.

Medication: _____

Dose: _____   Refills: 0   1   2   3

Administration directions: _____

This medication is intended to be given:

Daily ☐
On an as needed basis ☐ _____

This medication is most effective and most likely to produce the desired effect:

Immediately ☐
After 4 to 6 weeks ☐ Expected date of therapeutic response: _____

This medication is recommended:

With a behavior modification program ☐ or as a solitary recommendation ☐

This medication is recommended:

Long term ☐ or short term ☐ or to be determined based on response ☐

A weaning or gradual dose reduction program is recommended. Be sure to contact your veterinarian before discontinuing this medication. ☐

Baseline blood work is recommended prior to starting the medication. A health screen should be conducted minimally every 6 months or as directed while your pet is on medication.

☐ CBC
☐ Serum chemistry profile (age and health appropriate)
☐ Urinalysis

Next follow up examination or consultation: _____

Please do not hesitate to call if you have any questions or concerns about your pet's medication. Contact your veterinarian at: _____

Client signature: _____ Date: _____

Introducing a New Cat into a Household

Debra Horwitz and Amy Pike

When bringing home a new cat, planning ahead can help ensure a smooth transition. Whether you are bringing home your first cat or adding a new cat to your feline household, these instructions will make things go easier and facilitate a successful transition and integration of your new feline friend.

General Introduction Advice

- At least 72 hours prior to introduction, place Feliway diffusers throughout the home.
- Confine the new cat in a separate room especially created for the transition period to your home. Make sure to provide all necessary resources including a litter box, food, water, climbing tower or vertical perching area, hiding places, scratching posts, and toys.
- If you already have a resident cat, initially limit all visual access between the cats (a solid door will suffice). Eventually when visual access is desired, this can be achieved by using a screen door, several baby gates stacked on top of one another, or a hook on the top of the door to prevent it from opening wide enough to allow physical contact.
- If you only have one cat, allow the cat to have daily time outside of the transition room if so desired by the cat. This can be several hours at a time, but encourage the cat to return to their safe transition area for some part of every day. For kittens this may be prudent while owners are not home or sleeping until the kitten is more reliable and trained.
- Once the new cat, and existing feline residents if applicable, seem comfortable, the door can remain open to allow the new cat to come and go whenever it wishes. The resident cats must also have safe hiding places that they can access.

Introducing a New Cat to Resident Cats

- Cats identify each other by personal odors. Therefore, we want to help create a common scent profile between the resident cat(s) and your new feline. Take a towel and rub each resident cat, then the new cat, and then leave that towel in the newcomer's transition room. Next, repeat the process beginning with the new cat and then the resident cat and leave the towel outside the transition room. Rubbing should be concentrated on the location of the scent glands: face, back and tail. This can be done daily or several times a week for several weeks.
- Create a play area at the confinement door so the cats can play with one another. Use two toys attached to a string, rope or thick ribbon (providing neither cat has a history of ingestion of string). The string should freely flow back and forth underneath the door; use toys large enough that they will not slide under the door to the opposite side.
- High-value treats and rewards, such as toys, can be offered to the new cat and resident cats on either side of the closed door. Favored foods, such as canned food, can also be used to provide positive associations. However, once the door is open to any extent and the cats can see and smell each other easily, feeding in close proximity should not be done.
- Once the new addition appears comfortable with its surroundings, the resident cats can be confined to another room and the new cat allowed out of confinement to explore the rest of the home.
- Structured interactions:
  - All cats should be kept physically separated from one another through the use of harnesses and leads, carriers, wire crates, or the placement of baby gates, screen mesh, or hooks on the tops of doors.
  - Maintain a distance that allows each cat to relax and be comfortable.
  - Engage the cats in a favored activity during this time, such as playing with a prized toy or eating a high-value treat.
  - Keep initial sessions short, preferably less than 5 minutes.
  - Have daily sessions and over time slowly decrease the distance between the cats when each appears comfortable, relaxed and shows no aggressive displays (hissing, ears back, or pupils dilated).
  - The final phase is supervised contact without the use of physical separation. At the first sign of aggressive indicators (hissing, ears back) try to break up the interaction by blocking visual access using cardboard or a pillow. Alternatively, a thick heavy blanket can be gently placed over one of the cats involved in the conflict to end the interaction.
  - Owners should never attempt to handle an aggressively aroused cat without the use of the blanket to avoid injury if the cat redirects its aggression toward the humans.
  - If aggressive encounters occur, return to nonvisual introductions for several days and then begin to allow short visual encounters once again.
  - If there are no aggressive encounters, gradually increase the amount of time the cats are in supervised contact with one another and then slowly phase out the supervision.

- Have realistic expectations: successful introductions can take months and some cats may become good friends, while others learn to coexist peacefully.

It is important that all introductions are done safely and positively. If aggression occurs between the cats, introductions are taking place too quickly or inappropriately. Negative interactions can delay integration into the home. Consult with your veterinarian or a veterinary behaviorist if you are unsure how to proceed after an aggressive episode.

Managing Normal but Unwanted Behavior

Jacqui Ley

Cats do lots of nice things. The purr, they generally like to be patted, they are playful, and they like to hang out with us. But may cats do things that make living with them frustrating, especially when they miss the litter box or want to go out late at night. Many problematic behaviors are actually normal for cats but do not fit in with what people want. Hunting, being active at night, and ambushing people are all difficult to live with but normal behaviors. Understanding normal cat behavior and making some changes can make it easier to live with cats.

The *Real* Domestic Cat

The domestic cat developed from a desert dwelling small cat. Cats are solitary hunters with their prey being small mammals, birds, amphibians, reptiles, and larger insects. Like its prey, the cat is active at dawn and dusk. They are not easy to categorize as either a social or solitary species, with some cats happy in groups and others intolerant of other cats. Cats are territorial and mark their territory with urine spray marks, feces, and claw marks. Young cats tend to leave their mother's territory and travel until they find a safe place where they can settle that has plenty of food and potential mates.

So what can be done to help manage some of the more challenging behaviors of cats?

First we have to recognize the behavior as being normal. The cats are not being naughty or nasty or evil or anything else negative. Rather, they are trying to perform behaviors that are hard wired. By being aware that our cats may want to do these things, you can be prepared with alternative and more acceptable activities.

Dawn and Dusk Playtimes

These sessions are characterized by running around the house, jumping on and off the bed repeatedly, climbing curtains, and knocking things off shelves all while vocalizing loudly. They commonly take place in the early morning or very late at night.

Management approaches:
1. Be prepared. Have filled food dispensing toys available for your cat so they can "hunt" for their breakfast or dinner. To preserve your sleep, look for toys that are quiet.
2. Tire your cat out with plenty of exercise before bed time. Enticing it to chase a toy on a string, fetch a ball (yes, some cats will deign to play fetch), or other games will help your cat use up some energy especially if it has slept or been confined all day. If you are tired after a day at work, find toys such as fishing rod style toys that mean maximum fun for your cat with minimal movement from you.
3. If your cat is confined, pay attention to the activities you leave it during the day. Ditch the food bowls and hide food and food dispensing toys around the areas where your cat lives so it must move to find its food. Leave toys that are safe for it to play without supervision (e.g., a ping pong ball in the bath tub) so your cat has something to chase and pounce on while you are away.
4. Teach your cat to sleep in another room. This may be the opposite of why you got your cat; many people like their cat to snuggle on their bed with them. However, if you are constantly being woken up by your cat you will both end up frustrated.

Ambushing People

This is a fabulous game for many young cats as the humans (especially the little ones) squeal and run. It can actually be quite a dangerous game especially if the humans have mobility or other health problems.

Management approaches:
1. Be prepared. Young cats, especially young male cats have lots of energy. They are drawn to moving things and will often return to the same hiding places. So, identify the "danger zones" in your home. Have some small toys ready and throw them ahead of you so your cat has something to chase and pounce upon.
2. Confine your cat if young children or elderly people are moving around the house and you cannot supervise. The confinement is not a punishment so the area needs to be pleasant for your cat. Make sure there is a bed, water, food, toys, and a toilet for the cat.
3. See points 2 and 3 above: leave lots of fun activities for your cat.
4. Reward calm, friendly behavior by your cat with treats. This is an alternative strategy if throwing a toy makes your cat too excited. Drop some treats as you approach the ambush area and encourage your cat to come and collect them.

Hunting

Cats hunt. It is not great to deal with the results of their hunting and they can have some impact on the wildlife in their immediate area. Minimizing hunting can be done.

Management approaches:
1. Confining cats prevents them hunting, but attention to their environment is needed so they do not develop other unwanted behaviors. There are many good cat enclosure design companies that can help

you design an interesting and safe enclosure for your cat(s).

2. Bells, whistles, reflectors on the cat's collar can all help but some cats learn to get around these. But they are also the cheapest means to stop or reduce hunting.

3. A neoprene cat bib has been shown in university research to prevent hunting as the cat cannot get its feet forward to grab the prey. Some cats will adapt to wearing the bib (www.catbib.com.au).

Managing Your Cat's Painful Degenerative Joint Disease (Arthritis)

Richard Gowan

Although arthritis is a chronic disease condition that cannot be cured, there are several treatments and environmental modifications that you can do to make your cat more comfortable. Cats need easy access to their favorite sleeping spots and to high areas to perch. Managing their pain and making simple environmental changes allows them to fulfill their needs and ensures an excellent quality of life. While it is important to focus on the physical outcomes, it is often the changes to emotions and the well-being of your cat that are just as important in measuring quality of life. You are the most important individual to judge these improvements in your cat!

What You Can Do at Home

- Place food and water dishes in easily accessible areas to avoid jumping.
- Raise food and water dishes 3 to 4 inches from the floor.
- Add ramps or stairs to provide cats with easier access to favorite sleeping areas.
- Add intermediary points to lower the height and effort required to jump up and down from perches or beds.
- Provide comfortable bedding. This may include a heated cat bed.
- Provide multiple litter boxes in easily accessible locations.
- Provide litter boxes with one or more low sides.
- Provide regular play and gentle exercise to help maintain muscle and joint strength.
- Safe weight loss in overweight cats will improve joint function and mobility, and reduce pain.

Treatment Options

- Never use medication without a veterinarian's authorization. Human medications such as acetaminophen (Tylenol) or ibuprofen can kill cats!
- Your veterinarian can design a treatment plan specifically for your cat to ensure that your feline companion is as comfortable as possible.
- Prescribed veterinary medications can be safe and effective in reducing the joint and muscle pain that your cat experiences.

- There are numerous nonpharmaceutical arthritis supplements. Your veterinarian is best able to advise you as to whether they are effective and safe.
- Reducing obesity will reduce the stress on a cat's joints. For safe and healthy results, weight loss plans should be directed and monitored by your veterinarian.

The following table can help to assess responses to treatment. Please select three of your cat's physical activities and two nonphysical behaviors that you consider important to its quality of life. Examples of physical activities are jumping onto the bed or playing; examples of nonphysical behaviors include sleeping comfortably, grooming, and eating.

Physical Activities to Monitor	Normal	Slightly Below Normal	Worse Than Normal	Markedly Worse Than Previously	Unable to Perform Anymore
1.					
2.					
3.					

Nonphysical Parameters to Monitor	Normal	Slightly Below Normal	Worse Than Normal	Markedly Worse Than Previously	Unable to Perform Anymore
4.					
5.					

You should complete these observations before and after starting any treatment. This can help your veterinarian to assess the response to treatment and understand what you consider as important to your cat's quality of life. Rechecking your cat periodically based on your veterinarian's recommendation is very important. This allows your veterinarian to adjust medical management for your cat, monitor for common senior cat health conditions, and to establish health trends specific to your cat. Degenerative joint disease is just one of many conditions that commonly afflicts senior cats, but your cat can live a comfortable and quality life with appropriate treatment.

My Cat is Healthy—Or is it?*

Ilona Rodan

Cats are fascinating creatures and are important family members. But they are not small dogs and they are **not** small people! They differ from people and dogs in that they are not pack animals bur rather solitary hunters. As a relatively young species with approximately 10,000 years' history, they retain many of the behaviors of their wild ancestors, the African Wildcat. Being solitary hunters, they have adapted to appear strong and healthy when they may not be.[2] They also may not like another cat in the household, but they will rarely fight.[3,4] These behaviors are all designed to prevent injury by prey or another cat. Even though many now live in wonderful homes, they still maintain these behaviors.[2]

Cat owners know their cats better than anyone, and as a cat owner, you are in a position to significantly impact the health and happiness of your cat. Paying attention to the things mentioned in this handout can help you to recognize if there is a problem early on.

If your cat shows a change in its normal routines or behaviors, it is time for a check-up. *Herman always loved to jump and climb, and raced up and down the stairs faster than the fastest Olympic skier (well, maybe). His behavior changed, and although he still climbed the steps pretty quickly, he was much slower going down. He also didn't go to his high perches anymore. His owner saw him looking at a perch and hesitating as to whether he should jump. Although the owner wasn't sure whether he was just getting old, she brought him in for a checkup. Herman was diagnosed with severe arthritis in his knees and shoulders, and treatment was started after making sure he was otherwise healthy. His owner called me a few weeks later to say that Herman was back up on his favorite high spots, and everyone had to move aside when the "zoom-cat" went up and down the stairs! Herman's family was so happy to have the Herman back that they loved and knew so well.*

There are some important **changes** in a cat's normal patterns of behavior, as well as displays of abnormal behavior, that can indicate that there is pain and sickness.[5–9]

Changes in normal behaviors might include:
- Appetite: decrease or increase.
- Grooming: overgrooming in one or more areas or not grooming so that mats are forming.
- Sleep: sleeping more or not as well.
- Activity: decrease or increase.
- Vocalizing: yowling and keeping you up at night when they never did; not meowing for treats or food as usual.
- Play: decreased.

Abnormal behaviors might include:
- Accidents outside the litter box, either over the edge or in another place. This can involve either urine or feces or both, but it is more usual to be one or the other.
- Aggressive with you or another pet. This may occur with touching or handling or at any time.
- Getting on counters to get human food when they didn't previously.
- Destroying furniture.

Another very useful tip for increasing your awareness of subtle changes in your cat's health is to place a picture of your cat on the refrigerator or in another location where you can see it frequently. Each year, take a new photograph and put it alongside the previous one. Seek veterinary care if you notice a significant difference between the photos. Years can go by and we don't notice the subtle changes, unless they are staring us in the face. The pictures of my own cat, Watson, who I adored and did everything for, were only put side by side after his death (see next page). Watson was receiving nine medications a day for multiple conditions (he loved getting medication with treats). Unfortunately, the drug needed for his arthritis was contraindicated with the other medications he needed, and it was extremely difficult for me to make the decision to let him go. However, I would have made that decision a lot earlier if I had seen the photos together and noticed the changes.

Please contact your veterinarian if you notice any of these signs. Usually these can be avoided with routine preventive check-ups, which can identify other problems, such as hidden kidney or thyroid disease or dental disease before any signs occur. The combination of veterinary care and your detective work ensures the best for your cat. Herman's family are happy that they can keep him comfortable for much longer and improve his quality of life.

---

*In memory of her beloved Watson.

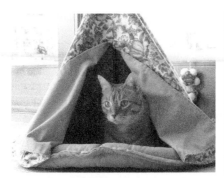

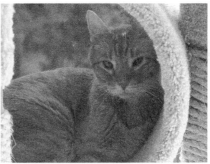

Watson, 4 years

Watson, 16 years

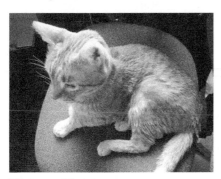

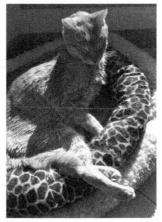

Watson, 17 years
Note the curling of his feet
and muscle loss as
compared to when Watson
was 16 years old

Watson, 17.5 years, just
before he was euthanized

REFERENCES

1. Driscoll CA, Menotti-Raymond M, Roca AL, et al. The Near Eastern origin of cat domestication. *Science*. 2007;317:519–523.
2. Bradshaw JWS, Casey RA, Brown SL. *The Behaviour of the Domestic Cat*. 2nd ed. Wallingford: CABI Publishing; 2012.
3. Griffin B, Hume KR. Recognition and management of stress in housed cats. In: August J, ed. *Consultations in Feline Internal Medicine*; vol. 5. St Louis: Elsevier; 2006:717–734.
4. Notari L. Stress in veterinary behavioural medicine. In: Horwitz D, Mills D, eds. *BSAVA Manual of Canine and Feline Behavioural Medicine*. 2nd ed. Gloucester: British Small Animal Veterinary Association; 2009:136–145.
5. Sparkes AH, Heiene R, Lascelles BD, et al. ISFM and AAFP consensus guidelines: long-term use of NSAIDs in cats. *J Feline Med Surg*. 2010;12:521–538.
6. Robertson SA, Lascelles BDX. Long-term pain in cats: how much do we know about this important welfare issue? *J Feline Med Surg*. 2010;12:188–189.
7. Benito J, Gruen ME, Thomson A, et al. Owner-assessed indices of quality of life in cats and the relationship to the presence of degenerative joint disease. *J Feline Med Surg*. 2012;14:863–870.
8. Lascelles BDX, Hansen BD, Thomson A, et al. Evaluation of a digitally integrated accelerometer-based activity monitor for the measurement of activity in cats. *Vet Anaesth Analg*. 2008;35:173–183.
9. Bennett D. Osteoarthritis in the cat: 1. How common is it and how easy to recognize. *J Feline Med Surg*. 2012;14:65–75.

Pheromonatherapy

Theresa DePorter

How Do I Know How to Apply a Pheromone Product for My Cat?

To be optimally effective, a pheromone should be placed in a location where the cat may inhale the pheromone either while in a relaxed state or when it is actively investigating and seeking a pheromone message from the environment. Pheromones are available in a variety of formulations that may be applied in various locations. This guide will help you to determine which application is most suitable for your cat, your home, and your cat's individual behavior concern.

Location

Resting Areas

While comfortable, relaxed and at ease, a cat will sniff and investigate pheromone messages in the environment. These messages may be left by another cat, by themselves, or in the form of commercial products. It can be beneficial to provide a diffuser in an area where your cat sleeps, rests, and is comfortable in order to reduce overall stress and anxiety. This will help to promote flexibility, adaptability, and coping skills. The diffuser must be operational, plugged in continuously, and not obscured by furniture so that the pheromone can diffuse into the environment.

Signposts

Cats may provide a signal in a specific location to leave an important message in the environment. Natural examples of such signposting include bunting, scratching, or urine marking. Application of a spray or a diffuser in the location where a cat may express or interpret such communications may reduce the inclination and need to convey such messages.

Formulation

Spray

A pheromone spray may be applied in a resting area, in a carrier, on bedding, or on a new surface or object preventatively. Any surface or substrate which has been previously urine marked, bunted, or scratched may be treated with a pheromone spray to change the pheromone message conveyed.

Wipes

Similar to the spray, a wipe may be used to deposit pheromone in a specific location.

Diffuser

A diffuser may be located in a resting area or in a new area which is unfamiliar to the cat or in a location in which undesired bunting, scratching, or urine marking has occurred.

Hand Gel or Spray

This may be applied to the veterinary professional's hands prior to an interaction to reduce associated stress or anxiety.

Behavior Concerns

Undesirable behaviors in cats may be normal or occur as a result of stress or anxiety. For example, scratching is a normal and typical feline behavior and the manifestation may vary widely between individuals. However, many cats will scratch with greater intensity, frequency, and on more surfaces during periods of stress, distress, strained social interactions, or even fear/anxiety. First, consider if your cat's problematic behaviors are normal, as these types of problems are unlikely to be alleviated by pheromones. Displays of undesirable behaviors as a result of stress or anxiety may be reduced in intensity, severity, and frequency proportionally to the successful reduction of such negative emotions.

Case Example

Lily and Max are housemate cats that do not get along. Max chases Lily so she hides in the den. Max has been urine marking on the front windows when he sees a cat in the garden. Max sleeps in the master bedroom.

Recommendations

- Feliway Spray around window
- MultiCat Diffuser in the master bedroom
- Feliway Diffuser in the den
- Feliway wipe inside carrier before veterinary visits

Playing With Your Cat

Jacqui Ley

Exercise and play are essential for maintaining a healthy body weight and a healthy mind. However, play and exercise are often ignored when it comes to managing our cats' health. This may be because cats are often left to their own devices inside or outside and maybe because cats play differently compared with people and that other common household pet, the dog. Cats can be enticed to play when you know the tricks for keeping them interested.

Most people know that cats are efficient hunters, capturing small rodents, birds, amphibians, and reptiles. They are classed as ambush hunters; that is they sneak up close to their prey then rush and try and grab it. The activity is over very quickly—either they caught the prey or they didn't. This is very different from the way people hunted—when we used to hunt we took a long time stalking, attempting to kill or at least wound our quarry, before chasing it over long distances to catch it. The activity may have taken many hours. So when people play we often play long, repetitive games. This means when we play with our cats, we tend to want to play long games, but they believe a good game is a short, fast game.

Many people also don't realize that cats evolved in an environment where they were hunted as well as being the hunter. This is why cats are cautious creatures that often pause before committing to an activity.

So what does this mean in relation to getting cats to play and exercise?

1. Cats play in short bursts. They may spend time considering if they will engage in a game, but when they play it is for a short time. For many cats, 2 to 5 minutes is fine, then they have had enough.
2. They are also more interested in playing with objects than playing with other cats or people.

These aspects of normal cat behavior need to be respected when playing with our pet cats and it is therefore advisable to:

1. Use toys that are small and furry or feathered. Smaller toys tend to be preferred over larger toys. Think mouse-sized.
2. Change the game or the toy every 2 to 5 minutes to keep your cat engaged and interested.
3. Hide small toys in climbing frames, on shelves, and other places the cat can access, as the novelty of these may encourage solo object play.
4. Only leave safe toys out for your cat to play with unsupervised. No strings or sharp things. Also make sure any electrical cords and curtain or blind cords are protected from inquisitive feline paws and teeth.
5. Toys don't have to be expensive. Balls of scrunched up paper, paper airplanes, ping pong balls in the bathtub, and cardboard boxes are all great toys that cost very little.
6. Be aware that laser pointers may lead to frustration as the cat never gets to "catch" the light. Always finish the game by having the cat "catch" some treats or a toy.

Senior Health and Behavior: Early Reporting is the Best Medicine

Gary M. Landsberg and Sagi Denenberg

With advances in veterinary medicine and nutrition, and the care provided by responsible and dedicated owners, cats are now living longer than ever. However, to maintain health and well-being, pet owners must remain vigilant in monitoring their pet's health and behavior and report any changes as soon as they are noticed. The following guidelines aim to help maintain your pet's quality of life, and perhaps even increase longevity.

1. Keep a lookout for any change in your pet's behavior no matter how subtle. Behavioral signs are often the first or only sign of emerging health concerns including sensory loss (e.g., hearing or sight), pain, illness, or cognitive dysfunction syndrome. Prompt reporting of any change in your cat's behavior is essential for early diagnosis.

2. Many diseases can be improved, controlled, or have their progression slowed. However, the best success is often achieved early in the course of disease, before complications develop. For instance, the progression of kidney disease might be slowed with dietary therapy alone. However, if the cat is not treated until the kidney disease is advanced, there may be no healthy kidney tissue left to save. Similarly, the diagnosis and treatment of diabetes mellitus (sugar diabetes) and thyroid disease are most easily treated if caught early, before complications develop. Therefore early diagnosis offers the best chance of early therapy.

3. Cognitive dysfunction is the pet equivalent of early Alzheimer's disease. Signs might include a decline in awareness, learning and memory, and behavior changes including disorientation, an increase in vocalization, changes in the pet's social behavior with family or other pets in the home, waking at night, house soiling, and an increase in anxiety.

4. As with other diseases, cognitive dysfunction might be controlled or slowed with early intervention through increased enrichment, dietary therapy, or cognitive supplements. However, if brain aging is sufficiently advanced, the damage may be too extensive to improve.

5. Since medical conditions can cause some or all of the signs of cognitive dysfunction, examination and diagnostic testing are needed to diagnose these conditions, and specific treatment to manage these conditions can then be identified. Ruling out medical causes is an important step in the diagnosis cognitive dysfunction.

6. Pain can cause or contribute to a wide range of behavioral signs including a decrease in play and sociability as well as an increase in aggression. In addition, the initial signs of pain may be a change from normal behavior or a decline in activity levels. Effective treatments are available. Therefore it is essential for the welfare of your pet to report any change in behavior to ensure prompt diagnosis and early intervention.

7. Use the checklist below to monitor your pet's health and if any of these signs develop, report them to your veterinarian so that the cause can be determined and any necessary treatment promptly initiated.

Feline Cognitive Questionnaire

Pet's Name: Age: Date:

Key: 0 = none; 1 = mild; 2 = moderate; 3 = severe

	When Did Signs Begin	Score
A: Disorientation—Awareness—Spatial Orientation		
– Gets stuck or can't get around objects		
– Stares blankly at walls or floor		
– Can't find leaves/dropped food		
– Goes into wrong side of door; walks into door/walls		
– Aimless vocalization		
B: Altered Social Interactions		
– Decreased interest in petting / avoids contact		
– Decreased greeting behavior		

(Continued)

	When Did Signs Begin	**Score**
– In need of constant contact, over-dependent, "clingy"		
– Altered relationship with other household pets—less social		
– Altered relationship with other household pets—fear/anxiety		
– Aggression		
– Toward family members		
– Toward unfamiliar people		
– Toward family pets		
– Toward unfamiliar pets		
– Other		
C: Response to Stimuli		
– Decreased response to auditory stimuli (sounds)		
– Increased response, fear, phobia to auditory stimuli		
– Decreased response to visual stimuli (sights)		
– Increased response, fear, phobia to visual stimuli		
– Decreased responsiveness to food/odor		
D: Sleep–wake Cycles; Reversed day/night schedule		
– Restless sleep/waking at nights		
– Increased daytime sleep		
E: Learning and Memory—House soiling		
– Indoor elimination at unacceptable locations in the home		
– Apparent inability to find the location of the litter box		
F: Activity Increased/Repetitive/Anxiety		
– Pacing/wanders aimlessly		
– Increased vocalization		
– Excessive grooming		
G: Activity—Apathy/Depressed		
– Decreased interest in food/treats		
– Decreased exploration/activity		
– Decreased interest in social interactions/play		
– Decreased self-care, e.g., grooming		
H: Learning and Memory—Work, Tasks, Commands		
– Decreased ability to perform tasks		
– Decreased responsiveness to commands and tricks		
– Inability/slow to learn new tasks (retrain)		

Modified from Landsberg G, Hunthausen W, Ackerman L: Behavior Problems of the Dog and Cat, ed 3, Philadelphia, Saunders, 2013.

Setting up a Home for Cats

Jacqui Ley

Cats are inquisitive, playful animals that evolved to spend their time hunting small prey while avoiding getting eaten themselves. Nowadays, not many things eat cats in our homes but plenty of things can hurt them. Increasingly cats are being confined to their owner's homes or properties for their own safety and the safety of local wildlife. Many cats are expected to live in close proximity to other cats that they may or may not like.

Setting up your home to provide for your cat or cats is not hard once you know what cats need.

Cats are territorial. They are a bit like the average teenager—they like to have a space that is theirs where they feel safe. For the cat, not the teenager, the space needs to have a bed, a view, a toilet, and food and water. This is called the home or core territory and cats do not share this with other cats unless they have formed a strong social bond. Other areas of the house or property may be used and shared with other cats. Each cat will have a preference for how much time they want to spend in the company of other cats and people.

Cats also need something to do. Sitting at home is boring—especially if you can't use Facebook. There is some thought that chronic boredom may be a factor in feline obesity amongst confined cats. Cats are evolved to find, stalk, and hunt prey so have a need to move at least a little every day.

So what to do:

1. Recognize that your cat or cats vary in how much feline company they can tolerate and enjoy. Consider this before adding further cats to your household. You may want lots of cats but your cat or cats may really be happy with the way things are.

2. Observe your cats to identify which cats are bonded; who gets along with whom and who need to be separated. Use the table below to identify bonded behavior between your cats. These cats may form a social group and can share core territory. You may also find you have one cat that can move between groups. This cat is very useful in providing companionship for cats that may need to be confined.

3. Each cat or group of bonded cats needs their own territory. This is the place that only those cats go and all other cats stay out. This may mean different cats have access to different rooms in the house or the cats may divide a large room between themselves. If your home is unsettled with lots of arguments between your cats, house soiling, or spraying problems, you may want to consider permanent separation of some of your cats to help manage the problem. If the situation is very stressful for the cats, rehoming one or more of the cats may be the best situation.

4. Supply your cats with adequate resources and make sure that they are distributed well throughout the home. This means more feeding locations, water stations, toilet facilities, sleeping and resting places, and exits from rooms. By increasing the resources available for the cats, they can avoid each other and avoid conflicts.

5. When there is more than one cat in a household, it is not uncommon to have house soiling problems. This may occur because there are not enough suitable litter boxes for every cat or because one or more cats is prevented from using the boxes by other cats. Having litter boxes in more than one part of the house can really help, as can making sure there is always a second exit (a back door, so to speak). And lastly, cleanliness. No one likes a dirty toilet, least of all cats.

6. If you have cats that do not get along, create a time-share arrangement for common areas of the house and yard. This mimics how cats in colonies manage and allows you to spend time with each cat or group of cats. Cats may already have a system in place. If one cat or group of cats is in a common area, then the other group of cats or cat is either confined in its core territory or somewhere else, such as outside. Each can use the area, just at different times.

7. If you have one cat that is making life really difficult for other cats, it may help to put a bell on the difficult cat. The other cats will hear it coming and can move away, minimizing conflicts.

8. Provide toys and climbing frames, cardboard boxes and tunnels, and other interesting and intriguing things with which your cats can play. Change them around and hide toys and ping pong balls and treats in them. Make your cat or cats hunt for their food. They will enjoy it and clever use of easy-to-wash food dispensing toys will make it easy for you to add into your routine.

9. Set aside time in your day to spend doing stuff that your cat likes. This may be playing games or grooming or petting or just hanging out. It isn't all about us—we need to be doing what cats like too.

When we invite cats into our homes we need to make sure we provide them with the things they need to thrive. Small changes may help your cat or cats live fuller lives.

Behavior	Description	My cats that do this are...
Show greeting behavior	Approach each other eagerly after absence, tails up and may make a greeting trill. Sniff noses and rub along each other.	
Allogrooming	Lick each other. One cat may do most of the grooming but sometimes both cats will groom each other.	
Allorubbing	Rub against each other. This could be part of the body or the entire body.	
Co-sleeping	Sleep curled up or intertwined or on top of each other. Always in close contact.	
Spending time together	Generally bonded cats can be found in the same area, maybe sitting or lying together or walking around together. They may work as a team to scare off intruder cats.	

Should I Adopt Another Cat?

Debra Horwitz and Amy Pike

Adding a cat to a household can be an exciting time for pet owners, but it can be fraught with stress for the owner, the resident cat(s), and the new cat if the household situation and composition cannot support the addition. The following questionnaire can help you determine whether or not your household is able to support a new feline friend.

If you are able to answer mostly "True" to the following series of statements, then a new cat would be a welcome addition to your family.

Any "False" answers should be discussed in depth with your veterinarian or a veterinary behaviorist prior to bringing home a new cat. It may be possible to make changes or accommodations that would facilitate bringing in a new cat despite the current situation.

	True	False
With my household layout, I have the ability to physically separate a new cat from the resident cat(s) until proper introductions have been made.		
I have the time needed in my day for proper introductions to take place.		
I have the capability to invest at least the next several weeks or months to facilitate gradual introductions.		
I have time to provide attention, care, and training to another cat.		
I can provide litter boxes spread throughout the house, including all levels of a multistoried home.		
I am willing and able to provide for as many litter boxes as there are cats in the house, plus one (N + 1 rule of thumb), but possibly more.		
Several weeks prior to adoption, I can plug in numerous Feliway diffusers throughout the home.		
I am willing to try different litter substrate types if needed.		
I am willing to, or already do, provide multiple feeding stations and water bowls throughout the home.		
I provide enough vertical resting perches throughout the home to accommodate my resident cat(s) and a new addition.		
I have plenty of space available for each cat to have its own core area and location away from the other cats if needed.		
I am willing to provide numerous toys and enrichment for all the cats.		
I have enough hiding places for each cat to have their own.		
I am willing to make each of the cats wear a quick-release collar with a bell so the cats can hear the approach of another cat.		
I do not currently own a cat that is aggressive towards other cats.		
If I have a shy/timid cat, I do not plan to adopt an active/aggressive cat.		
If I have an elderly cat, I do not plan to adopt a highly energetic or rambunctious cat.		
I am willing to accept that if introduction of the new cat does not go well, I need to keep each cat in the household permanently physically separated from one another.		

Social Behavior

Jacqui Ley

You may have been told that cats are solitary creatures that will take you for granted and give you little in return. They are portrayed as solitary animals that don't like other cats and can be aggressive and difficult to handle. Is this right? As with so many things there is some truth in these ideas but it is certainly not the full story and by understanding the way that cats live and their social behavior you can gain a much better appreciation of your feline friend.

Cats cannot be neatly classified as a social species or a solitary species as they are able to live along a continuum from solitary to living in high density colonies.

Cats: Not Solitary but not Really a Social Species

Cats are small hunters who prey upon small animals such as mice, rats, small birds, lizards, frogs, and fish. The prey usually provides just enough for one meal for a cat. Cats are also ambush hunters. They sneak up then pounce on their prey. What this means is that cats hunt by themselves and so spend a lot of time alone. This has led to people considering them to be solitary animals.

As well as being predatory, cats are also territorial. This means that they have an area where they live and hunt and they defend this from other cats. They are intolerant of cats that they are not related to or do not know well, and as a result it is unusual for them to readily accept a new cat into their home. The size of the territory varies with the availability of food, water, resting places, and potential mates. While cats that are living in the wild may have very large territories, cats living with people often have very small territories within which their resources are concentrated. Even though the size of the territory is small, cats still need to defend it and to safeguard their access to their resources.

Cats give every impression that they are a solitary species—until you see them interact with people and cats with whom they have relationships. They sniff noses and rub against other cats or rub around a person's legs. Cats will groom other cats with which they have a bond. Studies have shown that cats are a species that can live alone or with other cats but they are not a truly social species like dogs or humans. The fundamental difference is that they do not need social contact in order to survive and as a result they do not have behaviors that allow them to repair relationships when there is conflict.

Unlike dogs and children, cats do not like feline visitors and they do not like play dates with other people's cats.

Cats live in a matriarchal society and the groups of cats most likely to form bonds are mothers and their female kittens. Bonds also form between other cats who are related to one another or between individuals that are raised together from an early age and, although females are thought to be more inherently sociable with one another, both neutered males and females form social bonds if the circumstances are right. If you are planning on having more than one cat, a pair of kittens from the same litter appears to give the best chance of a good social bond between them, and certainly the younger cats are when they start to live together, the greater the chance that they will live harmoniously together.

In multicat households with unrelated cats, it is possible for good social bonds to become established, but you need to be prepared for the fact that this may not happen. If the cats in a household do not bond, they need to have separate access to food, water, toilets, resting places, and their owners. This can be arranged by having several locations for food, water, and toilets. Timesharing, that is allowing the one cat (or group of cats) to have access to a shared area for a time then confining them and allowing another cat (or group of cats) to then have access, can be used to give the cats access to the owners and shared parts of the house. This mimics how cats naturally organize themselves. It is also important to remember that cats are solitary feeders and even when the cats get on very well with each other, they would appreciate the opportunity to eat alone.

Kittens are social early on in their lives but from about 8 weeks of age, they start to show less social play and more objected-directed play. This is because they have to concentrate on learning their most important skill—hunting for food. By the time they reach social maturity at between 2 and 3 years of age, their interest in social play can be negligible. So don't be surprised when your cat becomes a little less interested in playing with you or with its sibling or housemate, and encourage the maintenance of social interaction with you through stroking (rubbing) and grooming your cat, allowing it to rest and sleep on your knee or beside you, and talking to it. Remember that object play should be encouraged throughout their lives, so invest in some suitable cat toys and continue to enjoy play time with your feline companion.

Feline Social Behavior

How do you recognize if your cats are bonded to each other or recognize that your cat has bonded with you? In the feline world, close relationships are characterized by the presence of tactile contact between them. Grooming and rubbing of each other are classified as affiliative behaviors, and bonded cats spend time close to and in close contact with each other. You may find your cats snuggled down in the same bed, tangled all together, and engaging in bouts of mutual grooming. You may also find your cat sitting or lying on you or touching you whenever you sit down. When you (or your cat) return home, your cat may greet you with a trill and approach you with their tail up. Your cat may then sniff at you and then bunt and rub its body along your legs. Responding to social bonding behaviors helps strengthen the bonds between individual cats and between cats and humans.

Recognizing when cats are bonded and when they are not will help you to know which cats can be confined together and which need to be separated.

Cats are a fascinating species that refuses to be easily categorized by humans. While they are solitary hunters and territorial, they are not a solitary species. They are able to form social bonds but lack the behaviors to repair bonds when they break. Recognizing social bonding behavior between cats and behavior directed towards humans can help manage cats so they feel safe and so that you get the very best out of the relationship with your pet.

Training Your Cat to Love Medications

Ilona Rodan

One of the biggest problems cat owners have is when their cat needs medication. You've seen the veterinarian and technician do it and it seems easy, but when you try at home, your cat may become frightened, run away or hide, and struggle and accidentally scratch or bite you if they are very scared. You cannot imagine how you will be able to do this day after day, whether it is short-term or long-term. The good news is that it doesn't need to be a challenge!

Learning to give oral medication is an important step. Fortunately there are tricks to maintain the wonderful relationship you have with your cat while treating it. In fact, for me and my cats, it has become one of the most fun parts of the day!

The easiest methods are to find a treat or food that your cat really likes and mix or hide the medication within. Instead of forcing your cat to take it, call "Treat" and this now becomes a fun way to medicate. If your cat does not need medication, this is still a great time to start. Start by giving a treat as below once daily. Give to all cats if possible because a cat will become suspicious if the other cats don't get it!

Examples of "treats" which work to hide medications, written in order of ease per author:

- Pill Pockets (several different flavors, although chicken is the most popular with my patients)
- Canned food or Fancy Feast enough to hide powder or well-crushed pill (some pills are bitter so this method may not work for certain medications. Be sure to check with your veterinarian)
- Cheese in a can: Cheez Whiz, Easy cheese, or other
- Pill paste or Pill Masker
- Anything else your cat likes to eat that is not toxic (poisonous foods for cats include onions or onion powder, grapes or raisins, and chocolate)
- Bonita fish flakes

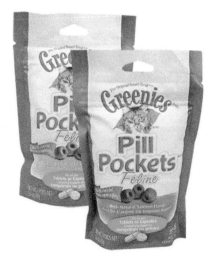

For the Stubborn or Allergic Cat and for Training Before Medication Is Needed

Some cats will never fall for hiding medication into food and others have food allergies and cannot have these tasty treats. The good news here is that it is very easy to train a cat as long as the rewards are highly desirable for them.

Start by training a cat to sit by taking a favorite treat or food and holding it close to the cat's nose and slowly moving it up over the head. As the head goes up, the bottom goes down. Say "sit" calmly when the bottom goes down and reward immediately with the treat. Do this once or twice a day until your cats learn the pairing of the word "sit" and the behavior of sitting. Never get impatient and don't do it too frequently or your cat will be suspicious of your behavior.

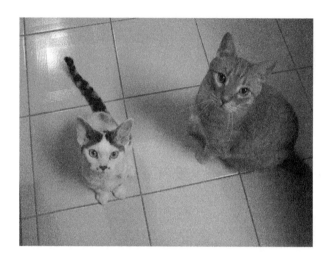

The next step is to quietly and calmly come from the side or behind and massage your cat's face or muzzle. Give a treat. If your cat is not interested, do it again tomorrow until it becomes routine. If you are already brushing your cat's teeth, the next step will be easy. Hold the cat's muzzle and slightly open the mouth. Give a treat. The next step will be to cradle your cat—my preference is with them on the floor turned away from me but with their hind end gently between my legs to keep them in place. Again reward this behavior. Another option is to use a towel to swaddle your cat. The first video demonstrates this. Always remember to give your cat a treat if there are still problems.

Pictures and videos make this clearer and here are some good suggestions:

- How to Give a Cat Medication
  https://www.youtube.com/watch?v=KFeF-x7akWs
- Giving Oral Medications to a Cat
  http://www.vetmed.wsu.edu/ClientED/cat_meds.aspx

- Examining and Medicating the Eyes of the Cat
  http://www.vetmed.wsu.edu/ClientED/cat_eyes.aspx
- Examining and Medicating the Ears of the Cat
  http://www.vetmed.wsu.edu/ClientED/cat_ears.aspx
- How to Medicate a Cat, A Cat Clinic, Germantown, MD
  https://www.youtube.com/watch?v=MWKUTxtiJ5U

Some cat owners may still have challenges depending on their cat or their own health. Having a technician come in to medicate your cat or bringing your cat to the veterinarian for medications are all options. If you are still having problems, please don't hesitate to contact your veterinarian for other options.

Transporting Your Cat Made Easier

Martha Cannon

Does it Make a Difference What Type of Carrier Is Used?

There are many carriers on the market. There are a couple of things to consider when buying one to make sure it is the best design for you, your cat, and your veterinarian.

Things to Look for in a Carrier

- A carrier in which the top half is easily removed via big clips. Sometimes the cat can remain in the carrier during the examination, which makes it feel secure.

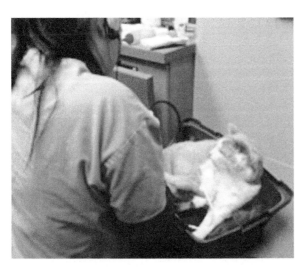

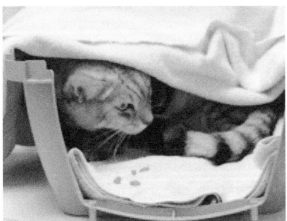

- A large top opening, with additional opening on the side. "Top-loaders" are much easier for lifting the cat in or out.

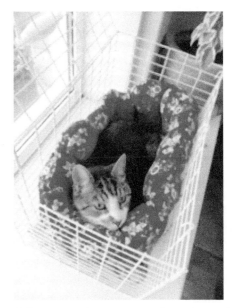

- A solid tray type bottom—much easier to clean if there is a bathroom "accident."

Things to Avoid in a Carrier

- Little pegs that allow the top to lift off; they are too easily broken or lost.
- A small front-opening door or one where the hinge is quite central; the cat becomes trapped behind the door when it opens!
- Wicker baskets; these can be very hard to clean if soiled.

Options

Some cats like mesh so they can see what's outside. Others like to tuck themselves away in the dark. If you want to see what type of traveler your cat is, it is good to borrow a hard-sided carrier, which comes apart in the middle, and then a wire mesh carrier, which can be covered or uncovered, and see which your cat prefers. You may be able to borrow these from fellow cat owners or from your veterinary practice.

Other Top Tips

- Incontinence liners or "puppy pads" to keep things tidy!
- Feliway spray—a calming pheromone. Ask us for further advice on either.

Getting Your Cat Into the Carrier

- Keeping the carrier readily visible and accessible in your home and putting treats inside helps train your cat to see the carrier as a safe place.
- Ideally your cat should enter the carrier voluntarily but if you do need to move it in or out, remember to do so carefully so that your cat does not become alarmed.

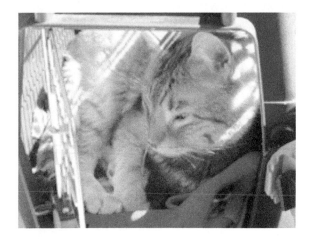

Adjusting to Car Rides

- When traveling with your cat in the car, always put the cat in a carrier or other protected container. Hold the carrier into place with the seat belt or place it on a flat surface on the floor. This is safer for both you and your cat.
- To make your cat more comfortable when riding in the car, take the cat to places other than the veterinary practice!
- Start with short journeys at first, then gradually extend the length of the drive.
- Because cats travel best on an empty stomach, do not feed your cat for several hours before traveling.
- After each successful car trip, reward your cat with positive attention and treats.

Pleasant Veterinary Trips

- To make your cat feel at home, bring the cat's favorite treats and toys with them.
- When at home, practice regular care routines like grooming, nail trimming and teeth brushing, touching the cats face, ears, feet, and tail. This should help your cat adjust to the veterinary practice and any needed home care.
- Make trips to the veterinary practice for visits involving no examinations or procedures, such as checking the cat's weight. It gives the staff a chance to interact with your cat in a nonthreatening way.
- Using a pheromone spray or wipe (Feliway) in your cat's carrier about 15 minutes before travel can make them feel more relaxed.

Understanding Our Commitment to Minimize Your Cat's Stress

Eliza Sundahl

Thank you for coming to our practice! You may find our approach to your cat's veterinary visit different from your previous experiences. We recognize that cats will probably be fearful when they come to the veterinarian and we will try to decrease your cat's anxiety with the steps we take during your visit.

There are some basic principles that can be helpful to understand in order to optimize the veterinary visit from a feline perspective. We know that kittens are more tolerant of experiencing new things and handling change than adult cats. Young animals (like people) don't seem to get as stressed about the unexpected. But as your cat gets older, changes in where they are and what is happening around them can create a great deal of anxiety. They get signals about their environment from their eyes and ears, but their sense of smell is also a very important signaling system. As a matter of fact, it's so important that many behaviorists say that "cats move through clouds of smell," creating another dimension to their landscape. When you're a small animal that is both a predator as well as another creature's prey, changes in your stable environment usually mean that you need to be alert to trouble or threat. Visits to the veterinary practice constitute a significant change and can be a significant challenge for a cat.

Cats will display a spectrum of responses to a stressful environment just like people do. Some people can cope with challenges and the unexpected much easier than others. It is the same with cats. Usually cats will seek out a hiding place so that they can stay hidden from view. A confident cat may sense that it can handle a situation and not display any anxious behaviors. Others may freeze and not move or react very much when they are handled. It is important to remember that these cats are still really scared. Some cats will lick themselves or fidget in some way to console themselves. And just as some people are going to be more likely to lash out under stress than others, cats that have exhausted their coping mechanisms will often become aggressive. Allowing them to stay hidden while at the veterinary practice or distracting them with toys or treats can help cats avoid escalating fear.

You are an important part of making your cat's visit less stressful. We will give you resources that will explain how you can help prepare for a visit. For example, choosing the right kind of carrier is very important. Being dragged, pulled, or tipped out of a carrier can be very scary and it starts the visit off with a cat already more fear-aroused. When we can remove the top half of a hard-sided carrier, your cat can stay hidden under a towel while we perform most of our examination. Allowing them to cope in this manner can prevent them from progressing into more fear and aggression.

There are other techniques that can be employed to allow your cat to cope better with their visit to the veterinary practice. Our doctors and staff have studied these techniques and use them to try to make your cat's visit as comfortable as possible. We hope that this also means **your** visit will be more comfortable too.

What are Feline Odontoclastic Resorption Lesions?*

A.J. Tsugawa

Feline odontoclastic resorption lesions (FORLs) are a common (20% to 75%) dental disease in cats over 4 years of age. In this disease, cells known as odontoclasts, which originate in the bone marrow or spleen, migrate and attach to the external surface of the tooth root (portion of the tooth within the tooth socket) and resorb (i.e., destroy) the root surface. The odontoclasts are cells that are normally involved in the process of turning over "baby" teeth before the permanent teeth erupt. Although it is not known why, these cells remain active in the adult cat. Over time, the root(s) of the teeth are completely destroyed, and in the latter stages of the disease, only the crown (portion of the tooth above the gumline) or portions of the crown remain. In many cats, the end-stage affected tooth is observed as missing.

FORLs were previously and incorrectly referred to as a feline cavity. We now know that cavities and FORLs are distinctly different diseases. Cavities are caused by bacteria, and FORLs, although their true cause is unknown, are not a bacterial disease. Many potential causes for this disease have been investigated, but to date, the true cause of the disease remains elusive, and is one of the current "hot" topics of research in the field of veterinary dentistry.

What Are the Clinical Signs of FORLs?

Cats with FORLs are often identified by the chief clinical sign of teeth "chattering," sensitivity upon eating/chewing (i.e., dropping food or preferentially chewing on one side of the mouth). Patients suffering with FORLs may also salivate profusely. This suggests that there is significant oral pain. On examination, the veterinarian will identify either missing teeth or teeth where portions of the tooth crown are missing. In areas where portions of the crown are missing, the gums are usually observed to cover the missing area, and a red spot is noticed on the crown. The teeth with early FORLs cannot be identified on gross examination, because the disease is localized to the root surface, and can only be documented by radiographs. Symptomatic cats are usually those that have teeth with partially missing tooth crowns and where the disease process has moved beyond the root surface. In other cats, despite the severe gross clinical appearance of the lesion, the cat remains unaffected in its behavior pattern: eating, gaining weight, and appearing content.

What Tests Are Needed?

Only the end-stage lesions involving the tooth crown can be identified readily on clinical examination, the remainder of lesions must be diagnosed by dental x-ray images. Due to a high percentage of cats affected by this disease, cats over the age of 4 years are recommended to have dental x-ray images as a screening test for the disease when having their teeth cleaned.

What Treatment Is Needed?

FORLs are believed to be a painful disease in the cat, and cats with documented disease should be treated. The primary treatment for this disease is extraction of the affected teeth. When FORLs were believed to be similar to cavities, the lesions or defects in the crown were filled, similar to human cavities. As the disease was further investigated, and follow-up was performed on teeth that had been filled, it became clear that despite our best efforts the filled teeth continued to resorb.

Extraction and crown amputation with intentional root retention are the only currently accepted methods of therapy. The latter is a procedure where the crown of the affected tooth is removed with a bur; leaving the resorbing roots buried in the bone to continue resorbing to completion. The crown amputation procedure alleviates the clinical signs of disease because the exposed and sensitive portion of the tooth is removed. This procedure, however, is limited to affected teeth that have been appropriately x-rayed and have severe tooth root resorption. Teeth with severe root resorption are difficult or impossible to extract, and significant damage to the surrounding bone may result from overzealous attempts at extraction.

Prognosis

The prognosis following extraction or crown amputation of affected teeth is good, but affected cats will always have a predisposition to the development of additional lesions. Follow-up visits on an annual basis are recommended for FORL screening.

---

*From Tsugawa AJ: Feline odontoclastic resorption lesions (FORLs). In: Ettinger SJ, Feldman EC, editors: Textbook of Veterinary Internal Medicine, ed 7, St Louis, 2011, Elsevier.

449

What Care Does Your Cat Need?

Ilona Rodan

Cats are beloved pets and family members. They make us laugh, are fun and affectionate, and wonderful companions to millions of people. Unfortunately, the veterinary care they receive has declined over the past two decades. This is not for a lack of love, but instead because of the following reasons:

- The perception that cats are self-sufficient, which is not true. See "The 10 Subtle Signs of Sickness"
- Lack of recognition of medical needs—even the indoor cat has had an increase in medical conditions and parasites over the past several years[1]
- Free or inexpensive adoptions giving the misperception that cats are inexpensive pets to own
- Cat and owner stress associated with the veterinary visit

Cats are not self-sufficient, but rather their signs of sickness are subtle, and consist of changes to their normal behavior.

The 10 Subtle Signs of Sickness

1. Inappropriate elimination*
2. Changes in interaction
3. Changes in activity
4. Changes in sleeping habits
5. Changes in food and water consumption
6. Unexplained weight loss or gain
7. Changes in grooming
8. Signs of stress
9. Changes in vocalization
10. Bad breath

*More appropriately termed "house soling."
Developed by James Richard and Ilona Rodan for Boehringer Ingelheim.

Because cats are adept at hiding illness, cats are often sicker than dogs by the time they are brought to a veterinarian. Also, it is a fact that many veterinarians prefer working with dogs and find cat diseases more challenging to diagnose and treat.[2]

The best thing that you can do for your cat is to recognize the subtle signs of sickness and seek veterinary care early on, in addition to finding a veterinarian that has expertise in finding clues through a thorough medical history and feline physical examination. You can find a good veterinarian for your cat by searching for a Cat Friendly Practice* in the United States or Cat Friendly Clinic in other countries** and/or a board certified feline practitioner. Make sure also to find a veterinarian that understands feline behavior, because many behavior problems are a consequence of feline stress or illness and a misunderstanding of the cat, which may result in surrender and/or euthanasia.

Keeping Your Cat Healthy Throughout Its Life

The goals of feline healthcare are to prevent disease and detect early signs of pain and illness. It is a team approach between you and your veterinarian. Your cat's age or life stage, breed, and individual traits, as well as home environment and other pets in the home, are all taken into consideration.

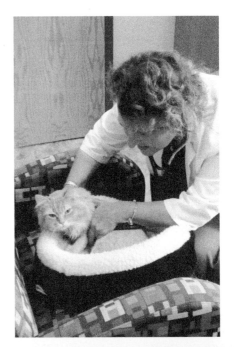

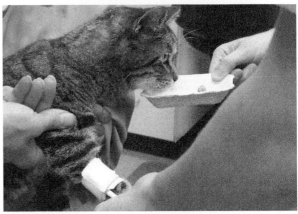

- **Examinations and routine health screening**
  - These should be carried out every 6 to 12 months because cats demonstrate subtle signs of disease and pain as changes in health occur quickly and signs are difficult to detect

- In senior cats (7 years and older) and those with chronic conditions, a minimum interval of 6 months is recommended
- Routine health screening uncovers disease in many apparently healthy cats[3]
- **Behavior counseling to prevent and treat behavior problems**
  - Please let us know your concerns
- **Weight management and nutritional counseling**
  - 58% of cats in the United States are overweight or obese
- **Oral health**
  - 80% of cats have dental disease by 3 years of age
- **Parasite control**
  - This is necessary for all cats because even totally indoor cats can get parasites

- **Vaccination**
  - Our practice individualizes vaccines to your cat's needs
- **Viral testing**
  - Feline leukemia virus and feline immunodeficiency virus testing is needed in kittens and more frequently in some cats depending on lifestyle
- **Microchipping**

With a combination of veterinary and home care, many cats can live into their late teens or even twenties. Between routine veterinary visits, you can help your cat by contacting us if there are any changes in your cat no matter how subtle and if you have any questions about your cat's behavior. We welcome your questions and are honored to help you take care of your *purrfect* pet!

ADDITIONAL RESOURCES

* Cat Friendly Practice through American Association of Feline Practioners, http://catfriendlypractice.catvets.com/

** Cat Friendly Clinic through International Cat Care, http://www.icatcare.org/cat-campaigns/cat-friendly-clinic

REFERENCES

1. Banfield Pet Hospital. State of pet health 2011 report, vol 1. Portland, Ore: Banfield Pet Hospital; 2011.
2. Bayer Healthcare/American Association of Feline Practitioners. Veterinary Care Usage Study III: feline findings. http://www.bayerdvm.com/show.aspx/news-release-bvcus-iii-feline-findings, Accessed June 6, 2015.
3. Paepe D, Verjans G, Duchateau L, et al. Routine health screening: findings in apparently healthy middle-aged and old cats. *J Feline Med Surg.* 2013;15:8–19.

What Is My Cat Trying to Say? Information for Owners About Cat Body Language

Jacqui Ley

Communication is not easy and it is even harder when the other party is another species! Understanding cat communication can make living with your cat more harmonious. Just like us, cats use several different methods of communication. They may use their body to tell us something immediately, use their voice to send a message over a longer distance, or use claw marks, spray marks, and feces to leave longer-lasting messages. This handout will cover some of the body signals that cats use to communicate their needs and how they are feeling.

Communication signals are not nearly as simple as they appear when they are described in books or even this handout. This is because the individual may use more than one type of signal to send a message. They may use their body and combine this with vocalization to make the message less ambiguous and, because communication is dynamic, the signals being sent will change in relation to the signals being received from the other party. If you want to learn more about your cat, the best thing you can do is spend time watching it to learn what different combinations of signals mean.

Cats use all of their body to communicate how they are feeling. It is true that they do not speak as we do, but you can gain information about what a cat is thinking by watching its body language. To get a feel for the emotional state of a cat it is necessary to consider the position of the cat's body, the orientation if its ears, the height and activity of the tail, and the size of the pupils in the eyes. Below are some descriptions of how cats use their bodies to send messages and then brief descriptions of how they use signals in combination to send clearer messages.

Cat Body Language

Posture

In general cats that are fearful hold their body low to the ground. Friendly or confident cats approach with their bodies held in a more relaxed posture. A cat that wants to frighten another cat or person away will arch its back and stand as tall as it can to look bigger and more scary. This is the classic "Halloween Cat" posture that you may have seen on cards and decorations.

Tail

Cat tails give a good indication of the cat's mood. The relaxed cat moves with its tail level with its back. A confident cat or a cat greeting a familiar person or cat (or dog) will generally hold its tail vertically. A cat that is getting grumpy, especially with being handled, will swish its tail from side to side. This movement is very different from the tail wag of a dog. A cat with a strongly swishing tail should be avoided.

Ears

Cats, in general, have pricked or upright ears and changes in their position give a good indication of what the cat is interested in and of the cat's mood. For breeds with lots of hair (longhaired cats) or with folded ears, the positions of the ears are a little harder to see, but the same rules apply. When cats are concentrating on someone or something, they hold their ears facing forward. A cat that is unsure or a bit anxious holds its ears rotated to the side. Cats in pain may also do this. A cat that is aggressive will flatten its ears back and down against its skull so they cannot be seen. Cats also have the enviable ability to rotate their ears separately and they will do this if something catches their attention or they are trying to monitor more than aspect of their environment at the same time.

Eyes

The eyes of cats are large, with some breeds being selected for incredible jewel-toned golds, greens, and blues. Apart from being beautiful, cats' eyes allow them to see in very dim light, while the slit shape of the pupil (the black part of the eye) helps cut out brighter light so they can see in daylight. In dim light, the pupil opens up and may almost fill the eye. The size of the pupil also gives an indication of the cat's level of arousal. As the cat becomes more aroused its pupils become larger. Arousal could be related to the cat defending itself, being frightened, hunting, or playing. Unless there is a medical problem causing the pupils to remain dilated, the size of the pupil tells us that the cat is not relaxed and resting. However, it does not give information about the emotional motivation for the cat's arousal.

Fur

Cats are able to fluff their fur up and do this when they want to frighten away another cat, person, or other animal. Fluffing their fur or pilo-erection makes the cat look larger.

Position

Cats also send messages by their position in the environment. A cat that is unhappy about the activities of another cat may block the other cat's access to resources such as the litter box, the house, or favored sleeping areas.

Complex Signals

As we all know, communication is not simple. Some signals are not specific; for example, large pupil size just tells us the cat is aroused but doesn't tell us if it is in a playful or aggressive mood. Other signals may not be received; yowling at another cat through a closed window doesn't convey as much information as body posture, ear position, and tail position. To make sure messages get through, several signals may be sent together. Cats use body language and vocalizations to signal how they are feeling and what their intentions are. Being able to recognize these complex signals will let you know when you can approach your cat and when it would like to be left alone.

Greeting Behavior

When cats recognize an approaching cat or person or dog they may give a greeting meow or trill. Often they will raise their tail to the vertical, while at other times it may be held lower. Once the cat has come into proximity to the individual it will sniff the other party and often bunt, that is, rub its cheek scent glands along the other cat or person. The cat is mixing its scent with the smell of the individual to freshen up the group smell.

Neutral Behavior

The cat that is relaxed may look at another cat or a person and then squint its eyes shut in a blinking action. This indicates that it does not object to being approached. In contrast, when cats are not interested in social contact but not frightened either, they may turn their head away. In both cases, the cat does not approach the other party.

Distance-Increasing Behavior

Some signals are combined to send the message "Go Away." They increase the distance between the cat and other individuals, especially if the cat cannot leave the area or is in its own territory.

The cat that is on the offensive may first stare at the individual to which it objects. It may approach the other individual and once close, begin to give a low growl. The cat's tail may be held at body height and swish from side to side. Its ears may be swiveled out to the sides. If the other party doesn't leave, the cat may progress to aggressive behavior. Or if the threat behavior is not working, the cat may decide it is better to retreat rather than risk a fight.

The cat that is uncertain may attempt to bluff its way out of trouble using a defensive threat. When approached by something or someone it finds frightening the cat may hiss and crouch down. If the threatening individual does not stop, the cat may stand up with its back arched and its tail in a downward curve. It may flatten its ears against its skull and fluff its fur out all over its body. This makes the cat appear twice its actual size. Pretty scary if you are not expecting it!

If an encounter progresses to a fight, the forefeet are used to strike and there may be wrestling using a combination of the forefeet to grapple, the hind feet to scratch, and the teeth to bite. The cats may give a very loud vocalization referred to as a shriek or give a pain cry. If one cat breaks away, the other may continue to pursue it or may remain in the area of the fight and spend time bunting objects and leaving important scent signals to warn off the other cat should it return.

Cat communication is complex. It takes time to learn what your cat is trying to communicate but it is not impossible. Time spent watching cats is never wasted as you will be learning how they communicate and like to interact with others.

What We Learn When We Examine Your Cat*

Martha Cannon

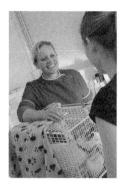
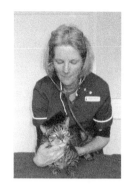
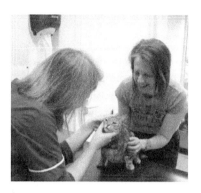
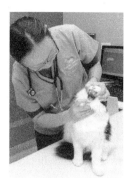

Cats can't tell us where it hurts or why they don't feel right. So we have to do some detective work to piece together the clues and find out what is wrong. You know your cat better than anyone, so we ask you for as much information as you can give us about their well-being, any signs of ill health, and any changes in their behavior that will help to tell us whether they are well and happy, or whether there is a problem. Then we use the physical examination to give us more information and to look for hidden problems.

The Examination

The examination has two parts: the "hands off" and the "hands on" parts.

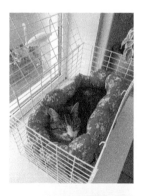
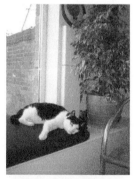
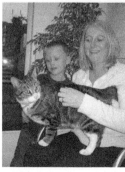
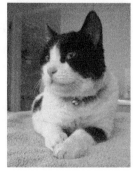

Hands Off Examination

As soon as you and your cat enter the room, the veterinarian starts assessing the cat from a distance. We do this while we are saying Hello; and while you are telling us how your cat is doing at home.

You and your cat may not be aware of this part of the examination, but we are looking at the way your cat breathes, sits, stands, and walks; how it reacts to its new environment and to any noises it hears.

What We Are Looking At

Demeanor: Is the cat alert and as aware of its surroundings as it should be? If not, is that because it is feeling too ill to react normally, or because it is in pain? Or is it not seeing or hearing as well as it should?

At rest: When the cat is sitting in the carrier, or at rest in the room, we are looking to see if it is sitting in a natural position. Is it underweight or overweight, and does its coat have a normal shine? Is there any increase in breathing noise, rate, or effort? Are the cat's eyes and nose clean, are the ears pricked up, and is the face symmetrical?

Movement: We encourage the cat to walk around the room. This helps the cat feel at ease, but it is also a valuable part of the "hands off" examination.

Is the cat lame or weak? Is it holding its tail in a normal position? Can it find its way around or is there a problem with its vision or co-ordination? Does it want to explore, or find a hiding place, or is it feeling too ill or weak to want to move?

Hands On Examination

This starts with a brief top to toe check of the major body systems, followed by a more detailed look at any areas that are giving trouble:

Head and Neck: Are the ears, eyes and nose clean? Are the whites of the eyes white, and are the pupils

---

*This handout has been modified with permission from the Oxford Cat Clinic.

symmetrical and responding to light? Do the backs of the eyes look normal? Are the insides of the mouth and the eyelids a healthy pink? Does the breath smell (more than usual!), and are the teeth and gums clean and healthy?

> Are the lymph nodes in the neck a normal size, is their any pain when the throat is gently handled; does this trigger any coughing or retching?

> In older cats we also feel the neck carefully to see if either of the thyroid glands are enlarged.

The Skin and Fur: Is the coat shiny with no "dandruff"? Are there any bald patches or any scabs under the fur? Are there dark black flecks in the coat indicating that the cat has fleas?

Chest: We watch the cat to see if the breathing is more rapid or labored than it should be. Then we use a stethoscope to listen to the heart and to the lungs, although if the cat is purring we won't be able to hear anything very useful!

> The *heart beat* should be regular and at a rate of between 120 and 180 beats per minute. Each heart beat has two sounds separated by a tiny pause. A heart murmur is a faint sound that fills the gap between the two heart sounds and indicates turbulent blood flow within the heart.

> *Lung sounds* should be faint, but just audible over all parts of the chest. Louder lung sounds can indicate bronchitis, pneumonia, or heart failure. Absence of lung sounds means there is something between the lungs and the chest wall—it might be fluid, or tissue, or free air but whatever it is it shouldn't be there.

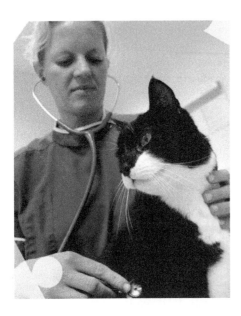

Tummy: When we examine the cat's tummy we can feel the outline of the larger internal organs—the liver,

kidneys, spleen, intestines, and bladder. We can check that each is the right size and can identify any sites of internal pain. We also feel all round the abdomen to identify any lumps that might indicate cancer.

WARNING: If your cat is overweight we won't be able to feel all these things.

What Can We Do to Help?

Most cats don't like being at the veterinary practice, and they don't like being examined. We understand this and always try to minimize their stress:

Little Things Can Make a Big Difference

We have longer than standard appointments so that we can give your cat time to adjust to us, and we can take a little extra time to handle your cat with the utmost care.

Coming out: We encourage your cat to come out of the carrier by themselves, or we take the carrier apart so that we don't need to haul your cat out of its safe spot.

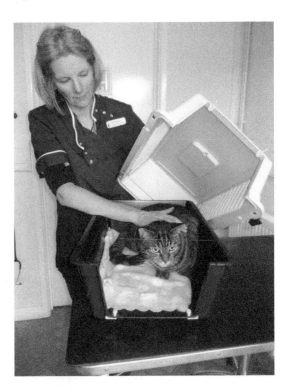

In the room: We allow your cat time to explore the room and if the table is too frightening we examine your cat on the window seat, on the floor, or even on your lap (if you and your cat are comfortable with that).

The examination: Cats don't like being stared at, so we do as much as we can with your cat facing away from us, and when we need to look at the face we look from the side not head-on.

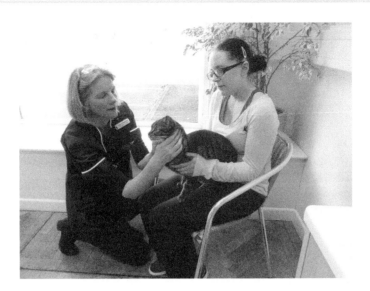

We avoid doing uncomfortable things when we can, so we only look down the ears when our initial external check tells us we need to. Likewise we only take your cat's temperature if its behavior suggests a fever, and we use the slimmest, quickest, and most comfortable thermometer that we can!

When Your Cat Needs Hospitalization

Ilona Rodan

We understand that it can be upsetting to have your cat hospitalized, worrying about whether it will get better and how it will cope away from home. We strive to help your cat get well so that it can return home as soon as possible, and to address its medical needs and comfort with tender nursing care and a comfortable environment while hospitalized.

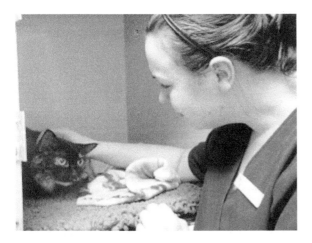

Our practice has a hospitalization ward that is set up to meet all your cat's needs: a comfortable bed to rest within and a hiding area for shy cats. Fresh food and water as well as a clean litter box are all provided and refreshed at least twice daily. We make sure that the environment is as quiet and comfortable as possible, and try our best to provide a consistent caretaker for your cat to become familiar with. Cats recovering from anesthesia will have a comfortable and warm, safe hospitalization cage until it is safe for them to move around more.

Familiarity helps cats feel safe, and we welcome you to bring your cat's favorite cat bed or blanket, foods, and small toys. You are also welcome to visit your cat as well. Many cats do better when their people visit, and we provide visiting privileges during regular business hours.

Should Your Cat Be Hospitalized?

At our facility, we recognize that most cats do better in their familiar home·environment. Many of our patients are treated on an outpatient basis, but there are times when hospitalization, medical observations, or treatments that cannot be done at home need to be done at the veterinary practice. We take the following into consideration:

- The severity of the medical condition
- Whether the same treatments can be done at home
- How the cat will respond to hospitalization

If it is in the best interest of your cat to be hospitalized, that recommendation will be made. Some instances are anesthetic procedures, a need for intravenous fluids to treat severe dehydration or low blood pressure, treatment of hypothermia (low body temperature), breathing difficulties, and monitoring of vital signs (e.g., heart rate).

Many veterinary practices prefer to keep patients until they start eating. This is commonly done with dogs. However, some cats will never eat in the veterinary practice, and so we may recommend getting them home earlier and ask you to bring them for a recheck within the next day or longer based on the veterinarian's discretion for the individual patient.

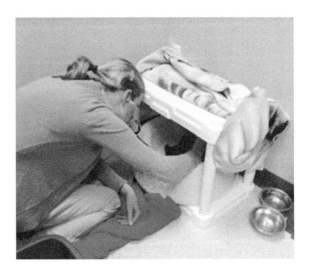

If your cat needs urgent or critical care after hours, we will recommend that your cat be taken to a 24-hour care facility that we work with closely.

Cat-Only Wards That Meet Your Cat's Needs

Our practice has cat-only wards, recommended to prevent fear caused by hearing, smelling, or seeing dogs. Cats may also become frightened if they see an unfamiliar cat, so we provide separate spaces where cats cannot see other cats. We take every precaution to keep your cat as comfortable as possible. Private rooms are available for cats that are anxious or meow loudly.

Warmth is important for the hospitalized patient. Traditional stainless steel cages are cold and noisy. At our facility, we provide cages that have laminate surfaces and are furnished with soft and warm bedding. Your cat will have space for the following:

- Comfortable bedding

- Hiding place if desired—this is important in an unfamiliar environment to prevent fear and allow a safe and quiet place to rest
- Vertical space if well enough to jump or climb
- Food
- Water
- Litter box

Supporting You and Your Cat

Your cat will receive the best care in as comfortable and respectful an environment as possible. We welcome you to come in to see where your cat will stay and to visit during business hours. Remember, your cat will be most comfortable if he or she has the familiarity of items from home—feel free to bring a cat bed, blanket, a favored toy or food.

A veterinarian will provide you with an update on your cat's well being at least once a day and you are welcome to call or e-mail our technicians for additional updates. Just like you, we want the best for your cat.